Nutrition in Public Health
Principles, Policies, and Practice

Nutrition in Public Health
Principles, Policies, and Practice

Arlene Spark

Hunter College,
New York U.S.A.

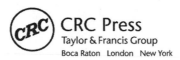

CRC Press
Taylor & Francis Group
Boca Raton London New York

CRC Press is an imprint of the
Taylor & Francis Group, an **informa** business

CRC Press
Taylor & Francis Group
6000 Broken Sound Parkway NW, Suite 300
Boca Raton, FL 33487-2742

© 2007 by Taylor & Francis Group, LLC
CRC Press is an imprint of Taylor & Francis Group, an Informa business

International Standard Book Number-10: 0-8493-1473-9 (Hardcover)
International Standard Book Number-13: 978-0-8493-1473-5 (Hardcover)

Library of Congress Cataloging-in-Publication Data

Spark, Arlene J.
 Nutrition in public health : principles, policies, and practice / author, Arlene Spark.
  p. ; cm.
 "A CRC title."
 Includes bibliographical references and index.
 ISBN-13: 978-0-8493-1473-5 (hardcover : alk. paper)
 ISBN-10: 0-8493-1473-9 (hardcover : alk. paper)
 1. Nutrition policy--United States. 2. Nutrition--United States. 3. Public health--United States. 4. Diet in disease. I. Title.
 [DNLM: 1. Nutritional Status--United States. 2. Health Promotion--United States. 3. Nutrition Policy--United States. QU 145 S736n 2007]

 TX360.U6S63 2007
 363.8'5610973--dc22   2007003464

Visit the Taylor & Francis Web site at
http://www.taylorandfrancis.com

and the CRC Press Web site at
http://www.crcpress.com

Dedication

———

To Hannah and Arthur, Dani, Harrison, and Justin, and very definitely
— Dan

Table of Contents

Preface

Immediately after deciding to embark on writing this book, I did exactly what any other public health nutritionist in the Internet age would do — a Google search to determine the availability of other books, and also journals, dedicated to nutrition in public health. I identified six books with "community nutrition" in the title but only two books and a single journal devoted exclusively to public health nutrition. I found myself asking why I should not be reticent to add yet another book to what already seemed like a crowded field. Is nutrition and public health sufficiently mature for three new books in that many years? I believe the answer to that question is a resounding, unequivocal "Yes!." Three books and a journal dedicated to a topic that unarguably holds the key to the primary and secondary prevention of some of the major causes of premature death in the United States must still be considered woefully inadequate.

The purpose of *Nutrition in Public Health: Principles, Policies, and Practice* is to provide public health professionals with an overview of the field, with a focus on the federal government's role in determining nutrition policy and practice. The book was written with the conviction that an understanding of government and a familiarity with the demographic profile of the United States population are necessary in order to appreciate nutrition in public health today.

The principles of public health nutrition are presented in the first half of the book. These eight chapters examine the population of the United States, nutritional epidemiology, food and nutrition surveys for monitoring the public's health, programs to reduce disparities in the prevalence of diet-related chronic disease, weight control challenges and solutions, and an examination of special populations — breastfeeding mothers, people with HIV and AIDS, and prison inmates.

The nutrition policy of the United States is addressed in the two chapters that deal with food and nutrition politics and dietary advice.

The last third of the book deals with practicing public health nutrition. These five chapters present the tools for conducting a food and nutrition assessment of a community, designing and carrying out a social marketing campaign, and writing a grant proposal. Programs to promote food security and to ensure the safety of the food supply are also discussed.

Acknowledgments

My sincerest thanks to all the people who helped bring this project to fruition: my current and former students (as every college professor readily admits, our students teach us far more than we could ever teach them by forcing us to organize our thoughts, sharpen our arguments, and critically examine all sides of an issue); my Hunter College colleagues and friends in the Urban Public Health Program and in the Nutrition and Food Science track; the City University of New York Food And Nutrition faculty (we call ourselves *CUNY FAN*); my cohorts in nutrition from New York City and throughout the United States; and the generous and knowledgeable public health nutritionists I have met online. Specifically, I must single out the following individuals:

- Margaret Meehan, M.A., M.P.H., R.D., Hunter College '06, and editor *par excellence.*
- Hunter College colleagues Nicholas Freudenberg, Dr. P.H. for his insight on correctional health in particular but, much more, for his overall inspiration as a leader in public health; epidemiologist Philip Alcabes, Ph.D., M.P.H., for his irreverent view of the world as well as his review of the epidemiology chapter; and environmental health scientist Jack Caravanos, Dr. P.H., who set me straight on GIS.
- Former Hunter College students, Fania Yanberger, J.D., who provided guidance on the legal materials, especially the sections about GM foods; Qalvy Grainzvolt, B.S., a Metropolitan Opera supernumerary who cheerfully supplied the opera quotations; and Nicole Bourdon, who discovered that low-income African American and Hispanic women read magazines that contain more advertisements for low-quality food than their white counterparts.
- Barbara Wakeen, M.A., R.D., L.D., C.C.F.P., owner of Correctional Nutrition Consultants, and Marge Bolella, M.S., R.D., of the New York State Department of Corrections for their advice about nutrition in correctional health.
- Meredith Johnston, Archivist at the Child Nutrition Archives, and Beth King, Acting Director of Technology Transfer, both at the National Food Service Management Institute, for their ability to retrieve primary sources of information about the genesis of the National School Lunch Program, including obscure typed reports that were originally disseminated through carbon copies.
- Margo Wooton, Director of Public Policy at the Center for Science in the Public Interest, who allowed some of her activist materials to be included in Chapter 10.
- Michael Ochs, formerly the Richard F. French Music Librarian at Harvard University, who trolled the JSTOR database of journal articles and Social Science Citation Index for quotations I failed to cite correctly.
- CRC Press staffers Randy Brehm, Gail Renard, and Patricia Roberson.

Any errors, omissions, and shortcoming in this book are, of course, my own.

Arlene Spark, EdD, RD, FADA, FACN
Demarest, NJ

The Author

Arlene Spark was educated at the City College of New York and Columbia University Teachers College. After majoring in English at City College, she worked as a narcotics caseworker with the New York City Department of Social Services and then as a home economics teacher at a correctional facility for men and women who had been incarcerated on drug-related charges. Her home economics experience led her to Columbia, where she earned degrees in public health nutrition, community nutrition education, and nutrition education. Dr. Spark started teaching on the college level while she was still in graduate school. The first course she taught was community nutrition, and she has been teaching it ever since. She is now an associate professor at Hunter College in the City University of New York, where she coordinates the tracks in nutrition and food science (undergraduate curriculum), public health nutrition (MPH curriculum), and the dietetic internship. Arlene Spark has been a nutritionist for 35 years. She was in the first cohort of registered dietitians to become board certified in pediatric nutrition. She is a fellow of the American Dietetic Association and of the American College of Nutrition. She has worked at the American Health Foundation and New York Medical College, where she directed nutrition in preventive cardiology and pediatric gastroenterology. She lives in Demarest, New Jersey, with Daniel Ochs, M.D.

1 Nutrition in Public Health

What's in a name? That which we call a rose by any other name would smell as sweet.

William Shakespeare's *Romeo and Juliet*, ca. 1594

1.1 PUBLIC HEALTH

In this chapter, we will introduce and describe a variety of processes, professionals, regulations, and regulatory agencies involved in the promotion of public health. Included is a brief historical overview of the development of attitudes about public welfare in this field, and their influence on the institutions and policies responsible in the U.S. for protecting the public and encouraging health through good nutrition. According to The Future of Public Health, a landmark report released two decades ago by the Institute of Medicine (IOM), the mission of public health is to "assure conditions in which people can be healthy."[1] This mission is carried out through organized, interdisciplinary efforts that address the physical, mental, and environmental health concerns of communities and populations at risk for disease and injury.

1.1.1 CORE FUNCTIONS AND ESSENTIAL SERVICES

The IOM report identified three core functions of public health — *assessment*, *policy development*, and *assurance*. Each of these core functions is realized through the provision of two or more essential (or key) public services.

- The purpose of *assessment* and monitoring of the health of communities and populations at risk is to identify health problems and priorities, and evaluate health services. Assessment and monitoring are carried out through the systematic collection, analysis, and dissemination of information about the health of the community in order to:

  1. Identify health problems in the community
  2. Evaluate effectiveness, accessibility, and quality of personal and population-based health services

- In collaboration with community and government leaders, *public health policies are formulated* in order to solve local and national health problems and priorities that have been identified. Comprehensive public health policies serve the public interest by their ability to:

  3. Support individual and community health efforts
  4. Inform, educate, and empower people about health issues
  5. Mobilize community partnerships to identify and solve health problems

- *Assurance* sees to it that all populations have access to appropriate and cost-effective care, including health promotion and disease prevention services, and evaluation of the effectiveness of that care. This oversight assures that the public receives the services promised to them, which is designed to:

  6. Assure a competent public health and personal healthcare workforce
  7. Ethically manage self, people, and resources

8. Enforce laws and regulations that protect health and ensure safety
9. Link people to needed personal health services and assure the provision of healthcare when otherwise unavailable

Research for new insights and innovative solutions is the tenth essential public health service identified by the IOM. Research serves as an umbrella over all the other essential services.

1.1.2 KEY RESPONSIBILITIES

The public's health is achieved through the application of health promotion and disease prevention technologies and interventions designed to improve and enhance quality of life. These responsibilities include the ability to:

- Prevent epidemics and the spread of disease
- Protect against environmental hazards
- Prevent injuries
- Promote and encourage healthy behaviors and mental health
- Respond to disasters and assist communities in recovery
- Assure the quality and accessibility of health services

1.1.3 TRAINING IN PUBLIC HEALTH

In the U.S., credible training in public health is offered through master of public health (MPH) degree programs that have been accredited by the Council on Education in Public Health (CEPH).[2] Whereas the MPH is the primary professional public health degree, other graduate degrees that also designate preparation for public health practice in a community setting that are considered to be equivalent to the MPH include the degrees of master of health administration (MHA), master of health services administration (MHSA), master of health science (MHS), and master of science in public health (MSPH).

At a minimum, CEPH-accredited degree-granting programs must offer training in five areas of knowledge that are basic to public health.

- *Biostatistics* — collection, storage, retrieval, analysis, and interpretation of health data; design and analysis of health-related surveys and experiments; and concepts and practice of statistical data analysis
- *Epidemiology* — distributions and determinants of disease, disabilities, and death in human populations; the characteristics and dynamics of human populations; and the natural history of disease and the biologic basis of health
- *Environmental health sciences* — environmental factors including biological, physical, and chemical factors that affect the health of a community
- *Health services administration* — planning, organization, administration, management, evaluation, and policy analysis of health and public health programs
- *Social and behavioral sciences* — concepts and methods of social and behavioral sciences relevant to the identification and solution of public health problems.

The study of nutrition is conspicuously absent from the fundamental areas of knowledge CEPH requires for accrediting public health programs and schools. In a sense, the tail wags the dog. As CEPH does not explicitly call for nutrition, schools and programs are not required to offer it in their curricula. Therefore, one goal of this book is to provide an overview of nutrition in public health for public professionals whose training lacked sufficient preparation in this important area.

1.2 NUTRITION IN PUBLIC HEALTH

Although the phrases "nutrition in public health," "nutrition and public health," and "public health nutrition" sound as if they are synonymous, subtle but important differences exist among these phrases.

On the one hand, "nutrition *and* public health" suggests the coexistence of the fields of nutrition and public health, although not necessarily as equal partners.

On the other hand, "nutrition *in* public health" refers to the discipline of nutrition that functions as a branch of the vast field of public health.

Closely related to "nutrition in public health" is "public health nutrition," which refers to the population-focused branch of public health that monitors diet, nutrition status and health, and food and nutrition programs, and provides a leadership role in applying public health principles to activities that lead to health promotion and disease prevention through policy development and environmental changes. This definition of public health nutrition represents a distillation of the competencies for public health nutrition that were suggested by national and international leaders in the field.[3,4,5]

Nevertheless, I use all three phrases interchangeably in this book.

1.2.1 NUTRITION IN COMMUNITY HEALTH

The term *nutrition in community health* refers to nutrition as a component of the community health branch of public health; "nutrition and community health" connotes the coexistence of nutrition and community health; and "community nutrition" refers to the branch of public health that focuses on promoting the health of individuals, families, and communities by providing quality services and community-based programs tailored to the unique needs of different communities and populations. Community nutrition comprises health promotion programs, policy and legislative initiatives, primary and secondary prevention, and healthcare across the life span. These three phrases are also used interchangeably in this book.

1.3 PUBLIC HEALTH NUTRITION

Public health nutrition is a professional discipline with its own body of knowledge and relevant skills. Imbedded in the practice of public health nutrition are services and activities to assure conditions in which people can achieve and maintain nutritional health. This array of services and activities includes:

- Surveillance and monitoring of nutrition-related health status and risk factors
- Community- or population-based assessment, program planning, and evaluation
- Leadership in community- and population-based interventions that collaborate across disciplines, programs, and agencies
- Leadership in addressing the access and quality issues around direct nutrition services for populations.[6]

1.3.1 SURVEILLANCE AND MONITORING

Nutrition monitoring is a complex system of activities that provides information about the dietary, nutritional, and related health status of Americans, the relationships between diet and health, and the factors affecting dietary and nutritional status. On the national level, surveillance and monitoring are carried out through a wide array of surveys conducted by the National Center for Health Statistics (NCHS) in the U.S Department of Health and Human Services (HHS) and by the U.S. Department of Agriculture (USDA).[7] Data from these surveys are used in public health nutrition policymaking in the areas of food safety, food fortification, food labeling, dietary guidance, tracking progress toward nutrition and health objectives, and setting nutrition research priorities. Some surveys, such as those in the behavioral risk factor surveillance systems (BRFSS), have state components, which can be used for state-level monitoring endeavors. These surveys are discussed in Chapter 5.

Monitoring the nation's food availability and consumption is one of the responsibilities of the USDA. Researchers at all levels of government have access to the USDA's food composition databases. In 2006, the USDA released nationwide dietary intake data for the years 2003–2004 that were collected in "What We Eat in America" (WWEIA), the dietary interview component of the National Health and Nutrition Examination Survey (NHANES) 2003–2004. NHANES and WWEIA are additional surveys discussed in Chapter 5.

1.3.2 ASSESSMENT, PROGRAM PLANNING, AND EVALUATION

Assessment is the foundation for developing and implementing program planning. Assessment also serves as a baseline for program evaluation. In public health nutrition, assessment may be based on data obtained from national and statewide surveys as well as from information obtained from local community food and nutrition assessments. These topics are discussed in Chapter 12.

1.3.3 PUBLIC HEALTH NUTRITIONISTS

Public health nutritionists are engaged in public health nutrition activities. They have data analysis skills and are proficient in community development, program planning, program management, program evaluation, budget development, and policy analysis and development.[8] Public health nutritionists include midlevel planners, researchers, and teachers, administrators, and directors of research and training programs. Public health nutritionists also function as macro planners, decision makers, and heads of governmental sectors. Although active communication among public health nutritionists and community nutritionists is highly valued, it is most likely that midlevel planners, researchers, and teachers will interact most with professionals at the community level and with upper-level public health nutritionists.[9]

Public health nutritionists provide leadership in assessing the need for public health nutrition campaigns planning, and evaluating them. They are also responsible for assuring compliance with laws and regulations regarding the provision of community nutrition services and assuring competence of the nutrition workforce.

Public health nutrition professionals are employed by the public (that is, government or tax-supported) sector, as opposed to being employed by the private (for-profit) sector. Table 1.1 compares the scope of practice of community vs. public health nutritionists. Box 1.1 contains a discussion of community and public health nutrition as separate branches of public health.

1.3.3.1 Training Public Health Nutrition Professionals

A review of domestic and international graduate and postgraduate programs in public health nutrition reveals an array of objectives and competencies the various programs want their graduates to attain. For example, Harvard established five broad objectives to guide their doctoral-level training of students in public health nutrition. Outlined in this section are the objectives Harvard identified for training their public health nutritionists along with the chapters in this book that focus on each of the objectives.

- To acquire detailed knowledge regarding the biological basis of nutrition and the mechanisms by which diet can influence health (Chapter 6 and Chapter 7)
- To develop the ability to translate research into practice through skills in nutrition surveillance, policy (Chapter 10), program planning and evaluation (Chapter 12), management, oral and written communication, and information dissemination (Chapter 14)
- To gain an interdisciplinary perspective on public nutrition (Chapter 15) in both its domestic and international context
- To develop the necessary quantitative skills in biostatistics required for the evaluation of diet and disease relationships in epidemiologic studies (Chapter 4)
- Attain skills in developing research proposals that require the integration of knowledge about human nutrition with epidemiologic concepts in order to improve diet and activity and reduce disease risk in populations (Chapter 16)

TABLE 1.1
Scope of Practice of the Community Nutritionist and the Public Health Nutritionist

	Community Nutritionist	Public Health Nutritionist
Focus	Focuses on issues that affect the whole population rather than the specific dietary needs of individuals	Focuses on issues that affect the whole population rather than the specific dietary needs of individuals
Emphasis	Emphasizes promoting health and preventing disease in populations and groups	Emphasizes promoting health and preventing disease in populations
Target population	The population is circumscribed to a local level that may consist of homogenous groups of people	The population includes a wide spectrum of people and needs
Practice	The practice of community nutrition may include the delivery of nutrition programs and services	The practice of public health nutrition may include the assessment for and design, management, and evaluation of nutrition programs and services
Supervision	Community nutrition programs and services may be delivered by professionals and also by paraprofessionals who are trained and supervised by professionals	Public health nutritionists may train and supervise community nutritionists
Rules	Community nutritionist adheres to laws and policies; suggests policy	Public health nutritionist enforces laws; creates policy
Employment	Community nutritionists may be employed at the city or county levels, and by local nonprofit and for-profit agencies that deliver nutrition services. Community nutritionists may also be self-employed	Pubic health nutritionists may be employed at the federal, state, county, and city levels

Box 1.1 Community Nutrition and Public Health Nutrition as Separate Branches of Public Health

Unquestionably, public health nutrition encompasses a broader domain than community nutrition. Nevertheless, almost a decade's worth of community nutrition textbooks mischaracterizes public health nutrition as a component of community nutrition.

The problem, as I see it, may be traced to the American Dietetic Association (ADA), whose House of Delegates recognizes six domains of professional practice — *community nutrition*, clinical nutrition, consultation and business practice, food and nutrition management, education, and research. Subsumed under each domain are specialized practice groups. To illustrate: classified under "community nutrition" are the areas of developmental and psychiatric disorders, hunger and environmental nutrition, food and culinary professionals, gerontological nutritionists, nutrition education for the public, vegetarian nutrition, and public health nutrition. This can only be described as a hodgepodge. It appears that as new subspecialties arose they were classified under community nutrition if they did not otherwise belong under the headings of clinical nutrition, management, and so on.

To regard the community as greater than the public is an inherently flawed view. The practice of cataloguing public health nutrition *under* community nutrition distorts the inherent logic of conceiving of the public as being a broader domain than the community. This is not just an issue of semantics. Community nutrition and public health nutrition are complementary disciplines; they are not hierarchical.

It is not my intention to denigrate the ADA, which is constantly challenged by the need to respond to a rapidly changing healthcare landscape. Classifying public health nutrition under community nutrition is just one example where ADA has fallen behind. Because of the organization's obligation to address what their leaders perceive as more pressing concerns, the logical fallacy represented by subsuming public health nutrition under community nutrition persists and has been repeated countless times. (Boyle and Holben, 2006: " … community nutrition is the broader of the two terms"; Obert, 1986, " … community nutrition is used here in a very broad sense to include all nutrition programs in which there is community interaction.")

In terms of career ladders, one may move from working as a community nutritionist in a local comprehensive primary care clinic to the position of senior public health nutritionist at the county level. Having moved from community to county indicates the ability to handle a much broader range of responsibilities and with it more authority and certainly a higher salary. But that move describes a switch from one job title to another. While some of the skills needed to work on the county level may have been honed in the community, new skills will be needed on the county level and other skills will no longer be practiced.

My point is that each area — community nutrition and public health nutrition — is its own specialty, and each is a separate, albeit connected, branch of public health. Similarly, the titles "community nutritionist" and "public health nutritionist" describe different sets of required skills and competencies and certainly a different scope of authority.

Sources:

American Dietetic Association. House of Delegates Governance Structure to Move the Profession Forward. June 23, 2006. Available at: http://www.eatright.org/ada/files/Gov_Structure_1_HOD_BG_FINAL_06-23-06.pdf. Accessed January 10, 2007. Boyle, M.A. and Holben, D.H. *Community Nutrition in Action: An Entrepreneurial Approach, Fourth Edition.* Belmont, CA: Wadsworth/Thomson, 2006. Obert, J.C. *Nutrition in the Community, Second Edition.* New York: Wiley, 1986.

1.3.3.1.1 Training and Credentials in the U.K.

The Nutrition Society of the United Kingdom (U.K.) publishes Standards of Competency in Public Health Nutrition (the U.S. does not have such a document). In the U.K., a nutritionist trained in public health who has recently graduated from an accredited program becomes an associate public health nutritionist (Assoc PHNutr). A full registrant who has professional experience is designated a registered public health nutritionist (RPHNutr). Public health nutritionists from the U.K. (with the credential RPHNutr) meet the Nutrition Society's competency standards. The U.K. provides specialist competencies in public health nutrition congruent with each of the U.K.'s essential public health services,[10] which are similar to those of the U.S. The document is available on the Nutrition Society Web site.[11]

1.4 COMMUNITY NUTRITION

Community nutrition focuses on the delivery of nutrition services in the areas where people live and work. Community nutritionists are engaged in the direct delivery of nutrition services in the community. The *community nutritionist* must have expertise in nutrition education and individual counseling for high-risk clients as well as experience in program planning, implementation, and evaluation. *Nutrition in the community* refers to tax-supported and private food and nutrition programs implemented for the purpose of decreasing the prevalence of undesirable nutrition-related conditions as well as increasing food security in the community. Nutrition in the community also includes the local environment that affects food choices, such as the availability of well-stocked supermarkets, the food environment in schools, businesses that support breastfeeding mothers, as well as nutrition services provided by tax-supported, nonprofit and for-profit entities, such as school meals, the Special Supplemental Nutrition Program for Women, Infants, and Children, local food stamp offices, congregate feeding programs for the elderly, and home delivered meals for the frail elderly and others who are housebound.

Both public health nutrition and community nutrition focus on issues that affect the whole population rather than the specific dietary needs of individuals. The emphasis for each is on promoting health and preventing disease. The population included in community nutrition is circumscribed to a local level. In contrast, the population under the aegis of public health nutrition is much broader.

1.4.1 COMMUNITY NUTRITIONISTS

Community nutritionists are largely employed by the public sector. Increasingly, however, nonprofit organizations (such as the United Way and Second Harvest) and for-profit healthcare organizations, such as health maintenance organizations and hospital outpatient departments, are employing community nutritionists to provide services to community groups. In addition, self-employed community nutritionists provide consultation services to the Special Supplemental Nutrition Program for Women, Infants, and Children programs and senior centers that are required to have a credentialed professional (such as a registered dietitian or licensed nutritionist) provide nutrition education and approve menus.

1.4.2 TRAINING COMMUNITY NUTRITION PROFESSIONALS

The Commission on Accreditation in Dietetics (CADE, the credentialing arm of the American Dietetic Association) requires that certain competencies are met by students who train in dietetic internships with a community emphasis.[12] They must be able to:

- Manage nutrition care for diverse population groups across the life span
- Conduct outcome assessment/evaluation of a community-based food and nutrition program
- Develop community-based food and nutrition programs
- Participate in nutrition surveillance and monitoring of communities
- Participate in community-based research
- Participate in food and nutrition policy development and evaluation based on community needs and resources
- Consult with organizations regarding food access for target populations
- Develop a health promotion/disease prevention intervention project
- Participate in waived point-of-care testing, such as hematocrit and cholesterol levels
- Conduct general health assessment, such as blood pressure and vital signs

1.5 GOVERNMENT'S ROLE IN NUTRITION IN PUBLIC HEALTH

The field of public health nutrition is fueled by the public largesse. As a result, every discussion about nutrition in public health must include reference to its funding sources in the federal government. To appreciate public health nutrition, it is therefore necessary to understand the organizational structure of the U.S. government, including its various departments and agencies that oversee public health nutrition programs. The following section provides a brief overview of the federal government. The federal government has enormous influence over public health nutrition. As noted in the next section, federal agencies are discussed in each chapter of this book.

1.5.1 FEDERAL GOVERNMENT

The structure and responsibilities of the federal[13] government are defined by the U.S. Constitution. Its first three articles establish the legislative branch (Article I), the presidency (Article II), and the judiciary (Article III). An organizational chart of the U.S. government appears in Figure 1.1.

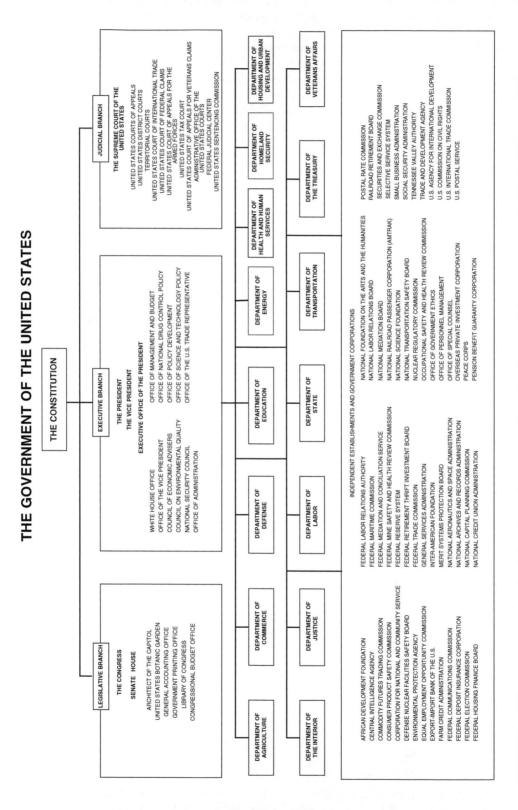

FIGURE 1.1 U.S. government organizational chart. (From Government of the United States. *U.S. Government Manual, 2006–2007 Edition*, p. 22.) Available at: http://bensguide.gpo.gov/files/gov_chart.pdf. Accessed August 22, 2006.

"Federal," which also means "national," refers to the government of the U.S. as distinct from those of the individual states. A federal government is one in which power is divided between one central and several regional authorities. In a federal system such as that of the U.S., the governments often evolved from confederations. (Example: the 13 original colonies).

1.5.1.1 The U.S. Constitution

As defined by the U.S. Constitution (1787), the federal government consists of three branches:

- *The executive branch* — comprised of the president, vice president, and executive departments and independent agencies — is responsible for enforcing the laws of the U.S.
- *The legislative branch or Congress* — made up of the Senate and the House of Representatives — is responsible for making the laws which govern the country
- *The judicial branch* — consisting of the federal courts such as the Supreme Court, court of claims, court of customs, circuit courts of appeal, and district courts — is responsible for interpreting the laws and ensuring that the rights of the people are protected.

1.5.1.2 The Bill of Rights

Just as important as the governmental structure established by the Constitution are the personal freedoms guaranteed by the Bill of Rights and the 13th, 14th, and 15th constitutional amendments. Approved by the First Congress in 1789 and ratified by the states in 1791, the first ten amendments to the Constitution, known collectively as the Bill of Rights, assure basic individual liberties essential to a free and democratic society. In the aftermath of the Civil War, the 13th, 14th, and 15th Amendments (1865–1870) continued the mission of the Bill of Rights by abolishing slavery, by assuring citizens due process in actions taken under state governments, and by taking the first steps toward providing suffrage for all adults. These Constitutional guarantees stand as a bulwark against governmental abuses. The Constitution has been amended 17 additional times since the Bill of Rights, most recently in 1992 (see Box 1.2).

Box 1.2 Constitutional Amendments, 1791–1992

Collectively, amendments one through ten are known as The Bill of Rights. They were signed in 1791.

1. "Freedom of speech, religion, assembly, and the press" protects the people's right to practice religion, to speak freely, to assemble (meet), to address the government and of the press to publish. *Rules regarding food advertising fall under this amendment.*
2. Protects the right to own guns. There is debate whether this is a right that protects the state or a right that protects individuals.
3. Guarantees that the army cannot force homeowners to give them room and board.
4. Protects the people from the government's improperly taking property, papers, or people without a valid warrant based on probable cause (good reason).
5. Protects people from being held for committing a crime unless they are properly indicted, that they may not be tried twice for the same crime, that you need not be forced to testify against yourself, and from property being taken without just compensation. It also contains due process guarantees.
6. Guarantees a speedy trial, an impartial jury, that the accused can confront witnesses against them, and that the accused must be allowed to have a lawyer.

7. Guarantees a jury trial in federal civil court cases. This type of case is normally no longer heard in federal court.
8. Guarantees that punishments will be fair and not cruel, and that extraordinarily large fines will not be set. Rules regarding correctional health fall under this amendment. A jail's failure to attend to the medical needs of its detainees may subject it to liability under U.S. law. In *Estelle v. Gamble,* a case involving medical care in the Texas prison system, the U.S. Supreme Court held that deliberate indifference to the serious medical needs of prisoners is "unnecessary and wanton infliction of pain" in violation of the Eighth Amendment's prohibition of cruel and unusual punishment. (A higher standard of medical care may apply to pretrial detainees, who are entitled under the due process clause of the Fourteenth Amendment to be free from all punishment; in any event, a pretrial detainee's rights should never be less than those of a convicted prisoner.)
9. A statement that other rights aside from those listed may exist, and just because they are not listed doesn't mean they can be violated.
10. States that any power not granted to the federal government belongs to the states or to the people.
11. More clearly defines the original jurisdiction of the Supreme Court concerning a suit brought against a state by a citizen of another state.
12. Redefines how the President and Vice President are chosen by the Electoral College, making the two positions cooperative, rather than first and second highest vote-getters. It also ensures that anyone who becomes Vice President must be eligible to become President.
13. "Abolition" abolished slavery.
14. "The right to vote" ensured that all citizens of all states enjoyed not only rights on the federal level, but on the state level, as well. It removed the three-fifths counting of slaves in the census. It ensured that the U.S. would not pay the debts of rebellious states. It also had several measures designed to ensure the loyalty of legislators who participated on the Confederate side of the Civil War.
15. Ensures that race cannot be used as a criterion for voting.
16. Authorizes the U.S. to collect income tax without regard to the population of the states.
17. Shifts the process of selecting senators from the state legislatures to the people of the states.
18. Also known as "Prohibition," abolished the sale or manufacture of alcohol in the U.S.; amendment repealed by the 21st Amendment.
19. Also known as "Suffrage," ensures that sex cannot be used as a criterion for voting.
20. Set new start dates for the terms of the Congress and the President, and clarifies how the deaths of presidents before swearing-in would be handled.
21. Repealed the 18th Amendment.
22. Set a limit on the number of times a president could be elected: two 4-year terms. It has one exception for a vice president who assumes the presidency after the death or removal of the president, establishing the maximum term of any president to 10 years.
23. Grants the District of Columbia (Washington, D.C.) the right to three electors in presidential elections.
24. The "poll tax" amendment ensures that no tax can be levied as a requirement to vote for any federal office.
25. Clarifies even further the line of succession to the presidency and establishes rules for a president who becomes unable to perform his duties while in office.
26. Ensures that any person 18 or over may vote.
27. Requires that any law that increases the salary of legislators may not take effect until after an election.

From time to time, amendments to the Constitution are cited in this book. For example, the First Amendment is examined during the discussion about advertising that appears in Chapter 7 (Weight Control Challenges and Solutions), and the 14th Amendment is referred to in a discussion about healthcare for inmates, which is presented in Chapter 8 (Special Populations).

1.5.1.3 The Legislative Branch of the Federal Government

The U.S. Congress is the legislative body of the federal government. It is bicameral (consisting of two bodies), comprising the House of Representatives and the Senate. The House of Representatives has 435 members, each representing a congressional district and serving a 2-year term. House seats are apportioned among the states by population. Each state has two senators, regardless of population. There are 100 senators, serving staggered 6-year terms. Both senators and representatives are chosen through direct election.

The U.S. Constitution vests all legislative powers of the federal government in the Congress. The powers of Congress are limited to those enumerated in the Constitution; all other powers are reserved to the states and the people. Through acts of Congress, Congress may regulate interstate and foreign commerce, levy taxes, organize the federal courts, maintain the military, declare war, and exercise certain other "necessary and proper" powers.

The House and Senate are coequal houses. However, there are some special powers granted to one chamber only. The Senate's advice and consent is required to confirm presidential nominations to high-level executive and judicial positions, and for the ratification of treaties. Bills for raising revenue must originate in the House of Representatives, and only the House may initiate any impeachment proceedings.

Congress meets in the U.S. Capitol in Washington, D.C. Reckoned according to the terms of Representatives, the 109th Congress was in session from 2005 through 2006. The 110th Congress meets from 2007 through 2008, and so on. THOMAS, named in honor of Thomas Jefferson and invoked throughout the book, is a powerful interactive tool used for obtaining information about bills proposed and laws that have been enacted.

The legislative mandates for incorporating cultural competence into all pubic health programs are discussed in Chapter 9 (Cultural Competence). Congress relies on epidemiology to help determine where to allocate limited resources, as discussed in Chapter 4 (Epidemiology).

1.5.1.4 The Executive Branch of the Federal Government

The power of the executive branch is vested in the president, who also serves as commander-in-chief of the armed forces. In order for a person to become president, he or she must be a native-born citizen of the U.S., be at least 35 years of age, and have resided in the U.S. for at least 14 years. Once elected, the president serves a term of 4 years and may be re-elected only once.

The president appoints the cabinet and oversees the various agencies and departments of the federal government. The tradition of the cabinet dates back to the beginnings of the presidency itself. One of the principal purposes of the cabinet (drawn from Article II of the Constitution) is to advise the president on any subject relating to the duties of their respective offices. The cabinet includes the vice president and the heads (usually known as "secretaries") of the 15 executive departments — Agriculture, Commerce, Defense, Education, Energy, Health and Human Services, Homeland Security, Housing and Urban Development, Interior, Justice (headed by the Attorney General), Labor, State, Transportation, Treasury, and Veterans Affairs. Also included in the cabinet are the administrator of the Environmental Protection Agency, the director of the Office of Management and Budget, the director of the National Drug Control Policy, and the U.S. trade representative.

In terms of nutrition in public health, the two most important cabinet departments — and the government agencies referred to most frequently in this book — are the U.S. Department of Agriculture (USDA) and the U.S. Department of Health and Human Services (HHS). In addition to USDA and HHS, occasional allusions appear to the Departments of Defense, Education, Homeland

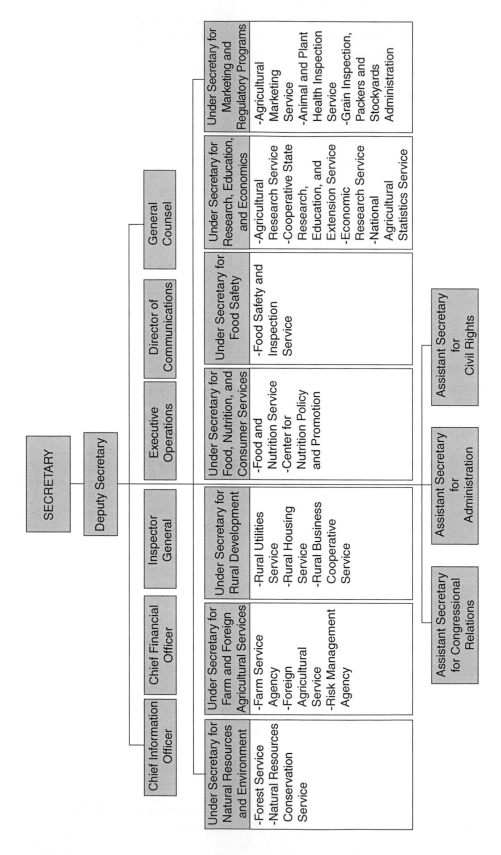

FIGURE 1.2 U.S. Department of Agriculture organizational chart. From http://www.usda.gov/img/content/org_chart_enlarged.jpg.

Security, Interior, and Justice (DOJ). For example, the Department of Defense Fruit and Vegetable Program is discussed in Chapter 14, and nutritional issues in the Justice Department's correctional health system are discussed in Chapter 8 (Special Populations).

1.5.1.4.1 Department of Agriculture

The U.S. Department of Agriculture (USDA) organizational chart appears in Figure 1.2. At least six USDA offices within three agencies have a profound effect on public health nutrition policy and practice see Box 1.3. These are the Food and Nutrition Service (FNS) and Center for Nutrition Policy and Promotion (CNPP) within Food, Nutrition, and Consumer Services (FNCS); Food Safety and Inspection Service (FSIS) within Food Safety; and Agricultural Research Service (ARS), Economic Research Service (ERS), and Cooperative State Research, Education, and Extension Service (CSREES) within Research, Education, and Economics.

1.5.1.4.1.1 Food, Nutrition and Consumer Services

The Food and Nutrition Service (FNS) administers the USDA food assistance programs, which serve one in six Americans, and represent the nation's commitment to the principle that no one in the U.S. should fear hunger or experience want. The goals of the programs are to provide needy persons with access to a more nutritious diet, to improve the eating habits of the nation's children, and to help America's farmers by providing an outlet for distributing foods purchased under farmer assistance authorities. FNS works in partnership with the states in all its programs. State and local agencies determine most administrative details regarding distribution of food benefits and eligibility of participants, and FNS provides commodities and funding for additional food and to cover administrative costs. FNS administers the following food assistance programs. FNS food and nutrition assistance programs are discussed in Chapter 13 (Promoting Food Security).

The Center for Nutrition Policy and Promotion (CNPP) coordinates nutrition policy in the USDA and provides overall leadership in nutrition education for the American public. It also coordinates with HHS in the review, revision, and dissemination of the Dietary Guidelines for Americans, the federal government's statement of nutrition policy formed by a consensus of scientific and medical professionals. Chapter 11 (Food and Nutrition Guidance) examines the food guidance system and dietary guidelines developed and maintained by CNPP.

1.5.1.4.1.2 Food Safety

The Food Safety and Inspection Service (FSIS) regulates the processing and distribution of meat and meat products, poultry and poultry products, and egg products, to ensure that those products moving in intrastate, interstate, and foreign commerce are wholesome, unadulterated, and properly labeled and packaged. Chapter 15 (Food Safety and Defense) describes the role of FSIS in protecting the food supply from unintentional and intentional contamination.

1.5.1.4.1.3 Research, Education, and Economics

The Agricultural Research Service (ARS) conducts research and provides information access and dissemination to ensure safe food and to assess the nutritional needs of Americans. The Economic Research Service (ERS) provides decision makers with economic and related social science information and analysis in support of the USDA's goals of enhancing the protection and safety of U.S. agriculture and food, and improving U.S. nutrition and health. Research from the ARS and ERS is cited throughout the book.

The Cooperative State Research, Education, and Extension Service (CSREES) links the research and education resources and activities of the USDA with academic and land-grant institutions throughout the nation. CSREES's partnership with the land-grant universities is critical to effective shared planning, delivery, and accountability for research, higher education, and extension programs. CSREES provides research, extension, and education leadership through economic and community systems; families, 4-H, and nutrition; and competitive research, education, and extension programs. CSREES, a major source of funds for demonstration projects and experiments in public health and nutrition, is discussed in Chapter 16 (Grant Writing).

Box 1.3 Selected USDA Agencies that Influence Public Health Nutrition Policy and Practice

- Agricultural Research Service (ARS) serves as the USDA's principal in-house research agency.
- Center for Nutrition Policy and Promotion (CNPP) strives to improve the health and well-being of Americans by developing and promoting dietary guidance that links scientific research to the nutrition needs of consumers.
- Cooperative State Research, Education and Extension Service (CSREES) works with land-grant universities and other public and private organizations to advance a global system of extramural research, extension, and higher education in the food and agricultural sciences.
- Economic Research Service (ERS) functions as the USDA's principal social science research agency.
- Food and Nutrition Service (FNS) increases food security and reduces hunger in partnership with cooperating organizations by providing children and low-income adults access to food, a healthy diet, and nutrition education in a manner that supports American agriculture and inspires public confidence.
- Food Safety and Inspection Service (FSIS) enhances public health and well-being by protecting the public from food borne illness and ensuring that the nation's meat, poultry, and egg products are safe, wholesome, and correctly packaged.

1.5.1.4.1.4   Library

USDA's National Agricultural Library (NAL) ensures and enhances access to agricultural information. The NAL administers the Food and Nutrition Information Center (FNIC, http://www.nal.usda.gov/fnic/about.shtml), which serves as a source of food and nutrition information for nutrition and health professionals, educators, government personnel, and consumers.

1.5.1.4.2   Department of Health and Human Services

The Department of Health and Human Services (HHS) organization chart appears in Figure 1.3. All 11 agencies in this department interface with nutrition, but particularly noteworthy are the Centers for Disease Control and Prevention (CDC), the Food and Drug Administration (FDA), and the National Institutes of Health (NIH), the Administration on Aging (AoA) and the Indian Health Service (HIS). Highlighted in Box 1.4 are the institutes and offices within the NIH that serve as the custodians of funds that support the preponderance of nutrition-related research in human health and disease.

1.5.1.4.2.1   Centers for Disease Control and Prevention

As indicated in Figure 1.4, the CDC consists of six coordinating centers and an institute. In terms of public health and nutrition, the most important units in the CDC are located within its Coordinating Center for Health Information and Service, especially the National Center for Health Statistics (NCHS) and the Coordinating Center for Health Promotion, especially the National Center for Chronic Disease Prevention and Health Promotion and the National Center for Birth Defects and Developmental Disabilities (NCBDDD).

Many programs under the jurisdiction of the CDC are discussed throughout this book. For example, Chapter 14 (Social Marketing and Communication) looks at Verb™ (which was defunded in 2006), the Diabetes Education Program, WISEWOMAN (Well-Integrated Screening and Evaluation for Women Across the Nation), and the National Bone Health Campaign. That chapter also contains a section about the folic acid education efforts of the NCBDDD. Chapter 5 (Food and Nutrition Surveys) examines surveys conducted by the National Center for Health Statistics (NCHS), whereas Chapter 7 presents the NCHS growth charts.

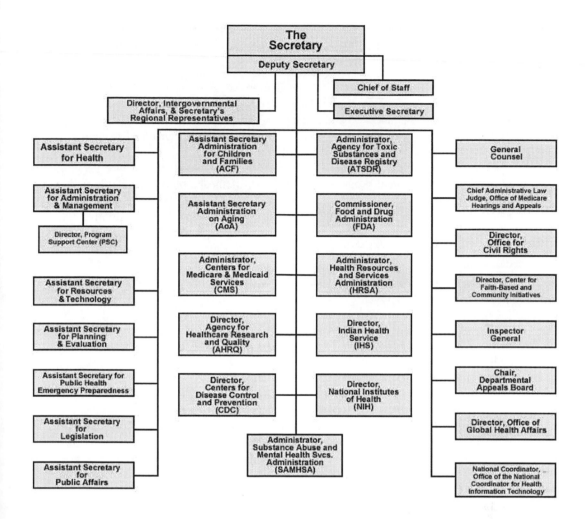

FIGURE 1.3 U.S. Department of Health and Human Services organizational chart. From HHS Grant Awards. Fiscal Year 2004. Available at: http://taggs.hhs.gov/AnnualReport/FY2004/documents/TAGGS_2004_Annual_Report.doc. Accessed August 22, 2006.

1.5.1.4.2.2 Food and Drug Administration

FDA's mission is to promote and protect the public health by helping safe and effective products reach the market in a timely way, to monitor products for continued safety after they are in use, and to help the public get the accurate, science-based information needed to improve health. As discussed in Chapter 15, FDA safeguards the nation's food supply by making sure that all ingredients used in foods are safe; that food is free of contaminants such as disease-causing organisms, chemicals, or other harmful substances; new food additives are safe; the safety of dietary supplements are monitored as well as the content of infant formulas and medical foods; and food labels are regulated.

1.5.1.4.2.3 Indian Health Service

IHS is responsible for providing federal health services to American Indians and Alaska Natives. The IHS is the principal federal healthcare provider and health advocate for Indian people. Its goal is to raise their health status to the highest possible level. The IHS currently provides health services to approximately 1.5 million American Indians and Alaska Natives who belong to more

---

Box 1.4 Selected NIH Institutes and Agencies that Fund Nutrition Research

- *National Cancer Institute* (NCI), established in 1937, addresses suffering and deaths due to cancer. Through basic and clinical biomedical research and training, NCI conducts and supports research aimed at preventing cancer before it starts, identifying at the earliest stage, cancers that do develop, eliminating cancers through innovative treatment interventions, and biologically controlling those cancers that cannot be eliminated so they become manageable, chronic diseases.
- *National Heart, Lung, and Blood Institute* (NHLBI), establish in 1948, provides leadership for a national program in diseases of the heart, blood vessels, lung, and blood; blood resources; and sleep disorders. Since October 1997, the NHLBI has also had administrative responsibility for the NIH Woman's Health Initiative. The institute plans, conducts, fosters, and supports an integrated and coordinated program of basic research, clinical investigations and trials, observational studies, and demonstration and education projects.
- *National Institute on Aging* (NIA), established in 1974, leads a national program of research on the biomedical, social, and behavioral aspects of the aging process, the prevention of age-related diseases and disabilities, and the promotion of a better quality of life for all older Americans.
- *National Institute of Allergy and Infectious Diseases* (NIAID), established in 1948, supports research aimed at understanding, treating, and ultimately preventing the myriad infectious, immunologic, and allergic diseases.
- *National Institute of Diabetes and Digestive and Kidney Diseases* (NIDDK), established in 1948, conducts and supports basic and applied research and provides leadership for a national program in diabetes, endocrinology, and metabolic diseases; digestive diseases and nutrition; and kidney, urologic, and hematologic diseases. Several of these diseases are among the leading causes of disability and death; all seriously affect the quality of life of those who have them.
- *National Center for Complementary and Alternative Medicine* (NCCAM), established in 1999, explores complementary and alternative medical (CAM) practices in the context of rigorous science.
- *National Center on Minority Health and Health Disparities* (NCMHD), established in 1993, promotes minority health and leads, coordinates, supports, and assesses the NIH effort to reduce and ultimately eliminate health disparities. In this effort NCMHD conducts and supports basic, clinical, social, and behavioral research, promotes research infrastructure and training, fosters emerging programs, disseminates information, and reaches out to minority and other communities with a disparity of health needs.

---

than 557 federally recognized tribes in 35 states. American Indian and Alaska Native communities, which suffer a disproportionately high rate of type 2 diabetes when compared with other populations in the U.S. and throughout the world, are discussed in Chapter 3 (The Population of the U.S.).

1.5.1.4.2.4   National Institutes of Health

NIH is the federal focal point for medical research in the U.S. The NIH, comprising 27 separate institutes and centers, is one of eight health agencies of the Public Health Service. The NIH National Library of Medicine (NLM) collects, organizes, and makes available biomedical science information to scientists, health professionals, and the public. The library's Web-based databases, including

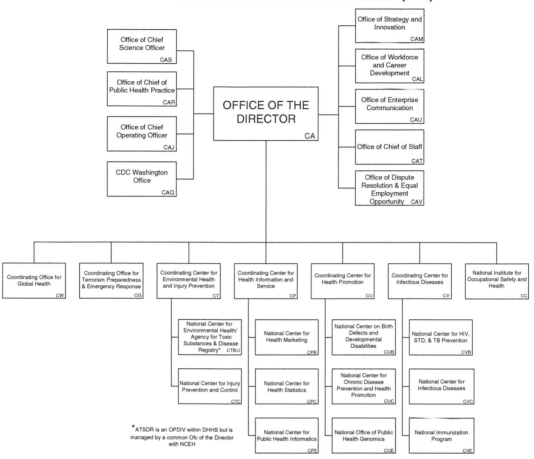

DEPARTMENT OF HEALTH AND HUMAN SERVICES
CENTERS FOR DISEASE CONTROL AND PREVENTION (CDC)

FIGURE 1.4 Centers for Disease Control and Prevention organizational chart. From http://www.cdc.gov/maso/pdf/CDC.pdf.

PubMed/Medline and MedlinePlus, are used extensively around the world. Grants administered by NIH are discussed in Chapter 16. Programs administered by the National Heart, Lung, and Blood Institute (NHLBI), such as *We Can!*, are discussed in Chapter 14, and the National Weight Control Registry, a program funded by the National Institute of Diabetes and Digestive Diseases, is examined in Chapter 7. Chapter 6 (Health Disparities) contains discussions of WISEWOMAN and *We Can!* (Ways to Enhance Children's Activity and Nutrition). Four NIH institutes (NHLBI, NIDDK, the National Institute of Child Health and Human Development, and the National Cancer Institute) collaborate on supporting *We Can!*

1.5.1.4.2.5   Administration on Aging
AoA's mission is to help society prepare for an aging population and to develop a comprehensive, coordinated, and cost-effective system of long-term care that helps elderly individuals to maintain their dignity in their homes and communities. The agency serves as one of the nation's largest providers of home- and community-based care for older persons and their caregivers. As such, Chapter 13 contains a discussion of AoA-administered congregate and home-delivered meals programs and other nutrition services that are carried out in a variety of settings.

1.5.1.5 The Judicial Branch of the Federal Government

The judicial branch hears cases that challenge or require interpretation of the legislation passed by Congress and signed by the president. It consists of the Supreme Court and the lower federal courts. Appointees to the federal bench serve for life or until they voluntarily resign or retire. The Supreme Court is the most visible of all the federal courts. The number of Justices is determined by Congress rather than the Constitution, and since 1869, the Court has been composed of one chief justice and eight associate justices. Justices are nominated by the president and confirmed by the Senate.

1.6 NUTRITION IN PUBLIC HEALTH — THE BOOK

The title of this book — *Nutrition in Public Health* — represents my view that nutrition is a component of the broad field of public health. As someone who trained in public health nutrition, I certainly had my colleagues in mind when writing this book, but public health nutritionists make up only a small fraction of the public health workforce engaged in nutrition. This book contains information that is useful to everyone who addresses food and nutrition issues as part of their public health duties — epidemiologists, grant writers, community health educators, public health nurses, public health physicians, and public health dentists, as well as nutritionists.

In particular, *Nutrition in Public Health* was designed to serve as a resource guide, reference book, textbook, roadmap, as well as a key to demystifying access to online information about nutrition in public health.

Nutrition in Public Health may be used as the following:

- Resource guide for public health and community nutritionists
- Reference book for nonnutritionist public health professionals who address food and nutrition issues as part of their duties
- Textbook for traditional and online courses in community and public health and nutrition
- Compendium of government-financed food and nutrition programs, surveys, and research tools for public health professionals who must assess the need for and design, manage, and evaluate nutrition programs and services
- Guide to accessing online information about topics related to nutrition in public health

1.6.1 NUTRITION IN PUBLIC HEALTH ONLINE

This book takes considerable advantage of the Internet.

1.6.1.1 Distance Education and Electronic Enhancements for Traditional Instruction

This is the first book devoted to nutrition in public health that has been developed for use in distance education courses as well as in the traditional classroom setting. The CRC Press Web site contains all the references included in this book, more than three quarters of which are linked to free full texts of the documents cited. *Nutrition in Public Health* relies heavily on government documents and reports, therefore, many of the sources referred to in the book are in the public domain and freely available online in their full-text versions.

A large proportion of the journal articles cited were chosen because they, too, are available in free full-text format. The occasional peer-reviewed journal article that is not freely available may be accessed through the college or teaching hospital's full-text electronic journal holdings.

1.6.1.1.1   *Interactive Database*

The almost universal availability of the Internet has revolutionized education and research. Public health practitioners and students may retrieve data from myriad interactive databases of national surveys and have the information instantly compiled into camera-ready tables, charts, and maps.

The Centers for Disease Control and Prevention (CDC), in particular, has released many online interactive databases. Wide-ranging Online Data for Epidemiologic Research (WONDER)[13] is one of CDC's databases highlighted in *Nutrition in Public Health.* WONDER makes the information resources of the CDC available to public health professionals and the public at large. For example, access to the widely-quoted Behavioral Risk Factor Surveillance System[14] (BRFSS) is available through WONDER.

Through THOMAS,[15] one can perform a quick search of the text of proposed and enacted legislation from the 101st Congress (1989–1990) to the current legislature by word/phrase or bill number. Several important pieces of legislation (such as Healthy Lifestyles and Prevention America Act [the HeLP America Act] of 2005) were still in committee when this book went to press. As recently as 1995, it would have been unproductive for me to discuss pending legislation, because of the difficulty for the reader to determine the bill's current status. Now, however, I can simply advise the reader to conduct a THOMAS search to find out if the bill became law, or if not, what its current status is. *Nutrition in Public Health* and its readers benefit from THOMAS, which makes it possible — literally, in seconds — to obtain current information about the federal legislation that is discussed in the book. Because of the power of the Internet, what was previously a frustrating circumstance has become easily achievable in a moment.

1.7   CONCLUSION

Nutrition in public health — the practice of nutrition within the public health arena — is a complex undertaking. Fueled by taxpayer dollars, public health involves all levels of government, from numerous agencies at the federal level to small, community-based organizations. Public health practitioners are specially trained, achieving competency in biostatistics, epidemiology, environmental health, health administration, and/or the social and behavioral sciences. In addition, public health nutritionists, while seeking to improve the health of populations through improved nutrition, must also be proficient in community development; program planning, management, and evaluation; budget development; and policy analysis and development.

The Internet opens up a vast world of resources to support this enterprise from access to legislative databases to scholarly articles to online access to other, like-minded organizations. I trust you will enjoy your exploration of this fascinating, rapidly changing field.

1.8   ACRONYMS

ADA	American Dietetic Association
AoA	Administration on Aging
CADE	Commission on Accreditation for Dietetics Education
CDC	Centers for Disease Control and Prevention
CNPP	Center for Nutrition Policy and Promotion
CSREES	Cooperative State Research, Education, and Extension Service
DHHS	Department of Health and Human Services
ERS	Economic Research Service
FDA	Food and Drug Administration
FNCS	Food, Nutrition and Consumer Services
FNIC	Food, Nutrition and Information Center
FSIS	Food Safety and Inspection Service
IHS	Indian Health Service

NCBDDD	National Center for Birth Defects and Developmental Disabilities
NCHS	National Center for Health Statistics
NHLBI	National Heart, Lung, and Blood Institute
NIDDK	National Institute of Diabetes and Digestive and Kidney Diseases
NIH	National Institutes of Health
NLM	National Library of Medicine
ARS	Agricultural Research Service
USDA	U.S. Department of Agriculture
We Can!	Ways to Enhance Children's Activity and Nutrition!
WIC	Special Supplemental Nutrition Program for Women, Infants, and Children
WISEWOMAN	Well-Integrated Screening and Evaluation for Women Across the Nation

REFERENCES

1. Institute of Medicine. *The Future of Public Health.* Washington, D.C.: National Academy Press, 1988. Box 13. Available at: http://darwin.nap.edu/books/030905625X/html/44.html. Accessed August 27, 2006.
2. Council on Education in Public Health (CEPH). Accreditation Criteria Public Health Programs. Amended June 2005. Available at: http://www.ceph.org/i4a/pages/index.cfm?pageid=3350. Accessed August 31, 2006.
3. Johnson, D.B., Eaton, D.L., Wahl, P.W., and Gleason, C. Public health nutrition practice in the United States. *Am Diet Assoc.* 101, 529–534, 2001.
4. Hughes, R. Definitions for public health nutrition: a developing consensus. *Public Health Nutr.* 6, 615–620, 2003.
5. Australian Public Health Nutrition Academic Collaboration: http://www.health.gov.au/internet/wcms/Publishing.nsf/Content/pherp-innovations-2.htm.
6. Johnson, D.B., Eaton, D.L., Wahl, P.W., and Gleason, C. Public health nutrition practice in the United States. *Am Diet Assoc.* 101, 529–534, 2001.
7. Interagency Board for Nutrition Monitoring and Related Research. Bialostosky, K., Ed. *Nutrition Monitoring in the United States: The Directory of Federal and State Nutrition Monitoring and Related Research Activities.* Hyattsville, MD: National Center for Health Statistics. 2000. Available at: http://www.cdc.gov/nchs/data/misc/direc-99.pdf. Accessed August 31, 2006.
8. Johnson, D.B., Eaton, D.L., Wahl, P.W., and Gleason, C. Public health nutrition practice in the United States. *Am Diet Assoc.* 101, 529–534, 2001.
9. Solon, F.S. Developing a national training pyramid. *Food Nutr Bull.* 18(2), June 1997. Available at: http://www.unu.edu/unupress/food/V182e/begin.htm#Contents. Accessed October 22, 2004.
10. The Nutrition Society. Standards of competency in public health nutrition. Specialist registration in public health nutrition. Available at: http://www.nutritionsociety.org/documents/20060410section3.pdf. Accessed August 27, 2006.
11. Map of Specialist Competencies in Public Health Nutrition on the Standards in Public Health. Available at: http://www.nutritionsociety.org/documents/20060411section3professionalphnguidance2004.pdf. Accessed August 27, 2006.
12. Commission on Accreditation for Dietetics Education. *Am Diet Assoc.* Foundation Knowledge and Skills and Competency Requirements for Entry-Level Dietitians. Available at: http://www.eatright.org/ada/files/2002rdfksc.pdf. Accessed August 27, 2006.
13. CDC. Wide-ranging Online Data for Epidemiologic Research (WONDER). Available at: http://wonder.cdc.gov/welcome.html. Accessed August 27, 2006.
14. CDC. Youth Risk Behavior Surveillance System (YRBSS). Available at: http://www.cdc.gov/HealthyYouth/yrbs/index.htm. Accessed August 27, 2006.
15. The Library of Congress. THOMAS. Available at: http://thomas.loc.gov/. Accessed August 29, 2006.

2 Preventing Disease or Promoting Health?

The most sophisticated and effective healthcare in the world cannot produce results as good as simply remaining healthy in the first place.

Robert G. Evans

2.1 INTRODUCTION

In June 2005, the *New York Times* reported on the sudden upsurge of obesity in Mexico. The article noted that obesity is increasing throughout developing nations as fast foods displace home cooking and urbanized populations cease to participate in any physical activity — a pattern well-established in the U.S. and echoed in other Westernized countries.[1] Along with obesity arrive increases in hypertension, cardiovascular disease (CVD), type 2 diabetes, and a host of other ills. Taking obesity as emblematic of most health issues confronting developed and developing nations,* we can ask what the role of public health should be in the relationship between the individual and the environment, both natural and built.

During the past century, public health has become increasingly dominated by technological advances and epidemiology. Yet scientific knowledge is only one of several elements fundamental to effective public health practice. Such knowledge must be combined with engagement in civil society and social movements to result in effective action.[2]

This chapter suggests we need a broader-based interpretation of effective public health in the U.S., with health promotion as its overarching theme. We can no longer develop effective public health measures by relying solely on Koch's postulates that equate one germ with one disease.[3]

Modern diseases of cancer, heart disease, and obesity do not fit this paradigm. Accepting that the health of an individual arises from the health of the society and of the environment, if the practice of public health is to be effective, the ideology of health promotion must pervade all fields impacting the public good — from environmental protection to healthcare.

2.1.1 TOWARD A DEFINITION OF HEALTH

Health is an amorphous concept. The word derives from the Greek word meaning "whole" and is defined as "wholeness, being whole, sound or well."[4] This idea of wholeness is open to wide-ranging interpretation and can be seen to refer to the health of the individual, the community, or the nation.

Historically, health was often synonymous with the health of the state (whose needs were a steady supply of soldiers or laborers well enough to fight or work), control of overpopulation, protection of the elite, and environmental stability.[5] Many developments in public health have arisen from the poor physical state of military recruits. At present, U.S. Army recruiters worry that potential soldiers are too overweight to fight.[6]

---

* The HIV/AIDS epidemic, for example, differs significantly from obesity as a health issue and occupies a different place in a health-promotion model of public health. See the discussion of tuberculosis in Section 2.7.3, Would a Health Promotion Model Neglect the Reality of Disease?

In 1948, the World Health Organization (WHO) defined health as "a state of complete physical, mental, and social well-being and not merely the absence of disease or infirmity."[7] Critics of the definition suggest that for the definition of "health" to be a useful guiding principle, it must refer to a less idealistic state that can be agreed upon as an achievable level of well-being.[8] Although WHO's intent may have been intentionally ambitious, it is also worth examining a more restrictive definition of health.

Seedhouse's "foundations theory of health," which ultimately results in individual achievement of human potential, posits four basic building blocks for all people, and a fifth block that varies due to personal characteristics and circumstances. Briefly, the first four blocks represent:

1. Basic needs such as food, shelter, and clothing
2. Access to as much information as possible about all factors affecting one's life
3. The skill and confidence needed to assimilate this information
4. The understanding that one does not operate in isolation but as part of one's physical and societal surroundings

The fifth block differs for each individual, depending on the additional support needed in difficult circumstances. This block becomes necessary when a life problem, such as an adverse medical event or the loss of a job or home, diminishes or destroys the ability of the four primary building blocks to support a person's present way of life.[8] Particularly valuable about this definition is that it does not rely on biology alone and thus not on traditional medicine. Rather, it places the individual within a context and provides the individual with the information, skills, and socialization needed to negotiate the environment in attempting to fulfill his or her potential.

Unfortunately, the foundations theory is limited in that it does not incorporate the role of an individual's environment on his or her health. A health promotion model, conversely, is based on the ideal of providing a healthy environment within which the individual operates.

2.2 BRIEF REVIEW OF THE HISTORY OF PUBLIC HEALTH

The history of public health in developed countries reveals origins far different from the contemporary practice of public health in the U.S., which has perhaps been sidetracked by a focus on medical intervention and an infatuation with technical solutions. It has been observed that while "public health has evolved into a subdivision of medicine with minimal and subordinate inclusion of the ancillary disciplines of engineering and the social sciences ... *health has been improved by many non-medical factors* — economic prosperity, town planning, architecture, religious and humanitarian charity, the power of organized labor, and even broader political changes resulting in the greater availability of political or economic rights ... " (italic emphasis added).[5]

One of the earliest roles of public health was in reaction to an epidemic crisis, an effort undertaken only when the public believed action would make a difference.[5] Classically, the reaction to an epidemic had been abject resignation. Medieval Christian Latin countries — in the face of the plague and leprosy — became activist, although the actions taken, such as quarantine and pogroms, by no means benefited everyone. A populace acting precipitously and independently (such as by burning groups of its citizens to death) threatened civil and ecclesiastical institutions. It is in institutional responses to such actions that public health emerges as a form of public authority.[5]

Another early role of public health in Western societies was to regulate communities for the common good. This policing function included enforcing rules for sanitation and construction, caring for the poor, regulating work hours, conducting markets and the quality of the goods sold, maintaining population statistics, and regulating medical practice — activities still within the purview of public health. Interestingly, whereas regulation of medical practice served the interests of established practitioners, it was done under the guise of maintaining the quality of public medical care,[5] a stance hauntingly reminiscent of the American Medical Association's.

During the course of the 19th century, public health became less a means of supporting the state than a right of citizenship. Public health grew less reactive and regulatory and more oriented toward the goal of reducing rates of morbidity and mortality.[5] This new focus on prevention paralleled and stimulated the growth in knowledge of the means of prevention. Yet during the first half of the 19th century, although France was the scientific leader in public health, sadly researchers could not envision how to translate their findings into preventive legislation. Whereas Britain embraced sanitation — comprehensive systems of water and sewerage — as a means not only to improved health, but for a "prettier," happier, and better world, significantly, the U.S. remained alone among Western nations in adhering to a policy that an individual's health was solely a private matter.[5]

The 20th century (1880–1970; described by Hamlin as the "Golden Age of Public Health") led to expanded public health regulation of an individual's life — home, work, family relations, recreation, sex — beyond that of the previous century's medical police. That it proved eminently successful in reducing morbidity and mortality was generally seen by its citizens as an appropriate and desirable role of the state. This social contract is reciprocal in that the state can then expect its citizens to strive to be healthy.

With the emergence of cancers and other chronic illnesses, such as type 2 diabetes, with no single preventive strategy, the question arose as to how far reaching were the health obligations of the liberal state to its citizens. Because many of these newly prominent diseases were not infectious, they did not disrupt the community or state in the same manner as the Black Death or impure drinking water, decreasing the value of the reactive and policing approaches to public health. Yet, these diseases do interfere with fulfillment of human potential — and citizens can justly demand attention by the state.[5]

Presently, the "problem of the relationship between the institutions of public health and the citizenry on whose behalf they claim to act is the greatest challenge currently facing public health in the developed world."[5] It is from this perspective that I suggest the role of public health demands a paradigm shift. A strictly reactive, policing, or preventive approach to public health ignores the current health conditions confronting individuals, if not worldwide, certainly in the U.S. and other developed countries. A holistic or systems approach accepts that health does not exist in a vacuum and that the health of a society's physical environment, culture, and economics manifests itself in the individual health status of its citizens.

2.3 DISEASE PREVENTION

Why doesn't disease prevention suffice as a model for public health? What is the relationship between public health, the health of the individual, and disease prevention? A focus on disease prevention assumes exposure to causative factors of disease; in other words, by the time a disease prevention model is implemented, it is already too late. Health promotion preempts disease; it shifts the concentration of effort, positing a state of health (or wholeness) as the norm, as something to be supported and encouraged, rather than a state of disease, of something that must be battled. Thus, although disease prevention and health promotion are often conjoined, I would argue that the two are distinct activities with distinct motivations and goals.

Disease prevention is incontrovertibly the overriding approach to health in the U.S. as evinced by a search of articles available on PubMed and Medline in 2005, retrieved using a limited set of search strings (see Table 2.1).

More than five times as many articles deal with disease prevention as with health promotion. Although 5 articles describe some form of research on promoting a healthy weight, over 3,000 deal with obesity prevention. Promoting nonsmoking got 5 hits, smoking cessation, 10,662. Combined, increasing physical activity and physical activity appeared in 18,954 articles, whereas just 3 diseases partly resulting from lack of activity appeared in 450,626 articles.

TABLE 2.1
Number of Articles Retrieved Using Various Search Strings (2005)

Search String	Number of Articles Retrieved
Health promotion	28,314
Disease prevention	151,841
Promoting healthy weight	5
Obesity prevention	3,498
Promoting nonsmoking	5
Smoking cessation	10,662
Increase fruit and vegetable consumption	50
Reduce fat intake	55
Increase physical activity	242
Physical activity	18,712
Diabetes mellitus	171,137
Cardiovascular disease	27,725
Hypertension	241,764

Clearly, the disease prevention paradigm is not working as effectively to enhance the health of our nation as we would hope. The 6 leading causes of death in the U.S. in 2002 were heart disease, cancer, chronic lower respiratory disease, accidents, and diabetes. None of these diseases cause widespread panic as would a raging epidemic, require policing as would an unsafe water supply, or are preventable by a vaccine. Yet, of these, all but accidental death (and, arguably, even this) would benefit from a health promotion model.

Because the nature of the predominant health issues confronting our society has changed, so must public health change the way in which it confronts these issues. Although diseases such as heart disease and diabetes can be attributed in part to lifestyle choices, cancer can often be attributed to environmental causes, although many remain unidentified or speculative. Even "lifestyle choices" are driven by economic conditions such as poverty or environmental conditions such as lack of sidewalks in suburban neighborhoods.

The public health workforce and infrastructure are unprepared to meet these challenges. "In most developed countries, public health has narrowed in focus and to a large extent, is driven by the research agenda of academic epidemiologists and biomedical scientists. Its focus has often been on what can be measured easily, such as cholesterol or blood pressure, rather than on the immensely more complex issues of the broader social forces that also affect health, directly or indirectly, such as economic transitions."[2] A strictly quantitative approach to health neglects many of the causes of lack of health. In short, the public health activities induced by a disease prevention model are inadequate.

2.4 CURRENT HEALTH BEHAVIORS OF THE U.S. ADULT POPULATION

Only a small portion of the U.S. population adheres to a healthy lifestyle. Four healthy lifestyle characteristics (HLCs) — nonsmoking, healthy weight, fruit and vegetable consumption, and regular physical activity — taken together can serve as a single healthy lifestyle indicator. Using data from the 2000 Behavioral Risk Factor Surveillance System, which surveyed more than 153,000 adults age 18–74 by phone, researchers determined that only 3% of U.S. adults practiced all 4 health behaviors.[9]

A subsequent study, using the same 4 HLCs, examined data from the third National Health and Nutrition Examination Survey (1988–1994) (NHANES III), with a pool of 16,176 adults 21 and older.

They found that 6.8% of the population engaged in all four healthy lifestyle factors and concluded, "there is a long road to travel" before a preponderance of Americans adopt a health lifestyle.[10]

Berrigan et al, using 5 HLCs — they added low alcohol consumption — found that 6% of U.S. adults adhere to a healthy lifestyle and 5% follow none of the recommendations at all.[11] These findings were further corroborated by a study of people with and without coronary heart disease (CHD), using three HLCs: nonsmoking, fruit and vegetable consumption, and physical activity. Among those without heart disease 5% adhered to all 3 behaviors; among those with heart disease 7% adhered to all 3 behaviors (adopting a healthier lifestyle subsequent to a heart incident).[12]

These studies make abundantly clear that the vast majority of the American public does not engage in healthy lifestyle practices. Yet, as discussed in Chapter 10, dietary guidelines for Americans — developed jointly by the Department of Health and Human Services (HHS) and the U.S. Department of Agriculture (USDA) — have been available in one form or another since 1980.[13] Of note, these guidelines were intended for healthy Americans — and thus adhere to a health promotion model. Yet there are very few healthy Americans according to any of the definitions offered thus far. The guidelines, although exemplary in many ways, may be an instance of "too little, too late."

The original impetus for the guidelines was the 1977 Dietary Goals for the U.S., also known as the McGovern report, issued by the Senate Select Committee on Nutrition and Human Needs. This report was particularly distressing to certain special-interest groups because of its recommendation for Americans to reduce their consumption of meat, soft drinks, and total calories.[14] In addition, the involvement of the USDA in developing dietary guidelines is considered by many to be in direct conflict with its goal of promoting agriculture, which can be interpreted as a goal to increase consumption.[15] Awareness of both these issues — the negative impact of lobbying by private industry and potential conflicts of interest of government agencies — must be maintained when developing a health promoting ideology.

Furthermore, the questionable efficacy of these guidelines and the accompanying MyPyramid in producing a healthy population — regardless of their scientific/ quantitative accuracy — indicates that tossing them out into the public arena without simultaneously providing a supportive environment in which to follow them is basically futile.

2.5 DISEASE PROMOTION

Compounding the inadequacies of disease prevention in our society are activities that are directly disease promoting. As my colleague Freudenberg notes, "Inadequate housing is associated with a variety of physical and mental problems."[16] Homelessness or overcrowding results from a number of disease-promoting policies including reduced federal support for low-income housing, conversion of low-income housing to middle- or upper-income housing, increases in the number of people living in poverty or having low-wage jobs, and deinstitutionalization of the mentally ill without compensating community mental health services.[16]

Further, whereas the last 25 years have seen environmental conditions in the United States as a whole improve, air, lead, particulate matter, and other forms of pollution in urban communities continue to be associated with increased rates of illness and death. Almost one fifth of the country's population lacks health insurance.[16]

Disease promotion is induced by activities of the tobacco industry, gun manufacturers, the alcohol industry, illicit drug dealers, and producers of high-fat, low-nutrient value foods,[16] many of whom freely lobby our policymakers and ruthlessly advertise to our children.

Urban dwellers often feel unsafe in their own neighborhoods because of real or perceived potential for crime, whereas suburbanites, deprived of sidewalks, also feel unsafe, deterred from physical activity by fear of speeding traffic. Our urban and suburban designs cry out for rethinking to encourage children to walk to school and play in playgrounds, and adults to jog, cycle, or otherwise include physical activity in their daily routines.

2.6 HISTORY OF HEALTH PROMOTION

Generally, a broader-based interpretation of health promotion has international origins, which the U.S. would be well advised to review.

WHO, established in 1948, attempted to define health and to make explicit the role of governments in the health of their citizens. In 1978, a combined conference of WHO and the United nationals International Children's Emergency Fund (UNICEF) in Alma Ata, U.S.S.R., with 134 nations present, confirmed WHO's original definition of health and expanded it to note that people are affected by their social, economic, and natural environments. This declaration led to the development in 1981 of the Global Strategy for Health for All by the Year 2000.* The major components of this strategy include equity in health; health promotion; preventive activity in primary healthcare settings; cooperation between government, communities, and the private sector; and increased community participation.[17]

The Alma Ata Declaration failed to provide an identifiable framework for action, spurring a series of international conferences on health promotion. The first, held in Ottawa in 1986, resulted in the Ottawa Charter for health promotion, a comprehensive document, some of whose ideas are similar to those addressed in this chapter, including the idea that "health promotion is not just the responsibility of the health sector."[18] The conference's call to action for WHO and other international organizations seems to have fallen on deaf ears.

The Second International Conference on Health Promotion was held in Adelaide, Australia, in 1988 and produced the Adelaide Recommendations on Healthy Public Policy. The Third International Conference on Health Promotion in 1991 in Sundsvall, Sweden, resulted in the Sundsvall Statement on Supportive Environments. In 1997, the Fourth International Conference on Health Promotion in Jakarta, Indonesia, prepared the Jakarta Declaration, which lists 5 priority areas for action: promote social responsibility for health, increase investments for health development, consolidate and expand partnerships for health, increase community capacity and empower the individual, and secure an infrastructure for health promotion.[17,19]

Mexico City hosted the Fifth Global Health Promotion Conference in 2000, which focused on how health promotion improves the lives of socially and economically disadvantage people. The ministers of health from 87 countries, including the U.S., signed a ministerial statement that included a pledge to "draw up a country-wide plan of action to monitor progress made in incorporating strategies which promote health into national and local policy and planning." [17,20]

The documents arising from these conferences contain sensitive analyses, impressive goals, and sweeping calls to action. Yet, HIV/AIDS rages throughout much of Africa and the obesity epidemic is spreading from the U.S. through developed nations and into developing ones. Individual nations are not acting upon the ideas and philosophies espoused by these conference findings.

For instance, Steps to a HealthierUS (discussed in Chapter 10), purports to move the U.S. from a disease care system to a healthcare system (an idea in agreement with a health promotion perspective). Yet, the online brochure describing the initiative states that "policy makers, the health community, and the public must come together to establish programs and policies that support *behavior changes*, encourage *healthier lifestyle choices*, and reduce disparities in healthcare"[21] (emphasis added). In other words, two of the three goals of this initiative are based solely on personal choices and none acknowledge the impact of the physical, social, political, or commercial environments on individual health.

2.6.1 ROLES OF HEALTH PROMOTION

How does an emphasis on health promotion change our perception of the appropriate activities of public health? How do we go about promoting health promotion? How do we make it fundamental to various fields outside of public health — for example, in town planning, where children can no

---

* Clearly, this didn't quite work out.

longer walk safely to school, or in architecture, where inadequately thought-through designs result in sick-building syndrome.

Public health cannot be seen as isolated within its own self-contained bubble, apart from other fields of study in the way, for example, pure mathematics might be considered distinct. Rather, public health must become a component of urban planning, architecture, engineering, legislation, and so on. The concept of environment refers to more than just the physical arena in which people live, work, and play, but also includes social, economic, and cultural dimensions.[22]

2.6.2 PUBLIC HEALTH PRACTITIONERS

Grounding public health in health promotion recognizes and appreciates that numerous professions — law, engineering, human relations personnel, public service, and so on — are currently, though perhaps unwittingly, engaged in public health. That "many disciplines are needed to understand the links between the underlying and proximal determinants of health"[2] is as much a potential strength of public health as it is a weakness. The goal would then be to make explicit the ideal of health promotion in fields of study as disparate as law, engineering, architecture, and city planning. Exposing students of these fields to the concepts of public health and health promotion is fundamental to achieving a true paradigm shift. It cannot be left to happenstance. Expanding the definition of who is a public health worker increases the ability of the public health workforce to meet current challenges.

2.7 HEALTH PROMOTION IN ITS CURRENT INCARNATION

Different individuals and organizations have developed their own definitions of health promotion, interpreting the term to match their agendas and philosophies, often equating the term with health education. Yet, the traditional preventive approach to health education has limited effectiveness.[22]

Currently, health promotion gasps for life as an almost irrelevant subset of disease prevention. Health promotion is a phenomenon that takes place almost entirely outside the 10 to 20 min available for a clinical encounter (longest for babies and for the elderly) and targets specific health risks or behaviors. Health promotion includes nutrition counseling and advice; smoking cessation education; weight loss and weight management education; prenatal education; health risk assessment; sexually transmitted disease (STD) prevention; stress management education; and substance abuse counseling.[23] This pale attempt at health promotion in which physicians might play only a very small role is the wrong mindset, and many of the programs listed arise from a disease prevention perspective, not health promotion. Surely, a smoking cessation or substance abuse program, for example, is not health promoting in the same manner as a nutrition education program, nor is a nutrition education through a program at a local clinic health promoting in the same manner as it would be if provided within the flow of elementary school education.

The ecological approach[24] — portraying itself as a systems approach — is not broad-based enough. Although its supporters believe "grass-roots health promotion efforts wield many advantages over larger national or supranational efforts" and consider them an important health promotion principle, without national and supranational efforts such grass-roots efforts are attempting to slay giants. Confronting asthma among children in the South Bronx will always pit David against Goliath — with David's slingshot sometimes hitting its mark after prodigious effort — until Goliath agrees that situating a preponderance of bus stations, transfer stations, and waste incinerators and their ilk in low-income neighborhoods is not a health promoting policy.

This is in no way meant to denigrate grass-roots programs, without which the health status of our nation would be further diminished. Nor does it predict their demise, yet it is intended to suggest a shift in perspective whereby the goals of grass-roots programs would be supported by the system at large.

2.7.1 TOWARD IMPROVED HEALTH PROMOTION

Freudenberg suggests 10 ways, some overlapping, to promote health, specifically in urban environments but applicable as well to suburban, ex-urban, and rural environments.

1. Give access to quality primary care.
2. Increase health knowledge (this, presumably, would contribute to the next point).
3. Reduce risky behaviors.
4. Increase social support (not clear how this differs from item 9 and possibly 5).
5. Reduce stigma and marginalization.
6. Advocate health-promoting policies.
7. Improve urban physical environments (a direct result of item 6 in the right environment).
8. Meet basic needs (not clear how this differs from item 10).
9. Create supportive social environments (essentially the same as 4).
10. Reduce income inequality.

Although Freudenberg does not prioritize these strategies, a health promotion model embracing all of these goals would absolutely reprioritize them, placing advocacy of health-promoting policies at the top of the list and access to quality primary healthcare toward the bottom as the first would reduce the need for the second.

Interestingly, two of these strategies directly coincide with the first two of the four primary building blocks for health discussed at the beginning of this chapter (see Section 2.1.1). These include building the first block 1 (to meet basic needs item #8 here) and the second block of access to information (item #2 here), as well.

2.7.2 EXAMPLES OF HEALTH PROMOTION ACTIVITIES

North Karelia: A comprehensive community program for health promotion was initiated in Finland in 1972 after a *petition by the local population* was submitted to the government, asking that something be done to reduce high cardiovascular disease (CVD) rates in the area (emphasis added).[25] The government had failed the population in helping to provide a health-promoting environment. Although the aims of the program were to improve detection and control of hypertension, reduce smoking, and improve dietary habits, an intriguing by-product of the intervention, in addition to improved health in neighboring townships due to "leakage," was the creation of new food products such as a sausage that substituted mushrooms for some meat and fat and low-fat milk (at no increase in cost), as well as increased consumer demand for these products. As the authors note, "The environment is often a determining influence on behavior and may be a direct influence on health."[25]

Note that the population, knowing their health was at risk, had to ask the government to intervene in helping them create a health-promoting environment rather than a disease-promoting environment (or even a disease-preventing one). Thus, health requires a coordinated systems approach and cannot be relegated piecemeal to small community-based organizations.

New York City; tobacco control measures: Although cigarette smoking remains the leading cause of preventable death in the U.S., a disease-prevention rather than a health-promotion perspective on public health gives rise to escalating wars of advertising by tobacco companies and counter-intelligence by community-based organizations, nationwide organizations such as the American Heart Association (AHA), and private foundations. As long as health-promoting policies such as limitations on advertising for known causes of cancer are denigrated as contrary to the First Amendment and freedom of speech, defensive disease-prevention actions such as increases in taxes on cigarettes, the Smoke-Free Air Act passed in 2002, and nicotine-dependence guidelines for physicians are imperative. Of these, the cigarette tax was most effective in reducing smoking, disproportionately affecting low-income users, yet exposing 67,000 fewer nonsmokers to the negative health impact of exposure to cigarette smoke.[26] Meanwhile, Kelley Brownell's proposed tax on junk food is derided as a "Twinkie tax" by the ultraconservative Center for Consumer Freedom.

Lifestyle compared to medication interventions: Herman et al.'s study of the cost-effectiveness of lifestyle modification compared with metformin in preventing type 2 diabetes perfectly exemplifies the fundamental difference between health promotion and disease prevention.[27] Whereas both interventions were effective in comparison to a placebo, the lifestyle intervention (health promoting) outclassed the drug (disease preventing) in terms of delaying onset, reducing absolute incidence, and cost per quality of life year.

Lifestyle intervention increased life expectancy by 0.5 years, metformin by 0.2 years. Associated morbidities such as blindness, end-stage renal disease, amputation, stroke, and coronary heart disease were decreased by greater percentages with lifestyle rather than metformin intervention. Overall, the lifestyle intervention provided greater health benefits at lower cost than the metformin intervention.[27]

2.7.3 Would a Health Promotion Model Neglect the Reality of Disease?

Health promotion cannot, ultimately, be naive. It would be irresponsible for a health promotion perspective to neglect the reality of disease and the need for clinical and social interventions. Health education as well as treatment are components of health promotion. However, their need would be reduced by a truly health promoting model.

In his article "The Consumption of the Poor: Tuberculosis in the 21st Century," Paul Farmer details the occurrence of tuberculosis in three separate individuals. Of the first, Jean Dubuisson, Farmer writes, " ... Jean is a member of [Haiti's] only truly productive class: the rural peasantry. But membership in that class brought certain 'birthrights.'" As a subsistence farmer, Jean belongs to the poorest class in the hemisphere and is thus ensured the "right" not to attend school, to lack electricity or safe drinking water, and to have little access to medical care. He also has no role whatsoever in running the country he and those like him support.[28]

A health promotion model, whatever we want to make of the economic abuse of small farmers throughout the world, would not permit lack of education, lack of safe water, denial of medical care, and political disenfranchisement. These are fundamental to the concept of health promotion.

Corina Bayona, a Peruvian woman who migrated from an unforgiving countryside to a sprawling slum, typifies Latin Americans living with multidrug-resistant tuberculosis. Although Peru has been praised for its improved tuberculosis control program, Corina was sick and infectious for at least six years during which she worked, taking crowded buses across Lima twice a day.[28] Throughout the course of her illness, Corina was frequently upbraided for noncompliance rather than receiving help (or at the very least sympathy) because she did not have the time to travel to distant clinics or could not afford the medicines prescribed or remained untreated because of a health workers' strike.[28]

Perhaps most egregious of all, in the U.S., Calvin Loach — a Vietnam vet, an African American, and an injection-drug user — received inappropriate care and was eventually "lost to follow-up." Farmer cites a 1991 study conducted at Harlem Hospital that found nearly 90% of patients did not complete their drug therapy for TB. The New York City Department of Health's overview for 1992 observed that the TB case rate in central Harlem of 222 per 100,000 exceeded that of many Third World countries.[28]

Farmer wisely contends that even if we lack the means to reduce poverty and social inequalities, "few data ... support the hypothesis that there are insufficient means to cure all tuberculosis cases, everywhere."[28] As we move toward a health promotion model, it is imperative to persist in disease treatment and prevention and avoid a blame-the-victim mentality. Yet the causes of Jean, Corina, and Calvin's illnesses, are rooted not in disease but in social displacement and economic deprivation. In 1923, Allen Krause had observed "More or less poverty in a community will mean more or less tuberculosis, so will more or less crowding and improper housing, more or less unhygienic occupations and industry." [28]

Without a health promotion model, although TB itself might be eradicated (as was smallpox) — vindicating a model based on Koch's postulates — other diseases or TB itself will recur with continued displacement of populations, with devaluation of agricultural workers, with overcrowding.

Although Haiti and Peru are poorer countries than the U.S. (Haiti significantly more so than Peru) the poor face similar problems in all three countries. Thus, it is not a matter of money but of political will.

2.7.4 HEALTH PROMOTION IS POLITICAL

Health promotion is inherently political[8] Although I don't fully accept this analysis of two hypothetical health promotion plans — one encouraging people to smoke, the other encouraging people to stop smoking — Seedhouse's point that there are facts, there are opinions masquerading as facts, and that many health promotion strategies are value-driven is well-taken. He writes that "in all cases [whether consciousness-raising about social injustice or non-smoking strategies] it is political philosophy (however implicit) which fires health promotion." [8]

This understanding is also evident in Freudenberg's sixth strategy — advocating health-promoting policies. He notes that public health strategies for policy change encompass legislative and electoral advocacy, media campaigns, and law suits.[16] A recent law suit, initiated by two teenage girls, cited McDonald's as responsible for their obesity. Although the suit was dismissed by the courts, it not only raised public awareness of the invasive role of fast foods in their lives and the relationship between what they eat and health but spurred the fast food industry to recognize, at least on a very fundamental level, its degree of responsibility in the health of their consumers.

2.8 PUBLIC POLICY

Freudenberg writes that the Jakarta Declaration of 1997 noted that trends such as urbanization threaten "the health and well-being of millions of people."[16] Urbanization is far more than a trend, it is a direct result of governmental policies — such as supporting agribusiness, mono-cropping, and exportation rather than small, local farmers. Such policies deprive subsistence farmers of their land, driving them into overcrowded cities where the spread of disease is rampant. Thus, public-health practitioners need to acknowledge the political nature of the process of developing health policy and act accordingly.[2]

This is not to suggest, however, that our current policies are completely devoid of a health-promoting ideology. In fact, a number of policies codified as federal, state, or local law have been instituted throughout the course of our history. The following provide examples of positive health-promoting policies:

- Theodore Roosevelt's creation of national parks, 1900–1901
- Poultry Products Inspection Act, 1957
- Federal Meat Inspection Act, 1967
- Egg Products Inspection Act, 1970
- Clean Water Act, 1987 (a reauthorization of a 1972 act)
- Clean Air Act, 1990
- American with Disabilities Act, 1990

- Healthy People 2000 and Healthy People 2010
- Senate Appropriations Committee's $2 million expansion of the USDA Fruit and Vegetable Snack Program, 2005

There is, however, no unified approach with a consistent philosophical base. These policies are enforced under the aegis of many different agencies, are often not perceived as public health initiatives *per se* and are frequently undermined by monetary interests of private industry such as meat packing and oil.

2.9 HEALTH PROMOTION AND UNIVERSAL HEALTHCARE

Healthcare is an important component of health promotion. Farmer asks, "As a global economy is 'restructured,' is there no room for alternative strategies of development — alternative visions of providing healthcare to the poor?" He notes that the pharmaceutical, insurance, and healthcare industries as well as international agencies (particularly financial institutions) increasingly determine who has access to effective medical care. Refreshingly, he contends that the power of technological advancement stems not merely from the wonders of science but from the power of moral persuasion. We can insist on certain measures not because they are "cost-effective" but because they are the best we can do for the sick.[28]

However, healthcare should not receive the undue focus as a solution that it currently receives. Universal healthcare, although imperative, is not a substitute for a health promotion paradigm. In fact, one could argue that the weaker the health promotion ethos within a society, the greater the need for healthcare — poor health being a logical outcome of poor health promotion.

On a more detailed level, evaluation of health education programs and responsibility for their implementation and effectiveness are key aspects of health promotion. McMenamin et al.'s study of "health promotion" in physician practice groups found that with each additional reporting requirement there was a 37% increase in the odds of offering some type of health promotion program.[23]

2.10 ROLE OF THE INDIVIDUAL IN PUBLIC HEALTH

The role of personal responsibility in achieving health cannot be overlooked or overemphasized. Traditionally, public health in the U.S. has taken a market approach, limiting government responsibility for public health and placing the burden of health improvement on the individual.[2] Certainly, given the reality of a health-promoting environment, it would be up to the individual to make the choice to be healthy. Most of us are outsiders some of the time, not compelled by the need to behave according to the "rules," whether by being overly lazy or daring, or by consuming less than the recommended five fruits and vegetables every day or more than the recommended shot (or two, for men) of alcohol.[8]

But the U.S. is nowhere near an ideal, health-promoting society where the healthier choice would be the easier choice, and health cannot be left solely to personal responsibility. Low-income people, for example, eating a less than optimal diet, may very well be aware of what they should be eating but cannot get it or cannot afford it. In a society with health promotion as its overriding agenda, access to fresh, good quality produce would be comparable to access to saturated fats and added sugars that are easily and cheaply available today.

In our present society, "Even those diseases most closely linked to lifestyle choice could be attributed to the broader social environment ... To expect disciplined personal behavior from alienated people living in a stressful world would be unrealistic, and the institutions of public health should recognize this ... How absurd, for example, for a state to subsidize the production of tobacco and the addiction to it of people in other nations, whilst blaming its own citizens for smoking."[5] How absurd it would be to blame Jean Dubuisson, Corina Bayona, or Calvin Loach for contracting tuberculosis.

2.11 A NEW DEFINITION OF PUBLIC HEALTH'S ROLE

The goal of health promotion should be fundamental to, and pervasive across, disciplines, with the ultimate goal being a healthy and enabling environment. Collective action is justified because health is both an end in itself — a human right — as well as a prerequisite for achieving human potential.[2,8] Public health must acknowledge the direct impact of environmental and socioeconomic circumstances on decisions individuals make about health.[2,22] A health-promoting environment enables the individual to make choices, although these will not always be what a public health practitioner or another informed citizen might define as "healthy."

A health-promoting society is one with strong public policy initiatives, constant evaluation of policy, universal healthcare, the ability to see beyond market-driven imperatives, and a clearly articulated definition of health.

2.12 CONCLUSION

The need to shift the focus of public health in the U.S. from disease prevention to one of health promotion — as described both here and in documents produced by bodies such as the WHO and international conferences on health promotion — is a vital and fascinating topic, which deserves further exploration. The observations in this chapter are but the tip of the iceberg, raising more questions than they answer.

Public health can no longer be relegated to a minor role as a subset of medicine; the practitioners of medicine must recognize that health has long been improved by nonmedical factors in addition to scientific and technological advances. Although universal healthcare is imperative, it alone cannot serve as a substitute for a health-promoting approach to public health.

The change in the nature of diseases most affecting society — from germ-based to environmentally-based — must be reflected in the practice of public health. The current health behaviors of the U.S. adult population indicate that the disease-prevention model of public health is ineffective at best, destructive at worst. Public health in the U.S. must develop a unified approach with a consistent philosophical base, coordinated among the numerous government agencies whose efforts impact the public health.

As a call for action, two changes affecting public policy and professional education in the U.S. are suggested. First, just as an environmental impact statement must be prepared prior to construction of bridges, dams, and tunnels, a health impact statement should be written for housing projects, employment and unemployment policies, healthcare plans, the building of roadways, agricultural policies, and so on. Second, awareness of public health issues must influence the practice of professions from politics to transportation. Therefore, public health and health promotion must become a part of the core curriculum of numerous professional programs throughout the country.

2.13 ACRONYMS

AHA	American Heart Association
AMA	American Medical Association
CHD	Coronary heart disease
CVD	Cardiovascular disease
HLC	Health lifestyle characteristic
HHS	United States Department of Health and Human Services
NHANES	National Health and Nutrition Examination Survey
STD	Sexually transmitted disease
UNICEF	United Nations International Children's Emergency Fund
USDA	United States Department of Agriculture
USSR	Union of Soviet Socialist Republics
WHO	World Health Organization

REFERENCES

1. Malkin, E. Mexico confronts sudden surge in obesity. *New York Times*. June 29, 2005.
2. Beaglehole, R., Bonita, R., Horton, R., Adams, O., and McKee, M. Public health in the new era: improving health through collective action. *Lancet*. 363, 2084–2086, 2004.
3. Robert Koch (1843–1910) is considered as one of the founders of bacteriology.
4. www.etymonline.com/index.php?1=h&p=4. Accessed June 26, 2005.
5. Hamlin, C. The history and development of public health in developed countries. In Detels, R., McEwen, J., Beaglehole, R., and Tanaka, H., Eds. *The Oxford Textbook of Public Health*. 4th ed. The Scope of Public Health. Oxford University Press. Oxford. 2002, pp. 21–37.
6. Marchione, M. Recruiters worry that new soldiers are too fat to fight. KATU 2 News. Portland, OR. June 29, 2005. www.katu.com/printstory.asp?ID=78068. Accessed July 1, 2005.
7. WHO definition of health. www.who.int/about/definition/en. Accessed June 26, 2005.
8. Seedhouse, D. *Health Promotion: Philosophy, Prejudice, and Practice*. John Wiley and Sons. New York. 1997.
9. Reeves, M.J. and Rafferty, A.P. Healthy lifestyle characteristics among adults in the United States. *Arch Intern Med*. 165, 854–857, 2005.
10. Ford, E.S., De Proost Ford, M.A., Will, J.C., Galuska, D.A., and Ballew, C. Achieving a healthy lifestyle among United States adults: a long way to go. *Ethn Dis*. 11, 224–231, 2001.
11. Berrigan, D., Dodd, K., Troiana, R.P., Krebs-Smith, S.M., and Barbash, R.B. Patterns of health behavior in U.S. adults. *Prev Med*. 36, 615–623, 2003.
12. Miller, R.R., Sales, A.E., Kopjar, B., Fihn, S.D., and Bryson, C.L. Adherence to heart-healthy behaviors in a sample of the U.S. population. *Prev Chron Dis*. 2(2), A18, April 2005. Epub 2005 March 15. Available at: http://www.pubmedcentral.nih.gov/articlerender.fcgi?tool=pubmed&pubmedid=15888229. Accessed September 1, 2006.
13. Appendix I: History of dietary guidelines for Americans. www.health.gov/dietaryguidelines/dga95/12DIETAP.HTM. Accessed July 1, 2005.
14. www.anaturalway.com/dietary_goals3.html. Accessed July 1, 2005.
15. Nestle, M. *Food Politics*. University of California Press. Berkeley, CA. 2002.
16. Freudenberg, N. Health promotion in the city: a review of current practice and future prospects in the United States. *Ann Rev Public Health*. 21, 473–503, 2000.
17. Web site to provide information, resources, and support to people involved in health promotion in Australian Capital Territory (ACT). www.healthpromotion.act.gov.au/whatis/history/default.htm. Accessed July 2, 2005.
18. Ottawa Charter for Health Promotion, 1986. www.who.dk/AboutWHO/Policy/20010827_2v. Accessed July 2, 2005.
19. The Jakarta Declaration on Health Promotion into the 21st Century. www.ldb.org/iuhpe/jakdec.htm. Accessed July 2, 2005.
20. World Health Organization. Mexico Ministerial Statement for the Promotion of Health. www.who.int/healthpromotion/conferences/previous/mexico/statement/en. Accessed July 3, 2005.
21. Steps to a HealthierUS. www.healthierus.gov/steps/steps_brochure.html. Accessed July 3, 2005.
22. Tones, K. Health promotion, health education, and the public health. In Detels, R., McEwen, J., Beaglehole, R., and Tanaka, H., Eds. *The Oxford Textbook of Public Health*. 4th ed. The Scope of Public Health. Oxford University Press. Oxford. 2002, pp. 829–863.
23. McMenamin, S.B., Schmittdiel, J., Halpin, H.A., Gillies, R., Rundall, T.G., and Shortell, S.M. Health promotion in physician organizations: results from a national study. *Am J Prev Med*. 26, 259–264, 2004.
24. Richard, L., Potvin, l., Kishchuk, N., Prlic, H., and Green, L.W. Assessment of the integration of the ecological approach in health promotion programs. *Am J Health Promot*. 10, 318–328, 1996.
25. McAlister, A., Puska, P., Salonen, J., Tuomilehto, J., and Koskela, K. Theory and action for health promotion: illustrations from the North Karelia project. *AJPH*. 72, 43–49, 1982.
26. Frieden, T.R., Mostashari, F., Kerker, B.D., Miller, N., Hajat, A., and Frankel, M. Adult tobacco use levels after intensive tobacco control measures: New York City, 2002–2003. *Am J Public Health*. 95, 1016–1023, 2005.
27. Herman, W.H., Hoerger, T.J., Brandle, M., Hicks, K., Sorenson, S., Zhang, P., et al. The cost-effectiveness of lifestyle modification or metformin in preventing type 2 diabetes in adults with impaired glucose tolerance. *Ann Intern Med*. 142, 323–332, 2005.
28. Farmer, P.E. The consumption of the poor: tuberculosis in the 21st century. *Ethnography*. 1(2), 183–216, 2000.

3 The U.S. Population — Looking Forward from the Past

The United States is getting bigger, older, and more ethnically diverse.[1]

3.1 INTRODUCTION

U.S. demographics are undergoing striking changes that will affect the practice of public health in the immediate and distant future. These changes include an increase in the number of people who live in poverty, are older, belong to ethnic or racial minority groups, have disabilities, and have diverse sexual orientations. These demographics will influence definitions of aging, health, and illness and will challenge current prevention and treatment models.

Although the diversity of the U.S. population in the 21st century is one of its greatest assets, this richness is often overshadowed by the reality that health disparities with respect to income level are pervasive. Racial and ethnic minority populations, in general, belong to a lower-income strata than the majority population. It must be recognized, however, that race and ethnicity are frequently only proxies for education and income. Education and income as indicators of socio-economic status (SES) are the most potent determinants of how people access and respond to healthcare services. Concentrating mainly on race and ethnicity runs the risk of minimizing the importance of SES on health.[2] Although the government programs discussed in Chapter 6 focus on eliminating the gap in health disparities between minority and majority populations, an equally compelling case can be made for guaranteeing that all children receive an education that will assure they will be able to hold well-paying jobs, live in comfortable neighborhoods, follow a healthy lifestyle, and afford quality medical care.

Diversity is and will continue to be a major factor in the development and delivery of primary and secondary preventive health services in the U.S. The world's 210 nations are well represented in the U.S. population, with more than 65 different categories of racial and ethnic combinations that are continually blending and merging. In addition, because mobility is such an ingrained feature of our society, cultural diversity has expanded into all regions of the country, predominantly the inner cities and coastal areas, but also throughout the Midwest, suburbs, and small towns.[3]

This chapter highlights information from the 2000 census regarding the major racial and ethnic groups represented in the U.S. as well as health issues public health practitioners can expect to confront.

3.2 MINORITY POPULATIONS, IMMIGRATION, AND MIGRATION

The study of immigration to and migration within the U.S. extends well beyond the scope of this book. Ideally, however, one needs to consider at least the following questions to appreciate the minority populations discussed in this chapter:

- What happened to Native Americans as successive waves of immigrants arrived from other nations?
- When and why did each immigrant group come to the U.S.?
- Where did the groups settle, both initially and in subsequent migrations?

- How were the immigrants received by the then citizens of the country?
- How did U.S. government policies and programs affect immigration patterns?
- How did U.S. government policies and programs affect immigrants' assimilation into the life of the nation?
- What role did the distribution of resources (natural and artificial) play in the immigration and subsequent migration patterns of immigrants?
- How did economic conditions impact immigrants' experiences?
- How did cultural heritage affect an immigrant's place of settlement?
- What impact did immigrant cultural traditions have on the U.S.?
- What impact do American traditions have on immigrants?

3.2.1 IMMIGRATION AND NATIONALITY ACT OF 1965

The Immigration and Nationality Act of 1965 ended U.S. immigration quotas based on national origin, race, or ancestry. Starting in the mid-1960s, the main factor for selection became the occupation of the applicant, with preference given to persons having special occupational skills, abilities, or training, particularly those who already had relatives living in the U.S. The effects of the 1965 act were immediate and significant, resulting in a demographic turning point in U.S. history and a shift in the origins and occupations of immigrants to the country. Since 1965, immigration to the U.S. has moved away from western and northern Europe. Southern European, Asian, and Caribbean immigrants now comprise a larger proportion of immigrants than previously. This shift in major sending countries to those of lesser economic development has had a profound effect on the composition of the U.S. immigrant population. Mexico, for example, now leads the list of sending countries, followed by the Philippines, India, China, and Vietnam. These countries are much less prosperous than those favored by the old national origin system replaced in 1965.

One of the unintended consequences of the 1965 legislation was that the labor market skills of successive groups of new immigrants (as measured by wages and education) gradually declined relative to those of native-born workers. Not surprisingly, immigrants from less prosperous countries tend to be less educated and less skilled than earlier immigrants from the more developed European nations. Asian immigrants, large numbers of whom were professionals before arriving in the U.S., are a major exception.[4]

3.3 THE U.S. CENSUS BUREAU

The U.S. Census Bureau is a division of the U.S. Department of Commerce, the agency within the executive branch of the federal government that promotes international trade, economic growth, and technological advancement. The Census Bureau is responsible for collecting and providing relevant data about the nation's people and economy. In addition to population, the bureau conducts a host of other surveys: collecting information about housing; retail merchandise; personal, business and transport services; international trade; local, state and federal government agencies; education; and transportation.

3.3.1 CENSUS BACKGROUND

Article I, Section 2 of the Constitution of the U.S. (subsequently modified by the 14th Amendment) calls for a decennial census. The origin of this mandate was a political compromise during the post–Revolutionary War era arising from the conflict between the sparsely populated southern states (Georgia, North Carolina, South Carolina, and Virginia) and the more heavily populated northern states (Connecticut, Delaware, Maryland, Massachusetts, New Hampshire, New York, New Jersey, Pennsylvania, and Rhode Island). The southern states wanted equal representation in the national legislature, whereas the northern states believed that their larger populations justified greater power. Two compromises settled this dispute: (1) the establishment of the bicameral U.S. legislature in which the states are equally represented in the Senate and are represented according to population in the House of Representatives, and (2) a slave counted as three fifths of a person when determining population (later modified by the 14th Amendment).

The first national U.S. census was conducted in 1790 and counted 3.9 million inhabitants. With the growth of the country, the needs for different kinds of information about the people changed. The original census included only these three items:

- Name of head of family.
- Number of persons in household. (In 1850, the census included inquiries on social issues, such as taxation, churches, poverty, and crime.)
- Number of persons in the household who match these descriptions: free white males 16 years and upward, free white males under 16 years, free white females, all other free persons (by gender and color), and slaves.

3.3.2 Uses of the Census

The fundamental reason for conducting the decennial census is to apportion the number of members of the House of Representatives to which each of the 50 states is entitled. Apportionment is the process of dividing the 435 seats in the U.S. House of Representatives according to the size of the population, among the 50 states. Using equal portions, each state is assigned one congressional seat; the remaining 385 seats are then allocated based on the population of each state. Based on the Census 2000 apportionment, each member of the U.S. House of Representatives represents an average population of almost 650,000 (actually 646,952).[5]

Census data are also used by the federal and state governments to allocate almost $200 billion every year to local governments for a wide variety of public purposes, including the allocation of state Community Development Block Grant (CDBG) funds (see Box 3.1). The census also provides all levels of government with information needed to design, implement, and evaluate programs and to enforce laws. Public and private agencies and corporations use census data for such diverse purposes as marketing, analysis of social and economic trends, and estimating the size of the target population for program planning. Because public health initiatives are greatly affected by federal and state funding, it is important to understand how census data is collected.

Box 3.1 State Administered Community Development Block Grants

State Administration

Because states are in the best position to know and to respond to the needs of local governments, Congress amended the Housing and Community Development Act of 1974 (HCD Act) in 1981 to give each state the opportunity to administer Community Development Block Grants (CDBG) funds for nonentitlement areas. Nonentitlement areas include those units of general local government that do not receive CDBG funds directly from HUD as part of the entitlement program (entitlement cities and urban counties). Nonentitlement areas are cities with populations of less than 50,000 (except cities that are designated principal cities of metropolitan statistical areas) and counties with populations of less than 200,000.

The state CDBG program has replaced the Small Cities program in states that have elected to participate. Currently, 49 states and Puerto Rico participate in the program. HUD continues to administer the program for the nonentitled counties in the State of Hawaii because the state has permanently elected not to participate in the state CDBG program.

Program Objectives

The primary statutory objective of the CDBG program is to develop viable communities by providing decent housing and a suitable living environment and by expanding economic opportunities, principally for persons of low and moderate incomes. The state must ensure that at least 70% of its CDBG grant funds are used for activities that benefit low- and moderate-income persons over a one-, two-, or three-year time period selected by the state. This general objective is achieved by granting "maximum feasible priority" to activities which benefit low- and moderate-income families or aid in the prevention or elimination of slums or blight. Under special circumstances, states may also use their funds to meet urgent community development needs. A need is considered urgent if it poses a serious and immediate threat to the health or welfare of the community and has arisen in the past 18 months.

Roles and Responsibilities of HUD, States, and Localities

States participating in the CDBG program award grants only to units of general local government that carry out development activities. Annually each state develops funding priorities and criteria for selecting projects. HUD's role under the state CDBG program is to ensure state compliance with federal laws, regulations, and policies.

Participating states have three major responsibilities:

- Formulating community development objectives
- Deciding how to distribute funds among communities in nonentitlement areas
- Ensuring that recipient communities comply with applicable state and federal laws and requirements

Local governments have the responsibility to consider local needs, prepare grant applications for submission to the state, and carry out the funded community development activities. Local governments must comply with federal and state requirements.

Eligible Activities

Communities receiving CDBG funds from the state may use the funds for many kinds of community development activities including, but not limited to:

- Acquisition of property for public purposes
- Construction or reconstruction of streets, water and sewer facilities, neighborhood centers, recreation facilities, and other public works
- Demolition
- Rehabilitation of public and private buildings
- Public services
- Planning activities
- Assistance to nonprofit entities for community development activities
- Assistance to private, for-profit entities to carry out economic development activities (including assistance to microenterprises)

The state may use $100,000, plus up to 50% of the costs it incurs for program administration, with a maximum of 3% of its CDBG allocation. The state may expend up to 3% of its CDBG allocation on technical assistance activities. However, the total the state spends on both administrative and technical assistance expenses must not exceed 3% of the state's allocation.

Distribution of Funds

HUD distributes funds to each state based on a statutory formula that takes into account population, poverty, incidence of overcrowded housing, and age of housing. Neither HUD nor states distribute funds directly to citizens or private organizations; all funds (other than administration and the technical assistance funds set aside) are distributed by states to units of general local government.

Source: U.S. Department of Housing and Urban Development, Homes and Communities: Community Planning and Development. State Administered CDBG. Available at: http://www.hud.gov/offices/cpd/communitydevelopment/programs/stateadmin/. Accessed August 27, 2006.

Box 3.2 Calculating Disease Rates

A *rate* is a statistical term that describes the force of a disease in a population. It includes the number of new cases of disease in the numerator and the number of persons at risk of the disease within a period of time in the denominator. A disease rate is calculated by dividing the number of cases of the disease in the numerator by a census-generated denominator. For example, if there were 100 new cases of cancer among 100,000 people over the course of 1 year, the rate of cancer would be expressed as 100 cases per 100,000 persons at risk per year.

Public health policy decisions and needs assessments are predicated on interpretations and conclusions drawn from combining the results from many surveys. The use of current estimates of population characteristics is necessary to make estimates of disease, injury, disability, and behaviors of interest to public health, as well as their distributions. Often, these estimates require population denominators that are derived from the census (see Box 3.2).

Information on race and housing available from the census are used by public and private organizations to identify areas where groups may need special services and to plan and evaluate education, housing, health, and other programs that address these needs. Census information can help identify where residents might need services of particular importance to certain racial or ethnic groups, such as screening for hypertension and diabetes.

3.3.3 POPULATION PROFILE OF THE U.S. IN THE 20TH CENTURY

In April 2001, the Census Bureau announced that the total population of the U.S. was 281,421,906 as of April 1, 2000 (see Figure 3.1). The true population of the U.S. in 2000 is known only to within 5 million persons.[6] Nevertheless, comparing the beginning and the end of the 20th century, the U.S. in 2000 was much more racially and ethnically diverse than in 1900. At the beginning of the century, just one out of eight Americans was of a race other than white (12.5%), but by 2000, the proportion was one out of four (25%). These and other noteworthy shifts in the U.S. population are summarized in Table 3.1.

The decade-to-decade trend illustrated in Figure 3.2 highlights the increasing diversity of the U.S., developing predominantly in the second half of the century. In particular, people of races other than white or black (in other words, Asian and Pacific Islander, American Indian and Alaska Native, two or more races, or other races) represented less than 1% of the U.S. population between 1900 and 1960, compared to 12.5% by 2000.

3.3.4 THE 2000 CENSUS

A copy of the short form of the 2000 census questionnaire mailed to all households in 2000 appears in Figure 3.5 at the end of this chapter. The questionnaire asks for each household member their name, sex, age, and relationship to person filling out the form, and whether they are of Hispanic origin and race. The person completing the form is also asked whether their housing unit is owned, mortgaged, rented, or rent-free. The subcategories for Spanish/Hispanic/Latino listed in the census are Mexican, Mexican American, Chicano, Puerto Rican, Cuban, and Other Spanish/Hispanic/Latino. The questions in the census questionnaire (excluding names) result in the data categories listed in Figure 3.1: sex and age, race, Hispanic or Latino and race, household relationships, household type, household occupancy, and household tenure.

From 1960 through 2000, the decennial census consisted of two parts: (1) the short form, which counted the population and (2) the long form, which obtained demographic, housing, social, and economic information from a 1-in-6 sample of households. Information from the long form is used

Subject	Number	Percent	Subject	Number	Percent
Total population....................	281,421,906	100.0	**HISPANIC OR LATINO AND RACE**		
			Total population........................	281,421,906	100.0
SEX AND AGE			Hispanic or Latino (of any race)...............	35,305,818	12.5
Male................................	138,053,563	49.1	Mexican...............................	20,640,711	7.3
Female.............................	143,368,343	50.9	Puerto Rican..........................	3,406,178	1.2
			Cuban................................	1,241,685	0.4
Under 5 years	19,175,798	6.8	Other Hispanic or Latino	10,017,244	3.6
5 to 9 years	20,549,505	7.3	Not Hispanic or Latino	246,116,088	87.5
10 to 14 years	20,528,072	7.3	White alone...........................	194,552,774	69.1
15 to 19 years	20,219,890	7.2			
20 to 24 years	18,964,001	6.7	**RELATIONSHIP**		
25 to 34 years	39,891,724	14.2	Total population........................	281,421,906	100.0
35 to 44 years	45,148,527	16.0	In households...........................	273,643,273	97.2
45 to 54 years	37,677,952	13.4	Householder..........................	105,480,101	37.5
55 to 59 years	13,469,237	4.8	Spouse	54,493,232	19.4
60 to 64 years	10,805,447	3.8	Child................................	83,393,392	29.6
65 to 74 years	18,390,986	6.5	Own child under 18 years..........	64,494,637	22.9
75 to 84 years	12,361,180	4.4	Other relatives	15,684,318	5.6
85 years and over..................	4,239,587	1.5	Under 18 years	6,042,435	2.1
			Nonrelatives	14,592,230	5.2
Median age (years)..................	35.3	(X)	Unmarried partner.................	5,475,768	1.9
			In group quarters.......................	7,778,683	2.8
18 years and over..................	209,128,094	74.3	Institutionalized population...........	4,059,039	1.4
Male................................	100,994,367	35.9	Noninstitutionalized population	3,719,594	1.3
Female.............................	108,133,727	38.4			
21 years and over..................	196,899,193	70.0	**HOUSEHOLD BY TYPE**		
62 years and over..................	41,256,029	14.7	Total households.......................	105,480,101	100.0
65 years and over..................	34,991,753	12.4	Family households (families)...................	71,787,347	68.1
Male................................	14,409,625	5.1	With own children under 18 years..........	34,588,368	32.8
Female.............................	20,582,128	7.3	Married-couple family	54,493,232	51.7
			With own children under 18 years	24,835,505	23.5
RACE			Female householder, no husband present.....	12,900,103	12.2
One race...........................	274,595,678	97.6	With own children under 18 years..........	7,561,874	7.2
White............................	211,460,626	75.1	Nonfamily households	33,692,754	31.9
Black or African American	34,658,190	12.3	Householder living alone	27,230,075	25.8
American Indian and Alaska Native..........	2,475,956	0.9	Householder 65 years and over..........	9,722,857	9.2
Asian............................	10,242,998	3.6			
Asian Indian	1,678,765	0.6	Households with individuals under 18 years	38,022,115	36.0
Chinese.........................	2,432,585	0.9	Households with individuals 65 years and over ..	24,672,708	23.4
Filipino..........................	1,850,314	0.7			
Japanese.........................	796,700	0.3	Average household size..................	2.59	(X)
Korean..........................	1,076,872	0.4	Average family size....................	3.14	(X)
Vietnamese........................	1,122,528	0.4			
Other Asian [1]	1,285,234	0.5	**HOUSING OCCUPANCY**		
Native Hawaiian and Other Pacific Islander....	398,835	0.1	Total housing units.......................	115,904,641	100.0
Native Hawaiian........................	140,652	-	Occupied housing units	105,480,101	91.0
Guamanian or Chamorro..................	58,240	-	Vacant housing units...................	10,424,540	9.0
Samoan..........................	91,029	-	For seasonal, recreational, or		
Other Pacific Islander [2]	108,914	-	occasional use....................	3,578,718	3.1
Some other race	15,359,073	5.5			
Two or more races	6,826,228	2.4	Homeowner vacancy rate (percent)............	1.7	(X)
			Rental vacancy rate (percent).................	6.8	(X)
Race alone or in combination with one					
or more other races: [3]			**HOUSING TENURE**		
White................................	216,930,975	77.1	Occupied housing units	105,480,101	100.0
Black or African American	36,419,434	12.9	Owner-occupied housing units	69,815,753	66.2
American Indian and Alaska Native.............	4,119,301	1.5	Renter-occupied housing units	35,664,348	33.8
Asian	11,898,828	4.2			
Native Hawaiian and Other Pacific Islander......	874,414	0.3	Average household size of owner-occupied units.	2.69	(X)
Some other race	18,521,486	6.6	Average household size of renter-occupied units.	2.40	(X)

- Represents zero or rounds to zero.   (X) Not applicable.
[1] Other Asian alone, or two or more Asian categories.
[2] Other Pacific Islander alone, or two or more Native Hawaiian and Other Pacific Islander categories.
[3] In combination with one or more of the other races listed. The six numbers may add to more than the total population and the six percentages may add to more than 100 percent because individuals may report more than one race.

FIGURE 3.1 Profile of the general demographic characteristics of the U.S. population according to the 2000 census. (From U.S. Department of Commerce. Profile of General Demographic Characteristics 2000. 2000 Census of Population and Housing. Table DP-1. U.S. Census Bureau. Available at: http://www.census.gov/prod/cen2000/dp1/2kh00.pdf. Accessed August 27, 2006.)

to administer federal programs and distribute billions of federal dollars. Census 2000, therefore, not only counted a population of 281.4 million residents, but also sampled the socioeconomic status of the population. The U.S. Census Bureau releases extensive statistics on the nation's population, all free and accessible online. Topics cover a broad range:

- Demographics (age, sex, race, and ethnicity)
- Social characteristics (education, marital status, household and family situation, fertility, place of birth, disability, language use and proficiency, and computer ownership and use)
- Economic characteristics (income and poverty, labor force status, occupation, benefit program participation, and wealth)
- Migration and commuting

TABLE 3.1
Noteworthy Shifts in the U.S. Population, 1900 to 2000

Most of the Population at the Beginning of the 20th Century	Most of the Population at the Beginning of the 21st Century
Lived in the Northeast or the Midwest	Lives in the South or the West
Lived in nonmetropolitan areas	Lives in metropolitan areas
Male	Female
Under 23 years old	At least 35 years old
White	White (but has more nonwhite neighbors)
Rented a home	Owns a home
Lived in a household with four or more other people	Lives alone or in a household with one or two other people

Source: Based on Hobbs, F., Stoops, N., U.S. Census Bureau, Census 2000 Special Reports, Series CENSR-4, *Demographic Trends in the 20th Century*, Washington, D.C., 2002.

As discussed in Section 3.3.5, in 2010, the American Community Survey (ACS) will replace the census long form.

3.3.4.1 Race and Ethnicity

All federal agencies that collect and report data on race and ethnicity follow the standards stated in *Standards for Maintaining, Collecting, and Presenting Federal Data on Race and Ethnicity* (1997).[7] The Office of Management and Budget (OMB), the federal agency that defines standards for government publications, accepted the recommendation made by the Interagency Committee for the Review of the Racial and Ethnic Standards that two separate questions, one for race and one for ethnicity or Hispanic origin, be used whenever feasible to provide flexibility and ensure data quality. Therefore, race and Hispanic origin (known as ethnicity) are considered by the Census Bureau to be distinct concepts that require separate questions in their surveys (see Box 3.3).

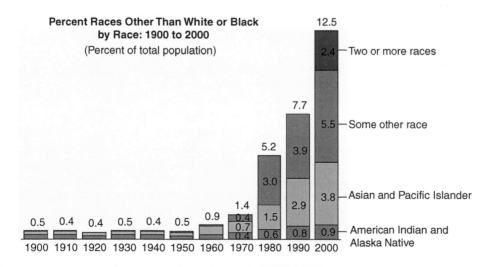

FIGURE 3.2 Total population by race and population of races, excluding white and black: 1900 to 2000. (From Hobbs, F. and Stoops, N., U.S. Census Bureau, Census 2000 Special Reports, Series CENSR-4, *Demographic Trends in the 20th Century*. Figures 3.1 and 3.2. Washington, DC, 2002. Available at: http://www.census.gov/prod/2002pubs/censr-4.pdf. Accessed June 8, 2006.)

Box 3.3 Census Bureau Reference Information on Race and Hispanic Origin

The Census Bureau maintains extensive online reference information on the concepts of race [www.census.gov/population/www/socdemo/race.html] and *Hispanic origin.* [www.census./gov/population/www/socdemo/hispanic.html].

In general, the Census Bureau defines *ethnicity* or *origin* as the heritage, nationality group, lineage, or country of birth of an individual or of the individual's parents or ancestors before their arrival in the U.S. Hispanic or Latino is considered a designation of ethnicity, not race; people of Hispanic or Latino origin may be of any race.

The Census Bureau's definition of *race* generally reflects a social definition of the concept that is recognized in this country and does not conform to any biological, anthropological, or genetic criteria. The Census 2000 question on race included 15 separate response categories, as well as three areas where respondents could write in a more specific race. The response categories and write-in categories for race and ethnicity classification have been consolidated by the OMB into these six basic categories:

- White
- Black, or African American
- American Indian and Alaska Native
- Asian
- Native Hawaiian and "Other Pacific Islander"
- Some other race

Table 3.2 presents the population of the U.S. by race and Hispanic origin for the year 2000 and with projections through 2050.

People may select more than one racial identification. In the 2000 census, 2.4% of the total U.S. population self-identified with more than one racial and/or ethnic group. Beyond showing the total number of people reporting two or more races, the Census Bureau uses two other approaches to present data for people reporting more than one race.[8]

- Reflecting the 57 possible combinations of the six race groups mentioned previously, these detailed categories can be combined, if desired, to show more than one use.
- Showing the number of times a respondent reports one of the six race categories either alone or in combination with the other five race categories: the category "black or African American alone or in combination with one or more other races" includes all people who reported only black or African American and people who reported Black or African American in combination with any of the other five race categories. Individuals will be counted only once. However, in tabulation approaches including the six race groups alone or in combination with one or more other races, respondents will be tallied in each of the race groups they reported. For example, people who reported "Asian and black or African American" would be counted both in the "Asian alone or in combination" population as well as in the "black or African American alone or in combination" population. Consequently, the total of the six alone or in combination groups exceeds the total population whenever some people in a group of interest reported more than one race.

3.3.4.1.1 White Populations

The term *white* refers to people having origins in any of the original natives of Europe, the Middle East, or North Africa. Whites represent about 70% of the U.S. population. They belong to a variety

TABLE 3.2
U.S. Population Projections by Race and Hispanic Origin: 2000–2050

Population	2000	2010	2020	2030	2040	2050
Total	282,125	308,936	335,805	363,584	391,946	419,854
White alone	228,548	244,995	260,629	275,731	289,690	302,626
Black alone	35,818	40,454	45,365	50,442	55,876	61,361
Asian alone	10,684	14,241	17,988	22,580	27,992	33,430
All other races[a]	7,075	9,246	11,822	14,831	18,388	22,437
Hispanic (of any race)	35,622	47,756	59,756	73,055	87,585	102,560
White alone, not Hispanic	195,729	201,112	205,936	209,176	210,331	210,283

	Percentage Change					
Population	2000–2050	2000–2010	2010–2020	2020–2030	2030–2040	2040–2050
Total	48.8	9.5	8.7	8.3	7.8	7.1
White alone	32.4	7.2	6.4	5.8	5.1	4.5
Black alone	71.3	12.9	12.1	11.2	10.8	9.8
Asian alone	212.9	33.3	26.3	25.5	24.0	19.4
All other races[a]	217.1	30.7	27.9	25.5	24.0	22.0
Hispanic (of any race)	187.9	34.1	25.1	22.3	19.9	17.1
White alone, not Hispanic	7.4	2.8	2.4	1.6	0.6	0.0

	Percent of Total Population					
Population	2000	2010	2020	2030	2040	2050
Total	100.0	100.0	100.0	100.0	100.0	100.0
White alone	81.0	79.3	77.6	75.8	73.9	72.1
Black alone	12.7	13.1	13.5	13.9	14.3	14.6
Asian alone	3.8	4.6	5.4	6.2	7.1	8.0
All other races[a]	2.5	3.0	3.5	4.1	4.7	5.3
Hispanic (of any race)	12.6	15.5	17.8	20.1	22.3	24.4
White alone, not Hispanic	69.4	65.1	61.3	57.5	53.7	50.1

Note: Resident population in thousands.

[a] Includes American Indian and Alaska Native alone, Native Hawaiian and Other Pacific Islanders alone, and those identified officially as Two or More Races.

Source: Based on U.S. Census Bureau, International Data Base, Table 094. Available at: http://www,census.gov/ipc/ www. idbprint.html. Accessed August 27, 2006.

of ethnic groups with distinct languages, dialects, and cultures. Some have been in the U.S. for many generations, whereas others are recent immigrants. Whites represent both extremes of socio-economic and health status. Their health status is used as the baseline against which other racial and ethnic groups are measured.

3.3.4.1.2　Hispanic or Latino Populations

Hispanic connotes an ethnic group; the Hispanic population includes people who may be of any race. The 1980 census was the first to include a separate question on Hispanic origin, asked of every individual in the U.S. Census information indicates that the Hispanic population more than doubled in size from 14.6 million in 1980 to 35.3 million in 2000, representing an increase from 6.4 to 12.5% of the total population. High levels of immigration coupled with relatively high fertility levels contributed to this rapid growth.

Box 3.4 Spanish/Hispanic/Latino

Hispanic and *Latino* are sometimes used interchangeably, although they do not have the same meaning. *Hispanic* is the term chosen by U.S. government agencies in 1970 as a convenient label that could be applied to all people from the Spanish-speaking countries of the central and southern parts of the Western Hemisphere (Mexico and the lands annexed by the U.S. in the 19th century: Puerto Rico, Cuba, the Dominican Republic) and from Spain. That catchall label has a particular and evolving meaning only in the U.S. context in which it was created and is applied. *Latino*, on the other hand, refers to people whose ancestral lineage connects to Latin America, but not to Spain.

Source: del Pinal, J., Singer, A. Generations of diversity: Latinos in the United States. *Population Bulletin,* 52(3): 1–48, 1997. Washington, D.C.: Population Reference Bureau, Inc.

The Hispanic population in the U.S. is far from homogenous. For example, some Hispanics speak only Spanish, whereas others speak no Spanish at all. Hispanic Americans come from many countries and cultures, making the differences between and within the Hispanic ethnic groups sometimes as great as their similarities. Although most of this population are of Mexican origin, the remainder includes at least 20 other national origin groups. About 10% of the Hispanic population is of Puerto Rican background, with about 3% each of Cuban, Salvadoran, and Dominican origins. The remainder are of some other Central American, South American, or other Hispanic or Latino origin (see Box 3.4).

Although Hispanics share many aspects of a common heritage, such as language and emphasis on extended family, Hispanic cultures vary significantly by country of origin. The health profiles of Hispanics vary according to their region of origin. Hispanics of all races represent the largest minority population in the U.S., accounting for 12.5% of the population. Spanish was the language spoken by almost of those speaking a language other than English at home.[9]

3.3.4.1.2.1   Mexican Immigrants

Current Mexican migration to the U.S. dates back to World War II when Mexico contributed to the war effort by providing temporary agricultural labor. The Bracero program (1942–1964) provided the U.S. with short-term temporary migrant workers to offset labor shortages faced during the war and its aftermath (see Box 3.5). An estimated 4.5 million Mexican workers came to the U.S. during this period. At its height in the late 1950s, more than 500,000 workers migrated each year. The number of Mexicans who left Mexico for the U.S. continued to increase steadily even after the Bracero program ended. During the 1980s, the intentions of many migrants shifted from a sojourner mentality to that of settler. By the 1990s, the phenomenon became one of permanent moves rather than reiterative and temporary ones. From the 1980s to the 1990s, Mexican immigration grew from 200,000 to 300,000. The Bracero system left a permanent legacy in the U.S., as Mexican migrants tend to be mainly selected from middle-to-lower segments of Mexico's socioeconomic structure.[10]

3.3.4.1.3   Black or African American Populations

The term *black* (or *African American*) refers to people having origins in any of the black racial groups of Africa. Blacks comprise 12% of the population and have a long history in the U.S. Some have been in the country for many generations, whereas others are recent immigrants from Africa, the Caribbean, and the West Indies. Blacks generally experience poorer health than the American population as a whole, with a shorter life expectancy and higher infant mortality rates. The infant mortality rate in 2001 for African Americans was more than twice as high as for whites (13.3 per 1,000 live births vs. 5.7 per 1,000 live births for whites). The prevalence of hypertension in blacks is higher than in any other racial or ethnic group. Overall, African Americans are more likely to develop cancer and have the highest cancer death rate. African American women have the highest mortality rates from breast cancer of any racial or ethnic group.

Box 3.5 The Bracero Program

The Mexican migrant worker has been the foundation for the development of the rich American agricultural industry, and the El Paso–Ciudad Juárez border region has played a key role in this historic movement. One of the most significant contributions to the growth of the agricultural economy was the creation of the Bracero Program in which more than 4 million Mexican farm laborers came to work in the fields of this nation. The braceros converted the agricultural fields of America into the most productive on the planet.

Mexican peasants were hardworking, skilled agricultural laborers. Yet, despite the fact that two million peasants lost their lives in the Mexican Revolution of 1910, the government failed to provide them the resources needed to improve their lives. By the late 1930s when the crop fields began yielding low harvests and employment became scarce, the peasant was forced to look for other means of survival.

The occurrence of this grave situation coincided with the emergence of a demand for manual labor in the U.S. brought about by World War II. On August 4, 1942, the U.S. and the Mexican government instituted the Bracero Program. Thousands of impoverished Mexicans abandoned their rural communities and headed north to work as braceros.

The majority of the braceros were experienced farm laborers who came from places such as La Comarca Lagunera, Coahuila, and other important agricultural regions of Mexico. They stopped working their land and growing food for their families with the illusion that they would be able to earn a large amount of money on the other side of the border.

Large numbers of bracero candidates arrived by train to the northern border, altering the social environment and economy of many border towns. Ciudad Juárez, Chihuahua, across from El Paso, TX, became a historic recruitment site and substantial gathering point for the agricultural labor force.

The following excerpt from the *El Paso Herald Post* (April 28, 1956) illustrates the movement: "More than 80,000 braceros pass through the El Paso Bracero Center annually. They're part of an army of 350,000 or more that marches across the border each year to help plant, cultivate, and harvest cotton and other crops throughout the United States."

The bracero contracts were controlled by independent farmers' associations and the Farm Bureau. The contracts were in English and the braceros would sign them without understanding their full rights and the conditions of employment. When the contracts expired, the braceros were required to turn in their permits and return to México. The braceros could return to their native lands in case of an emergency only with written permission from their boss.

The braceros labored tirelessly, thinning sugar beets, picking cucumbers and tomatoes, and weeding and picking cotton. They became the foundation for the development of North American agriculture.

Despite their enormous contribution to the American economy, the braceros suffered harassment and oppression from extremist groups and racist authorities.

By the 1960s, a large number of "illegal" agricultural workers, along with the introduction of the mechanical cotton harvester, destroyed the usefulness of the bracero program under which more than 3 million Mexicans entered the U.S. to labor in the agricultural fields. It ended in 1964. The U.S. Department of Labor officer in charge, Lee G. Williams, had described it as a system of "legalized slavery." The following note describes its last day:

BRACEROS CROSS TO UNITED STATES

With the crossing of 526 braceros through the Santa Fe Street Bridge Tuesday night, current contracting of Mexican laborers for work in U.S. farms ended, officials of the National Railways of Mexico reported Wednesday. The railroad in charge of transporting the braceros to Juárez from all parts of the state disclosed that the number of workers contracted totaled

12,127. Of this number, only a few were sent back after failing to pass their physical examination at the Bracero center.

The *El Paso Times*
May 30, 1963

The braceros returned home. Unable to survive in their communities, however, they continue to cross the Río Bravo (or Río Grande) to work in the farms and ranches of this country. In the fields of West Texas and southern New Mexico, you will still find braceros. They are now known as chile pickers and continue to be one of the most exploited labor groups in the U.S.

Source: The Farmworkers Web site. The Bracero Project: the Bracero program. Available at: www.farmworkers.org/bracerop.html. Accessed August 27, 2006.

3.3.4.1.4   Asian American Populations

The term *Asian* refers to people having origins in any of the original natives of the Far East, Southeast Asia, or the Indian subcontinent (including Cambodia, China, India, Japan, Korea, Malaysia, Pakistan, the Philippine Islands, Thailand, and Vietnam). Asians represent both extremes of socioeconomic and health indices. Factors contributing to poor health outcomes include language and cultural barriers and stigma associated with certain conditions. Asians comprise 3.6% of the U.S. population.

3.3.4.1.5   American Indian and Alaska Native (AI/AN) Populations

The terms *American Indian* and *Alaska Native* refer to any of the original people of North, Central, or South America, and who maintain tribal affiliation or community attachment. They comprise about 0.9% of the U.S. population.

The Bureau of Indian Affairs (BIA) in the Department of the Interior administers and manages more than 55 million acres of land held in trust by the U.S. for American Indians, Indian tribes, and Alaska Natives (see Box 3.6), and provides education services to approximately 48,000 Native American students. In conjunction with the BIA, the Indian Health Service (IHS), an agency in the Department of Health and Human Services (DHHS), is supposed to uphold the federal government's obligation to AI/AN people to honor and protect the inherent sovereign rights of tribes.

Although the IHS currently provides health services to approximately 1.5 million AI/ANs who belong to more than 550 federally recognized tribes in 35 states, more than half the AI/AN population does not permanently reside on a reservation and therefore has limited or no access to IHS services. AI/ANs generally experience poorer health than the American population as a whole. For example, among AI/ANs age 18 and older, 63.7% of men and 61.4% of women have one or more cardiovascular disease risk factors such as hypertension, current cigarette smoking, high blood cholesterol, obesity, and diabetes.

3.3.4.1.6   Native Hawaiian and Other Pacific Islanders (NHOPI) Populations

The term *Native Hawaiian and Other Pacific Islanders* refers to people having origins in any of the original people of Hawaii, Guam, Samoa, or other Pacific Islands. Pacific Islanders include people with Polynesian, Micronesian, and Melanesian backgrounds, whose languages and cultures differ. NHOPIs generally experience poorer health than the American population as a whole. They comprise 0.1% of the U.S. population.

3.3.4.2 Gender

In addition to its total size, two of the most important characteristics of a population are its gender and age structure. According to the 2000 census, of the 281.4 million people in the U.S., 143.4 million were female and 138.1 million male. The former made up 50.9% of the population, down from 51.3% in 1990.

Box 3.6 Relationship between the Federal Government and Indian Tribes

The Indian Health Service (HIS) is responsible for providing health services to AI/ANs. These services to members of federally recognized tribes grew out of the special government-to-government relationship between the federal government and Indian tribes. This relationship, established in 1787, is based on Article I, Section 8 of the Constitution ("The Congress shall have the power ... to regulate Commerce with foreign Nations, and among the several States, and with Indian tribes ... ") and has been given form and substance by numerous treaties, laws, executive orders, and Supreme Court decisions. Known as the Marshall Trilogy, three cases — *Johnson v. McIntosh* (1823), *Cherokee Nation v. Georgia* (1831), and *Worcester v. Georgia* (1832) — defined the relationship of tribes with the U.S. government and established the doctrine of federal trust responsibility.

More than a century ago, trust fund accounts were established to compensate Indians for the use of their land. An 1887 law made the federal government responsible for collecting fees from anyone using tribal land, with the money to be held in trust. Some of these funds belong to about 300,000 individual Native Americans, others belong to about 1400 tribes.[1] The funds are managed by the Department of the Interior's Office of Special Trustee, Office of the Secretary. Prior to 1996 the trust funds were managed by the Bureau of Indian Affairs. Billions were paid by mining companies, ranchers, and others over the decades. Currently over $300 million is collected annually by the BIA. The agency is responsible for sending checks to Indian trust beneficiaries, many of whom rely on trust funds for basic necessities. The money was supposed to be given to the descendants of the original Indian land owners, but every audit since 1928 has found billions missing from the trust fund, in what may be the greatest financial scandal in the history of the U.S.[2]

Sources:

[1] Interpretation of Federal Financial Accounting Standards. Interpretation Number 1. Reporting on Indian Trust Funds in General Purpose Financial Reports of the Department of the Interior and in the Consolidated Financial Statements of the United States Government: An interpretation of SFFAS 7. n.d. Available at: http://www.fasab.gov/interpretations/intprt1.htm. Accessed September 26, 2004.

[2] A Continuing Shame. Editorial. *The New York Times*. September 26, 2004. Week in Review, p. 10.

Although male births outnumber female births by about 5%, males generally have higher mortality rates than females at every age. These higher mortality rates translate into women outnumbering men, starting at approximately 35 years of age. The "excess" of women is most pronounced at older ages. As in most countries of the world, older women outnumber older men in the U.S., and women's share of the older population increases with age.

The disparity between numbers of men and women is expressed as the *sex ratio* — the number of men per 100 women. Figure 3.3 depicts changes in the sex ratio between 1900 and 2000. Between 1990 and 2000, the male population grew slightly faster (13.9%) than the female population (12.5%). The excess female-to-male population dropped from 6.2 million to 5.3 million as male death rates declined faster than female rates and as immigration brought in more men.

In 2000, the average sex ratio among those 65 and older was 70 (70 men per 100 women), and ranged from 86 (at 65–69 years of age) to 41 (85 years and older). The older non-Hispanic white population's sex ratio mirrored that of the total older population in 2000. Most other groups had slightly higher sex ratios than the total older population. The two exceptions were older blacks and older Pacific Islanders. With a sex ratio of 61.4, the older black population displayed a greater shortage of men than all other groups, mainly as a result of higher mortality rates for black men than for black women.[11]

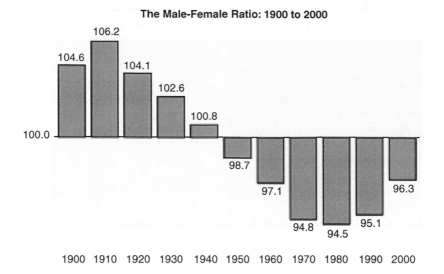

FIGURE 3.3 Changes in sex ratio: 1900 to 2000. (From Pennsylvania State College of Agriculture and Sciences. Resources, Census Data: Gender 2000, Census 2000 brief. Available at: http://ict.cas.psu.edu/ resources/Census/ PDF/C2K_Gender.pdf#search=%22u.s.%20census%20gender%22. Accessed August 27, 2006.)

Box 3.7 Administration on Aging: Mission and Services

The Administration on Aging (AoA), an agency in the U.S. Department of Health and Human Services, is one of the nation's largest providers of home- and community-based care for older persons and their caregivers. Their mission is to develop a comprehensive, coordinated, and cost-effective system of long-term care that helps elderly individuals to maintain their dignity in their homes and communities, and to help society prepare for an aging population.

Created in 1965 with the passage of the Older Americans Act (OAA), AoA is part of a federal, state, tribal, and local partnership called the National Network on Aging. This network, serving about 7 million older persons and their caregivers, consists of 56 state units and 655 area agencies on aging, 233 tribal and native organizations, two organizations that serve Native Hawaiians, 29,000 service providers, and thousands of volunteers. These organizations provide assistance and services to older individuals and their families in urban, suburban, and rural areas throughout the U.S.

Although all older Americans may receive services, the OAA targets those older individuals who are in greatest economic and social need: the poor, the isolated, and those elders disadvantaged by social or health disparities.

There are seven core services funded by the OAA:

- **Supportive services**, which enable communities to offer rides to medical appointments, and grocery and drug stores and provide house repair, chore running, and personal care help so that older persons can stay in their homes includes adult day care and information and assistance.
- **Nutrition services,** which include more than a meal. Since its creation, the OAA Nutrition Program has provided nearly 6 billion meals for at-risk older persons. Each day in communities across America, senior citizens come together in senior centers or other group settings to share a meal, as well as camaraderie and friendship. Nutrition services also provide nutrition education, health screenings, and counseling at senior centers. Homebound seniors are able to remain in their homes largely because of the daily delivery

of a hot meal, sometimes by a senior volunteer who is their only visitor. March 2002 marked the 30th anniversary of the OAA Nutrition Program, and AoA will be celebrating this successful community-based service throughout the year.

- **Preventive health services**, which educate and enable older persons to make healthy lifestyle choices. Every year, illness and disability that result from chronic disease affects the quality of life of millions of older adults and their caregivers. Many chronic diseases can be prevented through healthy lifestyles, physical activity, appropriate diet and nutrition, smoking cessation, active and meaningful social engagement, and regular screenings. The ultimate goal of the OAA health promotion and disease prevention services is to increase the quality and years of healthy life.

- **The National Family Caregiver Support Program (NFCSP)**, which was funded for the first time in 2000 and is a significant addition to the OAA. It was created to help the millions of people who provide primary care for spouses, parents, older relatives and friends. The program includes information to caregivers about available services; assistance to caregivers in gaining access to services; individual counseling, organization of support groups and training to assist caregivers in making decisions and solving problems relating to their care-giving roles, and supplemental services to complement care provided by caregivers. The program also recognizes the needs of grandparents caring for grandchildren and of caregivers of those 18 and under with mental retardation or developmental difficulties and the diverse needs of Native Americans.

- **Services that protect the rights of vulnerable older persons**, which are designed to empower older persons and their family members to detect and prevent elder abuse and consumer fraud as well as to enhance the physical, mental, emotional, and financial well-being of America's elderly. These services include pension counseling programs that help older Americans access their pensions and make informed insurance and healthcare choices, and long-term care ombudsman programs that serve to investigate and resolve complaints made by or for residents of nursing, board and care, and similar adult homes. AoA supports the training of thousands of paid and volunteer long-term care ombudsmen, insurance counselors, and other professionals who assist with reporting waste, fraud, and abuse in nursing homes and other settings. It also supports senior Medicare patrol projects, which operate in 47 states, and in the District of Columbia and Puerto Rico. AoA awards grants to state units and area agencies on aging, and community organizations to train senior volunteers how to educate older Americans to take a more active role in monitoring and understanding their healthcare.

- **Services to Native Americans**, which include nutrition and supportive services designed to meet the unique cultural and social traditions of tribal and native organizations and organizations serving Native Hawaiians. Native American elders are among the most disadvantaged groups in the country.

- **Eldercare Locator:** Additionally, AoA supports the Eldercare Locator, a national toll-free service to help callers find services and resources in their own communities or throughout the country. The number is 1–800–677–1116.

Source: Department of Health and Human Services, Administration on Aging: Mission. Available at: http://www.aoa.dhhs.gov/about/over/over_mission.asp. Accessed August 27, 2006.

3.3.4.3 Age

The U.S. population has grown older almost without interruption since the country's founding. For example, in 1900 only 4% of the U.S. population was age 65 or older. By 1980, the proportion in old age had nearly tripled to 11%.

Although, during the first half of the 20th century, the U.S. population was relatively young due to a high fertility rate, declining infant and childhood mortality rates, and high rates of net immigration, since 1950 the population has been aging rapidly. By the time all baby boomers will have reached age 65 in 2030, the Census Bureau projects that 20% of the population will be age 65 or older. Although the rate of population aging should then slow, the aged sector of the population will continue to rise slowly, reaching 23% by 2060.

By the year 2050, the percentage of the elderly in the U.S. population will surpass the figures currently observed in the oldest states. In 2000, the elderly made up 17.6% of the population of Florida. By 2050, 20% of the U.S. population will be comprised of elderly people. In essence, many of the challenges currently faced by the oldest states can be used to predict the health challenges the nation will face by the middle of the 21st century.[12]

3.3.4.3.1 Race and Ethnicity

As the older population grows larger, it will also grow more diverse, reflecting the demographic changes in the U.S. population as a whole. By 2050, programs and services for the elderly population will require greater flexibility to meet the needs of a more diverse population.

3.3.4.3.2 Longevity and Health

People in the U.S. are living longer and healthier lives than ever before. Average life expectancy at birth rose from 47.3 years in 1900 to 76.9 years in 2000. Today, heart disease, malignant neoplasms (cancer), and cerebrovascular diseases (stroke) are the leading causes of death among older Americans. Of the 1.8 million deaths in 2000 among people aged 65 and over, 8% were caused by cerebrovascular diseases, 22% by malignant neoplasms, and 33% by heart disease (see Figure 3.4). About 14 million civilian noninstitutionalized older people live with some type of disability. Disability is more likely to be experienced in older women (43%) than in older men (40%).[13]

3.3.4.3.3 Chronic Illnesses

Chronic diseases and impairments — among the leading causes of disability in older people — can negatively affect quality of life, lead to a decline in independent living, and impose an economic burden on the individual and the society at large. About 80% of seniors have at least one chronic health condition and 50% have at least two. Arthritis, hypertension, heart disease, diabetes, and respiratory disorders are some of the leading causes of activity limitations among older people.

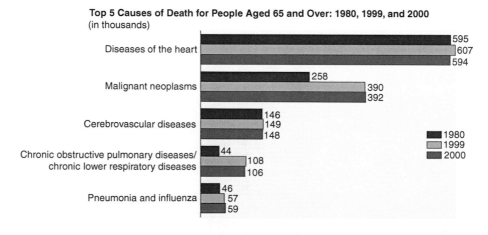

Top 5 Causes of Death for People Aged 65 and Over: 1980, 1999, and 2000 (in thousands)

FIGURE 3.4 Top 5 causes of death of people aged 65 and over. (From He, H., Sengupta, M., Velkoff, V.A., DeBarros, K.A. *U.S. Census Bureau, Current Population Reports, P23-209, 65+ in the United States: 2005.* U.S. Government Printing Office, Washington, DC, 2005. Available at: http://www.census.gov/prod/2006 pubs/ p23–209.pdf. Accessed August 18, 2006.)

The chronic diseases discussed in the following sections are either diet-related (hypertension, heart disease, stroke, diabetes, and osteoporosis) or they seriously compromise the individual's ability to shop, cook, and feed him or herself. The information provided is based on material compiled by the U.S. Census Bureau.[14]

3.3.4.3.3.1 Arthritis

Arthritis, encompassing more than 100 diseases and conditions that affect joints, surrounding tissues, and other connective tissues, is a leading cause of disability among older people. Although arthritis affects men and women of all ages, it is more common among older people, in general, and in women of all ages. In 1998–2000, in comparison with 2.2% of those between the ages of 18 and 44 years, 11.8% of people aged 65 to 74 years and 19.3% of people 75 years and older had activity limitations caused by arthritis and other musculoskeletal conditions.

3.3.4.3.3.2 Hypertension

Hypertension, another chronic condition, is prevalent among older adults. Activity limitations caused by heart and other circulatory diseases, including hypertension, increase with age. During the period 1998–2000, whereas about 0.5% of 18- to 44-year-olds suffered from heart disease or other circulatory conditions that limited activity, 11.1% of those 65 to 74 years old, and 17.1% of those 75 years and older also suffered this debility. Among older people, the prevalence of hypertension was higher among women and blacks than among men and whites. Among people 65 and older, prevalence of hypertension was highest among women aged 75 and over. Of these women, 85% had hypertension, compared with 71% of men.

3.3.4.3.3.3 Heart Disease and Stroke

Older women are more likely to have hypertension than older men, whereas the prevalence of coronary heart disease and stroke is higher among older men. During 1999–2000, 24.3% of older men and 15.4% of older women had coronary heart disease, with the prevalence higher among men in all older age groups. The incidence of both mild and more serious forms of coronary heart disease occurs at older ages in women than in men, with a lag of 10 or more years. During 1999–2000, 8.9% of older men and 7.6% of older women had a stroke. For the same period, older non-Hispanic blacks had a higher incidence of stroke (11.8%) than older Hispanics or non-Hispanic whites, with an incidence of 7.5% and 7.9%, respectively.

3.3.4.3.3.4 Diabetes

Diabetes also affects the health of older people and limits their ability to perform activities. The prevalence of diabetes-related limitations of activity was higher among those aged 65 to 74 (3.8%) and among those 75 and older (4.3%) than those aged 18 to 44. Among people 65 and older in 1999–2000, 15.1% of men and 13.0% of women reported having diabetes. The prevalence of diabetes was higher among older Hispanics (22.4%) and non-Hispanic blacks (22.8%) than among older non-Hispanic whites (12.5%). For additional information on diabetes, see Section 3.5.1.1 and Section 6.2.

3.3.4.3.3.5 Osteoporosis

Osteoporosis, another common chronic ailment among older people, reduces bone density and raises the risk for potentially disabling fractures. Hip fractures are particularly disabling and may increase the subsequent risk of mortality. Women are four times more likely than men to experience loss of bone density. The prevalence of osteoporosis and less severe osteopenia increases noticeably with age for both men and women, with a prevalence ten times greater among women.

3.3.4.3.3.6 Alzheimer's Disease

Alzheimer's disease (AD) is a progressive, degenerative disease that causes gradual but irreversible loss of brain cells and affects an estimated 4.5 million Americans. Although AD is not a part of normal aging, the risk of developing the disease increases with age. In 2000, 7% of those who had AD were

65 to 74 years, 53% were 75 to 84 years, and 40% were 85 or older.[15] The severity of AD also increases with age. In 2000, 17% of AD cases among people 65 to 74 years were classified as severe compared with 20% of cases among people aged 75 to 84 and 28% among those aged 85 and over.

The group of people at highest risk of AD, those aged 85 and over, is also the fastest-growing segment of the population. With the growing number of older people and the fact that the risk of AD increases as people age, AD is a growing public health concern. It is the major cause of dementia among older people and negatively affects their capacity to perform daily activities. The impact of AD is not limited to dementia and other health consequences. In addition to the cost of care (estimated to be about $100 billion every year), AD can create physical and emotional stress on caregivers (see Box 3.8). More than 7 out of 10 people with AD live at home, and 75% of them receive care from family members and friends. With the progression of the disease, families must often use long-term paid care. People with AD live for an average of 8 to 10 years, with an average lifetime cost per patient of $174,000.

Box 3.8 Alzheimer's Disease and the Caregiver

Alzheimer's disease and other forms of dementia do not affect just the patient. These diseases gradually rob patients of memory and other intellectual abilities, leaving them unable to perform routine tasks. As the disease continues to destroy brain cells, patients increasingly depend on family members or others to carry out simple tasks like shopping and getting dressed. Ultimately, most patients will need complete care, adding to the caregiver's burden.

Alzheimer's disease is the most common form of dementia, affecting up to 4 million Americans — and untold millions of family members and others who care for them. It is now recognized that caregivers need care themselves. The national Family Caregiver Alliance estimates that approximately 80% of the long-term care in the U.S. is provided without compensation, sometimes around the clock. Alzheimer's disease is not a typical disease model because the health and well-being of the caretaker is affected as well as the patient. Geriatricians who assume the care of an Alzheimer's patient also care for the caregiver.

Stress and Depression
According to the Alzheimer's Association, more than 80% of Alzheimer caregivers report that they frequently experience high levels of stress, and nearly half say they suffer from depression. The Family Caregiver Alliance estimates that caregiving spouses between the ages of 66 and 96 who are experiencing mental or emotional strain have a 63% higher risk of dying than people the same age who are not caregivers. Caregivers often experience feelings of guilt, believing they are not doing enough to help, it adds. Spouses and adult children feel grief and loss, not unlike a death in the family, except that instead of being sudden, the bereavement spans years. Alzheimer's is a progressively worsening disease, but the rate of progression from mild to advanced can vary widely, from 3 to 20 years. As Alzheimer's progresses, the loss of brain function itself will cause death unless the patient has one or more other serious illness.

The Child as Parent
For an adult child who cares for a parent with dementia, taking on the role of caregiver is a role reversal that needs adjustment. It can be a difficult transition for a child to take on the parenting and decision-making roles. The adult child might need to be empowered to step in and begin caring for the ailing parent — making sure the parent takes medication, for instance, or telling the parent he or she should not drive, and making difficult decisions about when the parent is no longer able to safely live alone.

These caregivers are often already juggling multiple responsibilities with their own spouses, children, and careers. In some cases, adult-child caregivers with siblings feel resentful if they must bear the brunt of their parent's care. An adult-child caregiver who is the only sibling living in the same city as the parent often feels isolated, overwhelmed, and underappreciated. This situation may be exacerbated when out-of-town siblings or other family members who see the parent infrequently may think the caregiver is exaggerating the extent of the Alzheimer's patient's decline. The out-of-town family members may feel guilty about not being able to help from a distance, and when they do visit, they may criticize or ask to change the care their parent is receiving.

Caregivers are often fatigued from carrying out their new responsibilities and neglect their own health. Concerns caregivers regularly express are loss of concentration due to their caregiving responsibilities and fear that they themselves might eventually get the disease. The warning signs of caregiver stress include anger, anxiety, denial, depression, exhaustion, health problems, irritability, decreased ability to concentrate, sleeplessness, and social withdrawal. Caregivers who regularly experience these conditions should be advised to seek help from their physician.

Financial Strain Heightens Burden
The presence of Alzheimer's disease often brings financial problems that can compound stress and depression. Caregivers often find additional responsibilities thrust on them, such as overseeing medications for their patient, knowing if or when the patient's care should be transferred to a nursing home, and taking on power of attorney duties along with living wills and advanced directives that specify whether terminal patients should undergo extreme measures to keep them alive. Sometimes caregivers resort to relinquishing paid employment for the uncompensated care of a loved one.

Respite Options
Because of the substantial responsibility of caring for a person with Alzheimer's disease, caregivers often seek respite. Respite options include adult day care services, in-home services, overnight and weekend services, and emergency care.

- Adult day services provide a planned program that includes a variety of health, social, and support services in a protective setting during daytime hours. This is referred to as a *community-based service* and is designed to meet the individual needs of functionally and/or cognitively impaired adults.
- In-home services offer a wide range of options, including companion services, personal care, household assistance, and skilled nursing care to meet the specific needs of those involved.
- Respite care facilities provide overnight, weekend, and longer stays for someone with Alzheimer's or a related dementia so a caregiver can have longer periods of time off. These facilities provide meals, help with activities of daily living, therapeutic activities to fit the needs of residents, and a safe and supervised environment. Examples of such facilities include nursing homes, residential care facilities, and assisted living facilities.
- Emergency respite is often offered in many nursing homes, residential care facilities, and assisted living facilities. Emergency respite care may be needed when a caregiver becomes ill or must go out of town unexpectedly, or if the care recipient is at risk of abuse or neglect.

3.3.5 AMERICAN COMMUNITY SURVEY

As expected, the once-a-decade data collection approach of a decennial census became obsolete with the advent of computer technology and the possibility of timely, easily available, up-to-date information. Thanks to the American Community Survey (ACS), which was fully implemented in 2005, the days of having to wait a decade for updated census figures are behind us. The ACS eliminates the need for the long form (used in four censuses, 1960–2000). The census short form (see Figure 3.5) will continue to produce the official count of the nation's population every 10 years, fulfilling the constitutionally mandated function of determining congressional apportionment.

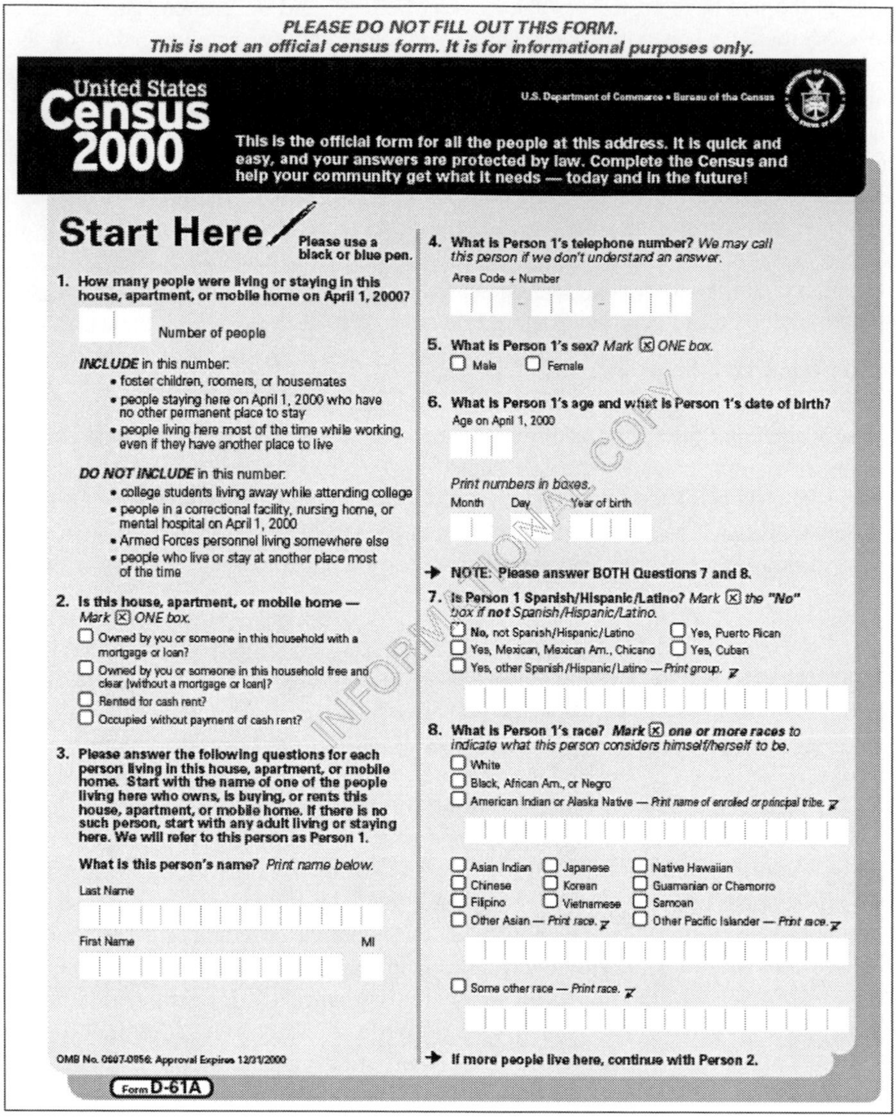

PLEASE DO NOT FILL OUT THIS FORM.
This is not an official census form. It is for informational purposes only.

United States Census 2000

U.S. Department of Commerce • Bureau of the Census

This is the official form for all the people at this address. It is quick and easy, and your answers are protected by law. Complete the Census and help your community get what it needs — today and in the future!

Start Here Please use a black or blue pen.

1. **How many people were living or staying in this house, apartment, or mobile home on April 1, 2000?**

   Number of people

   INCLUDE in this number:
   - foster children, roomers, or housemates
   - people staying here on April 1, 2000 who have no other permanent place to stay
   - people living here most of the time while working, even if they have another place to live

   DO NOT INCLUDE in this number:
   - college students living away while attending college
   - people in a correctional facility, nursing home, or mental hospital on April 1, 2000
   - Armed Forces personnel living somewhere else
   - people who live or stay at another place most of the time

2. **Is this house, apartment, or mobile home —** *Mark ☒ ONE box.*
   - ☐ Owned by you or someone in this household with a mortgage or loan?
   - ☐ Owned by you or someone in this household free and clear (without a mortgage or loan)?
   - ☐ Rented for cash rent?
   - ☐ Occupied without payment of cash rent?

3. **Please answer the following questions for each person living in this house, apartment, or mobile home. Start with the name of one of the people living here who owns, is buying, or rents this house, apartment, or mobile home. If there is no such person, start with any adult living or staying here. We will refer to this person as Person 1.**

   What is this person's name? *Print name below.*

   Last Name

   First Name MI

OMB No. 0607-0856: Approval Expires 12/31/2000

Form D-61A

4. **What is Person 1's telephone number?** *We may call this person if we don't understand an answer.*

   Area Code + Number

5. **What is Person 1's sex?** *Mark ☒ ONE box.*
   - ☐ Male ☐ Female

6. **What is Person 1's age and what is Person 1's date of birth?**

   Age on April 1, 2000

   Print numbers in boxes.

   Month Day Year of birth

→ **NOTE: Please answer BOTH Questions 7 and 8.**

7. **Is Person 1 Spanish/Hispanic/Latino?** *Mark ☒ the **"No"** box if **not** Spanish/Hispanic/Latino.*
   - ☐ No, not Spanish/Hispanic/Latino ☐ Yes, Puerto Rican
   - ☐ Yes, Mexican, Mexican Am., Chicano ☐ Yes, Cuban
   - ☐ Yes, other Spanish/Hispanic/Latino — *Print group.*

8. **What is Person 1's race?** ***Mark ☒ one or more races** to indicate what this person considers himself/herself to be.*
   - ☐ White
   - ☐ Black, African Am., or Negro
   - ☐ American Indian or Alaska Native — *Print name of enrolled or principal tribe.*
   - ☐ Asian Indian ☐ Japanese ☐ Native Hawaiian
   - ☐ Chinese ☐ Korean ☐ Guamanian or Chamorro
   - ☐ Filipino ☐ Vietnamese ☐ Samoan
   - ☐ Other Asian — *Print race.* ☐ Other Pacific Islander — *Print race.*
   - ☐ Some other race — *Print race.*

→ **If more people live here, continue with Person 2.**

FIGURE 3.5 2000 Census questionnaire (short form). (From U.S. Department of Commerce. Bureau of the Census. Public Information Office. Informational Short Form Questionnaire. Available at: http://www.census.gov/dmd/www/2000quest.html Accessed June 8, 2006.)

The ACS asks essentially the same questions as the previous long form, but because data collection is spread throughout the decade, rather than at a single point in time, it provides current information on a continuous basis. It is comprised of information on demographic characteristics, social welfare, education and health status, commuting patterns, crime patterns, and other important attributes of the U.S. population, as well as the interrelationships of these factors. Unlike other national surveys, the ACS provides information at the city and county level. Over a 5-year period, the survey's sample size will approximate that of the census long form, supporting the production of estimates for small and nonstandard geographical areas such

Person 2

Your answers are important!
Every person in the Census counts.

1. **What is Person 2's name?** *Print name below.*
   Last Name
   First Name   MI

2. **How is this person related to Person 1?** *Mark ⊠ ONE box.*
   - Husband/wife
   - Natural-born son/daughter
   - Adopted son/daughter
   - Stepson/stepdaughter
   - Brother/sister
   - Father/mother
   - Grandchild
   - Parent-in-law
   - Son-in-law/daughter-in-law
   - Other relative — *Print exact relationship.*

   If NOT RELATED to Person 1:
   - Roomer, boarder
   - Housemate, roommate
   - Unmarried partner
   - Foster child
   - Other nonrelative

3. **What is this person's sex?** *Mark ⊠ ONE box.*
   - Male
   - Female

4. **What is this person's age and what is this person's date of birth?** *Print numbers in boxes.*
   Age on April 1, 2000   Month   Day   Year of birth

→ NOTE: Please answer BOTH Questions 5 and 6.

5. **Is this person Spanish/Hispanic/Latino?** *Mark ⊠ the "No" box if not Spanish/Hispanic/Latino.*
   - No, not Spanish/Hispanic/Latino
   - Yes, Mexican, Mexican Am., Chicano
   - Yes, other Spanish/Hispanic/Latino — *Print group.*
   - Yes, Puerto Rican
   - Yes, Cuban

6. **What is this person's race?** *Mark ⊠ one or more races to indicate what this person considers himself/herself to be.*
   - White
   - Black, African Am., or Negro
   - American Indian or Alaska Native — *Print name of enrolled or principal tribe.*

   - Asian Indian
   - Chinese
   - Filipino
   - Other Asian — *Print race.*
   - Japanese
   - Korean
   - Vietnamese
   - Native Hawaiian
   - Guamanian or Chamorro
   - Samoan
   - Other Pacific Islander — *Print race.*

   - Some other race — *Print race.*

→ If more people live here, continue with Person 3.

Person 3

Census information helps your community get financial assistance for roads, hospitals, schools, and more.

1. **What is Person 3's name?** *Print name below.*
   Last Name
   First Name   MI

2. **How is this person related to Person 1?** *Mark ⊠ ONE box.*
   - Husband/wife
   - Natural-born son/daughter
   - Adopted son/daughter
   - Stepson/stepdaughter
   - Brother/sister
   - Father/mother
   - Grandchild
   - Parent-in-law
   - Son-in-law/daughter-in-law
   - Other relative — *Print exact relationship.*

   If NOT RELATED to Person 1:
   - Roomer, boarder
   - Housemate, roommate
   - Unmarried partner
   - Foster child
   - Other nonrelative

3. **What is this person's sex?** *Mark ⊠ ONE box.*
   - Male
   - Female

4. **What is this person's age and what is this person's date of birth?** *Print numbers in boxes.*
   Age on April 1, 2000   Month   Day   Year of birth

→ NOTE: Please answer BOTH Questions 5 and 6.

5. **Is this person Spanish/Hispanic/Latino?** *Mark ⊠ the "No" box if not Spanish/Hispanic/Latino.*
   - No, not Spanish/Hispanic/Latino
   - Yes, Mexican, Mexican Am., Chicano
   - Yes, other Spanish/Hispanic/Latino — *Print group.*
   - Yes, Puerto Rican
   - Yes, Cuban

6. **What is this person's race?** *Mark ⊠ one or more races to indicate what this person considers himself/herself to be.*
   - White
   - Black, African Am., or Negro
   - American Indian or Alaska Native — *Print name of enrolled or principal tribe.*

   - Asian Indian
   - Chinese
   - Filipino
   - Other Asian — *Print race.*
   - Japanese
   - Korean
   - Vietnamese
   - Native Hawaiian
   - Guamanian or Chamorro
   - Samoan
   - Other Pacific Islander — *Print race.*

   - Some other race — *Print race.*

→ If more people live here, continue with Person 4.

FIGURE 3.5 (Continued).

as school districts. In addition, given the sample size, information is available for specific demographic groups, including racial and ethnic groups, children, the elderly, people in specific occupations, people with specific health conditions, and people with various levels of educational attainment.[16,17]

Information provided by the ACS also includes topics ranging from housing values and educational attainment to commute times and language spoken at home. Data users can access this detailed annual demographic and housing data online, helping them make more accurate, timely, and informed decisions. Roughly 2.5% of the population (about 1 in 40 addresses) will participate in the survey each year. By comparison, 1 in 6 addresses received the Census 2000 long form.

The Census Bureau mails the mandatory survey to a rolling, random sample of about 3 million households throughout the country. The ACS is being conducted in all 3,141 counties,

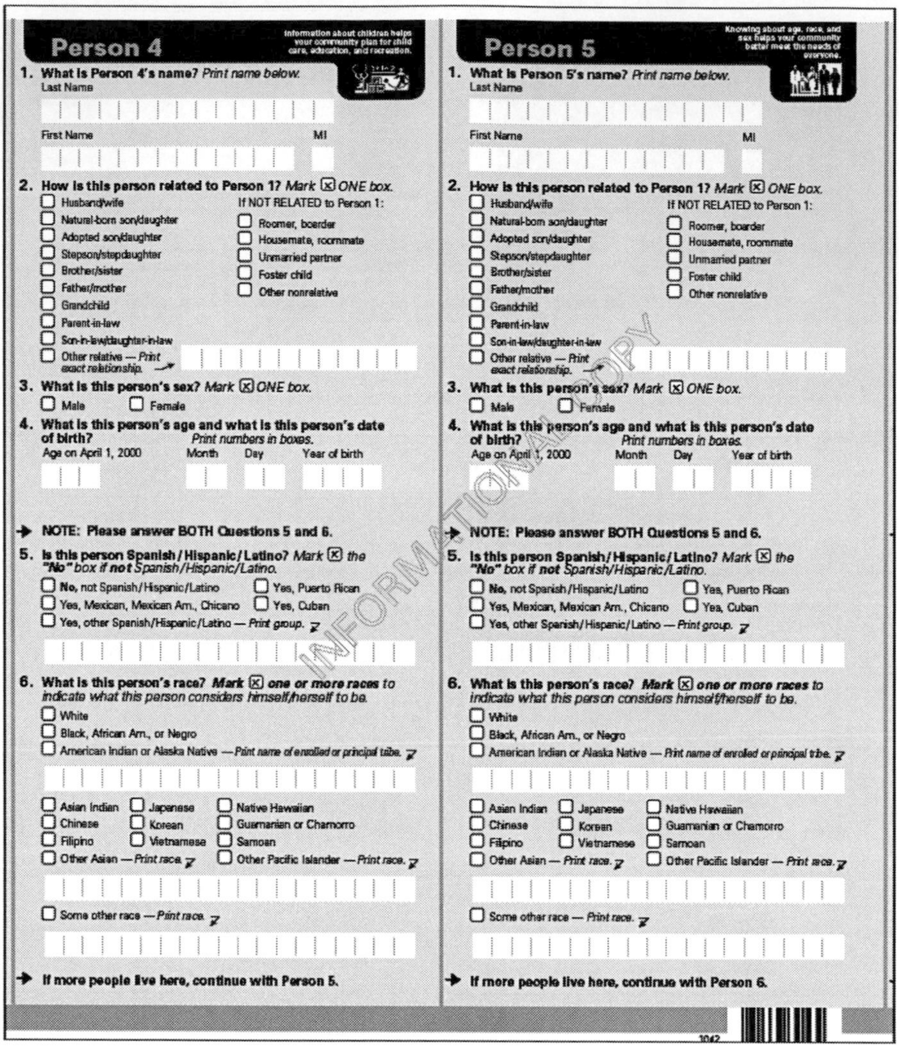

FIGURE 3.5 (Continued).

in American Indian and Alaska Native areas, Hawaiian homelands, and in Puerto Rico (250,000 housing units per month). It produces data for areas with populations of 65,000 or more. Starting in about 2008, data for areas of smaller populations (20,000 or more) will be released. Once data are collected, tabulations are released based on rolling 3-year averages annually for areas with populations between 20,000 and 65,000, and rolling 5-year averages annually for areas as small as census tracts[18] (see Box 3.9). The 2005 data provides estimates for over 8,000 geographic areas, including all counties and places with a population greater than 20,000.[19]

Addresses selected for the ACS will receive a letter from the Census Bureau director asking them to respond promptly to the survey. Attempts at follow-up interviews of a sample of nonresponders will be made first by phone and then by personal visit. As with the answers to other census questionnaires, federal law guarantees the confidentiality of ACS responses. People with

Person 6

Your answers help your community plan for the future.

1. **What is Person 6's name?** *Print name below.*
   Last Name
   First Name   MI

2. **How is this person related to Person 1?** *Mark* ☒ *ONE box.*
   ☐ Husband/wife
   ☐ Natural-born son/daughter
   ☐ Adopted son/daughter
   ☐ Stepson/stepdaughter
   ☐ Brother/sister
   ☐ Father/mother
   ☐ Grandchild
   ☐ Parent-in-law
   ☐ Son-in-law/daughter-in-law
   ☐ Other relative — *Print exact relationship.*

   If NOT RELATED to Person 1:
   ☐ Roomer, boarder
   ☐ Housemate, roommate
   ☐ Unmarried partner
   ☐ Foster child
   ☐ Other nonrelative

3. **What is this person's sex?** *Mark* ☒ *ONE box.*
   ☐ Male   ☐ Female

4. **What is this person's age and what is this person's date of birth?** *Print numbers in boxes.*
   Age on April 1, 2000   Month   Day   Year of birth

   → **NOTE: Please answer BOTH Questions 5 and 6.**

5. **Is this person Spanish/Hispanic/Latino?** *Mark* ☒ *the "No" box if not Spanish/Hispanic/Latino.*
   ☐ No, not Spanish/Hispanic/Latino   ☐ Yes, Puerto Rican
   ☐ Yes, Mexican, Mexican Am., Chicano   ☐ Yes, Cuban
   ☐ Yes, other Spanish/Hispanic/Latino — *Print group.*

6. **What is this person's race?** *Mark* ☒ *one or more races to indicate what this person considers himself/herself to be.*
   ☐ White
   ☐ Black, African Am., or Negro
   ☐ American Indian or Alaska Native — *Print name of enrolled or principal tribe.*

   ☐ Asian Indian   ☐ Japanese   ☐ Native Hawaiian
   ☐ Chinese   ☐ Korean   ☐ Guamanian or Chamorro
   ☐ Filipino   ☐ Vietnamese ☐ Samoan
   ☐ Other Asian — *Print race.*   ☐ Other Pacific Islander — *Print race.*

   ☐ Some other race — *Print race.*

   → **If more people live here, list their names on the back of this page in the spaces provided.**

   Form D-61A

Please turn to go to last page.

FIGURE 3.5 (Continued).

access to the answers take an oath to protect the confidentiality of the information they collect. Violators are subject to imprisonment and a substantial fine.

3.3.5.1 Uses of ACS Responses

State and local health departments as well as the U.S. Department of Health and Human Services use data on the following:

- *Age and residence* to plan programs for older people who are living alone
- *Language spoken at home and English fluency* to develop programs that target a diverse population
- *Grandparents responsible for grandchildren* to provide data to apply for grants
- *Income* to tailor products and services appropriately
- *Disability* to decide where to locate facilities and services for people with disabilities

Persons 7 – 12

If you didn't have room to list everyone who lives in this house or apartment, please list the others below. *You may be contacted by the Census Bureau for the same information about these people.*

Person 7 — Last Name

First Name   MI

Person 8 — Last Name

First Name   MI

Person 9 — Last Name

First Name   MI

Person 10 — Last Name

First Name   MI

Person 11 — Last Name

First Name   MI

Person 12 — Last Name

First Name   MI

The Census Bureau estimates that, for the average household, this form will take about 10 minutes to complete, including the time for reviewing the instructions and answers. Comments about the estimate should be directed to the Associate Director for Finance and Administration, Attn: Paperwork Reduction Project 0607-0856, Room 3104, Federal Building 3, Bureau of the Census, Washington, DC 20233.

Respondents are not required to respond to any information collection unless it displays a valid approval number from the Office of Management and Budget.

Thank you for completing your official U.S. Census 2000 form.

The "Informational Copy" shows the content of the United States Census 2000 "short" form questionnaire. Each household will receive either a short form (100-percent questions) or a long form (100-percent and sample questions). The short form questionnaire contains 6 population questions and 1 housing question. On average, about 5 in every 6 households will receive the short form. The content of the forms resulted from reviewing the 1990 census data, consulting with federal and non-federal data users, and conducting tests.

For additional information about Census 2000, visit our website at **www.census.gov** or write to the Director, Bureau of the Census, Washington, DC 20233.

FOR OFFICE USE ONLY

| A. JIC1 | B. JIC2 | C. JIC3 | D. JIC4 |

FIGURE 3.5 (Continued).

3.4 CENSUS INFORMATION ONLINE

All Census Bureau reports since 1996 are readily available online. In addition, personalized reports can be generated instantly by using the interactive features on the U.S. Census homepage. For example, one can compare the demographics of a state, city, or county with those of any

Box 3.9 Census Definitions

- **Census tract** — Small, relatively permanent statistical subdivision of a county averaging about 4,000 inhabitants.
- **Census block group** — At 600 to 3000 people, the census block group is the smallest geographic level for which data will be produced. Estimates for small numbers of people or areas are not published if there is a probability that an individual in that group can be identified.

other municipality in the nation, or with the entire U.S. QuickFacts provides data for cities and towns with more than 25,000 people. One can compare national, state, city, and county data for the categories listed in Table 3.3. Some of the items of interest to public health nutrition professionals include percentage of persons below poverty, per capita income, income per household, language other than English spoken at home, percentage of people aged at least 25 who are high school graduates, and percentage of population less than 18 years as well as more than 65 years.

3.5 U.S. POPULATION PROJECTIONS TO 2050

These projections are estimates of the population at future dates, calculating likely population changes based on assumptions about future births, deaths, and international and domestic migration. Projected numbers are based on an estimated population consistent with the most recent decennial census, projected forward.

As indicated in Table 3.2, the U.S. Census projects a 48% increase in the U.S. population for the first half of the 21st century, with the largest increases predicted for the Asian population, and the smallest for non-Hispanic whites. In particular, the percentage of the population that is non-Hispanic white is expected to decrease from just over of the total U.S. population in 2000 to just over 50% in 2050. During the same period of time, the percentage of the population that is Hispanic, of any race, is expected to double, from 12.6 to 24.4%. The black population is projected to increase from 12.7 to 14.6%. The Asian population will more than double, from 3.8 to 8.0%, as will the percentage of the total population that is identified as "all other races" (including American Indian and Alaska Native, Native Hawaiian and "Other Pacific Islander," and people who identify with two or more races), which is expected to increase from 2.5 to 5.3%.[20]

3.5.1 DISEASE FORECASTING BASED ON POPULATION PROJECTIONS

Projections of the incidence and prevalence of disease are important for public health planning. Disease projections can be estimated by combining prevalence data with population projections. To project the number of people with a chronic diet-related disease in 2050, the U.S. Census Bureau's age-, sex-, and race-specific population projections are multiplied by predicted disease prevalence rates for each subgroup. For example, the percentage of the population with Alzheimer's disease would be expected to increase concomitant with the increasing age of the population. The number of people with Alzheimer's disease in the U.S. population was estimated at 4.5 million in 2000, which is a prevalence rate of 16 per 1000 population. By 2050 the number of cases of Alzheimer's disease is expected to almost triple to 13.2 million,[21] which is a prevalence rate of 32 per 1000 population. Similar projections are possible for other chronic diseases, based on the projected population of the U.S. and the projected number of cases of a disease in a particular year.

3.5.1.1 Case in Point: Diabetes

Forecasts of the number of people with diabetes are needed to help policymakers prepare for changes in the demand for healthcare resources, and develop preventive and treatment interventions that target the populations with the largest expected increases in diabetes prevalence.

If recent trends in diabetes prevalence rates continue through 2050, changes in the size and demographic characteristics of the U.S. population will lead to dramatic increases in the number of Americans with diagnosed diabetes. The projected number of people with diagnosed diabetes will rise from 12.0 million in 2000 to 39.0 million in 2050, implying an increase in diagnosed diabetes prevalence from 4.4% in 2000 to 9.7% in 2050.[22] Because the size of the older population is expanding, the largest percentage increase in diagnosed diabetes will be among those aged 75 years and older.

TABLE 3.3
QuickFacts Data Categories

People QuickFacts

Population, 2005 estimate
Population, percent change, April 1, 2000 to July 1, 2005
Population, 2000
Population, percent change, 1990 to 2000
Persons under 5 years old, percent, 2004
Persons under 18 years old, percent, 2004
Persons 65 years old and over, percent, 2004
Female persons, percent, 2004
White persons, percent, 2004 (a)
Black persons, percent, 2004 (a)
American Indian and Alaska Native persons, percent, 2004 (a)
Asian persons, percent, 2004 (a)
Native Hawaiian and Other Pacific Islanders, percent, 2004 (a)
Persons reporting two or more races, percent, 2004
Persons of Hispanic or Latino origin, percent, 2004 (b)
White persons, not Hispanic, percent, 2004
Living in same house in 1995 and 2000, percent age 5+, 2000
Foreign-born persons, percent, 2000
Language other than English spoken at home, percent age 5+, 2000
High school graduates, percent of persons age 25+, 2000
Bachelor's degree or higher, percent of persons age 25+, 2000
Persons with a disability, age 5+, 2000
Mean travel time to work (minutes), workers age 16+, 2000
Housing units, 2004
Homeownership rate, 2000
Housing units in multiunit structures, percent, 2000
Median value of owner-occupied housing units, 2000
Households, 2000
Persons per household, 2000
Per capita money income, 1999
Median household income, 2003

Business QuickFacts

Private nonfarm establishments, 2003
Private nonfarm employment, 2003
Private nonfarm employment, percent change 2000–2003
Nonemployer establishments, 2003
Manufacturers shipments, 2002 ($1000)
Retail sales, 2002 ($1000)
Retail sales per capita, 2002
Minority-owned firms, percent of total, 1997
Women-owned firms, percent of total, 1997
Housing units authorized by building permits, 2004

Geography QuickFacts

Land area, 2000 (square miles)
Persons per square mile, 2000

However, the fastest growing group with diagnosed diabetes is expected to be among black males, followed by black females, white males, and white females.[23]

Forecasts of the number of people with diabetes help policymakers prepare for changes in the demand for healthcare resources and develop preventive and treatment interventions that target the populations with the largest expected increases in diabetes prevalence.

What does this mean for nutrition in public health?

- A larger healthcare workforce trained in medical nutrition therapy or certified as diabetes educators will help people with diabetes manage their condition.
- Feeding programs, such as the National School Lunch Program, the School Breakfast Program, the Child and Adult Care Feeding, and the Nutrition Program for the Elderly will offer food and services that meet the needs of a population with diabetes.
- Restaurants, particularly those located in areas with large elderly populations, will offer menu selections appropriate for people with diabetes.
- Programs targeting the populations most at risk will receive increased funding for preventive programs.
- Employee wellness programs will focus on weight management.
- Organizations that purchase healthcare benefits for their members or employees will insist that diabetes self-management education, medications, and supplies be included in the services provided, and managed care organizations will include these services and supplies in the basic plan available to all participants.
- Evaluation of school administrators will be tied to their providing healthy school environments, including the school food program.

3.6 CONCLUSION

Although the U.S. census was originally a political compromise used to apportion seats in the House of Representatives, it has become fundamental to our practice of government. The decennial census, augmented by the continuous ACS since 2005, provides a picture, in numbers, of who we are as a people. At first glance a perhaps overwhelming compendium of facts, the census upon closer inspection details our race, age, and gender composition. Through the census, we know where the preponderance of the population lives, what their occupations are, and which languages they speak. This information is used to allocate federal monies, project future population patterns, and determine public health priorities. Lacking the census, it would be impossible to understand the character of the U.S. population, to note and anticipate disease patterns, or to pursue the goal of eliminating health disparities.

3.7 ACRONYMS

ACS	American Community Survey
AI/AN	American Indian and Alaska Native
AD	Alzheimer's disease
AoA	Administration on Aging
BIA	Bureau of Indian Affairs
CDBG	Community Development Block Grants
DHHS	Department of Health and Human Services
FY	Fiscal year (October 1–September 30)
HIS	Indian Health Services
LBW	Low birth weight
NHOPI	Native Hawaiian and other Pacific Islanders
OMB	Office of Management and Budget
SES	Socioeconomic status

REFERENCES

1. Shrestha, L.B. The Changing Demographic Profile of the United States. CRS Report to Congress. The Library of Congress, Congressional Research Service. Order Code RL 32701. Available at: http://www.fas.org/sgp/crs/misc/RL32701.pdf. Accessed August 18, 2006.
2. Isaacs, S.L. and Schroeder, S.A. Class — The ignored determinant of the nation's health. *N Eng J Med.* 351, 1136–1142, 2004.
3. U.S. Department of Health and Human Services. Public Health Service. The Office of Minority Health. Assuring Cultural Competence in HealthCare: Recommendations for National Standards and an Out-comes-Focused Research Agenda. *Recommendations for National Standards and a National Public Comment Process.* Available at: http://www.omhrc.gov/clas/cultural1a.htm. Accessed August 2, 2004.
4. Smith, J.P. and Edmonston, B., Eds. Panel on the Demographic and Economic Impacts of Immigration, National Research Council. *The New Americans: Economic, Demographic, and Fiscal Effects of Immigration.* Washington, D.C.: National Academy Press, 1997.
5. U.S. Census Bureau. Congressional Apportionment. Available at: http://www.census.gov/population/www/censusdata/apportionment.html. Accessed June 12, 2006.
6. Cohen, J.E. World population in 2050: assessing the projections. In Little, J.S. and Triest, R.K., Eds. *Seismic Shifts: The Economic Impact of Demographic Change.* Federal Reserve Bank of Boston Conference Series. No. 46, June 2001. Available at: http://www.bos.frb.org/economic/conf/conf46/conf46d1.pdf. Accessed August 8, 2006.
7. Office of Management and Budget. *Revisions to the Standards for the Classification of Federal Data on Race and Ethnicity.* 1997. Available at http://www.census.gov/population/www/socdemo/race/ Ombdir15.html. Accessed August 5, 2004.
8. U.S. Census Bureau, 2004 American Community Survey. Available at: http://www.census.gov/. Accessed June 12, 2006.
9. Alba, F. Mexico: A Crucial Crossroads. March 2004. Available at: http://www.migrationinformation.org/Profiles/display.cfm?ID=211. Accessed June 11, 2006.
10. He, H., Sengupta, M., Velkoff, V.A., and DeBarros, K.A. U.S. Census Bureau, Current Population Reports, P23-209, 65+ in the United States: 2005. Washington, D.C., 2005. Available at: http://www.census.gov/prod/2006pubs/p23-209.pdf. Accessed August 18, 2006.
11. Shrestha, L.B. The Changing Demographic Profile of the United States. CRS Report to Congress. The Library of Congress, Congressional Research Service. Order Code RL 32701. Available at: http://www.fas.org/sgp/crs/misc/RL32701.pdf. Accessed August 18, 2006.
12. He, H., Sengupta, M., Velkoff, V.A., and DeBarros, K.A. U.S. Census Bureau, Current Population Reports, P23-209, 65+ in the United States: 2005. Washington, D.C., 2005. Available at: http://www.census.gov/prod/2006pubs/p23-209.pdf. Accessed August 18, 2006.
13. National Institute on Aging. New Prevalence Study Suggests Dramatically Rising Numbers of People with Alzheimer's Disease. http://www.nia.nih.gov/Alzheimers/ResearchInformation/NewsReleases/Archives/PR2003/PR20030818prevalence.htm.
14. National Research Council. *The American Community Survey: Summary of a Workshop.* Committee on National Statistics. Washington, D.C.: National Academy Press, 2001.
15. Cork, D.L., Cohen, M.L., and King, B.F., Eds. National Research Council. *Reengineering the 2010 Census: Risks and Challenges.* Committee on National Statistics. Washington, D.C.: National Academies Press, 2004.
16. U.S. Census Bureau. *American Community Survey. A Handbook for State and Local Officials.* December 2004. Available at: http://www.census.gov/acs/www/Downloads/ACS04HSLO.pdf. Accessed June 12, 2006.
17. U.S. Census Bureau. 2004 *American Community Survey.* Available at: http://www.census.gov. Accessed June 12, 2006.
18. U.S. Census Bureau, 2004, U.S. Interim Projections by Age, Sex, Race, and Hispanic Origin, http://www.census.gov/ipc/www/usinterimproj.
19. Hebert, L.E., Scherr, P.A., Bienias, J.L., Bennett, D.A., and Evans, D.A. Alzheimer disease in the U.S. population: prevalence estimates using the 2000 census. *Arch Neurol.* 60, 1119–1122, 2003.
20. Honeycutt, A.A., Boyle, J.P., Broglio, K.R., et al. A dynamic Markov model for forecasting diabetes prevalence in the United States through 2050. *HealthCare Manage Sci.* 6, 155–164, 2003.
21. Boyle, J.P., Honeycutt, A.A., Narayan, K.M., et al. Projection of diabetes burden through 2050: impact of changing demography and disease prevalence in the U.S. *Diabetes Care.* 24, 1936–1940, 2001. Available at: http://care.diabetesjournals.org/cgi/content/full/24/11/1936. Accessed: August 8, 2006.

4 Nutritional Epidemiology

Statistics are no substitute for judgment.

Henry Clay (1777–1852)

Nutritional epidemiology is defined as the study of the nutritional determinants of disease in human populations.[1] The function of nutritional epidemiology is to identify and study associations between diet and disease in defined populations. Although it originally focused on nutrient deficiency diseases, contemporary nutritional epidemiology concentrates on the study of heart disease, cancer, diabetes, osteoporosis, and neural tube defects (NTDs). These irreversible chronic conditions have multiple causes, long latency periods, occur with relatively low frequency (despite a substantial cumulative lifetime risk), and are associated with excessive as well as insufficient intake of nutrients and other food factors.[2] A major enterprise of nutritional epidemiology is to assess the efficacy of nutrition interventions, including nutrition education, and to develop diet assessment methods that enable public health officials and researchers to monitor dietary intake and other healthy-related behaviors of defined populations.

Epidemiological methods are widely applied in public health nutrition, and even practitioners who do not themselves carry out surveys will find that their public health practice is influenced by epidemiological observations. In this chapter we look at the types of studies used in nutritional epidemiology. Two landmark experimental studies in nutrition are included: Lind's (1747) experiment that demonstrated limes cure scurvy and Goldberger's (1914) experiments demonstrating that a diet containing animal products prevents and cures pellagra. We also examine some of the tools used to determine what people eat, including food frequency questionnaires and diet histories, and biochemical markers that indicate dietary intake.

4.1 STUDY DESIGNS IN NUTRITIONAL EPIDEMIOLOGY

Several types of research study designs are used in epidemiology. Their purposes are to (1) generate hypothesis, (2) describe relevant risk factors and health outcomes, or (3) study causal linkages between risk factors and diseases. The types of studies used in nutritional epidemiology include case studies and case series (what clinicians see), ecological studies (geographical comparisons), cross-sectional studies (survey, a "snapshot" in time), case-control studies (compare people with and without a disease), cohort studies (follow people over time to see who gets the disease), and randomized controlled trials (human experiments).

Study designs that help to generate hypotheses include case studies, case series, and ecological studies. Case studies are descriptions of individual cases of disease. Case series are descriptions of a series of similar cases of disease. Ecological studies are epidemiologic studies where risk factors and health outcomes are studied at population levels (hence, the data generated is in aggregates).

Cross-sectional surveys are "snapshots" of risk factors, health outcomes, and other relevant factors in a population.

4.1.1 USES OF DESCRIPTIVE STUDIES

- Provide data regarding the magnitude of disease load and types of disease problems in the community in terms of morbidity and mortality rates and ratios
- Provide clues to disease etiology, and help in the formulation of an etiological hypothesis
- Provide background data for planning, organizing, and evaluating preventive and curative services
- Contribute to research by describing variations in disease occurrence by time, place, and person

From the perspective of causal linkages, a weakness of these four types of studies is their lack of comparison groups. Although case studies and case series provide information about possible linkages, they cannot control for the effects of alternative explanations or confounding variables. However, cross-sectional surveys provide limited information about comparison groups at the time of data analysis.

Two common observational epidemiologic study designs used to examine causal linkages between risk factors and diseases are case-control studies and cohort studies.[3]

- In case-control studies, individuals with health outcomes (cases) are compared with individuals who have no evidence of health outcomes (controls). In this kind of study, effect sizes are calculated as ratios of likelihood (known as *odds ratios*) of exposure to the risk factors.
- In a cohort study, the investigator begins with two groups that are initially free of the health outcome. One of the groups is exposed to the risk factor of interest, whereas the other group is not. The incidences of health outcomes are followed prospectively. The incidence rates of the health outcomes are then compared among the exposed and nonexposed individuals. The effect size is expressed as the ratio (relative risk or rate ratio) of the incidence of disease among exposed vs. incidence of disease among nonexposed.

A case-control study is shorter and less expensive. It provides the possibility of studying different exposures for rare diseases. However, from the perspective of deriving causal inferences, it is less reliable than a cohort study because it cannot account for temporal sequence, and it is open to different types of biases. On the other hand, a cohort study, although a powerful design, is more expensive, and is open to problems of loss of study participants to follow-up. A cohort study is not suitable for studying diseases that take a long time to develop. However, given a set of exposures, multiple outcomes can be studied using a cohort study design. In nested case-control study designs, a case-control study is embedded ("nested") within a longitudinal prospective cohort study.

4.1.2 PROSPECTIVE VS. RETROSPECTIVE STUDIES

A prospective study watches for outcomes, such as the development of a disease, during the study period and relates this to other factors such as suspected risk or protection factor(s). The study usually involves taking a cohort of subjects and watching them over a long period. The outcome of interest should be common; otherwise, the number of outcomes observed will be too small to be statistically meaningful (indistinguishable from those that may have arisen by chance). All efforts should be made to avoid sources of bias such as the loss of individuals to follow-up during the study. Prospective studies usually have fewer potential sources of bias and confounding than retrospective studies. A retrospective study looks backwards and examines exposures to suspected risk or protection factors in relation to an outcome that is established at the start of the study. Most sources of error due to confounding and bias are more common in retrospective studies than in prospective studies.[4]

In the sections below, the strongest evidence comes from studies that are presented last.

4.1.3 CASE REPORTS AND CASE SERIES

These are simply descriptions of cases. They are useful because they may generate ideas for future epidemiologic investigations. Strongly suggestive anecdotal or clinical observations may indicate a possible causal relationship. Analytic epidemiology studies can then be designed to verify and quantify the risks, and to determine the role of confounding factors. Case reports or case series may be used to track toxicity reports of new foods or to document the beginning of an epidemic. A case series is of greater value than a case report because the series provides more documentation of evidence for the suggested hypothesis.[5]

Case reports are a type of descriptive epidemiology study frequently evaluated by the Center for Food Safety and Applied Nutrition (CFSAN). There are two principal avenues through which case reports come to CFSAN's attention — through reports published in the peer-reviewed medical literature and through reports captured in one or more of CFSAN's ongoing voluntary (also called "passive") adverse event monitoring systems, such as the Adverse Reaction Monitoring System (ARMS). ARMS collects spontaneous reports from consumers and health professionals regarding alleged adverse effects from food products. In addition, CFSAN receives adverse event reports linked to the products it regulates through FDA's MedWatch program.[6] As described in Box 4.1, the Food and Drug Administration (FDA) uses this reporting system to issue public health advisories regarding unsafe food and nutrition products.

4.1.4 ECOLOGICAL OR CORRELATIONAL STUDIES

Ecological studies examine the rate of disease of a population in a given geographical area based on average measures of exposure. In an ecological or correlational study, the unit of analysis is an aggregate of individuals, and information is collected on this group rather then on individual members. The association between a summary measure of disease and a summary measure of exposure is studied. Ecological studies are relatively quick and inexpensive. Because they often rely on data that have been routinely collected by government agencies for standard surveillance initiatives, ecological studies can provide a useful first look at relationships.

Box 4.1 Blue Discoloration and Death in Patients Receiving Enteral Feedings Tinted with FD&C Blue No. 1 Dye

In 2003 the FDA issued a public health advisory on the basis of several reports of toxicity, including death, temporally associated with the use of FD&C Blue No. 1 (Blue 1) in enteral feeding solutions. Blue 1 was administered in order to help in the detection and/or monitoring of pulmonary aspiration in patients being fed by an enteral feeding tube. Case reports received by the FDA indicated that seriously ill patients, particularly those with a likely increase in gut permeability (e.g., patients with sepsis), were manifesting blue discoloration of the skin, urine, feces, or serum and some developed serious complications such as refractory hypotension and metabolic acidosis. Because these events were reported voluntarily from a population of unknown size, it was not possible to establish the incidence of these episodes. Although the FDA was not at the time able to establish a cause-and-effect relationship between the reported serious and life-threatening patient outcomes and the use of the dye, nonetheless, given the seriousness of the potential complications, they notified health professionals of these case reports. The FDA continued to closely monitor reports of additional events, and they encouraged all health professionals to report any serious adverse events occurring with Blue 1-tinted enteral feedings to the FDA's MedWatch program at http://www.fda.gov/medwatch/.

Source: Food and Drug Administration. Center for Food Safety and Applied Nutrition. Reports of blue discoloration and death in patients receiving enteral feedings tinted with the dye, FD&C Blue No. 1. FDA Public Health Advisory. September 29, 2003. Available at: http://www.cfsan.fda.gov/~dms/col-ltr2.html. Accessed June 4, 2005.

Ecological and correlational studies do not examine the relationship between exposure and disease among individuals. They are useful for generating, rather than definitively testing, a scientific hypothesis. They may also be used for a preliminary evaluation of a new hypothesis to determine whether more extensive and expensive investigations are warranted.[7] Thus, the results of correlational studies would be insufficient to demonstrate a relationship without other types of data to support them.

4.1.4.1 Examples of Ecological Studies

As discussed by Willett in his *Nutritional Epidemiology* (1998),[8] ecological studies of migrant and other special populations have been widely used to differentiate between genetic and environmental determinants of neural tube defects (NTDs), whereas other ecological studies relate the intake of dietary factors to the incidence of coronary heart disease (CHD).

A genetic component in the etiology of NTDs had long been suspected because previously affected pregnancy and family history of an affected pregnancy are risk factors for subsequent NTDs. However, ecological studies demonstrated that rates of NTD varied by geographic area, in populations that migrate from areas of high to low incidence, among populations that are malnourished, and among populations that consume fortified cereals. Migration studies showed that groups that migrated from high-risk areas in Ireland to low-risk south of Britain and the U.S. manifest lower risks of a pregnancy with an NTD. An additional ecological study revealed, in retrospect, that an epidemic of NTDs appears to have occurred in Boston during the Great Depression. And finally, it was an ecological study that demonstrated the decline in the prevalence of NTDs after breakfast cereals in Dublin were fortified with folic acid and vitamin B_{12}.

Ancel Keys, M.D., was known worldwide for his landmark epidemiological seven countries study of Finland, Greece, Italy, Japan, the Netherlands, the U.S., and Yugoslavia, which demonstrated that the intake of saturated fat as a percentage of calories was strongly correlated with coronary death rates. His studies provided evidence that a diet rich in vegetables, fruits, and pasta and low in meat, eggs, and dairy products is associated with the reduced occurrence of CHD. In Keys' sample, the less industrialized countries manifested the low saturated fat intake and low incidence of CHD. In addition to differences in intake of saturated fat, the less- and more-industrialized countries also differed in terms of physical activity, obesity, and smoking. The percentage of energy from total fat had little relationship with CHD incidence or mortality, which led Willet as well as Keys to recommend a Mediterranean-style diet.[9]

Among men of Japanese ancestry, there is a gradient in CHD mortality increasing from Japan to Hawaii to California. A study of 11,900 Japanese men in Hiroshima and Nagasaki, Honolulu, and the San Francisco Bay Area of California was conducted to investigate this disease difference.[10] According to Willett,[11] when the investigators compared the saturated fat intake of Japanese men living in Japan, Hawaii, and California, the three populations were found to have saturated fat intakes as a percentage of calories of 7%, 23%, and 26%, respectively. With transition to the U.S., the men in the study manifested increases in mean serum cholesterol and weight (but not height) parallel to the observed changes in dietary saturated fat. Distributions of serum cholesterol, glucose, uric acid, and triglycerides were also examined. In every age group, the mean for each of the biochemical variables is lower for men in Japan than in Hawaii and California.[12] Examination of public health records indicated that age-adjusted CHD rates were consistently and significantly lower in Japan than in American Japanese.[13] This ecological study supports the hypothesis that an increased intake of saturated fat is associated with an increased risk of CHD.

4.1.4.2 Ecological Fallacy

A fallacy is an error in reasoning, usually based on mistaken assumptions. Researchers should be familiar with the fallacies they are susceptible to. Errors based on ecological studies occur when conclusions are drawn about individuals from data that are associated with groups. Relationships observed for groups necessarily hold for individuals. The ecological fallacy occurs when one makes conclusions about individuals based only on analyses of group data. For example, we know from ecological studies that a positive correlation exists between consumption of saturated fat and CHD across many nations. However it is not possible to infer that people with CHD actually had a high saturated fat intake. Thus, while we can conclude that saturated fat consumption is a risk factor for CHD, it would be an error of reasoning (an ecological fallacy) to further conclude that people with CHD actually had a high saturated fat consumption. Because ecological studies are not based on the actual exposure of individuals, they are less sophisticated than case-control and cohort studies, and results should be treated with caution.

4.1.5 Cross-Sectional or Prevalence Studies

Cross-sectional studies are those in which individuals are observed at a single point in time. These studies provide a snapshot of the health experience of a population at a given time. Such information can be very useful in assessing the health status and needs of a population. Some cross-sectional studies are surveys. Cabinet-level departments of the U.S. government conduct many important surveys. The Department of Agriculture and the Department of Health and Human Services oversee national food and nutrition surveys, some of which are discussed in Chapter 8. Whereas many of the surveys offer a representative overview of the health of the population, they cannot shed light on disease etiology.[14] Another cross-sectional survey that has a major impact on nutrition in public health is the diennial census, conducted by the Commerce Department's Census Bureau. Chapter 3 contains a discussion of the census.

Other cross-sectional studies include a biologic measurement of disease or of nutrient exposure. These studies provide information about disease prevalence and factors associated with that prevalence. Information is collected about dietary exposures for individuals so that in cross-sectional studies, unlike ecologic studies, it is known whether the individuals with the disease are those with the exposure. In other words, the presence or absence of disease and the presence or absence of suspected etiologic factors are determined in each member of the study population or in a representative sample at a particular time. An example is a study that linked calcium intake with blood pressure measurements in healthy populations. The calcium and blood pressure data indicated whether the individuals with higher blood pressure were those with lower intakes of calcium.[15]

The advantages of cross-sectional studies are that the people are contacted only once, so these studies are relatively inexpensive to conduct, and can be completed relatively quickly. But this also limits their usefulness. Cross-sectional studies reveal nothing about the temporal sequence of exposure and disease. It is not known whether the dietary exposure as measured is a consequence of the disease or a causal factor. In the calcium and blood pressure example, it is not known from cross-sectional data if individuals with higher blood pressure had altered their diets and their intake of calcium in response to a previous diagnosis of high blood pressure.[16] Also, cross-sectional studies can only measure disease prevalence, not incidence.[17]

4.1.6 Case-Control Studies

These retrospective studies look at the characteristics of one group of people who already have a certain health outcome (the cases) and compare them to a similar group of people who do not have the outcome (the controls). Such studies frequently include a biologic measurement of disease or of nutrient exposure. Case-control studies are designed to answer such questions as, "Do persons with osteoporosis (case subjects) consume diets that differ from those consumed by individuals without this disease (control subjects)?"

Whereas case-control studies can be done quickly and relatively inexpensively, they are less than ideal for studying diet because information is gathered from the past. People with illnesses often recall past behaviors differently from those without illness (known as *recall bias*), which subjects these studies to potential inaccuracies and bias. In addition, choosing appropriate controls is always biased unless they are a random sample of the population. Despite these challenges, carefully designed case-control studies can provide useful results.

The FDA, for example, often looks carefully at the results of case-control studies in the setting of outbreaks of foodborne disease to identify the food vehicle that was most likely responsible for transmitting the infectious agent. The results then can be used to help target specific food vehicles for microbiologic testing as a means of recovering the pathogen from the implicated food. In addition, results of case-control studies have been frequently used in safety evaluations at FDA, primarily to add further information to the overall assessment of safety.[18]

4.1.6.1 Examples of Case-Control Studies

A case-control study was carried out in Northern Ireland to compare dietary intake and biochemical indices of nutritional status in women following birth of a baby/termination of a pregnancy affected by NTDs and women with a normal baby. Dietary records and blood samples were obtained from 15 women who had been referred to the study following an affected pregnancy (subjects) and the same number of women whose pregnancy outcome was normal (controls). Although there was no statistically significant differences in nutrient intake between the two groups, but the subjects demonstrated a tendency for lower fruit and vegetable consumption compared to the controls. Blood tests revealed that levels of serum vitamin B_{12} were significantly lower in subjects, and activities of two of the nucleotide salvage pathway enzymes were significantly higher, findings that are consistent with other research on NTDs and the metabolism of folate and vitamin B_{12}. This early study suggested the need for a focus on vitamin status to prevent NTDs.[19]

Researchers conducted a case-control study of 462 confirmed pancreatic cancer cases and 4721 population-based controls to assess associations between specific and total carotenoid intakes and the risk of pancreatic cancer. Dietary intake was assessed by a self-administered FFQ. After adjustment for age, BMI, smoking, educational attainment, dietary folate, and total energy intake, lycopene, provided mainly by tomatoes, was associated with a 31% reduction in pancreatic cancer risk among men when comparing the highest and lowest quartiles of intake. Both beta-carotene and total carotenoids were associated with a significantly reduced risk among those who never smoked, suggesting that a diet rich in tomatoes and tomato-based products with high lycopene content may help reduce pancreatic cancer risk.[20]

Next to tobacco, saccharin may be the substance that has been most studied epidemiologically. Literally thousands of patients with bladder cancer have participated in case-control studies.[21] In 1972, the FDA removed saccharin from the list of Generally Recognized as Safe (GRAS) substances and issued an interim food additive regulation limiting the use of saccharin in foods. On the basis of subsequent studies demonstrating that saccharin caused bladder cancer in rats, Congress instituted product labeling requirements for saccharin-sweetened foods and beverages.

In 1977, the National Cancer Institute and the Food and Drug Administration conducted a case-control study to reveal the possible roles of the artificial sweeteners saccharin and cyclamate in human urinary bladder cancer. More than 500 hundred patients with confirmed bladder cancer and an equal number of matching controls participated. Questionnaires revealed no significant differences between subjects' and controls' previous intake of artificial sweeteners. As these findings persisted after simultaneous adjustment for the effects of smoking, occupation, age, diabetes mellitus, and a number of other potentially confounding factors, the researchers concluded that neither saccharin nor cyclamate is likely to be carcinogenic, at least at the moderate dietary ingestion levels reported by the patient sample.[22] The results of this study, together with findings of additional research with laboratory animals, convinced the FDA in December 2000 to remove the warning label that had been used on saccharin-sweetened foods since 1977 (Box 4.2).

4.1.7 Cohort Studies

Cohort or follow-up studies follow large groups of people over a long period of time. Researchers regularly gather information from the people in the study on a wide variety of variables, such as meat intake, physical activity level, and weight. Once a specified amount of time has elapsed, the

---

Box 4.2 Former Warning Label on Saccharin-Sweetened Foods and Beverages

"Use of this product may be hazardous to your health. This product contains saccharin, which has been determined to cause cancer in laboratory animals."

Source: National Institutes of Environmental Health Sciences. "Panel Recommends that Saccharin Remain on U.S. List of Carcinogens." October 31, 1997. Available at: http://www.nih.gov/news/pr/oct97/niehs-31.htm. Accessed February 11, 2007.

---

characteristics of people in the group are compared to test specific hypotheses, such as the link between carotenoids and glaucoma, or meat intake and prostate cancer.

Cohort studies generally provide more reliable information than case-control studies because they do not rely on information from the past. Cohort studies gather the information during a long duration of time, from before anyone develops the disease being studied. As a group, these types of studies have provided valuable information about the link between lifestyle factors and disease. Two of the largest and longest-running cohort studies of diet are the Harvard-based Nurses' Health Study (http://www.channing.harvard.edu/nhs/) and the Health Professionals' Follow-up Study (http://www.hsph.harvard.edu/hpfs/).

There are a number of disadvantages to prospective studies. They are time-consuming and expensive, because both large study populations and long periods of observation are required for definite results. Additionally, bias may be introduced in cohort studies if every member of the cohort is not followed. And, finally, the length of the study may be less than the latency period of the disease, e.g., if the study is stopped before old age, many important diseases such as cancer may be missed. Presented in Table 4.1 are the manor strengths and weaknesses of case-control vs. prospective cohort studies.

4.1.7.1 Retrospective Cohort Studies

A research study in which the medical records of groups of individuals who are alike in many ways but differ by a certain characteristic (for example, liveborn infants, stillbirths, and pregnancy terminations) are compared for a particular outcome (such as cases of NTDs). This type of investigation is also known as a *historic cohort study.*

The first recommendations about increasing intake of folic acid were made in 1992. In order to help reduce the incidence of NTDs in the U.S. in 1996 the FDA mandated that all breads and grains sold in the U.S. be fortified with folic acid by January 1998. However, other developed

---

TABLE 4.1
Strengths and Weaknesses of Case-Control vs. Prospective Cohort Studies

	Case-Control	Prospective Cohort
Strengths	Less expensive	More efficient for studying rare exposures
	Smaller number of people	Less bias in risk factor data
	Time to carry out study is shorter	May find associations with other diseases
	Suitable for rare diseases	Yields incidence rates as well as relative risk
Weaknesses	Incomplete information about past events	Large numbers of subjects required
	Biased recall of exposures may occur	Lengthy follow-up period
	Problems of selecting controls and matching variables	Attrition
	May yield only relative risk (odds ratio)	Changes in criteria and methods over time
		More expensive

countries (such as Norway, Finland, the Northern Netherlands, England and Wales, Ireland, France, Hungary, Italy, Portugal, and Israel) responded to the mounting mass education campaigns without fortifying the food supply. To evaluate the effectiveness of policies and recommendations on folic acid aimed at reducing the occurrence of NTDs, a retrospective cohort study was conducted of births monitored by birth defect registries in these countries. Researchers examined the incidences and trends in rates of NTDs before and after 1992 and before and after the year of local recommendations (when applicable). No detectable improvement in the incidence of NTDs was found. As recommendations alone did not seem to influence trends in NTDs up to six years after the confirmation of the effectiveness of folic acid in clinical trials, the researchers concluded that a reasonable strategy would be to quickly integrate food fortification with fuller implementation of recommendations on supplements, similar to the policy in the U.S.[23]

4.1.7.2 Prospective Cohort Studies

In prospective cohort studies, a population is assembled and then followed to see if those with the highest exposure to a particular factor develop particular conditions at a higher rate than those with lower exposure. Examples of this kind of study are the Framingham Study of cardiovascular disease, which began in 1948; the Nurses' Health Study I (NHS I), which has examined the effect of lifestyle factors on disease since 1976; the Health Professionals Follow-up Study; the Nurses' Health Study II (NHS II); and the Growing Up Today Study (GUTS), started in 1996, to follow children 9 to 14 years of age whose mothers participated in the NHS II.

Nutritional epidemiologic research at Harvard University primarily involves the investigation of dietary factors in the cause and prevention of cardiovascular disease, cancer, and other conditions. The development of methods to measure dietary intake in large populations has been fundamental to this work. A substantial effort has been devoted to the development, evaluation, and refinement of methods to measure various aspects of diet in the context of large epidemiologic studies. This has resulted in the development and validation of separate FFQs for women, men, and children. Although the FFQs developed for NHS II, HPFS, and GUTS have been demonstrated to provide reasonably accurate assessments of a wide spectrum of dietary factors, their validity has been questioned recently, as discussed in the section of this chapter that deals with biochemical indicators of dietary intake. Researchers at Harvard and elsewhere have been developing and evaluating biological markers of dietary intake, particularly using plasma and toenail samples, indicators that are primarily utilized in nested case-control studies using the large specimen banks collected prospectively as part of such ongoing studies as NHS II.

4.1.7.2.1 Framingham Study (1948–)

In 1948, the National Heart Institute (now the National Heart, Lung, and Blood Institute; NHLBI) established the longitudinal Framingham Heart Study to identify CVD risk factors (common factors or characteristics that contribute to a disease) by following its development in a large cohort who had not yet developed overt symptoms of CVD or suffered a heart attack or stroke. Since 1971, the study has been conducted under the aegis of Boston University. The original cohort consisted of 5209 men and women between the ages of 30 and 62 from the town of Framingham, Massachusetts. They began the first round of extensive physical examinations and lifestyle interviews that they would later analyze for common patterns related to CVD development. The original cohort consisted of respondents of a random sample of 2/3 of the adults, 30 to 62 years of age, residing in Framingham, Massachusetts, in 1948. (Approximately 20% of the original cohort was alive in 1998.) Since 1948, the subjects have continued to return to the study every 2 years for a detailed medical history, physical examination, and laboratory tests.

In 1971, the study enrolled a second-generation cohort of 5124 of the original cohort's adult children and their spouses to participate in similar examinations. The Offspring Study was initiated when the need for establishing a prospective epidemiologic study of young adults was recognized. As of 1998, there were approximately 4524 offspring surviving with only 20 lost to follow-up and 4 in whom survival status was unknown. The data collection forms for the examinations conducted in 1996–1998 and for the Offspring Study in 1995–1998 are available on the study's Web site http://www.nhlbi.nih.gov/about/framingham/index.html. A third generation (the children of the Offspring Cohort) of 3500 grandchildren of the original cohort is being recruited to further understand how genetic factors relate to cardiovascular disease. These participants are given an extensive cardiovascular examination similar to that of their parents and grandparents. Since its inception in 1949, more than 1300 published research articles have been produced by scientists working with data from the study. A bibliography (1950–2004) of these studies appears on the Web at http://www.nhlbi.nih.gov/about/framingham/biblio.htm. Highlights of some of the most significant diet-related milestones of the study are listed in Table 4.2.

4.1.7.2.2 Health Professionals Follow-Up Study (1986–)

The Health Professionals Follow-Up Study (HPFS) began in 1986 to evaluate a series of hypotheses about men's health relating nutritional factors to the incidence of serious illnesses, such as cancer, heart disease, and other vascular diseases. This all-male national longitudinal study was designed to complement the all-female NHS I and II, which examine similar hypotheses. In the beginning, a cohort of 51,529 men in health professions enlisted to participate in the study (58% dentists, 20% veterinarians, 8% pharmacists, 7% optometrists, 4% osteopathic physicians, and 3% podiatrists), 1% of whom are African American and 1.5% Asian American. (In other research, where ethnic background is a focus, the researchers over-sample ethnic groups in order to draw valid results.) The researchers selected health professionals in the belief that men who chose these types of careers would be motivated and committed to participating in a long-term project and would appreciate the necessity of answering the survey questions accurately. Every 2 years, study participants receive questionnaires with questions about diseases and health-related topics like smoking, physical activity, and medications taken. The questionnaires that contain FFQs are administered in 4-year intervals. Approximately 93% of the original cohort still participates. Since its inception, more than 100 published research articles have been produced by scientists working with data from the study.[24] Based on analysis of HPFS data to date:

TABLE 4.2
Some of the Most Significant Food- and Nutrition-Related Milestones in the Framingham Study

1960	Cigarette smoking found to increase the risk of heart disease.
1961	Cholesterol level and blood pressure found to increase the risk of heart disease.
1967	The risk of heart disease is found to be decreased by physical activity and increased by obesity.
1970	High blood pressure found to increase the risk of stroke.
1974	Overview of diabetes and its complications.
1976	Menopause found to increase the risk of heart disease.
1977	Effects of triglycerides and LDL and HDL cholesterol described.
1978	Psychosocial factors found to affect heart disease.
1987	High blood cholesterol levels found to correlate directly with risk of death in young men.
1988	High levels of HDL cholesterol found to reduce risk of death.
1990	Homocysteine identified as possible risk factor for heart disease.
1991	Heart disease risk prediction models produced.
1994	Lipoprotein (a) and apolipoprotein E found as possible risks factor for heart disease.
1996	Progression from hypertension to heart failure described.
1997	Report on the cumulative effects of smoking and high cholesterol on the risk for atherosclerosis.

Source: From Framingham Heart Study Research Milestones. Available at: http://www.nhlbi.nih. gov/about/framingham/timeline.htm. Accessed June 6, 2006.

- For every kilogram of weight gained, the risk of developing diabetes increased by 7.3%. Researchers prospectively examined the relations between changes in body weight and body fat distribution (1986–1996) and the subsequent risk of diabetes (1996–2000) among 22,171 men in the HPFS. A gain in abdominal fat was positively associated with risk, independent of the risk associated with weight change. Compared with men who had a stable waist, men who increased waist circumference by 14.6 cm or more had 1.7 times the risk of diabetes after controlling for weight gain. In contrast, men who lost more than 4.1 cm in hip girth had 1.5 times the risk of diabetes compared with men with stable hip circumference. In this cohort, 56% of the cases of diabetes could be attributed to weight gain greater than 7 kg, and 20% of the cases could be attributed to a gain in waist measurement exceeding 2.5 cm. The findings of this study highlight the importance of maintaining body weight and waist circumference to reduce the risk of diabetes.[25]
- Abdominal adiposity is associated with the incidence of symptomatic gallstone disease, and measures of abdominal adiposity, abdominal circumference, and waist-to-hip ratio predict the risk of developing gallstones independently of BMI. As part of the HPFS, men reported newly diagnosed symptomatic gallstone disease on questionnaires mailed to them every 2 years. The researchers prospectively studied measures of abdominal obesity in relation to the incidence of symptomatic gallstone disease in a cohort of 29,847 men who were free of prior gallstone disease and who provided complete data on waist and hip circumferences. Data on weight and height, and waist and hip circumferences were collected in 1986 and in 1987 through self-administered questionnaires. The researchers documented 1117 new cases of symptomatic gallstone disease. After adjustment for BMI and other risk factors for gallstones, men with a height-adjusted waist circumference >102.6 cm (40.4 in) had a relative risk (RR) of 2.29 compared with men with a height-adjusted waist circumference < 86.4 cm (34 in). Men with a waist-to-hip ratio > or = 0.99 had a RR of 1.78 compared with men with a waist-to-hip ratio < 0.89.[26]
- Low birth weight (LBW) is associated with an increased risk of hypertension and diabetes, and high birth weight (HBW) is associated with an increased risk of obesity, findings that support the hypothesis that early life exposures, for which birth weight is a marker, are associated with several chronic diseases in adulthood. The researchers examined the relation between birth weight (BW) and cumulative incidence of adult hypertension, incidence of noninsulin-dependent diabetes mellitus, and prevalence of obesity in a cohort of 22,846 men in the HPFS. BWs, medical histories, family histories, and other factors were collected by biennial mailed questionnaires. Compared with men in the referent birth weight category (7.0 to 8.4 lb), men who weighed < 5.5 lb had an age-adjusted odds ratio for hypertension of 1.26 and for diabetes mellitus of 1.75. Compared with men in the referent group, the age-adjusted odds ratio of being in the highest vs. the lowest quintile of adult BMI for men with BW > 10.0 lb was 2.08.[27]
- Data from the HPFS and NHS II do not support any overall association between coffee intake or alcohol intake and risk of pancreatic cancer. The researchers obtained data on coffee, alcohol, and other dietary factors using FFQs administered at baseline (1986 in the HPFS and 1980 in the NHS) and in subsequent follow-up questionnaires. Individuals with a history of cancer at study initiation were excluded from all of the analyses. During the study, 288 participants were diagnosed with pancreatic cancer. The data were analyzed separately for each cohort, and results were pooled to compute overall RR. Neither coffee nor alcohol intakes were associated with an increased risk of pancreatic cancer in either cohort or after pooling the results for > 3 cups of coffee/day vs. none, and for > or = 30 grams of alcohol/day vs. none. Similarly, no statistically significant associations were observed for intakes of tea, decaffeinated coffee, total caffeine, or alcoholic beverages.[28]

4.1.7.2.3   Nurses Health Studies (1976–)

The Nurses Health Studies are among the largest prospective investigations into the risk factors for major chronic diseases in women. Relations between diet, physical activity, weight gain, and risk of chronic diseases are studied. The first Nurses' Health Study (NHS I) was established by Dr. Frank Speizer in 1976 with funding from the National Institutes of Health (NIH). The original goals for the NHS I was to investigate the potential long-term consequences of the use of oral contraceptives in normal women. Registered nurses (RNs) were selected to be followed prospectively. It was anticipated that because of their nursing education, they would be able to respond with a high degree of accuracy to brief, technically-worded questionnaires and would be motivated to participate in a long-term study. Married RNs who were aged 30 to 55 in 1976, who lived in the 11 most populous states (California, Connecticut, Florida, Maryland, Massachusetts, Michigan, New Jersey, New York, Ohio, Pennsylvania, and Texas) and whose state nursing boards agreed to supply the study with their members' names and addresses were enrolled in the cohort if they responded to our baseline questionnaire. Approximately 121,700 RNs responded out of the 170,000 queried. Every 2 years cohort members receive a follow-up questionnaire with questions about diseases and health-related topics including smoking, hormone use, and menopausal status. Because it was recognized that diet and nutrition would play important roles in the development of chronic diseases, a first FFQ was collected in 1980, a second in 1984, and every 4 years thereafter. Dietary intake was measured by a FFQ (developed and validated by Willett and his colleagues at Harvard) that was administered in 1980, 1984, 1986, 1990, 1994, and 1998. Physical activity has been repeatedly assessed, and ongoing validation studies show it to be a valid measure. Quality of life (QOL) questions were added in 1992 and repeated every 4 years. Because certain aspects of diet cannot be measured by questionnaire, particularly minerals that become incorporated in food from the soil in which it is grown, the RNs submitted 68,000 sets of toenail samples between the 1982 and 1984 questionnaires. Similarly, to identify potential biomarkers, such as hormone levels and genetic markers, 33,000 blood samples were collected in 1989–1990 followed by second samples from 18,700 of these participants in 2000–2001. These samples are stored and used in case/control analyses. After 20 years of follow-up, more than 90% of participants in the NHS I responded to the 1998 follow-up questionnaire.

In 1989, with funding from the NIH, Walter Willett and his colleagues established the Nurses' Health Study II (NHS II) to study oral contraceptives and diet and lifestyle risk factors in a population younger than the NHS I cohort. The initial target population was women between the ages of 25 and 42 years in 1989; the upper age was to correspond with the lowest age group in the NHS I. A total of 116,686 women remained in the NHS II. Every 2 years, cohort members receive a follow-up questionnaire with questions about diseases and health-related topics including smoking, hormone use, pregnancy history, and menopausal status. In 1991, the FFQ was collected and subsequent FFQs are administered at four-year intervals. A two-page QOL supplement was included in the first mailing of the 1993 and 1997 questionnaires. Blood and urine samples from approximately 30,000 RNs were collected in the late 1990s. The response rates to NHS II questionnaires are at approximately 90% for each 2-year cycle. A newsletter detailing the progress of NHS I and NHS II is sent to each participant annually. http://www.channing.harvard.edu/nhs/history/index. shtml.

4.1.7.2.4   The Growing Up Today Study (1996–)

The Growing Up Today Study (GUTS) was established in 1996 to assess the predictors of dietary intake, activity, and weight gain during a 4-year period by recruiting children from 9 to 14 years of age of women participating in the Nurses' Health Study II (NHS II). Baseline questionnaires were mailed to the 13,261 girls and 13,504 boys whose mothers had granted consent to invite them to participate in GUTS. Approximately 68% of the girls and 58% of the boys returned completed questionnaires, thereby agreeing to participate in the cohort. The resulting cohort consisted of 6149 girls and 4620 boys who were 9 to 14 years old in 1996, residing through the country. All returned questionnaires in the fall of 1996 and again in 1997. Each child provided his or her current height and weight and a detailed assessment of typical past-year dietary intakes, physical activities, and recreational "inactivities" (TV, videos/VCR, and video/computer games). Because ongoing participation is crucial to the validity of cohort studies, no efforts were made to increase baseline enrollment from the nonresponders. Each child provided his or her current height and weight and a detailed assessment of typical past-year dietary intakes, physical activities, recreational "inactivities" (TV, videos/VCR, and video/computer games), and other behaviors and lifestyle patterns. Included was a validated FFQ designed specifically for children and adolescents. Follow-up questionnaires are sent annually for the duration of this national longitudinal study. The GUTS cohort is being followed from 2002 through 2007 to investigate determinants of binge eating, purging (i.e., use of vomiting or laxatives) and eating disorders of at least subsyndromal severity.[29]

Based on analyses of GUTS data through 2005:

- Infants who were fed breast milk more than infant formula, or who were breastfed for longer periods, had a lower risk of being overweight during older childhood and adolescence. In order to examine the extent to which overweight status among adolescents is associated with the type of infant feeding (breast milk vs. infant formula) and duration of breastfeeding, mothers of the children in the GUTS cohort were mailed a supplemental questionnaire in 1997. In the first 6 months of life, 9553 subjects (62%) were only or mostly fed breast milk, and 4744 (31%) were only or mostly fed infant formula. A total of 7186 subjects (48%) were breastfed for at least 7 months while 4613 (31%) were breastfed for 3 months or less. At ages 9 to 14 years, 404 girls (5%) and 635 boys (9%) were overweight.[30]
- Weight-related issues of parents are transmitted to their children, suggesting that peers, parents, and the media must be targeted for intervention to prevent children and adolescents from developing extreme concern with weight and unhealthy weight control behaviors.[31]
- For many adolescents, dieting to control weight is not only ineffective, but it may actually promote weight gain. Dieting to control weight, binge eating, and dietary intake were assessed annually from 1996 through 1998. In 1996, 25.0% of the girls and 13.8% of the boys were infrequent dieters and 4.5% of the girls and 2.2% of the boys were frequent dieters. Among the girls, the percentage of dieters increased over the following 2 years. During 3 years of follow-up, dieters gained more weight than nondieters. Among the girls, frequency of dieting was positively associated with increases in age; among the boys, both frequent and infrequent dieters gained 0.07 z scores of BMI more than nondieters. In addition, boys who engaged in binge eating gained significantly more weight than nondieters.[32]
- Although snack foods may have low nutritional value, they do not appear to be an important independent determinant of weight gain among children and adolescents.[33]
- Children who drank more than three servings a day of milk gained more in BMI than those who drank smaller amounts, but the added calories appeared responsible. Dietary calcium and skim and 1% milk were associated with weight gain, but dairy fat was not. The authors concluded that drinking large amounts of milk might provide excess energy to some children.[34]

4.1.8 META-ANALYSES

Meta-analyses are increasingly used to address the problem of the explosion of information in the scientific literature coupled with the pressure for timely, informed decisions in public health. A meta-analysis combines and analyzes the results of a (preferably) large number of previous reports to yield overall conclusions about a hypothesis. Unlike narrative scientific reviews of the literature, meta-analyses provide a quantitative synthesis of the available data. The technique is best used when examining studies addressing the same question and employing similar methods to measure relevant variables. Meta-analysis can be a valuable tool to aggregate relevant findings across studies and help to explain differences among studies. However, the strength of conclusions from meta-analyses can vary according to such factors as criteria for inclusion of studies, statistical methods used, and the type of studies being analyzed, i.e., observational vs. randomized clinical trials. Although meta-analysis restricted to RCTs is usually preferred to meta-analyses of observational studies, the number of published meta-analyses concerning observational studies in health has increased substantially.[35]

The role of meta-analyses for systematically combining the results of randomized clinical trials (RCT) to determine best practices in nutrition support has become routine.[36,37,38] However, meta-analyses are also conducted to study issues that determine nutrition practice in the community, such as examining the efficacy of school-based nutrition education,[39] determining the most effective means to promote breastfeeding[40] and weight management,[41] determining nutrition recommendations concerning fish consumption to decrease CHD mortality,[42] and so on.

Because of the inherent limitations of meta-analysis, it often serves not as primary evidence for a hypothesis but rather as a source of supporting evidence that can confirm the validity of data concerning a hypothesis, or may suggest avenues for new investigations. The results of a well-done meta-analysis may be accepted as a way to present the conclusions of disparate studies by using a common scale.[43] In order to conduct a meta-analysis, one must develop a research protocol that explains how the researcher will (1) identify criteria for the inclusion and exclusion of studies and avoid biases in this process, (2) decide whether the characteristics of study subjects, their interventions, and outcomes in each study are comparable, (3) use well-defined methods to extract data from the studies, (4) express the results of multiple studies in a consistent fashion, and (5) use statistical methods to assess the data.[44]

4.1.9 Controlled Trials

A controlled clinical trial is a human experiment in which people are assigned to receive one treatment or the other. This treatment is often a drug as clinical trials of drugs are required before being licensed for prescription. The treatment may also be a health intervention, such as a weight loss or smoking cessation program. Preferably the individual (and preferably also the health professional) are "blind" to which treatment a person receives, although this is not always possible. In clinical trials, the aim is to replicate the "real life" situation, so that the results obtained are as close as possible to what would happen if the treatment were used in the natural setting ("real life"). Clinical trials tend to be extremely expensive and are unsuitable for use in some situations. For example, it is not ethical to randomize people to heavy drinking in order to investigate the effects of alcohol. The "gold standard" of epidemiological studies is the *randomized controlled trial*. The superiority of the randomized controlled trial over designs is based on the fact that randomization controls are for unknown confounders.

4.1.9.1 Nonrandom Controlled Trials

We start our examination of controlled clinical trials by examining the nonrandom experiments of Lind (1716–1794) and Goldberger (1874–1929), whose studies represent seminal nutritional epidemiologic research.

4.1.9.1.1 Lind and Scurvy

The reputation of James Lind rests mainly on his conducting the first clinical trial in nutrition (1747), in which the potencies of a number of supposed antiscorbutic remedies were compared[45] (see Box 4.3). Lind took 6 pairs (n = 12) of scorbutic patients and provided each pair with 1 of 6 different standard treatments. The experiment demonstrated that citrus fruit was a more effective treatment for scurvy than the other therapies he administered.[46] As the patients receiving two of his six chosen interventions had such a dramatic recovery, he felt ethically obligated to end his trial and administer these treatments to all the remaining sailors.[47] Contemporary historians[48,49] claim that by the time Lind conducted his experiment, Woodall (1612) and Strother (1725), among others, had already established that fresh fruit prevented scurvy, but Lind's contribution was in recording the natural history of the disease and demonstrating through the use of controlled conditions of experimentation how scurvy might best be treated (and, indeed, prevented). The commendable features of Lind's experiment included his selecting participants who were similar at the beginning of the experiment (they were all scorbutic) and maintaining them throughout the experiment under the same general environmental and dietary conditions. The groups differed from each other only in respect to the type of treatment used. It remained for the antiscorbutic factor in (found in adrenal glands and plants) to be isolated and synthesized almost 200 years after Lind's experiments.

Box 4.3 In James Lind's Own Words, from His *Treatise on the Scurvy* (1753)

Clinical Description of Scurvy

"The first indication ... of this disease, is generally a change of colour in the face ... to a pale and bloated look ... Their ... aversion to motion degenerates soon into an universal lassitude, with a stiffness and feebleness of the knees upon using exercise with which they are apt to be much fatigued, and upon occasion subject to a breathlessness or panting. Their gums soon after become itchy, swell, and are apt to bleed upon the gentlest friction. Their breath is then offensive; and upon looking into their mouths, the gums appear of an unusual redness, are soft and spongy and ... putrid. They ... are prone to fall into haemorrhages from other parts of the body. Their skin at this time feels dry...and when examined, it is found covered with several reddish, bluish, or rather black and livid spots ... as it were a bruise ... Many have a swelling of their legs; which is first observed on their ancles [SIC] towards the evening, and hardly to be seen next morning; but ... it gradually advances up the leg, and the whole member becomes oedematous ... "

Description of Controlled Trial on the Treatment of Scurvy

"On the 20th of May 1747, I selected twelve patients in the scurvy, on board the Salisbury at sea. Their cases were as similar as I could have them. They all in general had putrid gums, the spots and lassitude, with weakness of the knees. They lay together in one place, being a proper apartment for the sick in the fore-hold; and had one diet common to all, viz. water gruel sweetened with sugar in the morning; fresh mutton-broth often times for dinner; at other times light puddings, boiled biscuit with sugar, etc., and for supper, barley and raisins, rice and currants, sago and wine or the like. Two were ordered each a quart of cyder a day. Two others took twenty-five drops of elixir vitriol three times a day ... Two others took two spoonfuls of vinegar three times a day...Two of the worst patients were put on a course of sea-water ... Two others had each two oranges and one lemon given them every day ... The two remaining patients, took ... an electary recommended by a hospital surgeon ... The consequence was, that the most sudden and visible good effects were perceived from the use of oranges and lemons; one of those who had taken them, being at the end of six days fit for duty ... The other was the best recovered of any in his condition; and ... was appointed to attend the rest of the sick. Next to the oranges, I thought the cyder had the best effects ..."

Source: From Dunn, P.M. James Lind (1716–94) of Edinburgh and the treatment of scurvy. *Arch Dis Child Fetal Neonatal Ed* 76,F64–F65, 1997. Available at: http://fn.bmjjournals.com/cgi/content/full/76/1/F64. Accessed June 9, 2005.

4.1.9.1.2 Vitamin C

In 1928 Hungarian-American biochemist Szent-Györgyi (1893–1986) isolated from the adrenal cortex, orange juice, and paprika (which was widely available in his native Hungary) a substance he named hexuronic acid. He subsequently sent large supplies of it to Paul Karrer (1889–1971) and Walter N. Haworth (1883–1950, the first British organic chemist) and his colleagues, who determined the structure of hexuronic acid and synthesized it in 1932. It was the first vitamin to be synthesized. Similarly, American biochemist Charles Glen King isolated vitamin C in 1931–1932 by studying the antiscorbic activities of guinea pigs with preparations from lemon juice. The chemical identity of King's active substance was almost identical to Szent-Györgyi's hexuronic acid. In the spring of 1932, first King and then 2 weeks later Szent-Györgyi's, published articles declaring that vitamin C and hexuronic acid were indeed the same compound. In 1937, Haworth shared the Nobel Prize in chemistry and Szent-Györgyi's received the Nobel Prize in Physiology or Medicine, in part, for their work on vitamin C. Controversy remains over whether King as well as Szent-Györgyi deserve equal credit for their work on the vitamin. King is not mentioned in the speech used to present Szent-Györgyi to the King of Sweden for the 1937 Nobel Prize in Physiology or Medicine.[50] King's research is referred to in Szent-Györgyi's Nobel Lecture (see Box 4.4), but he then goes on to intimate that King was not interested in collaborating.

4.1.9.1.3 Goldberger and Pellagra

Rarely encountered in the U.S. today, pellagra is defined by its classic triad of symptoms: dermatitis, diarrhea, and dementia (referred to as the three Ds of pellagra — a fourth D is death). In the beginning of the 20th century, pellagra was a leading cause of death in the southern U.S. Between 1900 and 1940, at least 100,000 individuals died of the disease. Women between the ages of 22 and 44 years, children between the ages of 2 and 10 years, and elderly people were the most frequent casualties. Most pellagrous patients were rural, poor, and lived in cotton mill villages; half of them were African American and more than two thirds were women. Also affected

---

Box 4.4 Excerpt from Szent-Györgyi's Nobel Lecture

… At the same time King and Waugh also reported crystals obtained from lemon juice, which were active antiscorbutically and resembled our hexuronic acid … Suddenly the long-ignored hexuronic acid moved into the limelight, and there was an urgent need for larger amounts of the substance, so that on the one hand its structural analysis could be continued and on the other its vitamin nature confirmed. However, in the course of our vitamin experiments we had used up the last remnants of our substance, and we had no chance of preparing the substance from adrenals, every other material was unsuitable for large-scale work … My town, Szeged, is the centre of the Hungarian paprika industry. Since this fruit travels badly, I had not had the chance of trying it earlier. The sight of this healthy fruit inspired me one evening with a last hope, and that same night investigation revealed that this fruit represented an unbelievably rich source of hexuronic acid, which, with Haworth, I re-baptized ascorbic acid. … It was still possible by making use of the paprika season, which was then drawing to a close, to produce more than half a kilogram, and the following year more than three kilogram of crystalline ascorbic acid. *I shared out this substance among all the investigators who wanted to work on it* [emphasis added]. I also had the privilege of providing my two prize-winning colleagues P. Karrer and W. N. Haworth with abundant material, and making its structural analysis possible for them.

Source: Szent-Györgyi, A. Oxidation, energy transfer, and vitamins. *Nobel Lecture,* December 11, 1937. Available at: http://nobelprize.org/medicine/laureates/1937/szent-gyorgyi-lecture.pdf. Accessed July 3, 2005.

Box 4.5 The Scientific Method

The scientific method consists of making observations, posing a question, formulating a hypothesis, testing the hypothesis, and drawing conclusions. Using the scientific method, Goldberger proved that pellagra is a noncommunicable disease caused by a faulty diet linked to the prevailing economic conditions in the South.

---

were thousands of institutional inmates. Pellagra was uncommon among children younger than 2 years of age, postpubertal adolescents, and active men.[51] The central figure in the U.S. government's efforts to combat this malady was Joseph Goldberger, M.D., a physician educated in New York City who specialized in infectious diseases. In 1914, the U.S. surgeon general appointed Goldberger to direct investigations into pellagra, which was widely considered to be an infectious disease and one that was becoming epidemic in orphanages, asylums, and mill towns. It seems reasonable to assume that he was selected for the project because of his expertise in infectious disease.[52]

Like the first cases of AIDS, pellagra was limited to populations towards whom there was public apathy, if not hostility. As the epidemic grew, concluding that pellagra was from malnutrition and poverty, rather than infection, would have forced acknowledging the existence of an underclass and taking steps to ameliorate their condition. Consequently, the investigation of the disease and introduction of preventive measures were impeded for years.

Following community observation that many of the afflicted people subsisted on a limited diet of pork fat, corn bread, and molasses, Goldberger challenged previous theories that pellagra was infectious, noting that it was more consistent with a dietary deficiency. To validate his hypothesis, Goldberger intervened in the diets of orphanages, asylums, and prisons both to cure and induce pellagra. Goldberger demonstrated that changing the diet — by including meat, dairy products, and legumes — decreased the incidence of pellagra. He also demonstrated that healthy volunteers could not be inoculated with the disease.

Goldberger conducted pellagra prevention experiments in two orphanages in Mississippi and a Georgia state sanitarium. Pellagra had been endemic in these institutions for several years. The diets at the three institutions were modified with a liberal intake of fresh animal foods and legumes beginning in the fall of 1914. By the following spring, there was only one case of recurrence among the 172 pellagrins from both the orphanages, and no new cases of pellagra occurred. In the Georgia sanitarium, after dietary modification there was no recurrence of pellagra among the 72 pellagrins, though the recurrence rate was 50% among controls. During the study period, the sanitary conditions of the orphanages and the asylum remained unchanged. With these studies, Goldberger was convinced that pellagra was a preventable dietary disease.[53]

In an experiment conducted at a state prison farm, he produced pellagra in convicts by feeding them a traditional, monotonous Southern diet. Goldberger persuaded authorities in Mississippi to allow 12 prisoners to volunteer to eat for 6 months an experimental diet that might induce pellagra. In return the prisoners would be released at the end of the experiment. The diet had abundant corn and other cereals but no meat or dairy products. (With hindsight we know that meat and dairy products can protect against pellagra because they supply the amino acid tryptophan, which is converted to niacin in the body.) After 5 months, 6 of the men had developed dermatitis on the scrotum and in a few cases, on the back of their hands. Goldberger was satisfied that this was pellagra, but the volunteers immediately fled after obtaining their release, and he could not demonstrate their condition to physicians who doubted whether he truly had produced the disease.[54]

Box 4.6 Goldberger's Observations

Goldberger observed that people who contracted pellagra subsisted on a limited diet of pork fat, corn bread, and molasses, whereas those who did not contract the disease had more varied diets. In the first experiment, he hypothesized that pellagra is caused by limited diets. His null hypothesis was that a restricted diet will not produce pellagra. Goldberger tested his hypothesis by feeding convicts the traditional, monotonous Southern diet, which produced pellagra. Thus, Goldberger concluded that pellagra is caused by eating a limited diet.

Upon observing that pellagra was contracted by prisoners (but not guards) and patients (but not nurses), Goldberger hypothesized that the disease is not contagious. His null hypothesis was that germs cause pellagra. To prove that pellagra was not infectious, Goldberger, his wife, and 14 associates ingested or were injected with urine, blood, skin scrapings, and feces from patients with pellagra. Pellagra did not develop in any of them, thus leading Goldberger to conclude that *pellagra is not a contagious disease.*[55] Table 4.3 summarizes Goldberger's use of the scientific method.

Next, Goldberger established the socioeconomic epidemiology of pellagra. Seven cotton mill villages in South Carolina were chosen. The entire population was screened for pellagra, and meticulous dietary data for all households were collected. Pellagrous households had restricted intake of animal protein. There was no association with consumption of corn or sanitary conditions to development of pellagra. Pellagrous households were all poor. The poverty and diet of those affected could be linked to cotton. Cotton was "king" among the cash crops: sharecroppers and tenant farmers cultivated cotton at the expense of other crops. Lack of diversification and the speculative nature of cotton prices during the Depression made the tenant farmer and the sharecropper vulnerable to poverty, poor diet, and pellagra. By now Goldberger concluded that pellagra was a socioeconomic malady, its occurrence in epidemic proportions in the South reflecting the extent of southern poverty. If poor diet resulting from poverty among Southern tenant farmers and mill workers was the root cause of pellagra, then the only real cure was social reform, especially changes in the land tenure system.[56]

TABLE 4.3
Goldberger's Use of the Scientific Method to Determine the Cause of Pellagra

Scientific Method	Pellagra Is Caused by Diet	Pellagra Is Not Infectious
Observation	Observed that people who contracted pellagra subsisted on a limited diet of pork fat, corn bread, and molasses, whereas those who did not contract the disease had more varied diets	Observed that prisoners contracted pellagra but not guards
Hypothesis	Hypothesized that pellagra is caused by limited diets. His null hypothesis was that a restricted diet will not produce pellagra	Hypothesized that the disease is not contagious. His null hypothesis was that germs cause pellagra
Test	Tested his hypothesis by feeding convicts the traditional, monotonous Southern diet, which produced pellagra	Tested his hypothesis by inoculating healthy volunteers with substances from pellagrins, which did not produce pellagra
Conclusion	Concluded that pellagra is caused by eating a limited diet	Concluded that pellagra is not contagious

4.1.9.2 Randomized, Nonblind Clinical Trial

The Multiple Risk Factor Intervention Trial (MRFIT) was a randomized, nonblind primary prevention trial, conducted at 22 U.S. clinical centers from 1973 to 1982 to test whether lowering elevated serum cholesterol and diastolic blood pressure and ceasing cigarette smoking would reduce coronary heart disease (CHD) mortality. From the 361,662 men 35–57 years of age who were screened, 12,866 volunteers were selected for the trial. All of the volunteers had one or more of three risk factors for CHD (elevated cholesterol, hypertension, cigarette smoking). Half of the participants were assigned to the special intervention group (SI) and half to the usual care (UC) group, and followed for 6–8 years. The SI group was advised to follow an eating pattern designed to result in a nutrient intake of 30–35% of calories from fat, with 10% (later 8%) from saturated and 10% from polyunsaturated fat, approximately 300 (later 250) mg of cholesterol, and modification of carbohydrates as needed for individual requirements. This group was also encouraged to cease cigarette smoking by a combination of techniques, including counseling and audiovisual aids. Hypertension management was based on a stepped-care program of weight reduction and medications. SI men had risk factor assessments every 4 months and annual examinations. Those in the UC group were referred to their personal physician or other source of care for such management of their risk factors as considered appropriate by these providers. Men in both groups returned for assessment of changes in risk factor levels annually for a medical history and physical examination. The primary endpoint was death due to CHD. An electrocardiogram was also obtained to identify nonfatal myocardial infarction as an additional endpoint.[57]

The 3 risk factors declined in both groups but the reductions were larger throughout the trial in the SI group, being significant at P < 0.01 at each annual visit. For example, after 6 years, 50% of SI men who were smokers had quit compared with 29% of the UC. Diastolic blood pressure fell in the two groups by 10.5 and 7.3, respectively. Plasma cholesterol fell in the two groups by 12.1 and 7.5 mg/dl, respectively, which primarily represented changes in low-density lipoprotein cholesterol (LDL-C) and not high-density lipoprotein cholesterol (HDL-C). The unexpected decline in cholesterol in the UC group and a smaller than predicted decline in the SI group meant that the SI-UC difference was about half of that expected. At the end of the follow-up period, the mortality rates were SI 41.2/1000 and UC 40.4/1000. The CHD death rates were 17.9 per 1000 in the SI group and 19.3 per 1000 in the UC group. Total mortality rates were 41.2 per 1,000 (SI) and 40.4 per 1,000 (UC). Neither death rates from CHD nor any other cause were reported as significantly different in the two groups. The researchers concluded that it is possible to apply an intensive long-term intervention program against three coronary risk factors with considerable success in terms of risk factor changes, but the overall results do not show a beneficial effect on CHD or total mortality from this multifactor intervention.[58]

Posttrial mortality surveillance of the 12,300 participants still living at the end of active intervention in 1982 continued through 1998. After 16 years, 370 SI and 417 UC men had died from CHD, which represents an 11.4% lower mortality rate for SI vs. UC men. Results for total mortality followed a similar pattern — 991 SI and 1050 UC men had died by the end of follow-up. Differences between SI and UC men in mortality rates from acute myocardial infarction, CHD, and all causes were greater during the posttrial follow-up period than during the trial. The researches conclude that these results demonstrate a long-term, continuing mortality benefit from the program.[59] Using the National Death Index, a mortality follow-up of the 361,662 men screened for the MRFIT was also continued thorough 1998.

4.1.9.3 Randomized Controlled Double-Blind Clinical Trials

Like cohort studies, these studies follow a group of people over time. However, with randomized trials, the researchers actually intervene to see how a specific behavior change or treatment, for example, affects a health outcome. They are called "randomized trials" because people in the study are randomly assigned either to receive or not receive the intervention. This randomization helps researchers hone in on the true effect the intervention has on the health outcome. However, randomized trials also have drawbacks, especially when it comes to diet. Although they are good at looking at topics like vitamin supplements and cancer, when the change in diet is more involved than taking a vitamin pill, participants begin to have trouble keeping to their prescribed diets. Such involved interventions can also become very expensive.

4.1.9.3.1 Neural Tube Defects

Czeizel and Dudas (1992) demonstrated that periconceptional vitamin use decreases the incidence of NTDs. They conducted a large (n = > 4000) randomized, controlled trial of women planning a pregnancy. Participants were randomly assigned to either the experimental group (vitamin supplement containing 12 vitamins, including 0.8 mg of folic acid; 4 minerals; and 3 trace elements) or the control group (trace-element supplement containing copper, manganese, zinc, and a very low dose of vitamin C daily). The trial was stopped early when six cases of NTDs were observed in infants born to women in the control group compared with no NTDs in the experimental group.[60]

4.2 DIETARY ASSESSMENT

The dietary assessment component of nutritional epidemiology focuses on the various approaches to collecting and analyzing dietary data. There are two functions of the dietary assessment component of nutritional epidemiology. The first is to determine the appropriateness of different assessment methods for specific applications, nutrients, and populations. The other is to determine what people eat.

How do we know what people eat? We can watch them, ask them, perform biochemical assays that indicate nutrient intake, or use a combination of these methods. As indicated in Table 4.4, each method has its strengths and weaknesses.

4.2.1 OBSERVATION

There are two methods used to determine what people eat by watching them. In the first method, a trained observer is assigned the task of estimating and recording everything eaten by up to several

---

TABLE 4.4
Strengths and Weaknesses of the Various Methodologies for Determining Food Intake

	Diet History	Dietary Recall	Food-Frequency Questionnaire	Food/Diet Record
Strengths	Does not alter usual diet Can provide data about eating habits	Quick and easy to administer Inexpensive Low respondent burden Does not alter usual diet	Quick and easy to administer Can be self-administered Inexpensive for large samples Machine-readable: low burden on researcher for analysis and data-entry Moderate respondent burden	Does not rely on memory Can provide data about eating habits Can provide detailed intake data
Weaknesses	Relies on respondent's memory High respondent burden High researcher burden Requires labor-intensive analysis data entry	Relies on memory Requires labor-intensive analysis data entry Frequent over- and underreporting Omissions of dressings and sauces can lead to low estimates of high-fat, sodium-rich foods	When self-administered, respondent must be literate Depends on ability of respondent to describe diet May not represent usual foods or portion sizes consumed by respondent	Requires high degree of cooperation Not appropriate for large surveys Requires labor-intensive analysis and data entry Act of recording may alter diet High respondent burden Respondent must be literate

Source: From Lee, R.D., Nieman, D.C. Measuring diet. *Nutritional Assessment*, 3rd ed. Boston, MA: McGraw-Hill, 2003, chap. 3.

people during a given meal. The second method is known as a plate waste study. The two most common types of plate waste studies are weighed and visual. In the weighed study, the amount of food consumed is calculated by subtracting the amount of food waste left after a meal from the amount of food served. Alternatively, the amount of waste can be visually estimated by subtracting the estimated plate waste from the weighed food served.[61] Using direct observation to determine what people eat is a laborious process that makes it impractical for working with large populations.

4.2.2 SELF-REPORT

Examples of surveys that provide information about an individual's dietary intake include 3- and 7-d diet records, 24-h recalls, and food frequency questionnaire (FFQ) checklists.

4.2.2.1 Diet Record (3-d, 7-d, etc.)

The diet record is a prospective tool that asks the individual to record everything he or she eats for a specified number of days. Diet records have been found to be superior to FFQs when estimating the amount of nitrogen (a marker for protein), potassium, and sodium consumed,[62] but the burden on the individual is high, making diet records impractical for large-scale studies. Additionally, food records require that subjects are literate and motivated. Nevertheless, the American Medical Association has posted a sample food diary and with instructions at http://familydoctor.org/299.xml.

4.2.2.2 24-H Recall

The USDA's 1994–1996 Continuing Survey of Food Intakes by Individuals (CSFII) uses 24-h dietary recalls to record food intake over 2 nonconsecutive days. Two sets of tables from ERS report food and nutrient intake and compare American's diets to recommendations of the Food Guide Pyramid and the 2000 *Dietary Guidelines for Americans*. Data is reported for Americans ages 2 and older, children ages 2–18, and seniors ages 60 and older. Average consumption/intake and the proportion of consumers meeting the recommendation are reported. Also reported is consumption/intake by location, from which dietary deficiencies can be linked to locations where foods are prepared. The ERS food consumption and nutrient intake tables are available at http://www.ers.usda.gov/briefing/DietAndHealth/data/.

4.2.2.3 Food Frequency Questionnaires and Checklists

A FFQ is a common method used to assess individual long-term dietary intake of foods and nutrients. FFQs are retrospective tools used to determine estimates of usual dietary intakes over time (typically 6 months to a year) of individuals belonging to groups. The questionnaires elicit a subjectively reported "usual frequency" of consuming an item from a list of foods. The FFQ lists specific foods and asks the subjects they eat them and if so, how often and how much. FFQs must be culture-specific, with different lists of foods appropriate for assessing diverse diets. Both short (60 food items) and long (100 food items) FFQs have been developed, but none assess current energy intake. Modified FFQs were designed for identification of people with high intake of dietary fat and/or low intakes of fiber, fruits, and vegetables. Some of these questionnaires were developed to identify potential candidates for enrollment into intervention research studies.[63] FFQs are often used in large cohort studies to place individuals into broad categories along a distribution of nutrient intake.

As the process required to develop an FFQ is laborious, time consuming, and costly, the development of FFQs usually require a major national effort or coordinated task force. Subsequently, FFQs are validated using serial 24-h recalls, food records or biomarkers as the gold standard. Three different versions of the FFQ have been developed at Harvard University. The original semiquantitative FFQ was created to be used as a self-administered, mailed questionnaire in the NHS. Questionnaires have also been developed for elderly[64] and youth/adolescent[65] populations.

4.2.3 BIOMARKERS

Asking people about their food intake results in self-reports that may be less than accurate. One way to verify self-reports is by the use of biomarkers. Biomarkers are external indicators that reflect food intake by measuring metabolites in urine and serum. Biomarkers have been identified to verify self-reported intake of protein, fatty acids, and fruits and vegetables, and of energy.[66] Doubly-labeled water (DLW) is currently the most widely-used and well-accepted biomarker. It provides an accurate measure in free-living subjects of their total energy expenditure and hence energy requirements, which is frequently underreported. The use of DLW is based on the principle of energy balance, i.e., if a person is weight-stable, then their energy expenditure, as measured by DLW, must be equal to their energy intake. Because of the high cost and sophisticated technology associated with DLW, it does not lend itself to routine use in clinical settings, but it is used for validating energy intakes obtained from other dietary intake methods.[67]

4.2.4 IMPROVING DIET AND PHYSICAL ACTIVITY ASSESSMENT MODALITIES

Diet and physical activity are lifestyle and behavioral factors that play a role in the etiology and prevention of many chronic diseases such as cancer and coronary heart disease. Both also play roles in preventing overweight/obesity and in maintaining weight loss. Therefore, diet and physical activity are assessed for both surveillance and epidemiologic/clinical research purposes. The measurement of usual dietary intake or physical activity over varying time periods or in the past, by necessity, has relied on self-report instruments. Such subjective reporting instruments are cognitively difficult for respondents, and are prone to considerable measurement errors that may vary among population subgroups and depend on the time frame considered and the characteristics of the respondents. As such, the National Cancer Institute (NCI), National Heart, Lung, and Blood Institute (NHLBI), National Institute on Aging (NIA), National Institute of Child Health and Human Development (NICHD), National Institute of Diabetes and Digestive and Kidney Diseases (NIDDK), National Institute of Mental Health (NIMH), National Institute of Nursing Research (NINR), and National Institutes of Health (NIH) Office of the Director (OD) Office of Diary Supplements (ODS) are interested in promoting innovative research to enhance the quality of measurements of dietary intake and physical activity. Therefore, through at least 2009 the NIH will accept proposals for the development of (1) novel assessment approaches; (2) better methods to evaluate instruments, (3) assessment tools for culturally diverse populations, (4) assessment methods to be used across various age groups including older adults, improved technology or applications of existing technology, and (5) statistical methods to assess or correct for measurement errors or biases.[68]

4.3 TECHNICAL SUPPORT

Various government agencies provide support for research that uses techniques in nutritional epidemiology (see Box 4.7).

- The Nutritional Epidemiology Program at the National Institute for Digestive Diseases and Kidney Disease (NIDDK) serves as a focus for the collection, analysis, ands dissemination of data on nutritional disorders and obesity.[69]
- The Nutritional Epidemiology Branch of the National Cancer Institute (NCI) develops and validates methods for nutritional epidemiology, including questionnaires, biologic measures, and analytic approaches, and develops national nutrition data resources, such as the Diet History Questionnaire (DHQ). The DHQ is a FFQ that consists of 124 food items and includes both portion size and dietary supplement questions. It takes about an hour to complete and was designed to be easy to use.[70]
- The Nutritional Epidemiology core at the University of North Carolina's NIH-funded Clinical Research Center provides research support to projects of young investigators.[71]

Box 4.7 Technical Support for Research Using Techniques in Nutritional Epidemiology

The Nutrition Epidemiology Program in the National Institute for Digestive Diseases and Kidney Disease (NIDDKD)[1] serves as a focus for the collection, analysis, and dissemination of data on nutritional disorders and obesity. The program:

- Identifies the data needed to address the scientific and public health issues in nutritional disorders and obesity
- Addresses the epidemiology of nutritional disorders of public health significance, with particular emphasis on national surveys and their follow-up.
- Promotes the timely availability of reliable data to pertinent scientific, medical, and public organizations
- Promotes the standardization of data collection and terminology in clinical and epidemiological research
- Collaborates with members of the scientific community to develop investigator-initiated research in the epidemiology of nutritional disorders and obesity. The program encourages research that addresses risk factors for disease occurrence and disease prognosis or natural history
- Supports databases and biological repositories that support clinical and epidemiological studies in nutritional disorders and obesity

The Nutritional Epidemiology Branch at the National Cancer Institute (NCI)[2] has several functions. The group:

- Assesses in human populations specific etiologic hypotheses concerning the relationships of diet, nutrition, and cancer that have been suggested by laboratory, epidemiologic, and clinical studies
- Tests for associations between dietary factors, hormones, and specific cancers, and generates hypotheses about the nature of relationships detected
- Develops and validates methods for nutritional epidemiology, including questionnaires, biologic measures, and analytic approaches
- Develops and utilizes national nutrition data resources
- Elucidates the basic biology of carcinogenesis through epidemiologic and multidisciplinary studies into nutritional determinants of cancer
- Collaborates with laboratory scientists to incorporate biologic measures into epidemiologic research designs to clarify dietary, nutritional, and related mechanisms of carcinogenesis. http://www3.cancer.gov/oma/hnc9c4.htm Cf also http://dceg.cancer.gov/nutri-overview.html

The Nutritional Epidemiology core at the University of North Carolina's Clinical Nutrition Research Center in the School of Pubic Health and the School of Medicine[3] provides research support for its center investigators and affiliated faculty through the following services:

- Grant development: choice of dietary assessment tools and write-up, choice of biomarkers and write-up, doubly-labeled water, carotenoids, tocopherols, Vitamin C, folic acid, fatty acids
- Database development: preparation of new nutrient/nonnutrient database, glycemic index, tocopherols, protease inhibitors, carotenoids
- Multimedia support: digital food photography, digital food library, audio recording, digital photography of baby and toddler foods for portion size

- Training in use of dietary assessment tools: Nutrition Data System (NDS), computerized nutrient analysis, Computer Assisted Self Interview (CASI) diet history, food frequency questionnaire (FFQ), 24-h recall, multiday records
- Software access: NDS, CASI, SIDE (for intake distribution estimation)
- Analysis: Nutrition Data System (NDS), CASI diet history interview, FFQ, 24-h recall, multiday records

Sources:

[1]U.S. Department of Health and Human Services. National Institutes of Health. National Institute of Diabetes and Digestive and Kidney Diseases. Programs Descriptions M-R. Nutritional Epidemiology http://www.niddk.nih.gov/fund/program/M-Rlist.htm#nutritionalepid. Accessed December 7, 2004.

[2]U.S. Department of Health and Human Services. National Institutes of Health. National Cancer Institute. Nutritional Epidemiology Branch homepage. Available at http://dceg.cancer.gov/nutri.html. Accessed December 7, 2004.

[3]University of North Carolina. Clinical Nutrition Research Center. Nutritional Epidemiology homepage. Available at http://www.cnrc.unc.edu/core_b.htm. Accessed December 5, 2004.

4.4 CONCLUSION

Nutritional epidemiology is fundamental to the practice of public health nutrition. Through the keen observational skills of its practitioners, numerous advances in public health have been made — from an appreciation of a clean water supply to an understanding of the relationship between food and nutrition, as in Lind's and Goldberger's studies. The history and development of epidemiology as a science is an engaging narrative and a continually evolving story, moving from an initial focus on deficiency diseases to our current spotlight on chronic diseases such as heart disease and diabetes.

Although the gold standard of research is often the randomized, controlled trial, other study designs are both possible and desirable. Longitudinal prospective studies, for example, though costly and cumbersome, are a powerful tool in the study of the effects of diet on health as these effects take years to manifest themselves. As technology continues to evolve and expand, it will prove a useful adjunct to the pursuit of nutritional epidemiology and our understanding of nutrition and health.

4.5 ACRONYMS

ARMS	Adverse Reaction Monitoring System
BMI	Body Mass Index
BW	Birth weight
CFSAN	Center for Food Safety and Applied Nutrition
CHD	Coronary heart disease
CSFII	Continuing Survey of Food Intake by Individuals
CVD	Cardiovascular disease
DHQ	Diet history questionnaire
DLW	Doubly-labeled water
ERS	Economic Research Service
FDA	Food and Drug Administration
FFQ	Food Frequency Questionnaire
GUTS	Growing Up Today Study
HDL-C	High-density lipoprotein cholesterol
HPFS	Health Professionals Follow Up Study
LBW	Low birth weight
LDL-C	Low-density lipoprotein cholesterol
MRFIT	Multiple Risk Factor Intervention Trial
NHLBI	National Heart, Lung, and Blood Institute
NHS I and II	Nurses Health Study I or II
NICHD	National Institute of Child Health and Human Development

NIDDK	National Institute for Diabetes and Digestive and Kidney Diseases
NIH	National Institutes of Health
NIMH	National Institute of Mental Health
NINR	National Institute of Nursing Research
NTDs	Neural Tube Defects
ODS	Office of Dietary Supplements
QOL	Quality of life
RR	Relative risk
SI	Special Intervention
UC	Usual care

REFERENCES

1. Langseth, L. *Nutritional Epidemiology: Possibilities and Limitations*. Brussels, Belgium: International Life Sciences Institute, 1996. Available at: http://europe.ilsi.org/file/Ilsiepid.pdf. Accessed June 13, 2005.
2. Willett, W. Overview of Nutritional Epidemiology. In *Nutritional Epidemiology*, 2nd ed. New York: Oxford University Press, 1998, chap. 1.
3. Kelsey, J.L., Whittemore, A.S., Evans, A.S., and Thompson, W.D. *Methods in Observational Epidemiology*, 2nd ed. New York: Oxford University Press, 1996.
4. FDA. Office of Food Additive Safety. *Redbook 2000. Technological Principles for the Safety Assessment of Food Ingredients*. July 2000. Updated October 2001, November 2003, and April 2004. Chapter VI.B: Epidemiology (October 2001). Available at: http://www.cfsan.fda.gov/~redbook/red-toca.html. Accessed June 6, 2005.
5. Sherry, B., Archer, S., and Van Horn, L. Descriptive epidemiologic research. In Monsen, E.R., Ed. *Research: Successful Approaches*, 2nd ed. Chicago, IL: American Dietetic Association, 2003, chap. 8.
6. FDA. Office of Food Additive Safety. *Redbook 2000. Technological Principles for the Safety Assessment of Food Ingredients*. July 2000. Updated October 2001, November 2003, and April 2004. Chapter VI.B: Epidemiology (October 2001). Available at: http://www.cfsan.fda.gov/~redbook/red-toca.html. Accessed June 6, 2005.
7. Langseth, L. *Nutritional Epidemiology: Possibilities and Limitations*. Brussels, Belgium: International Life Sciences Institute Europe, 1996. Available at: http://europe.ilsi.org/file/Ilsiepid.pdf. Accessed June 5, 2005.
8. Willett, W. Folic acid and neural tube defects. In *Nutritional Epidemiology*, 2nd ed. New York: Oxford University Press, 1998, chap. 18.
9. Willett, W.C. *Eat, Drink, and Be Healthy*. New York: Simon and Schuster Source, 2001.
10. Syme, S.L., Marmot, M.G., Kagan, A., Kato, H., and Rhoads, G. Epidemiologic studies of coronary heart disease and stroke in Japanese men living in Japan, Hawaii and California: introduction. *Am J Epidemiol*. 102, 477–480, December, 1975.
11. Willett, W. Diet and coronary heart disease. In *Nutritional Epidemiology*, 2nd ed. New York: Oxford University Press, 1998, chap. 17.
12. Nichaman, M.Z., Hamilton, H.B., Kagan, A., Grier, T., Sacks, T., and Syme, S.L. Epidemiologic studies of coronary heart disease and stroke in Japanese men living in Japan, Hawaii and California: distribution of biochemical risk factors. *Am J Epidemiol*. 102, 491–501, 1975.
13. Worth, R.M., Kato, H., Rhoads, G.G., Kagan, K., and Syme, S.L. Epidemiologic studies of coronary heart disease and stroke in Japanese men living in Japan, Hawaii and California: mortality. *Am J Epidemiol*. 102, 481–490, 1975.
14. Sherry, B., Archer, S., and Van Horn, L. Descriptive epidemiology research. In Monsen, E., Ed. *Research: Successful Approaches*, 2nd ed. Chicago, IL: American Dietetic Association, 2003, chap. 8.
15. Hamet, P. The evaluation of the scientific evidence for a relationship between calcium and hypertension. *J Nutr*. 125, 311S–400S, 1995.
16. Freidenheim, J.L. Study design and hypothesis testing: issues in the evaluation of evidence from research in nutritional epidemiology. *Am J Clin Nutr*. 69, 1315S–1321S, 1999.
17. FDA. Office of Food Additive Safety. *Redbook 2000. Technological Principles for the Safety Assessment of Food Ingredients*. July 2000. Updated October 2001, November 2003, and April 2004. Chapter VI.B: Epidemiology (October 2001). Available at: http://www.cfsan.fda.gov/~redbook/red-toca.html. Accessed June 6, 2005.

18. FDA. Office of Food Additive Safety. *Redbook 2000. Technological Principles for the Safety Assessment of Food Ingredients.* July 2000. Updated October 2001, November 2003, and April 2004. Chapter VI.B: Epidemiology (October 2001). Available at: http://www.cfsan.fda.gov/~redbook/red-toca.html. Accessed June 6, 2005.

19. Wright, M.E. A case-control study of maternal nutrition and neural tube defects in Northern Ireland. *Midwifery.* 11, 146–152, 1995.

20. Nkondjock, A., Ghadirian, P., Johnson, K.C., and Krewski, D. Canadian cancer registries epidemiology research group: dietary intake of lycopene is associated with reduced pancreatic cancer risk. *J Nutr.* 135, 592–597, 2005.

21. Morgan, R.W. and Wong, O. A review of epidemiological studies on artificial sweeteners and bladder cancer. *Food Chem Toxicol.* 23, 529–533, 1985.

22. Kessler, I.I. and Clark, J.P. Saccharin, cyclamate, and human bladder cancer: no evidence of an association. *JAMA.* 240, 349–355, 1978.

23. Botto, L.D., Lisi, A., Robert-Gnansia, E., et al. International retrospective cohort study of neural tube defects in relation to folic acid recommendations: are the recommendations working? *BMJ.* 330, 571, 2005. Epub 2005 February 18.

24. President and Fellows of Harvard College. School of Public Health. Health Professionals Follow-Up Study. About the Health Professionals Follow-Up Study. Available at: http://www.hsph.harvard.edu/hpfs/ Accessed December 19, 2004.

25. Koh-Banerjee, P., Wang, Y., Hu, F.B., Spiegelman, D., Willett, W.C., and Rimm, E.B. Changes in body weight and body fat distribution as risk factors for clinical diabetes in U.S. men. *Am J Epidemiol.* 159, 1150–1159, 2004.

26. Tsai, C.J., Leitzmann, M.F., Willett, W.C., and Giovannucci, E.L. Prospective study of abdominal adiposity and gallstone disease in U.S. men. *Am J Clin Nutr.* 80, 38–44, 2004.

27. Curhan, G.C., Willett, W.C., Rimm, E.B., Spiegelman, D., Ascherio, A.L., and Stampfer, M.J. Birth weight and adult hypertension, diabetes mellitus, and obesity in U.S. men. *Circulation.* 94, 3246–3250, 1996.

28. Michaud, D.S., Giovannucci, E., Willett, W.C., Colditz, G.A., and Fuchs, C.S. Coffee and alcohol consumption and the risk of pancreatic cancer in two prospective United States cohorts. *Cancer Epidemiol Biomarkers Prev.* 10, 429–437, 2001.

29. Activity, dietary intake, and weight changes in a longitudinal study of preadolescent and adolescent boys and girls. *Pediatrics.* 105(4), e56, April, 2000.

30. Gillman, M.W., Rifas-Shiman, S.L., Camargo, C.A. Jr., et al. Risk of overweight among adolescents who were breastfed as infants. *JAMA.* 285, 2461–2467, 2001.

31. Field, A.E., Camargo, C.C., Jr., Taylor, C.B., Berkey, C.S., Roberts, S.B., and Colditz, G.A. Peer, parent, and media influences on the development of weight concerns and frequent dieting among preadolescent and adolescent girls and boys. *Pediatrics.* 107, 54–60, 2001.

32. Field, A.E., Austin, S.B., Taylor, C.B., et al. Relation between dieting and weight change among preadolescents and adolescents. *Pediatrics.* 112, 900–906, 2003.

33. Field, A.E., Austin, S.B., Gillman, M.W., Rosner, B., Rockett, H.R., and Colditz, G.A. Snack food intake does not predict weight change among children and adolescents. *Int J Obes Relat Metab Disord.* 28, 1210–1216, 2004.

34. Berkey, C.S., Rockett, H.R.H., Willett, W.C., and Colditz, G.A. Milk, dairy fat, dietary calcium, and weight gain: a longitudinal study of adolescents. *Arch Pediatr Adolesc Med.* 159, 543–550, 2005. Available at: http://archpedi.ama-assn.org/cgi/content/full/159/6/543. Accessed June 8, 2005.

35. Stroup, D.F., Berlin, J.A., Morton, S.C., et al. Meta-analysis of observational studies in epidemiology: a proposal for reporting. Meta-analysis of Observational Studies in Epidemiology (MOOSE) group. *JAMA.* 283, 2008–2012, 2000.

36. Willett, W. Issues in analysis and presentation of dietary data. In *Nutritional Epidemiology,* 2nd ed. New York: Oxford University Press, 1998, chap. 13.

37. Brown, L. and Dattilo, A. Meta-analysis in nutrition research. In Monsen, E., Ed. *Research: Successful Approaches.* Chicago, IL: American Dietetic Association, 2003, chap. 11.

38. Tolley, E.A. and Headley, A.S. Meta-analyses: what they can and cannot tell us about clinical research. *Curr Opin Clin Nutr Metab Care.* 8, 177–181, 2005.

39. McArthur, D.B. Heart healthy eating behaviors of children following a school-based intervention: a meta-analysis. *Issues Compr Pediatr Nurs.* 21, 35–48, 1998.

40. Guise, J.M., Palda, V., Westhoff, C., Chan, B.K., Helfand, M., and Lieu, T.A. U.S. Preventive Services Task Force. The effectiveness of primary care-based interventions to promote breastfeeding: systematic evidence review and meta-analysis for the U.S. Preventive Services Task Force. *Ann Fam Med.* 1, 70–78, 2003. Available at: http://www.annfammed.org/cgi/content/full/1/2/70. Accessed June 9, 2005.

41. Mullen, P.D., Simons-Morton, D.G., Ramirez, G., Frankowski, R.F., Green, L.W., and Mains, D.A. A meta-analysis of trials evaluating patient education and counseling for three groups of preventive health behaviors. *Patient Educ Couns.* 32, 157–173, 1997.

42. He, K., Song, Y., Daviglus, M.L., Liu, K., Van Horn, L., Dyer, A.R., and Greenland, P. Accumulated evidence on fish consumption and coronary heart disease mortality: a meta-analysis of cohort studies. *Circulation.* 109, 2705–2711, 2004. Available at: http://circ.ahajournals.org/cgi/content/full/109/22/2705. Accessed June 9, 2005.

43. FDA. Office of Food Additive Safety. *Redbook 2000. Technological Principles for the Safety Assessment of Food Ingredients.* July 2000. Updated October 2001, November 2003, and April 2004. Chapter VI.B: Epidemiology (October 2001). Available at: http://www.cfsan.fda.gov/~redbook/red-toca.html. Accessed June 6, 2005.

44. FDA. Office of Food Additive Safety. *Redbook 2000. Technological Principles for the Safety Assessment of Food Ingredients.* July 2000. Updated October 2001, November 2003, and April 2004. Chapter VI.B: Epidemiology (October 2001). Available at: http://www.cfsan.fda.gov/~redbook/red-toca.html. Accessed June 6, 2005.

45. Hughes, R.E. James Lind and the cure of scurvy: an experimental approach. *Med Hist.* 19, 342–351, 1975. Available at: http://www.pubmedcentral.nih.gov/articlerender.fcgi?tool=pubmed&pubmedid=1102818. Accessed June 9, 2005.

46. Brown, S.R. *Scurvy: How a Surgeon, a Mariner, and a Gentleman Solved the Greatest Medical Mystery of the Age of Sail.* New York: Thomas Dunne Books (St. Martin's Press), 2003.

47. Doig, G.S. Interpreting and using clinical trials. *Crit Care Clin.* 14, 513–524, 1998.

48. Hughes, R.E. James Lind and the cure of scurvy: an experimental approach. *Med Hist.* 19, 342–351, 1975. Available at: http://www.pubmedcentral.nih.gov/articlerender.fcgi?tool=pubmed&pubmedid= 1102818. Accessed June 9, 2005.

49. Bartholomew, M. James Lind and scurvy: a revaluation. *J Marit Res.* January 2002. Serial online. Available at: http://www.jmr.nmm.ac.uk/server/show/conJmrArticle.3. Accessed May 8, 2005.

50. Hammarsten, E. The 1937 Nobel Prize in Physiology or Medicine Presentation Speech. December 10, 1937. Available at: http://nobelprize.org/medicine/laureates/1937/press.html. Accessed July 3, 2005.

51. Marks, H.M. Epidemiologists explain pellagra: gender, race, and political economy in the work of Edgar Sydenstricker. *J Hist Med Allied Sci.* 58, 34–55, 2003.

52. Klevay, L.M. And so spake Goldberger in 1916: pellagra is not infectious! *J Am Coll Nutr.* 16, 290–292, June, 1997.

53. Rajakumar, K. Pellagra in the United States: a historical perspective. *Southern Med J.* 93, 272–277, 2000. Available at http://www.medscape.com/viewarticle/410505_1. Accessed December 7, 2004.

54. Cooper, K.J. A short history of nutritional science: part 3 (1912–1944). Pellagra in the United States. *J Nutr.* 133, 3023–3032, 2003. Available online http://www.nutrition.org/cgi/content/full/133/10/3023?maxtoshow=&HITS=10&hits=10&RESULTFORMAT=&fulltext=pellagra&searchid=11. Accessed December 6, 2004.

55. Kraut, A.M. *Goldberger's War: The Life and Work of a Public Health Crusader.* New York: Hill and Wang, 2003.

56. Rajakumar, K. Pellagra in the United States: a historical perspective. *Southern Med J.* 93, 272–277, 2000. Available at http://www.medscape.com/viewarticle/410505_1. Accessed December 7, 2004.

57. Kjelsberg, M.O., Cutler, J.A., and Dolecek, T.A. Brief description of the multiple risk factor intervention trial. *Am J Clin Nutr.* 65, 191S–195S, 1997.

58. Multiple risk factor intervention trial. Risk factor changes and mortality results. Multiple Risk Factor Intervention Trial Research Group. *JAMA.* 248, 1465–1477, 1982.

59. The multiple risk factor intervention trial research group. Mortality after 16 years for participants randomized to the Multiple Risk Factor Intervention Trial. *Circulation.* 94, 946–951, 1996.

60. Czeizel, A.E. and Dudas, I. Prevention of the first occurrence of neural-tube defects by periconceptional vitamin supplementation. *N Engl J Med.* 327, 1832–1835, 1992.

61. Kirks, B.A. and Wolff, H.K. A comparison of methods for plate waste determinations. *J Am Diet Assoc.* 85, 328–331, 1985.

62. Daya, N.E., McKeown, N., Wong, M.Y., Welch, A., and Bingham, S. Epidemiological assessment of diet: a comparison of a 7-day diary with a food frequency questionnaire using urinary markers of nitrogen, potassium and sodium. *Int J Epidemiol.* 30, 309–317, 2001. Available at: http://ije.oxford-journals.org/cgi/content/full/30/2/309#R1. Accessed June 3, 2005.

63. Johnson, R.K. Dietary intake — how do we measure what people are *really* eating? *Obes Res.* 10, 63S–68S, 2002. Available at: http://www.obesityresearch.org/cgi/content/full/10/suppl_1/63S. Accessed June 3, 2005.

64. Shahar, D., Fraser, D., Shai, I., and Vardi, H. Development of a food frequency questionnaire (FFQ) for an elderly population based on a population survey. *J. Nutr.* 133, 3625–3629, 2003. Available at: http://www.nutrition.org/cgi/content/full/133/11/3625. Accessed June 4, 2005.

65. Rockett, H.R., Breitenbach, M., Frazier, A.L., et al. Validation of a youth/adolescent food frequency questionnaire. *Prev Med.* 26, 808–816, 1997.

66. Johnson, R.K. and Hankin, J.H. Dietary assessment and validation. In Monsen, E., Ed. *Research: Successful Approaches,* 2nd ed. Chicago, IL: American Dietetic Association, 2003, chap. 15.

67. Schoeller, D.A. Measurement of energy expenditure in free living humans by using doubly labeled water. *J Nutr.* 118, 1278–1289, 1988.

68. NIH. Improving Diet and Physical Activity Assessment (R01). Program Announcement (PA) Number: PAR-06-104. Release date: December 23, 2005. Available at: http://grants.nih.gov/grants/guide/pa-files/PAR-06-104.html. Accessed January 24, 2006.

69. U.S. Department of Health and Human Services. National Institutes of Health. National Institute of Diabetes and Digestive and Kidney Diseases. Programs Descriptions M-R. Nutritional Epidemiology http://www.niddk.nih.gov/fund/program/M-Rlist.htm#nutritionalepid. Accessed December 7, 2004.

70. Langserg, L. *Nutritional Epidemiology: Possibilities and Limitations.* Brussels, Belgium: International Life Sciences Institute, 1996. Available at http://europe.ilsi.org/file/Ilsiepid.pdf. Accessed June 13, 2005.

71. University of North Carolina. Clinical Nutrition Research Center. Nutritional Epidemiology home-page. Available at: http://www.cnrc.unc.edu/core_b.htm. Accessed December 5, 2004.

72. U.S. Department of Health and Human Services. National Institutes of Health. National Institute of Diabetes and Digestive and Kidney Diseases. Programs Descriptions M-R. Nutritional Epidemiology http://www.niddk.nih.gov/fund/program/M-Rlist.htm#nutritionalepid. Accessed December 7, 2004.

73. U.S. Department of Health and Human Services. National Institutes of Health. National Cancer Institute. Nutritional Epidemiology Branch homepage. Available at http://dceg.cancer.gov/nutri.html. Accessed December 7, 2004.

74. University of North Carolina. Clinical Nutrition Research Center. Nutritional Epidemiology homepage. Available at http://www.cnrc.unc.edu/core_b.htm. Accessed December 5, 2004.

5 Food and Nutrition Surveys for Monitoring the Public's Health

Epidemiology examines the distribution of disease in populations and the factors that influence or determine its distribution. Surveillance monitors changes and trends in factors related to disease in populations. Together, epidemiology and surveillance provide the background information necessary for public health interventions and programs.*

This chapter presents an overview of nutrition monitoring and related research activities carried out by the Department of Health and Human Services (HHS) and the U.S. Department of Agriculture (USDA), along with links to useful Web sites within these and other agencies. Nutrition monitoring activities in the HHS are conducted by the National Center for Health Statistics (NCHS) in the Centers for Disease Control and Prevention (CDC). Within the USDA, the Food Surveys Research Group (FSRG) implements food consumption surveys. (See Box 5.1.)

Health statistics provide critical information on where we stand as individuals and as a society. Statistics inform us about public health challenges and provide a basis for understanding existing problems. Health statistics are used to create a basis for comparisons between population groups as well as to demonstrate trends in health status and how they develop and change over time.

Surveys generate health statistics that form the cornerstone of nutrition monitoring. Estimates of dietary intake are an important part of monitoring the nutritional status of the U.S. population. Assessing dietary intake allows public health agencies and organizations to determine whether the population, or subgroups within the population, have adequate or excess intake of specific foods and nutrients. A food survey is a retrospective approach in which a statistical representation of the population's food consumption is surveyed by interviewers or via self-administered questionnaire.[1] The history of food consumption surveys through 2002 appears in Table 5.1.

The major food and nutrition survey that shapes nutrition policy in the U.S. is known as What We Eat in America–NHANES, an integration of two surveys: the Continuing Survey of Food Intake of Individuals (CSFII) and the National Health and Nutrition Examination Survey (NHANES). Other important surveys include the National Health Interview Survey (NHIS), Behavioral Risk Factor Surveillance System (BRFSS), Youth Risk Behavior Surveillance System (YRBSS), Pediatric Nutrition Surveillance System (PedNSS), Pregnancy Nutrition Surveillance System (PNSS), and Pregnancy Risk Assessment Monitoring System (PRAMS).

A strategic objective of HHS is to reduce the major threats to the health and well-being of Americans by focusing on the promotion of healthy behaviors, such as regular exercise and a healthy diet to reduce obesity and the incidence of chronic diseases such as diabetes.[2] Similarly, one of the USDA's objectives is to promote healthier eating habits and lifestyles. One actionable strategy to attain this objective is to continuously advance the science of nutrition by monitoring food and nutrient consumption.[3]

---

* Centers for Disease Control and Prevention. *Health Risks in America: Gaining Insight from the Behavior Risk Factor Surveillance System.* Revised edition. Atlanta: U.S. Department of Health and Human Services, 1997.

Box 5.1 Definitions: Nutrition Monitoring in HHS, CDC, and USDA

- *Nutrition monitoring* — intermittent assessment of dietary or nutrition status in order to detect changes in the nutritional status of a population
- *Nutrition surveillance* — continuous assessment of nutritional status for the purpose of detecting changes in trend or distribution in order to initiate corrective measures
- *Dietary status* — the condition of a population's or an individual's intake of foods and food components, especially nutrients
- *Nutrition assessment* — measurement of indicators of dietary status and nutrition related health status to identify the possible occurrence, nature, and extent of impaired nutritional status

TABLE 5.1
History of Food Consumption Studies in the U.S.

1935, 1942, 1948, 1955	USDA collects information about "household food use" through 7-d food recalls. These household level surveys include only food used in the home; they exclude information on the kinds and amounts of food obtained and eaten away from home. Information is not provided concerning how food is divided among individuals within households.
1965–1966	USDA collects information about "household food use" through 7-day food recalls. FDA funds a 24-h recall during one quarter of the study.
1977–1978	USDA collects information about "household food use" through 7-d food recalls. FDA funds a 24-h recall and a 2-d diet record of household members. The coordinated survey is designated the *Nationwide Food Consumption Survey* (NFCS).
1985–1986	USDA conducts the first *Continuing Survey of Food Intake of Individuals* (CSFII). The surveys include an all-income sample and a low-income sample. The all-income sample is nationally representative and includes about 1500 women 19 to 50 years in each year and their children 1 to 5 years (about 550 children in each year). A sample of 1100 men age 19 to 50 years of age is included in 1985 only. The low-income sample is nationally representative and includes about 2100 women in 1985 and about 1300 women in 1986 and about 1300 children 1 to 5 years in 1985 and 800 children in 1986. Food intake data are collected on 6 nonconsecutive days at intervals of approximately 2 months over a 1-year period. The first day of intake is collected using an in-person interview; subsequent data are collected by telephone, when possible. A 1-d dietary recall is used for all intakes.
1987–1988	USDA conducts the second NFCS, which is identical in design to the 1977–1978 NFCS (7-d household food use, 24-h recall, 2-d diet record of household members).
1989–1991	CSFII in which household members are interviewed for a 24-h recall and are asked to provide a food record for the following 2 d. Individuals who take part in the CSFII are asked to provide 3 consecutive days of dietary data. The first day's data are collected in a personal in-home interview using a 1-d dietary recall. The second and third days' data are collected using a self-administered 2-d diet record. Individuals identified as the main meal planners/preparers in the CSFII are contacted by telephone, if possible, about 6 weeks after collection of the dietary data and are asked to answer a series of questions about knowledge and attitudes toward diet, health, and food safety.
1994–1996	The CSFII 1994–1996, 1998 provides information on 2-d food and nutrient intakes by 20,607 individuals of all ages. The Diet and Health Knowledge Survey (DHKS) is a telephone follow-up to the CSFII. The two surveys are designed so that individuals' diet and health knowledge and attitudes can be linked with their food choices and nutrient intakes. The DHKS provides information on dietary knowledge and attitudes of 5765 individuals 20 years of age and over who provide at least 1 d of dietary intake data in the CSFII 1994–1996.

TABLE 5.1 (Continued)
History of Food Consumption Studies in the U.S.

1998	CSFII in which 2 nonconsecutive dietary recalls are secured for children less than 10 years of age. CSFII 1998 is conducted in response to the Food Quality Protection Act of 1996, which required the USDA to provide data from a larger sample of children for use by the Environmental Protection Agency in estimating exposure to pesticide residues in the diets of children. The CSFII 1998 adds intake data from 5559 children from birth through age 9 years to the intake data collected from 4253 children of the same ages participating in the CSFII 1994–1996.
1999–2001	In a survey designated Continuous NHANES, the Agricultural Research Services of USDA and the National Center for Health Statistics of HHS administer a 24-h dietary recall together with questionnaires about food consumption frequency and dietary supplement, antacid, and medication use.
2002	The CSFII and the dietary component of NHANES are integrated. The dietary intake methodologies developed by USDA and the sampling and data collection capabilities of NCHS are combined to create a survey that can link nutrition data to health status data. The combined survey collects data continuously.

Various health indicators measured over time provide information regarding our progress in attaining these admittedly broad objectives. Examples of such indicators include:

- Proportion of Americans age 18 and over who report engaging in physical activity 5 times a week for at least 30 min at a time
- Proportion of Americans defined as obese (by age group)
- Percentage of persons consuming fruits and vegetables five times per day
- Proportion of adults who report changes in their decisions to buy or use a food product because they read the food label
- Number of meals delivered to the homebound elderly

To detect change, whether improvement or deterioration, it is necessary to compare a baseline measurement with one or more follow-up measurements. This is precisely what surveys allow us to do. They give us the information to describe a variable at a single point in time. However, what is more useful is comparing data from at least two time periods, which indicates whether a change has occurred, and if so, in what direction. By comparing multiple time periods, we are able to detect trends. For example, NHANES and BRFSS provide estimates of obesity prevalence and indicate that the prevalence of obesity in the U.S. has been increasing since the 1980s. In this instance, we are clearly moving in the wrong direction.

5.1 NATIONAL CENTER FOR HEALTH STATISTICS

CDC's National Center for Health Statistics (NCHS) is the nation's principal health statistics agency, providing data to identify and address health issues. NCHS compiles statistical information to help guide public health and health policy decisions. Collaborating with USDA and other public partners, NCHS employs a variety of data collection mechanisms to obtain accurate information from multiple sources. This process provides a broad perspective to help understand the population's health, influences on health, and health outcomes.

NCHS carries out its mission of monitoring America's health by developing and implementing mechanisms for obtaining statistics. As the nation's principal health statistics agency, NCHS generates data to identify and address health issues. By collecting, analyzing, and disseminating data on the health status of U.S. residents, NCHS allows researchers, policymakers, public health practitioners, journalists, academics, and students to identify health problems, risk factors, and disease patterns; plan and assess public health programs; and compare populations, providers, and geographic areas.

Box 5.2 Accessing NHIS Questionnaires and Other Information

National Health Interview Survey (NHIS) questionnaires from 1962 to the present are available online at http://www.cdc.gov/nchs/about/major/nhis/quest_doc.htm. Data users can obtain the latest information about NHIS from the National Center for Health Statistics Web site: http://www.cdc.gov/nchs/nhis.htm. This Web site features downloadable public use data and documentation for National Health Interview Surveys, as well as important information about any modifications or updates to the data or documentation. Researchers may also wish to join the NHIS electronic mailing list at http://www.cdc.gov/subscribe.html. The listserve is made up of NHIS data users located around the world who receive electronic news about NHIS surveys (e.g., new releases of data or modifications to existing data), publications, conferences, and workshops).

Source: Adams, P.F., Dey, A.N., and Vickerie, J.L. Summary health statistics for the U.S. population: National Health Interview Survey, 2005. National Center for Health Statistics. Vital Health Stat 10(233). 2007. Available at: http://www.cdc.gov/nchs/data/series/sr_10/sr10_233.pdf . Accessed January 11, 2007.

Some of the surveys conducted by NCHS are designed to track changes in health and healthcare by allowing for comparisons across population groups. Other surveys support biomedical research by identifying research priorities and providing the mechanisms for epidemiologic studies of risk factors and outcomes. Still other surveys provide the justification for prevention programs by identifying health problems, targeting opportunities for interventions, and supporting program evaluation.

Many NCHS surveys examine issues relating diet to health and disease by tracking changes in food consumption, nutritional status, and the prevalence of diet-related chronic diseases. Nutrition information is provided by NHIS, BRFSS, YRBSS, PedNSS, and PNSS. Unarguably, however, the gold standard for nutrition surveys is NHANES, which can link food intake data to anthropometric, clinical, and biochemical indices, allowing researchers to explore relationships between diet and health status.

5.1.1 SOCIODEMOGRAPHIC DATA

To provide the broadest possible perspective on the health data obtained in the survey, each NCHS survey collects information on the sociodemographic characteristics of respondents, such as age, race, Hispanic origin, sex, education, income, employment, family size and relationships, and geographic region of residence. Demographic characteristics are collected primarily because they provide a context for the health data collected in the survey and because they help to explain interrelated trends in the survey data. Inequalities in health status and access to care — as well as the unequal burden of morbidity and mortality — for some racial and ethnic groups in the U.S. have made race and Hispanic origin among the most important demographic characteristics of interest to users of the NHIS.

5.1.2 NATIONAL HEALTH INTERVIEW SURVEY (NHIS)

The NHIS is the principal source of information on the health of the civilian, noninstitutionalized population of the U.S. and one of the major data collection programs of NCHS.[4] The NHIS is a cross-sectional household interview survey. Since 1957, its data have been used to monitor trends in illness and disability and to track progress toward achieving national health objectives, such as those of Healthy People 2010. NHIS data are also used by the public health research community for epidemiologic and policy analysis of such timely issues as characterizing those having various health problems, determining barriers to accessing and using appropriate healthcare, and evaluating federal health programs. The main objective of the NHIS is to monitor the health of the U.S. population through the collection and analysis of data on a broad range of health topics.

Box 5.3 BRFSS Questionnaires

Behavioral Risk Factor Surveillance System questionnaires from 1984 to the present are available online at: http://www.cdc.gov/brfss/questionnaires/questionnaires.htm. Beginning in 1997, the questionnaires became available in both Spanish and English.

Source: Behavioral Risk Factor Surveillance System Operational and User's Guide Version 3.0. December 12, 2006. BRFSS Operational and Users Guide 2. Available at: http://ftp.cdc. gov/pub/Data/Brfss/userguide.pdf. Accessed January 11, 2007.

Although the NHIS has been conducted continuously, its content has been revised roughly every 10–15 years. For example, a feature added for the 1995 sample design was the over-sampling of both black and Hispanic persons. In addition, the NHIS sample is now drawn from each state. Although the NHIS sample is too small to provide state level data with acceptable precision, its design facilitates the use of NHIS data with state-level telephone health surveys.

Sampling and interviewing are continuous throughout the year. Households selected to be interviewed each week are a probability sample representative of the target population annually. NHIS data are collected from approximately 40,000 households including about 100,000 persons. Survey participation is voluntary and the confidentiality of responses is assured under Section 308(d) of the Public Health Service Act. The annual response rate of NHIS is greater than 90% of the eligible households in the sample.

Data are collected through a personal interview conducted in the participant's household by interviewers employed and trained by the U.S. Bureau of the Census. The NHIS questionnaire is conducted using a computer-assisted personal interviewer (CAPI). The interviewer uses a laptop computer to enter responses directly into the computer during the interview. This computerized mode offers distinct advantages over the previous pencil and paper formats in terms of timeliness of the data and improved data quality. Since 2004, questionnaires have been available in Spanish as well as in English.

The NHIS questionnaire has three parts or modules similar to the questionnaires used in the adult and youth surveys in the BRFSS, discussed later in this chapter. These three parts include a basic module, a periodic module, and a topical module. The basic module functions as the core questionnaire. See Section 5.1.3 Behavioral Risk Factor Surveillance System for a description of these modules.

In 2000, the National Cancer Institute (NCI) funded a topical module about cancer control that covered tobacco use, diet (intake of fat, fruits, vegetables, legumes, and alcohol), drug use, family history of cancer, genetic testing, and sun avoidance behavior. An analysis of the results conducted by NCI researchers[5] revealed that, in general, intakes of fat, fruits, vegetables, and legumes were closer to recommendations among well-educated individuals, those engaged in other healthful behaviors, and underweight and normal weight individuals. As illustrated in Table 5.2, Latinos had higher intakes of fruits and vegetables, and generally a lower percentage of energy intake from fat than did non-Latino whites and non-Latino blacks.

5.1.3 Behavioral Risk Factor Surveillance System (BRFSS)

By the early 1980s, there was universal agreement that personal health behaviors play a significant role in premature morbidity and mortality. Although national estimates of health risk behaviors among U.S. adult population had been periodically obtained through surveys conducted by the NCHS, these data were not available on a state-specific basis. This deficiency was viewed as critical for state health agencies, which have the primary role of targeting resources to reduce behavioral risks and their consequent illnesses. Although national data may not be appropriate for any given state, state and local agency participation was critical to achieving national health goals. As a result, the CDC established the BRFSS[6] to collect state-level data that would provide the basis for monitoring state-level prevalence of the major behavioral risks among adults associated with

TABLE 5.2
**Intakes of Fruits and Vegetables, Fiber, and Fat according to the National
Health Information Survey, 2000**

	Latino		Black, Non-Latino		White, Non-Latino	
	Males	Females	Males	Females	Males	Females
Fruits/vegetables servings	6	4.8	5.4	4.4	5.4	4.5
Fiber (grams)	23	17	19	13	19	14
Fat (% of calories)	33.7	32.1	34.7	33.5	33.9	32

Source: From Thompson, F.E., Midthune, D., Subar, A.F., McNeel, T., Berrigan, D., Kipnis, V.
Dietary intake estimates in the National Health Interview Survey, 2000: methodology, results,
and interpretation. *J Am Diet Assoc.* 2005; 105: 352–363.

premature morbidity and mortality. The basic philosophy was to collect data on actual behaviors
— rather than on attitudes or knowledge — that would be especially useful for planning, initiating,
supporting, and evaluating health promotion and disease prevention programs.

Over the years, data from BRFSS have been used to monitor prevalence of high-risk health
behaviors, specific diseases, and use of preventive health services; dictate the design, focus, implementation, and evaluation of prevention health programs and strategies; and monitor progress toward
achieving local, state, and national health objectives.

To provide data that could be compared across states, CDC developed a core of standard
questions for states to incorporate into their own questionnaires, which are administered by telephone. By 1994, all states, the District of Columbia, and three territories were participating in the
BRFSS, making it the world's largest telephone survey. BRFSS maintains online interactive databases that include these variables: location (state or entire U.S.), year (1995–present), and category.
Categories include cholesterol awareness, nutrition, weight control, hypertension awareness, diabetes diagnosis, exercise, and average frequency of fruit and vegetable consumption each day.

All health departments must ask the core questions without modification; however, the optional
modules and additional questions are at the discretion of the state. The BRFSS questionnaire
comprises three parts, described as follows:

- The *core component* consists of a *fixed*, a *rotating*, and an *emerging* core. The fixed core is
  a standard set of questions asked by all states and includes queries about current behaviors
  that affect health (for example, tobacco use and women's health) and questions on demographic characteristics. The *rotating core* consists of two distinct sets of questions, each
  asked in alternating years by all states, addressing different topics. In the years that a rotating
  topic is not used in the core, it is supported as an optional module. The *emerging core* is a
  set of up to five questions added to the fixed and rotating cores. Emerging core questions
  typically focus on issues of a "late breaking" nature and do not necessarily receive the same
  scrutiny other questions receive before being added to the questionnaire. These questions
  form part of the core for 1 year and are evaluated during or soon after the year concludes
  to determine if they should be included as a regular component of subsequent surveys.
- The *optional modules* are sets of questions on specific topics (for example, smokeless
  tobacco) which a state can elect to use on its questionnaire. Although the modules are optional,
  CDC standards require that, if they are used, they must not be modified. Module topics have
  included questions on smokeless tobacco, oral health, cardiovascular disease, and firearms.
- The *state-added questions* are questions on topics of particular interest to an individual
  state that it may choose to add. In the past, categories of interest to public health
  nutritionists have included cholesterol, folic acid, food consumption, food handling, lead
  poisoning, physical activity, and weight control.

5.1.4 YOUTH RISK BEHAVIOR SURVEILLANCE SYSTEM (YRBSS)

YRBSS was launched by CDC in 1990 to monitor those health risk behaviors that contribute markedly to the leading causes of death, disability, and social problems among youth in the U.S. Objectives of YRBSS are to determine the prevalence and age of initiation of health-risk behaviors; assess whether health-risk behaviors increase, decrease, or remain the same over time; allow researchers to examine the occurrence of health risk behaviors among young people; provide comparable national, state, and local data; and monitor progress toward achieving Healthy People 2010 objectives.

YRBSS data are used at the national, state, and local levels in a variety of policy and program applications. YRBSS data can be used to describe risk behaviors, create awareness, set program goals, develop programs and policies, support health-related legislation, and seek funding.

The questionnaire is anonymous and self-administered, with either a computer-scannable booklet or answer sheet. It can be completed in one 45-min class period. The system includes national, state, and local school-based surveys of representative samples of 9th through 12th grade students. It is conducted every 2 years by CDC, usually during the spring semester. The national survey provides data representative of high school students in both public and private schools in the 50 states and the District of Columbia. To provide critical information on health risk behaviors among young people in high-risk situations and those in college, CDC also conducted national surveys among college students and adolescents in alternative schools. In 1995, the National College Health Risk Behavior Survey was administered to almost 5000 students. In 1998, almost 9000 students participated in the National Alternative High School Youth Risk Behavior Survey (see Box 5.4).

A voluntary component of the program is the provision of funding and technical support to states and major cities to conduct their own surveys. With technical assistance from CDC, state and local departments of education and health conduct a youth survey every 2 years. Sites can add or delete questions in the core questionnaire to meet the needs of their locale.

5.1.4.1 Nutrition-Related Questions

The nutrition-related questions used in the 2007 survey appear in Table 5.3. Respondents are asked about their current height and weight, dietary behaviors, alcohol use, and weight control strategies.

Box 5.4 The 1995 National College Health Risk Behavior Survey

Nationwide, 20.5% of college students were classified as being overweight based on body mass index (BMI) calculations. However, twice as many (41.6%) college students believed themselves to be overweight. At the time of the survey, 46.4% of college students were attempting weight loss — 59.8% of the females vs. 29.6% of the males.

Nationwide, for the 30 d preceding the survey:

- Almost one third (30.8%) of college students had dieted either to lose weight or to keep from gaining weight, 42.1% of the females vs. 16.7% of the males.
- Approximately half (53.6%) of college students had exercised either to lose weight or to keep from gaining weight, 62.6% of the females vs. 42.3% of the males.
- Of the female students, 7% had taken diet pills either to lose weight or to keep from gaining weight
- Of the female students, 4.2% had either vomited or taken laxatives to lose weight or to keep from gaining weight.

Source: Youth Risk Behavior Surveillance: National College Health Risk Behavior Survey — United States, 1995. *MMWR.* 1997 (November 14); 46(SS-6): 1–54.

TABLE 5.3
Some Diet-Related Questions in the 2005 Youth Risk Behavior Survey

Category	Question Number	Question
Health Status	6	How tall are you without your shoes on?
	7	How much do you weigh without your shoes on?
Dietary Behaviors	64	How do you describe your weight?
	65	Which of the following are you trying to do about your weight?
	66	During the past 30 d, did you exercise to lose weight or keep from gaining weight?
	67	During the past 30 d, did you eat less food, fewer calories, or foods low in fat to lose weight or keep from gaining weight?
	68	During the past 30 d, did you go without eating for 24 h or more (also called "fasting") to lose weight or keep from gaining weight?
	69	During the past 30 d, did you take any diet pills, powders, or liquids without a doctor's advice to lose weight or keep from gaining weight? (Do not include meal replacement products such as Slim Fast.)
Overweight and Weight Control	70	During the past 7 d, did you vomit or take laxatives to lose weight or to keep from gaining weight?
	71	During the past 7 d, how many times did you drink 100% fruit juices such as orange juice, apple juice, or grape juice? (Do not count punch, Kool-Aid, sports drinks, or other fruit-flavored drinks.)
	72	During the past 7 d, how many times did you eat fruit? (Do not count fruit juice.)
	73	During the past 7 d, how many times did you eat green salad?
	74	During the past 7 d, how many times did you eat potatoes? (Do not count french fries, fried potatoes, or potato chips.)
	75	During the past 7 d, how many times did you eat carrots?
	76	During the past 7 d, how many times did you eat other vegetables? (Do not count salad, potatoes, or carrots.)
	77	During the past 7 d, how many glasses of milk did you drink? (Include the milk you drank in a glass or cup, from a carton, or with cereal. Count the half-pint of milk served at school as equal to one glass.)

Source: 2005 State and Local Youth Risk Behavior Survey. Available at: www.cdc.gov/HealthyYouth/yrbs/pdfs/ 2005 highschoolquestionnaire.pdf. Accessed July 8, 2005.

- The *weight control* questions concern self-reported height and weight, self-perception of body weight status, and specific weight-control behaviors. Data on self-reported height and weight can be used to calculate body mass index and provide a proxy measure of whether high school students are overweight. Although overweight prevalence estimates derived from self-reported data are likely to be low, they can be useful in tracking trends over time. For example, prevalence trends from national surveys of adults using self-reported height and weight have been consistent with trend data from national surveys, such as NHANES, that use heights and weights measured by health professionals (referred to as *measured* heights and weights).
- The *dietary behaviors* questions assess food choices. Six of the questions address fruit and vegetable consumption, one addresses soda or pop consumption, and one addresses milk consumption. Although data are limited, an increased intake of fruits and vegetables appears to be associated with a decreased risk of overweight. Consumption of sugar-sweetened drinks, including soft drinks, appears to be associated with being at increased risk for overweight in children.

- The *physical activity* questions measure participation in physical activity, physical education classes, sports teams, television watching, and video game and computer use. The 2005 Dietary Guidelines for Americans recommends that youth engage in at least 1 h of physical activity on most, preferably all, days of the week. Television viewing and heavy use of computers and video games are associated with overweight and physical inactivity among adolescents and young adults.
- The *overweight and weight control* questions measure self-reported height and weight, self-perception of body weight status, and specific weight control behaviors. Data on self-reported height and weight can be used to calculate Body Mass Index (BMI) and provide a proxy measure of whether high school students are overweight. Although overweight prevalence estimates derived from self-reported data are likely to be low, they can be useful in tracking trends over time.
- The *alcohol use* questions measure lifetime and current use of alcohol, age of initiation, episodic heavy drinking, access to alcohol, and drinking on school property. Alcohol consumption among adolescents is associated with other risk behaviors, such as having unprotected sex and motor vehicle accidents. Heavy alcohol consumption is also associated with a nutrient-poor diet, which paradoxically, may be accompanied by overweight when drinking leads to an excess intake of calories.

5.1.4.2 Selected Results of the YRBSS

The 2005 National YRBSS survey was administered to a national probability sample of almost 14,000 public and private school students in 44 states, 4 territories, and 23 major cities. The school and student response rates were 78% and 86%, respectively; thus, there was an overall 67% response rate (the school response rate multiplied by the student response rate).

Results from the 2005 national YRBSS demonstrate that almost 10% of high school students reported regularly smoking cigarettes. Three-quarters had had at least one drink during their life (down from 80% in 1999). However, more than 40% had had at least one drink and one quarter had had at least five drinks in a row within the previous month.

Most of the risk behaviors associated with cardiovascular diseases and cancer in adults are initiated during adolescence. Almost 15% were overweight; two thirds had participated in an insufficient amount of physical activity; and more than 80% had not eaten at least 5 servings a day of fruits and vegetables during the 7 d preceding the survey. Consumption of fruits and vegetables includes 100% fruit juice, fruit, green salad, potatoes (excluding French fries, fried potatoes, or potato chips), carrots, or other vegetables.

Comprehensive information about the results of YRBSS can be found on CDC's Web site at www.cdc.gov/yrbss. The site includes a copy of the most recent questionnaire and item rationale; links to the Morbidity and Mortality Weekly Report Surveillance Summaries that highlight YRBSS data; the data and codebooks for the national YRBSS; related publications, journal articles, and fact sheets; and Youth Online (see Box 5.5).

Box 5.5 Youth Online

Youth Online provides results from national, state, and local YRBSS surveys conducted since 1991. This interactive Internet site http://apps.nccd.cdc.gov/yrbss/ produces statistical reports based on BRFSS data by location and by race/ethnicity, gender, school grade, and health topic for two locations or survey years. Visitors to the site can instantly create tables and graphs illustrating survey results, and develop reports that identify behaviors whose rates have changed significantly over time.

5.1.5 Pediatric Nutrition Surveillance System (PedNSS)

In 1973 the CDC's PedNSS [7,8] began monitoring growth indicators, hematologic test results, and breastfeeding practices for low-income infants and children who participate in publicly funded maternal and child nutrition and health programs. PedNSS provides a framework for gathering and analyzing state-specific information on the nutritional characteristics of low-income children. These data are useful to both health professionals who manage public health programs and those who are involved in the direct care of low-income children. The data can be used to identify prevalent nutrition-related problems, identify high risk groups, monitor trends, target resources for program planning, and evaluate the effectiveness of interventions.

The primary source of PedNSS data is the Women, Infants, and Children Supplemental Food Program (WIC); in 2001, 82% of the national PedNSS database was derived from WIC records. The Early Periodic Screening, Diagnosis, and Treatment program (EPSDT) and clinics funded by Maternal and Child Health Program (MCH) block grants also provide data for this program-based surveillance system. Data are collected on sociodemographic variables (ethnicity/race, age, geographic location), birth weight, anthropometric indices (BMI), biochemical indices (hemo-globin (Hgb) and/or hematocrit (Hct)), and breastfeeding practices. The indicators monitored by PedNSS are birth weight, childhood growth status, anemia, and breast-feeding patterns (see Box 5.6).

State health departments that choose to participate in PedNSS submit data to CDC on a monthly basis on computer disks. Surveillance participants receive, in turn, monthly reports that identify children at high nutritional risk. These data are analyzed semiannually and annually and summaries are returned for use in program planning, management, and evaluation of state and local maternal and child health programs and activities. Data analysis occurs at both CDC and the state level. CDC provides assistance to the participants on using and interpreting the data. For example, statewide and local data can be compared to the year 2010 targets. CDC encourages PedNSS participants to distribute appropriate sections of the summaries to individual counties, clinics, and programs.

PedNSS has expanded from an original five states in 1973 to 39 states and territories, 6 tribal governments, and the District of Columbia in 2002. In 2002, records were contributed for more than 5 million children from birth to 5 years of age. It is expected that future PedNSS develop-ments will continue to increase state capacity for nutrition surveillance. In 2002, 83% of the sample was enrolled in WIC. Efforts are being made to include children who participate in programs other than WIC.

Box 5.6 Definitions of PedNSS Indicators

- Low birth weight (LBW) is defined as weight at birth < 2,500 g; high birth weight (HBW) is > 4,000 g.
- Short stature is defined as the 5th percentile length-for-age for children < 2 years of age and height-for-age for children > 2 years of age, based on the 2000 CDC growth charts.
- Risk of overweight is defined as BMI-for-age 85–95th percentile in children > 2 years of age; overweight is BMI-for-age > 95th percentile in children > 2 years of age.
- Anemia is present when the Hgb or Hct is < 5th percentile of CDC's recommendations to prevent and control iron deficiency anemia.[*]
- Infant feeding practices data is collected for children under two years to assess the prevalence of those who were ever breastfed and of those who were breastfed at six months.

[*]CDC recommendations to prevent and control iron deficiency anemia in the United States. *MMWR Recomm Rep.* 47(RR-3), 1998.

Box 5.7 PedNSS and PNSS Training Modules

Online training modules for PedNSS and PNSS are available at: www.cdc.gov/pednss/how_ to/index.htm#Table%20of%20Contents.

Source: United States Department of Health and Human Services. Centers for Disease Control and Prevention. National Center for Chronic Disease Prevention and Health Promotion. Division of Nutrition and Physical Activity. "The Pediatric Nutrition Surveillance System (PedNSS) and the Pregnancy Surveillance System (PNSS)." Available at: http://0-www.cdc.gov.mill1.sjlibrary.org/pednss/index.htm. Page last updated June 12, 2006. Accessed January 11, 2007.

CDC will continue to be the focal point for technical assistance, consultation, and training to states, and for the collection, processing, analysis, interpretation, and use of PedNSS data. Online training modules for PedNSS and PNSS use case studies to explain how to read a table, review data quality, interpret the data, use it for program evaluation, and disseminate it in reports and facts sheets.

5.1.6 PREGNANCY NUTRITION SURVEILLANCE SYSTEM (PNSS)

PNSS[9] is a program-based public health surveillance system that monitors risk factors associated with infant mortality and poor birth outcomes among low-income pregnant women who participate in federally funded public health programs. Similar to PedNSS, PNSS uses existing data from WIC and MCH. A majority of the data are from the WIC program, which serves pregnant, breastfeeding, and postpartum women. Data on maternal health indicators include prepregnancy weight status, maternal weight gain, parity, interpregnancy intervals, anemia, diabetes, and hypertension during pregnancy. Data on maternal behavioral indicators include medical care, WIC enrollment, multivitamin consumption, smoking, and drinking. In addition, PNSS obtains indicators of infant health: birth weight, preterm births, full-term low birth weight (LBW), and breastfeeding initiation. PNSS provides nutrition surveillance reports for the nation defined as "all participating contributors" as well as for each contributor. A contributor may be a state, U.S. territory, or a tribal government. Each contributor can receive more specific reports by clinic, county, local agency, region, or metropolitan area.

The goal of PNSS is to collect, analyze, interpret, and disseminate data to guide public health policy and action. PNSS information is used to set priorities and plan, implement, monitor, and evaluate public health programs.

5.1.6.1 Selected Results from PedNSS and PNSS

Data from the 1989 and 2000 PedNSS were analyzed to document the state-specific prevalence of overweight and underweight and examine trends among 2- through 4-year-old children from low-income families. The study revealed that the number of states reporting a prevalence of overweight of more than 10% increased from 11 states (in 1989) to 28 states (in 2000). Trend analyses showed significant increases in overweight in 30 states and decreases in underweight in 26 states.[10]

Box 5.8 NHANES as Data Collection Mechanism

NHANES serves as the data collection mechanism for the joint Health and Human Services/U.S. Department of Agriculture effort to monitor the diet and nutritional status of Americans, providing information needed for food policy and dietary guidelines.

Source: United States Department of Health and Human Services. Centers for Disease Control and Prevention. National Center for Health Statistics. "National Health and Nutrition Examination Survey." Factsheet Updated October 16, 2006. Available at: http://www.cdc.gov/nchs/data/factsheets/nhanes.pdf. Accessed January 11, 2007.

Box 5.9 Integration of CSFII and NHANES into What We Eat in America

The year 2002 was the first year of full integration of two nationwide dietary intake surveys — the Continuing Survey of Food Intakes by Individuals (CSFII) conducted by USDA and NHANES conducted by DHHS.[1] The new integrated dietary component of the survey is called What We Eat in America and is the food and nutrition component of NHANES.

[1]Special issue on the Integrated CSFII-NHANES, *J. Nutr.* 133, 575S–634S, 2003. Available at: http://ods.od. nih. gov/News/Special_Issue_on_the_Integrated_CSFII-NHANES_Survey.aspx. Accessed July 12, 2005.

Source: United Stated Department of Agriculture. Agriculture Research Service. "What We Eat In America (WWEIA), NHANES: Overview." Last modified September 14, 2006. Available at: http:// www.ars.usda.gov/Services/docs.htm?docid=13793&pf=1&cg_id=0#intro. Accessed January 11, 2007.

From 1980 through 1991, the trends for LBW, low height-for-age (shortness), low weight-for-height (thinness), and high weight-for-height (overweight) were stable for all children monitored by the PedNSS, with the exception of Asian children, who were predominantly of Southeast Asian refugee background. In the early 1980s, the prevalence of LBW and short stature was higher among Asian children than among children of other racial or ethnic groups who were monitored. However, these prevalences declined steadily from 1980 through 1991. By 1991, the prevalences of LBW and shortness for Asian children were similar to those observed for children of other races/ethnic groups. Overall, low-income U.S. children had a slightly lower height-for-age than expected, indicating that some of these children were at a health and nutritional disadvantage. The prevalence of overweight varied among different racial/ethnic groups: Hispanic and Native American children had the highest prevalences of overweight. The 20–30% prevalence of anemia among low-income children monitored by the PedNSS was higher than among the general population. However, the prevalence of anemia declined more than 5% for most of the age- and race/ethnicity-specific groups that were monitored.[11]

PNSS and PedNSS data were analyzed to examine whether increasing duration of breastfeeding is associated with a lower risk of overweight in a low-income population of 4-year-olds in the U.S. Records that followed more than 12,000 child–mother pairs for 5 years indicate that the duration of breastfeeding shows a dose-response, protective relationship for risk of overweight only among non-Hispanic whites; no significant association was found among non-Hispanic blacks or Hispanics. Among non-Hispanic whites, the adjusted odds ratio of overweight to breastfeeding for 6 to 12 months compared to never breastfeeding was 0.70 (95% CI: 0.50–0.99) and for greater than 12 months vs. never was 0.49 (95% CI: 0.25–0.95). Breastfeeding for any duration was also protective against underweight (BMI-for-age below the fifth percentile). The researchers concluded that breastfeeding is associated with a reduced risk of overweight among non-Hispanic white children, and that breastfeeding longer than 6 months provides health benefits to children beyond the period of breastfeeding.[12]

5.1.7 PREGNANCY RISK ASSESSMENT MONITORING SYSTEM (PRAMS)

PRAMS is an ongoing state- and population-based surveillance system implemented in 31 states plus New York City. The system was designed to monitor selected maternal behaviors and experiences that occur before, during, and after pregnancy among women who deliver live-born infants. PRAMS employs a mixed mode data-collection methodology: up to three self-administered surveys are mailed to a sample of mothers, and nonresponders are followed-up with telephone interviews. Self-reported survey data are linked to selected birth certificate data and weighted for sample design, nonresponse, and noncoverage. From these are created the annual PRAMS analysis data sets that can be used to produce statewide estimates of different perinatal health behaviors and experiences among women delivering live infants. PRAMS data can also be used to identify racial, ethnic, and socioeconomic disparities in critical maternal health-related behaviors.

5.1.7.1 Selected Results from PRAMS

PRAMS data for 2000 indicate that the prevalence of multivitamin use four or more times per week during the month before pregnancy ranged from 25.0 to 40.7% across the 19 states surveyed. Thus, as measured by multivitamin use, at least 19 states are well below the Healthy People 2010 objective for folic acid consumption. State maternal and child health programs can use this data to monitor progress toward Healthy People 2010 objectives and evaluate adherence to guidelines for care. The data can be shared with policymakers to direct policy decisions affecting the health of mothers and infants.[13]

The following year, PRAMS surveyed women from eight states (Alabama, Colorado, Florida, Hawaii, Illinois, Maine, Nebraska, and North Carolina) about smoking during pregnancy, alcohol use during pregnancy, and breastfeeding initiation — behaviors for which substantial health disparities have been previously identified. Consistent patterns were observed among the eight states by age, race, ethnicity, education, and income level. Overall, the prevalence of smoking during pregnancy ranged from 9.0 to 17.4%, with the highest rates of smoking consistently reported among women who were younger (less than 25 years), white, American Indian, non-Hispanic (except in Hawaii), with a high school education or less, and with low incomes. The prevalence of alcohol use during pregnancy ranged from 3.4 to 9.9%. In seven states, in contrast to smoking, the highest prevalence of alcohol use during pregnancy was seen in women who were older (over 35 years), non-Hispanic, with more than a high school education, and with higher incomes. The prevalence of breastfeeding initiation ranged from 54.8 to 89.6%. The lowest rates of breastfeeding initiation occurred in women who were younger, black, with a high school education or less, and with low incomes. Prevalences of the behaviors among each population often varied by state, indicating the potential impact of state-specific policies and programs.

States can use PRAMS data to identify populations at greatest risk for maternal behaviors that have negative consequences for maternal and infant health and to develop policies and plan programs that target populations at high risk. Although prevalence data cannot be used to identify causes or interventions to improve health outcomes, they do indicate the magnitude of disparities and identify populations that should be targeted for intervention. The results of this study suggest a need for wider targeting than is often done to provide state and national agencies with the information necessary to create more effective public health policies and programs. Additionally, the data produced by this study can serve as a baseline for states to use in measuring the impact of policies and programs on eliminating the identified health disparities.[14]

5.1.8 OTHER DATABASES

In 1999, the NCHS created a database for dietary supplements, receiving additional support from the NIH Office of Dietary Supplements (ODS) in 2001. The database, using values declared on product labels rather than direct analysis as is done with foods, contains information taken from 4,000 product labels. These include dietary supplements such as nutrients and botanicals and calcium-containing antacids reported as consumed or ingested by participants in previous NHANES household interviews. This database is compatible with USDA's food databases and is used in national survey data collection efforts. The NCHS dietary supplement database and others such as those developed at the Pennsylvania State University and University of California, San Diego, are not currently available publicly. A main obstacle to their release is that in all cases the databases are constantly changing.[15]

5.1.9 NATIONAL HEALTH AND NUTRITION EXAMINATION SURVEY (NHANES)
BACKGROUND

In the 1950s, the NCHS National Health Examination Survey (NHES) was launched. However, in the late 1960s, with a burgeoning awareness of and concern about domestic hunger and other nutrition issues, it became apparent that the lack of a nutrition component in NHES seriously flawed the survey. In 1971, when a nutrition component was added, NHES expanded into NHANES.

Initially, NHANES was conducted episodically: NHANES I, from 1971 through 1974; NHANES II, from 1976 through 1980; and NHANES III, from 1988 through 1994. Since 1999, the survey has been conducted continuously, with results reported for 2-year cycles: NHANES 1999–2000 (sometimes referred to as NHANES IV), NHANES 2001–2002, NHANES 2003–3004, NHANES 2005–2006, NHANES 2007–2008, and so on. The current NHANES cycle names use years rather than Roman numerals.

5.1.9.1 NHANES Methodology

NHANES is a continuous, annual survey that collects data from a nationally representative sample of the civilian, noninstitutionalized U.S. population aged 2 months and older through in-home personal interviews, physical examinations in mobile examination centers (MECs), and mail follow-up food frequency questionnaires (FFQs). Certain groups are over-sampled to allow for more precise estimates of their populations. Over-sampled groups include adolescents 12–19 years, persons 60 or more years of age, African Americans, Hispanics, low-income persons, and pregnant women. The CSFII was integrated into NHANES in 2002.

NHANES III was the last of this series of surveys to be implemented before integrating NHANES and the Continuing Survey of Food Intake of Individuals (CSFII), described in Section 5.1.10.1. Nearly 34,000 people were interviewed in NHANES III, and more than 31,000 were examined. NHANES III over-sampled blacks, Mexican Americans, children under 5 years, and the elderly ($\geq$ 60 years). Data on weight and height were collected through direct physical examination of each individual in the MEC. Based on self-reported race and ethnicity, subjects were classified into non-Hispanic white, non-Hispanic black, Mexican American, and four other ethnic groups. The survey obtained food consumption measurements for 1 day through a 24-h recall, along with dietary, nutritional, and health status measurements. A nonrandom subsample of about 5% of respondents provided food consumption information for a second day to allow estimation of usual intakes.

NHANES IV began in 1999. Of the 13,156 persons eligible for the survey in 2001–2002, 80% (n = 10,477) participated in a physical examination at the MEC, three quarters of these participants had complete and reliable 1-d dietary interview data. Heights and weights were among the measurements obtained from more than 4000 adults and 4000 children in 1999–2000 and again in 2001–2002.

Diet-related conditions studied include cardiovascular disease, diabetes, kidney disease, obesity, oral health, and osteoporosis. As indicated in Box 5.10, MEC data collection includes physical examinations, a standardized dental examination, physiological measurements, and laboratory tests on blood and urine. People leave the MEC wearing a physical activity monitor. In addition, they are requested to allow a technician to visit their homes to ask a short set of questions, some of which relate to vitamin and mineral supplement use, and to collect a dust sample by vacuuming areas in the room where they sleep. The sample is then sent to a lab where it is tested for allergens.

Box 5.10 NHANES Health Examination Tests

Health Measurements by Participant Age and Gender
- Physician's exam — all ages
- Blood pressure — ages 8 years and older
- Body fat — ages 8–64 years
- Bone density — ages 8 years and older
- Oral health exam — ages 5 years and older
- Vision test — ages 12 years and older
- Hearing test — ages 12–19 years and 70 years and older
- Fitness test — ages 12–49 years
- Height, weight, and other body measures — all ages
- Ophthalmology exam for eye diseases — ages 40 and older

Lab Tests on Urine: 6 Years and Older
- Kidney function tests — ages 6 years and older
- Sexually transmitted disease (STD)
  - Chlamydia and gonorrhea — ages 14–39
  - Human immunodeficiency virus (HIV) — ages 18–49 (only if no blood is drawn)
- Exposure to environmental chemicals — selected persons ages 6 and older
- Pregnancy test — females 12–59 years and girls 8–11 years who have periods

Lab Tests on Blood: 1 Year and Older
- Anemia — all ages
- Cholesterol — ages 6 years and older
- Glucose measures — ages 12 years and older
- Infectious diseases — ages 2 years and older
- Kidney function tests — ages 12 years and older
- Lead — 1 year and older
- Cadmium — 1 year and older
- Mercury — ages 1–5 years and females 16–49 years
- Liver function tests — ages 12 years and older
- Nutrition status — 1 year and older
- Hormone tests — ages 6 years and older
- Prostate Specific Antigen (PSA) — males ages 40 and older
- Sexually transmitted diseases (STD)
  - Herpes type 1 and 2 — ages 14–49 years
  - Human immunodeficiency virus (HIV) — ages 18–49 years
  - Human papillomavirus (HPV) antibody — ages 14–59 years
- Exposure to environmental chemicals — selected persons ages 6 and older

Lab Tests on Water
- Environmental chemicals — 12 years and older

Other Lab Tests
- Vaginal swabs (self-administered) females ages 14–59 years
- Human papillomavirus (HPV) ages 14–59 years

Private Health Interviews
- Health status — all ages (parent answers for ages 11 and younger)
- Questions about drug and alcohol use — ages 12 years and older (no drug testing will be done)
- Nutrition — all ages
- Reproductive health — females ages 12 years and older
- Questions about sexual experience — ages 14–59 years
- Tobacco use — ages 12 years and older

After the Visit to the NHANES Mobile Examination Center
- Persons asked about the foods they eat will receive a phone call 3–10 d after their exam for a similar interview, all ages.
- A food questionnaire will be mailed to the participant's home. Adults and parents of children 2 years and older, are asked to complete this questionnaire and return it to our office in a prepaid envelope provided.
- Persons 6 years and older will be asked to wear a physical activity monitor at home for 7 d and return it to our office in a prepaid envelope provided. Parents or guardians will assist children 6–11 years old.
- Participants will be asked to allow a technician to visit their homes to ask a short set of questions and collect a dust sample by vacuuming areas in the room where they sleep. The dust sample will be sent to a lab where it will be tested for allergens.

- Persons who test positive for hepatitis C will be asked to participate in a brief telephone interview 6 months after the exam. Parents will respond for children.
- Men (ages 40 and older) with a high PSA test result will be called for a brief phone interview 6 months after the exam.

5.1.9.2 NHANES Dietary Measures

What We Eat in America forms the dietary interview component of the National Health and Nutrition Examination Survey. It consists of dietary recalls, a food frequency questionnaire (FFQ), and interview questions about the use of vitamin and mineral supplements.

Two 24-h recalls are collected for all respondents. The first recall is collected in-person at the MEC, and the second is obtained via a phone call within 10 d of the MEC interview. The automated multiple pass method (AMPM) is used to collect the recalls. This computerized protocol, developed by the USDA, collects interviewer-administered 24-h dietary recalls either in person or by telephone. The software program provides a series of questions or prompts to help skilled interviewers elicit precise information. Designed to enhance recall accuracy and reduce respondent burden, it is the primary instrument used to collect dietary intake data from individuals sampled in national surveys.[16]

A food frequency questionnaire (FFQ) is also sent to each participant through a survey mailed several days after the in-person data collection. Information about the use of nutrition supplements is obtained during the home interview.

The food intake data collected by NHANES can be linked to the health status data from other NHANES components, allowing researchers to explore relationships between dietary intakes and health status. For example, results from NHANES 1999–2000, conducted after the implementation of food fortification and educational efforts to increase folate consumption indicate these public health efforts have been effective in increasing folate status among U.S. women of childbearing age. Consumption of adequate quantities of folate in this population is essential in preventing neural tube defects such as spina bifida and anencephaly.

5.1.10 Food Surveys Research Group (FSRG)

The mission of FSRG is to plan, design, coordinate, and manage the USDA's nationwide food surveys.[17] Uses of FSRG survey data include assessment of dietary intakes, dietary trends, and food consumption economics; development of policies for food assistance, food labeling, and food safety programs; and implementation of dietary guidance and nutrition education programs.

FSRG monitors and assesses food consumption and related behaviors of the U.S. population by conducting surveys and providing the resulting information for food and nutrition-related programs and public policy decisions. FSRG surveys include nationwide food consumption surveys, diet and health knowledge surveys, Continuing Survey of Food Intake by Individuals, and a Supplemental Children's Survey.

Box 5.11 NHANES Food Intake Data

NHANES food intake data can be linked to health status data from other NHANES components, allowing researchers to explore relationships between dietary intakes and health status.

Source: United States Department of Health and Human Services. Centers for Disease Prevention and Control. National Center for Health Statistics. National Health and Nutrition Examination Survey. "DHHS-USDA Dietary Survey Integration - What We Eat in America." Page last reviewed January 11, 2007. Available at: http://www.cdc.gov/nchs/about/major/nhanes/faqs.htm. Accessed January 11, 2007.

**Box 5.12 The Proposed National Health, Nutrition,
and Physical Activity Monitoring Act**

In 2005, the *National Health, Nutrition, and Physical Activity Monitoring Act* was introduced in the House of Representatives as H.R. 2844. The purpose of the bill is to:

1. Amend the National Nutrition Monitoring and Related Research Act of 1990 to foster greater understanding of human dietary eating patterns and food intake, physical activity level, food security, dietary exposure, and nutritional status through 2015.
2. Provide timely information to public program managers and private sector decision makers to improve nutritional intake, physical activity, health, productivity and other measures of quality of life of Americans, based on scientifically established norms and the knowledge and experience developed under the National Nutrition Monitoring and Related Research Act of 1990 over the past decade.
3. Reauthorize the NCHS, CDC and the Agricultural Research Service to collect and analyze dietary, health, physical activity, diet, and health knowledge data.
4. Support other purposes.

Assignment: Check THOMAS to determine the status of this bill.

Source: U.S. House. 105th Congress, 1st Session. *H.R. 2844,* National Health, Nutrition, and Physical Activity Monitoring Act of 2005. *Congressional Record* ONLINE June 9, 2005. Thomas. Available at: http://thomas.loc.gov/cgi-bin/bdquery/z?d109:h.r.02844. Accessed January 11, 2007.

FSRG also maintains the FSRG listserv, an electronic distribution list for users of nationwide dietary data and databases. Subscribers receive e-mail announcements when data are released from What We Eat In America; for new releases of the Food and Nutrient Database for Dietary Studies; of new FSRG products, such as reports and research articles; and when FSRG sponsors activities, such as presentations at professional meetings and workshops on using dietary survey data.

5.1.10.1 Continuing Survey of Food Intake of Individuals

As indicated in Table 5.1, the first Continuing Survey of Food Intake of Individuals (CSFII) was conducted in 1985. It was originally conceived of as a smaller survey to fill in the gaps between the large Nationwide Food Consumption Surveys (NFCS) conducted every 10 years. The first of the surveys that evolved into the NFCS was conducted in the 1930s; more contemporary NFCS surveys were conducted in 1976–1977 and 1987–1988. The early CSFII in 1985 and 1986 focused on women 19 to 50 years of age and their children 1 to 5 years of age; one sample of men 19 to 50 years of age was also included. CSFII in 1989–1991 and 1994–1996 included all members of sample households. NFCS and the Household Food Consumption Surveys conducted in earlier years have been discontinued.

5.1.10.2 What We Eat in America

The USDA's 10th nationwide survey was called the 1994–1996, 1998 Continuing Survey of Food Intakes by Individuals. Using a 24-h dietary recall format, respondents were asked to provide information on all foods and beverages consumed on two nonconsecutive days. A total of 16,000 respondents provided day-1 data and more than 15,000 respondents provided data for both days. A 1998 supplement to the CSFII obtained similar data for 5559 children from birth through 9 years (i.e., until their 10th birthday), using the same methods as in 1994–1996.

The Diet and Health Knowledge Survey (DHKS) was initiated in 1989–1991 to collect information on attitudes and knowledge about diet and health among Americans. In 1994–1996, the DHKS was conducted as a follow-up telephone survey to the CSFII: respondents were a subset of persons participating in the CSFII. The CSFII and DHKS were designed so that individuals' attitudes and knowledge about healthy eating could be linked with their food choices and nutrient intakes. The CSFII and DHKS together were known as the What We Eat in America survey. DHKS is no longer funded.

5.2 NUTRITION MONITORING ACTIVITIES BY THE USDA

Individual food consumption can be estimated through direct observation, plate waste studies, interviews, and food records. The advantage of these prospective studies is that data collection does not depend on the respondent's memory. On the other hand, respondent burden is high. Retrospective food frequency questionnaires and 24-h dietary recalls, other ways of estimating food consumption of individuals, also pose a high respondent burden.

Determining intake of populations as a whole is another matter. For small groups, food consumption can be monitored by analyzing food frequency questionnaires or by menu analysis coupled with an analysis of wasted food. This is done by calculating the nutrient composition of a given menu, subtracting the nutrient composition of the food wasted, then dividing by the number of people who were served. Estimates of a group's food consumption can also be expressed in food supply and utilization data.

Every year, the USDA's Economic Research Service (ERS) measures the flow of raw and semi-processed food commodities through the U.S. marketing system. The series provides continuous data beginning in 1909. It is typically used to measure changes in food consumption over time and to determine the approximate nutrient content of the food supply. Food supply data, also known as "food disappearance data," reflect the amount of the major food commodities entering the market, regardless of their final use. The total amount available for domestic consumption is estimated by determining the residual after exports, industrial uses, seed and feed use, and year-end inventories are subtracted from the sum of production, beginning inventories, and imports. Consumption estimates derived from food disappearance data tend to overstate actual consumption because they include spoilage and waste accumulated through the marketing system and in the home. Conversion factors are needed to compensate for processing, trimming, spoilage, and shrinkage within the distribution system. Nevertheless, food disappearance data are useful as indicators of trends in consumption over time.[18]

5.2.1 AGRICULTURAL RESEARCH SERVICE

The Agricultural Research Service (ARS) funds six National Human Nutrition Research Centers (HNRCs) through its Human Nutrition Research Program. These centers conduct research targeted towards health, quality of life, prevention of chronic disease and promotion of a nutritious supply of food. They are:

- Beltsville Human Nutrition Research Center (BHNRC; established 1941), Beltsville, MD
- Grand Forks HNRC (established 1977), Grand Forks, ND
- Children's Nutrition Research Center (established 1979), Houston, TX
- Jean Mayer HNRC on Aging (established 1980), Boston, MA
- The Western HNRC (established 1980), Davis, CA
- Arkansas Children's Nutrition Center (established 1995), Little Rock, AR

The oldest and most comprehensive of the centers is in Beltsville, a suburb of Washington, D.C. BHNRC houses eight laboratories. (See Box 5.13.) *This center's* history of conducting food and human nutrition research began with the USDA and Atwater. Currently, most nutrition monitoring at the USDA is carried out through two laboratories within the BHNRC — the Community Nutrition Research Group and the Food Surveys Research Group — with input from the Nutrient Data Laboratory. These facilities are discussed in the following sections.

Box 5.13 The Beltsville Human Nutrition Research Center of the USDA's Agricultural Research Service

Units in the Beltsville Human Nutrition Research Center of the USDA's Agricultural Research Service:

Community Nutrition Research Group. Mission: to monitor and assess the capacity of communities to meet their food and nutrition needs for a better understanding of linkages between nutrition, agriculture, health, and community.

Food Surveys Research Group. Mission: to monitor and assess food consumption and related behavior of the U.S. population by conducting surveys and providing the resulting information for food and nutrition-related programs and public policy decisions.

Diet and Human Performance Laboratory. Mission: to determine the interrelationships of dietary intake of energy, fiber, fat and fatty acids, and selected fat soluble micronutrients to metabolic and physiological parameters in humans so that recommendations for intakes of these nutrients are consistent with life-long maintenance of health and optimum quality of life for the diverse population of adult Americans. Lack of knowledge of how lipids, carbohydrates, fiber, vitamins, other nutrients and alcohol interact in human metabolism limits our ability to predict how different intake patterns will affect an individual's health and well-being. This is especially important in developing recommendations for prevention of the most prevalent diseases, such as cancer, heart disease, hypertension, diabetes, and obesity. Understanding the relationship between energy metabolism and diet and body composition is critical to defining optimal dietary intakes of fat, carbohydrate, protein, fiber and other nutrients to prevent disease.

Food Composition Laboratory. Mission: to develop innovative measurement systems for the determination of food components that influence human health.

Human Studies Facility (HSF). Mission: to support the execution of human studies at the BHNRC. A state-of-the-art research complex significantly expands the HSF clinical research area. The core services within HSF include study volunteer recruitment, volunteer screening, study biological sample collection and processing, residence for long-term studies, and managing the dietary unit. The dietary unit is primarily designed for planning, preparing, and serving specialized controlled diets to independently living adults. Volunteers consume their meals (one to three times per day) in the dining room, following research guidelines. The dietary unit can accommodate studies with up to 90 volunteers per meal — either from one large study or from two or more simultaneous small studies. The HSF is operational year-round.

Nutrient Data Laboratory (NDL). Mission: to develop authoritative food composition databases and state of the art methods to acquire, evaluate, compile and disseminate composition data on foods available in the U.S. NDL and its predecessor organizations in USDA have been compiling and developing food composition databases for over a century. NDL has an interdisciplinary staff composed of nutritionists, dietitians, food technologists, and computer specialists.

Nutrient Requirements and Functions Laboratory. Mission: to determine human requirements, functions, and basic mechanisms of action for specific vitamins and minerals; develop methodology for assessment of mineral and vitamin nutrition in humans; and develop cost-effective cellular, molecular, and immunological methods for evaluating micronutrient requirements and functions, and the effect of nutritional status on immune function. A multidisciplinary research team investigates vitamins, minerals, and other components of the diet as they affect the health and well-being of the U.S. population. Special emphasis is placed on how nutrients interact to provide maximum benefit to the immune system. New criteria are established to quantify requirements for specific micronutrients and to define their mode of action through studies that include the use of animal models. Cooperative research programs with other laboratories and various institutions and organizations within and outside the U.S. are established.

Phytonutrients Laboratory. The mission: to delineate the metabolism in humans of phytonutrients that are present in foods, understand the roles of these compounds in health promotion, and provide information relative to the intake of fruits, vegetables, and grains for the diverse population of adult.

Source: U.S. Department of Agriculture. Agricultural Research Service. Beltsville Human Nutrition Research Center homepage. http://www.barc.usda.gov/bhnrc/. Accessed October 25, 2004.

5.2.2 NUTRIENT DATA LABORATORY

The USDA has borne primary responsibility for characterizing the nutrient content of the U.S. food supply for over 100 years. The first food composition tables[19] were published in 1891 by Atwater and Woods, who assayed the refuse, water, fat, protein, ash, and carbohydrate content of approximately 200 foods.

Today, the USDA's Nutrient Data Laboratory (NDL) is one of the eight units at BHNRC. NDL and its predecessor organizations have been compiling and developing food composition databases for over a century. The mission of NDL's interdisciplinary team of nutritionists, dietitians, food technologists, and computer specialists is to develop authoritative food composition databases and state-of-the-art methods to acquire, evaluate, compile, and disseminate composition data on foods available in the U.S.

The Laboratory develops and maintains the Nutrient Databank System (NDBS), along with many nutrient-specific and population-specific databases. The NDBS contains data for about 8000 foods and 115 components as well as tables for compounds of special interest.

5.2.2.1 Nutrient Database for Standard Reference

The principal database in the NDBS is known as Release* 17 of the USDA Nutrient Database for Standard Reference[20] (SR), a system designed specifically to collect and disseminate food composition data. It is only available in electronic form. A search tool enables the user to retrieve the nutrient content of foods directly from NDL's Web site. The SR can also be downloaded onto a personal computer, a personal digital assistant (PDA), or a CD-ROM purchased from the Government Printing Office. NDL's databases need constant revision as the food supply constantly changes. The completeness of analytical data varies from nutrient to nutrient.[21] This database is the successor to the Agriculture Handbook No. 8, Composition of Food, published in hard copy until 1992, but no longer available in print form.

5.2.3 NUTRITIVE VALUE OF FOODS, HOME AND GARDEN BULLETIN 72

Data from Release 13 of the USDA National Nutrient Database for Standard Reference was used to create the most recent edition of Nutritive Value of Foods, Home and Garden Bulletin 72 (HG-72), published in 2002. Since its first publication in 1960, this reference has been an important source of food composition data for consumers, as well as a useful educational tool for dietitians and other professionals. The current version of HG 72 contains data on almost 1300 foods typically consumed in the U.S., expressed in common household units. The nutrients and other food factors in the table are water, calories, protein, total fat, fatty acids (saturated, monounsaturated, and polyunsaturated), cholesterol, total dietary fiber, calcium, iron, potassium, sodium, vitamin A (in IU and RE units), thiamin, riboflavin, niacin, and ascorbic acid. (See Box 5.14.)

---

* *Release* and *version* are synonymous terms.

Box 5.14 Nutritive Value of Foods URL

Nutritive Value of Foods, Home and Garden Bulletin 72, is available at: http://www.nal.usda.gov/fnic/foodcomp/Data/HG72/hg72_2002.pdf.

Source: U.S. Department of Agriculture. Agricultural Research Service. Products and Services. Data sets prepared by USDA-ARS's Nutrient Data Laboratory. Last Modified: August 31, 2006. Available at: http://www.ars.usda.gov/Services/Services.htm?modecode=12-35-45-00. Accessed January 11, 2007.

Box 5.15 Activity: Investigate State and Regional Maps

Investigate state and regional food and nutrition maps at: http://www.ba.ars.usda.gov/cnrg/services/cnmapfr.html.

Source: Bliss, R.M. Putting community nutrition on the map. *Agricultural Research.* 2003;51(4):16-17.

Box 5.16 Sources of Food and Nutrition Indicators for CNMap

- Information on nutrient intakes, healthy eating patterns, physical activity, and body weight come from the USDA Continuing Survey of Food Intakes by Individuals (CSFII) 1994–1996, 1998, which is available on CD-ROM.[1] All weight estimates are based on body mass index (BMI) values computed from self-reported height and weight obtained from CSFII participants.
- The percentages of individuals meeting the Dietary Reference Intakes (DRI) are based on day-1 nutrient intakes from the CSFII and DRI values established during the period from the mid-1990s to 2002.[2]
- Pyramid servings groups (fruit, grain, vegetable, dairy, and meat) estimates are for individuals 2 years old and over who meet the minimum daily servings recommendations.[3]
- Information on farmers markets was obtained from the Agricultural Marketing Service.[4]
- Food stamp participation rate is a combination of information from the USDA Food and Nutrition Service food stamp participation totals[5] and the Bureau of the Census household totals.
- Hunger information comes from the Food Security Supplement of the Current Population Survey,[6] which is conducted by the Bureau of the Census for the USDA Economic Research Service.
- Demographic information was obtained from the Bureau of the Census' QuickFacts Web site,[7] which includes data for cities and towns with more than 25,000 people.

Income and poverty values are model-based estimates created by the Bureau of the Census.

[1] USDA Food Surveys Research Group. CD-ROM: CSFII 1994–1996, 1998 Data Set. Available at: http://www.barc.usda.gov/bhnrc/foodsurvey/Cd98.html. Accessed May 19, 2005.

[2] The DRI reports may be accessed via www.nap.edu; Dietary Reference Intakes for Calcium, Phosphorous, Magnesium, Vitamin D, and Fluoride (1997); Dietary Reference Intakes for Thiamin, Riboflavin, Niacin, Vitamin B6, Folate, Vitamin B12, Pantothenic Acid, Biotin, and Choline (1998); Dietary Reference Intakes for Vitamin C, Vitamin E, Selenium, and Carotenoids (2000); Dietary Reference Intakes for Vitamin A, Vitamin K, Arsenic, Boron, Chromium, Copper, Iodine, Iron, Manganese, Molybdenum, Nickel, Silicon, Vanadium, and Zinc (2001); Dietary Reference Intakes for Energy, Carbohydrate, Fiber, Fat, Fatty Acids, Cholesterol, Protein, and Amino Acids (2002/2005).

[3] USDA Community Nutrition Research Group. Pyramid Servings Database for USDA Survey Food Codes and summary tables for Pyramid Servings Intakes by U.S. Children and Adults, 1994–1996, 1998. Available at: http://www.barc.usda.gov/bhnrc/cnrg/. Accessed May 19, 2005.

[4] USDA Agricultural Marketing Service. Farmers Market homepage. Available at: http://www.ams.usda.gov/farmersmarkets. Accessed May 19, 2005.

[5] USDA Food and Nutrition Service. Food Stamp Program: Average Monthly Participation (Households). Available at: http://www.fns.usda.gov/pd/fsfyhh.htm. Accessed May 19, 2005.

[6] USDA Economic Research Service. Food Security in the United States. Available at: http://www.ers.usda.gov/data/ foodsecurity. Accessed May 19, 2005.

[7] U.S. Census Bureau. State and County QuickFacts. Available at: http://quickfacts.census.gov/qfd/index.html. Accessed May 19, 2005.

5.2.3.1 Food and Nutrient Database for Dietary Studies (FNDDS)

FNDDS, formerly known as the USDA Survey Nutrient Database, is designed for the coding and analysis of food consumption data. It includes comprehensive information that can be used to code individual foods and portion sizes and contains nutrient values for calculating nutrient intakes. FNDDS data are for foods as consumed; many of the foods in FNDDS are mixtures not available in the SR (described in Section 5.2.2.1). The SR is the source of the nutrient values for foods in FNDDS, including the mixed foods whose nutrient values are calculated by combining the SR data for separate ingredients.

The FNDDS portion weights are for the portion sizes survey respondents report. Therefore, FNNDS includes additional weights for common food portion sizes not available in the SR. The FNDDS can be used in research projects using What We Eat in America and other dietary research studies to code foods and amounts eaten and to calculate the amounts of nutrient and food components in those foods. To date, FNDDS has been used in What We Eat in America, NHANES 2001–2002, and NHANES 2003–2004; the Healthy Eating Index (HEI); the Pyramid Servings Database; the Food Commodity Intake Database; and the National Cancer Institute (NCI) Diet History Questionnaire.

5.2.4 FoodLink and Pyramid Servings Database

FoodLink is a research tool intended to be used in specialized analysis of USDA food surveys. It consists of databases and tables that link USDA food codes to information on ingredients and commodities. FoodLink's databases are regularly updated with recent NHANES codes. An example of the databases in FoodLink is the Pyramid Servings Database for USDA Survey Food Codes Version 2. The Pyramid Servings Database was designed to allow researchers to measure food intakes in terms of servings. Released in 2004, this database[22] provides:

- Servings data using recommended sizes from the USDA Food Guide Pyramid
- Pyramid servings food data files containing the number of Pyramid servings per 100 grams of food categorized into 30 Pyramid food groups
- Pyramid servings intake data files for CSFII, 1994–1996, 1998 and for What We Eat In America, NHANES 1999–2000, 2001–2002, and 2004–2005
- Revised servings data for lean meat, grams of discretionary fat, and added sugar
- Complete documentation on how the database was developed
- Food descriptions, data formats, and model programs to join the servings data with food intake

The adequacy of the U.S. population's food intakes can be assessed in terms of Pyramid servings. For example, Pyramid servings data indicate that, on average, diets in 1994–1996 were below recommendations for the fruit, dairy, and meat groups and near the bottom of recommended ranges for the grain and vegetable groups. Calories from fats and sugars exceeded recommendations.[23] Based on the 1999–2002 data for individuals 2 years of age and over, the average number of grain products servings was 6.8, only 12% of which (0.8 servings) were whole grains.[24] However, the 2005 Dietary Goals recommends that at least half of grain products come from whole grains.

5.2.5 COMMUNITY NUTRITION RESEARCH GROUP (CNRG)

The mission of CNRG is to monitor and assess the capacity of communities to meet their food and nutrition needs for a better understanding of linkages between nutrition, agriculture, health, and community.

5.2.5.1 Community Nutrition Mapping Project

CNRG's Community Nutrition Mapping Project (CNMap) is a comprehensive database to be used for community assessments, nutrition program planning, implementation and evaluation, and food safety research. It combines data from 1994–1996, 1998 CSFII, and other sources with state geographic codes to provide a picture of food and nutrition indicators at the regional and state levels.[25] As not all states were included in the CSFII, omitted states were assigned the values of the estimates for their geographical region (Northeast, South, Midwest, and West). To further develop the mapping procedure and to provide specific community level data, CNRG conducted small studies to document and analyze nutrition and health indicators in two counties in Alabama.[26] The methodological approach used in these studies may be used as a model for conducting similar local or statewide surveys of other regions. According to the CNRG, specific community level data will be available in the future.

This resource tool provides a series of tables and color-coded customized maps at community, county, state, and national levels that can gauge whether a community is at risk for food security or other nutritional problems. For example, users can look up the percentage of individuals in a given state who meet the recommended dietary allowance (RDA) for a specific nutrient and the percentage of those meeting recommended Food Guide Pyramid servings.

Anyone with access to the World Wide Web can access CNRG's interactive Map Gallery. Public health nutritionists, community nutritionists, policymakers, and other public health professionals can create profiles in CNMap to gauge whether a state may be at risk for food security or other nutritional problems. Currently, the statewide and regional information described as follows is available; eventually, specific community level data will also be accessible:

- *Nutrient intakes*: Percentage of individuals meeting REE/DRI for energy, calcium, folate, iron, magnesium, niacin, phosphorous, protein, riboflavin, selenium, thiamin, Vitamin A, Vitamin B6, Vitamin C, Vitamin E, zinc, copper, and carbohydrate. DRIs are based on both day-1 nutrient intakes from the CSFII and the DRI value established during the period 1998 to 2002.
- Percentage of individuals using supplements.
- *Healthy eating patterns*: percentage of individuals meeting the Pyramid serving recommendations for vegetables, fruits, grains, meat, and dairy.
- Percentage of individuals with intakes at specified levels for: less than 30% of calories from total fat, less than 10% of calories from saturated fat, less than 300 mg of cholesterol intake, and less than 2400 mg of sodium intake.

- *Food security indicators*: percentage of households receiving food stamps and percentage of households not experiencing hunger. Hunger information comes from the Food Security Supplement of the Current Population Survey conducted by the Bureau of the Census for the USDA's ERS.
- *Demographics*: Percentages of the population who are white, black, American Indian and Alaskan Native, Asian, Native Hawaiian and other Pacific Islander, or other race; percentage of the population that is of Hispanic origin; numbers of adults > 25 years of age who are high school graduates and college graduates; medium household income, in dollars; percentage of households below poverty; and percentage of children below poverty. Demographic information is obtained from the Bureau of the Census.
- *Physical activity and body weight indicators*: Percentage of individuals who exercise at least once monthly, percentage of individuals at a healthy weight, and percentages of overweight children and adults. All weight estimates are based on BMI values computed from self-reported height and weight obtained from CSFII participants. Individuals over 20 years old with BMI values of 25 and over are in the overweight and unhealthy weight categories; those with BMI values less than 19 are in the unhealthy weight class.

5.2.6 COORDINATED FEDERAL NUTRITION MONITORING

The National Nutrition Monitoring and Related Research Act of 1990* (NNMRRA) was enacted to establish a comprehensive, coordinated program for nutrition monitoring and related research to improve the assessment of the health and nutritional status of the U.S. population. NNMRRA called for the following: a program to achieve coordination of federal nutrition monitoring efforts within 10 years and assist states and local governments in participating in a nutrition monitoring network; an interagency board to develop and implement the program; and an advisory council to provide scientific and technical advice and evaluate program effectiveness.[27] The act also required that Dietary Guidelines be issued every 5 years and that the HHS (and the USDA) and review in advance any dietary guidance issued by the federal government for the general public (see Chapter 11).

As defined in NNMRRA,[28] nutrition monitoring and related research refers to those activities needed to provide timely information about the role and status of factors relevant to the contribution nutrition makes to the health of the people of the U.S., including:

- Dietary, nutritional, and health status measurements
- Food consumption measurements
- Food composition measurements and nutrient data banks
- Dietary knowledge and attitude measurements (KA)
- Food supply and demand determinations

After 10 years, the act expired and very little of the infrastructure required to maintain a fully coordinated system remains in place today. Nevertheless, some of NNMRRA's major activities are maintained under other legislative authorities.[29] For example, the Dietary Guidelines must be reviewed every 5 years, and full integration of CSFII (USDA) and NHANES (HHS) has been realized. Under this integrated framework, HHS is responsible for sample design and data collection, whereas the USDA is responsible for dietary data collection methodology, maintaining the databases used to code and process the data, and data review and processing.[30] (See Box 5.17.)

---

* P.L. 101–445

Box 5.17 NNMRRA Activity

Although NNMRRA was not approved in 2000, a complementary bill, HR 2844 (the National Health, Nutrition, and Physical Activity Monitoring Act of 2005) was introduced in Congress 5 years later. The intent of HR 2844 was to reauthorize NNMRRA, strengthen the combined DHHS and USDA nutrition monitoring and research activities, and ensure sufficient resources for a national nutrition monitoring system. Use THOMAS at http://thomas.loc.gov/ to read HR 2844 and determine if the bill ever moved out of committee for further action on the House floor.

Source: H.R. 2844. National Health, Nutrition, and Physical Activity Monitoring Act of 2005. Available at: http://thomas. loc.gov/cgi-bin/query/query. Accessed July 10, 2005.

5.3 CONCLUSION

Because good nutrition is fundamental to good health, knowing the nutritional status of the population is essential to the practice of public health. Surveys, food consumption data, and analysis of nutrient content are important tools in assessing the nutritional status of the general population and in pinpointing those segments of the population at risk for particular health problems and needing targeted outreach. What We Eat in America, the premier food and nutrition survey in the U.S., provides insight into the general population. However, because pregnancy and fetal well-being, infancy, childhood, and adolescence are key predictors of future health, a number of surveys focus specifically on these stages of the lifecycle.

The science of nutrition surveys is continuously evolving as our technology and our food supply change. The complexity of data gathering and dissemination — who should collect the data, how should it be collected, who should be surveyed, what knowledge is needed, how should the data be analyzed and used — involves federal, state, and local agencies. Although the CDC is the principal agency for data collection and analysis, the USDA also provides key information on the food supply and composition.

5.4 ACRONYMS

AMPM	Automated multiple pass method
ARS	Agricultural Research Service
BHNRC	Baltimore Human Nutrition Research Center
BMI	Body Mass Index
BRFSS	Behavioral Risk Factor Surveillance System
CAPI	Computer Assisted Personal Interviewer
CDC	Centers for Disease Control and Prevention
CI	Confidence interval
CNMap	Community Nutrition Mapping Program
CNRG	Community Nutrition Research Group
CSFII	Continuing Survey of Food Intake of Individuals
DHKS	Diet and Health Knowledge Survey
DRI	Dietary Reference Intakes
EPSDT	Early periodic screening, diagnosis, and treatment
ERS	Economic Research Service
FFQ	Food Frequency Questionnaire
FNDDS	Food and Nutrient Database for Dietary Studies
FSRG	Food Survey Research Group
Hct	Hematocrit
Hgb	Hemoglobin
HHS	Department of Health and Human Services
HNRC	Human Nutrition Research Centers
IU	International units

LBW	Low Birth Weight
MCH	Maternal and Child Health Program
MEC	Mobile Examination Center
NCHS	National Center for Health Statistics
NCI	National Cancer Institute
NFCS	National Food Consumption Surveys
NHANES	National Health and Nutrition Examination Survey
NHES	National Health Examination Survey
NHIS	National Health Interview Survey
NNMRRA	National Nutrition Monitoring and Related Research Act of 1990
PedNSS	Pediatric Nutrition Surveillance System
PNSS	Pregnancy Nutrition Surveillance System
PRAMS	Pregnancy Risk Assessment Monitoring System
REE	Resting Energy Expenditure
SR	Standard Reference
USDA	United States Department of Agriculture
WIC	Women, Infants, and Children Supplemental Food Program
YRBSS	Youth Risk Behavior Surveillance System

REFERENCES

1. Clydesdale, F. *Functional Foods: Opportunities and Challenges*. IFT Expert Panel Report. Released March 24, 2004. Available at: http://members.ift.org/NR/rdonlyres/20B9EBDD-93B9-4B1B-B37B-3CF15066E439/0/FinalReport.pdf. Accessed July 12, 2005.
2. HHS Strategic Plan FY 2004–2009. Available at: http://aspe.hhs.gov/hhsplan/. Accessed July 21, 2006.
3. U.S. Department of Agriculture. Strategic Plan for FY 2002–2007. September 2002. Available at http://www.usda.gov/ocfo/usdasp/pdf/sp2002.pdf. Accessed October 31, 2004.
4. The material about the NHIS is taken directly from the NHIS description on its web-site: http://www.cdc. gov/nchs/about/major/nhis/hisdesc.htm.
5. Thompson, F.E., Midthune, D., Subar, A.F., McNeel, T., Berrigan, D., and Kipnis, V., Dietary intake estimates in the National Health Interview Survey, 2000: methodology, results, and interpretation. *J Am Diet Assoc.* 105, 352–363, 2005.
6. CDC. Behavioral Risk Factor Surveillance System. Available at: http://www.cdc.gov/brfss/index.htm. Accessed July 10, 2005.
7. U.S. Department of Health and Human Services. Centers for Disease Control and Prevention. Pediatric Nutrition Surveillance System. Available at http://www.cdc.gov/nccdphp/dnpa/pednss.htm/. Accessed October 27, 2004.
8. Polhamus, B., Dalenius, K., Thompson, D., Scanlon, K., Borland, E., Smith, B., and Grummer-Strawn, L. *Pediatric Nutrition Surveillance 2002 Report*. Atlanta: U.S. Department of Health and Human Services, Centers for Disease Control and Prevention, 2004. Available at http://www.cdc.gov/nccd-php/dnpa/pdf/PedNSS_2002_Summary.pdf. Accessed October 27, 2004.
9. CDC. What is PNSS? Available at: http://www.cdc.gov/pednss/what_is/pnss/index.htm. Accessed March 6, 2005.
10. Sherry, B., Mei, Z., Scanlon, K.S., Mokdad, A.H., and Grummer-Strawn, L.M. Trends in state-specific prevalence of overweight and underweight in 2- through 4-year-old children from low-income families from 1989 through 2000. *Arch Pediatr Adolesc Med.* 158, 1116–1124, 2004. Available at: http://archpedi.ama-assn.org/cgi/content/full/158/12/1116. Accessed March 5, 2005.
11. Yip, R., Parvanta, I., Scanlon, K., Borland, E.W., Russell, C.M., and Trowbridge, F.L. Pediatric nutrition surveillance system — United States, 1980–1991. *MMWR CDC Surveill Summ.* 41, 1–24, 1992.
12. Grummer-Strawn, L.M. and Mei, Z. Does breastfeeding protect against pediatric overweight? Analysis of longitudinal data from the Centers for Disease Control and Prevention Pediatric Nutrition Surveillance System. *Pediatrics.* 113, e81–e86, 2004.
13. Williams, L.M., Morrow, B., Lansky, A., Beck, L.F., Barfield, W., Helms, K., Lipscomb, L., and Whitehead, N. CDC. Surveillance for selected maternal behaviors and experiences before, during, and after pregnancy. Pregnancy Risk Assessment Monitoring System (PRAMS), 2000. *MMWR Surveill Summ.* 52(11), 1–14, 2003.

14. Phares, T.M., Morrow, B., Lansky, A., Barfield, W.D., Prince, C.B., Marchi, K.S., Braveman, P.A., Williams, L.M., and Kinniburgh, B. Surveillance for disparities in maternal health-related behaviors — selected states, Pregnancy Risk Assessment Monitoring System (PRAMS), 2000–2001. *MMWR Surveill Summ.* 53(4), 1–13, 2004.

15. Dwyer, J., Picciano, M.F., Raiten, D.J., and Members of the Steering Committee. Food and dietary supplement databases for What We Eat in America–NHANES. *J Nutr.* 133, 624S–634S, 2003.

16. Bliss, R.M. Researchers produce innovation in dietary recall. *Agric Res.* 52(6), 10–12, 2004.

17. Moshfegh, A.J. Researchers produce innovation in dietary recall. *Agric Res.* 10–12, June, 2004.

18. Putnam, J. Major Trends in U.S. Food Supply, 1909–1999. *Food Rev.* 23, 8–15, 2000. Available at: http://www.ers.usda.gov/publications/foodreview/jan2000/frjan2000.pdf. Accessed July 12, 2005.

19. Atwater, W.O. and Woods, C.D. The Chemical Composition of American Food Materials. U.S. Department of Agriculture. Office of Experiment Station. Bulletin No. 28. 1896. Available at http://www.nal.usda.gov/fnic/foodcomp/Data/Classics/es028.pdf. Accessed October 30, 2004.

20. U.S. Department of Agriculture, Agricultural Research Service. 2004. USDA National Nutrient Database for Standard Reference, Release 17. Nutrient Data Laboratory HomePage, http://www.nal.usda.gov/fnic/foodcomp. Accessed October 20, 2004.

21. Dwyer, J., Picciano, M.F., Raiten, D.J., and Members of the Steering Committee. Food and dietary supplement databases for What We Eat in America–NHANES. *J Nutr.* 133, 624S–634S, 2003.

22. Cook, A.J. and Friday, J.E. *Pyramid Servings Database for USDA Survey Food Codes Version 2.0.* Beltsville, MD: USDA, ARS, Community Nutrition Research Group, 2002. Available at: http://www.ba.ars.usda.gov/cnrg/services/deload.html#Pyramid. Accessed May 20, 2005.

23. Cleveland, L.E., Cook, A.J., Wilson, J.W., Friday, J.E., Ho, J.W., and Chahil, P.S., Pyramid Servings Data: Results from USDA's 1994 Continuing Survey of Food Intakes by Individuals. ARS Food Surveys Research Group. March 10, 1997. Available (under "Releases"): http://www.barc.usda.gov/bhnrc/ foodsurvey/pdf/Pynet_94.pdf. Accessed July 13, 2005.

24. Cook, A.J. and Friday, J.E. Pyramid Servings Intakes in the United States 1999–2002, 1 Day. [Online]. Beltsville, MD: USDA, Agricultural Research Service, Community Nutrition Research Group, CNRG, Table Set 3.0, 2004. Available at: http://www.ba.ars.usda.gov/cnrg/services/ts_3-0.pdf. Accessed July 13, 2005.

25. Harris, E., Nowverl, A. Community Nutrition Mapping Project (CNMAP). On Line ARS Community Nutrition Research Group web site, January 2002. Available at: www.ars.usda.gov/research/publications/ publications.htm?seq_no_115=193062, Accessed August 25, 2006.

26. Center for Urban and Rural Research, Alabama A&M University; Alabama Cooperative Extension System. *Food and Nutrition Indicators: County Profiles of Madison County, Alabama and Jackson County,* Alabama. September 2002. Available at: http://www.ba.ars.usda.gov/cnrg/services/alabmcounty. pdf. Accessed May 19, 2005.

27. Moshfegh, A.J. The national nutrition monitoring and related research program: progress and activities. *J Nutr.* 124(9 Suppl.), 1843S–1845S, 1994.

28. 7 U.S.C. §5302 (National Nutrition Monitoring and Related Research Act, definitions).

29. Kuczmarski, M.F. and Kuczmarski, R.J. Nutrition monitoring in the United States. In Shils, M.E., Shike, M., Ross, A.C., Caballero, B., and Cousins, R.J., Eds. *Modern Nutrition in Health and Disease,* 10th ed. Philadelphia, PA: Lippincott Williams and Wilkins, 2006, chap. 106.

30. Dwyer, J., Ellwood, K., Moshfegh, A.J., and Johnson, C.L. Integration of the continuing survey of food intakes by individuals and the national health and nutrition examination survey. *J Am Diet Assoc.* 101, 1142–1143, 2001.

6 Prevalence of Diet-Related Chronic Diseases: Disparities and Programs to Reduce Them

Injustice anywhere is a threat to justice everywhere.

Martin Luther King, Jr. (1929–1968)

Type 2 diabetes, end-stage renal disease, heart disease and stroke, cancer, and fetal alcohol syndrome (FAS) comprise the constellation of diet-related chronic conditions that affect racial and ethnic minority populations to a greater extent than the general population. As indicated in Box 6.1, all of these diseases are more prevalent in African Americans than in whites. In addition, FAS and type-2 diabetes are particularly prevalent among Native Americans, while the death rate from stomach cancer is substantially higher among Asians and Pacific Islanders, including Native Hawaiians, than among other populations. This chapter focuses on cardiovascular disease, diabetes, and cancer. We examine public health initiatives taken to reduce the burden of these diet-related chronic conditions, especially for health disparity populations (see Box 6.2).

6.1 THE LEADING DIET-RELATED CHRONIC DISEASES

The profile of diseases contributing most heavily to illness, disability, and death among Americans changed dramatically during the last century. Today, chronic diseases — such as cardiovascular disease (CVD) (primarily heart disease and stroke), cancer, and diabetes — are among the most prevalent, costly, and preventable of all health problems. Long-term illness and disability from these diseases result in extended pain and suffering and decreased quality of life for millions of Americans. The following sections look more closely at each of these conditions.

6.1.1 DIET AND CHRONIC DISEASE PREVENTION

Collectively, CVD, cancer, and diabetes account for two thirds of all deaths in the U.S. and about $700 billion in direct and indirect costs each year. The common causes of these chronic illnesses — physical inactivity, poor diet, and obesity — are not unique to any one of these conditions but are shared by each of them. These shared risk factors provide opportunities for prevention. Focusing attention on a limited number of risk factors and screening tests holds the potential to achieve greater progress in health promotion and disease prevention. Simplified, easily understood recommendations designed to reduce individual risk for CVD, cancer, and diabetes could become a unifying force for action and advocacy for communities and organizations as well as for individuals, their families, and clinicians.[1]

6.1.1.1 General Prevention Guidelines

In 2004 the American Cancer Society (ACS), the American Diabetes Association (ADA), and the American Heart Association (AHA) reviewed strategies for the prevention and early detection of cancer, CVD, and diabetes. The organizations launched a collaborative initiative to: (1) create national commitment to prevention and to improvement in primary prevention and early detection, (2) promote greater public awareness about healthy lifestyles, (3) support and initiate legislative action that results in more funding for and access to primary prevention programs and research,

Box 6.1 Health Disparities in Diet-Related Diseases

Fetal Alcohol Syndrome (FAS). FAS is a preventable condition that is six times more prevalent among African Americans than whites. Some Native American tribes have 33 times the incidence of FAS found in whites.

Heart Disease. There exists a disproportionate burden of death and disability from cardiovascular disease in minority and low income populations. The prevalence of coronary heart disease in African Americans has increased steadily since the early 1970s, with mortality 40% higher for African Americans than whites.

Stroke. Stroke is the third leading cause of death in the U.S., killing approximately 150,000 Americans every year. The incidence of stroke is disproportionately high in African Americans, where the mortality rate is nearly 80% higher than in whites.

Cancer. Cancer is the second most common cause of mortality in the U.S. Many minority groups suffer disproportionately from cancer, and disparities exist in both mortality and incidence rates. The death rate from stomach cancer is substantially higher among Asian and Pacific Islanders, including Native Hawaiians, than among other populations.

Type 2 Diabetes. Diabetes affects nearly 16 million Americans and leads to more than 300,000 deaths annually. It is also the leading cause of end stage renal disease (ESRD), peripheral neuropathy, adult blindness, and amputation. The prevalence of diabetes in African Americans is nearly 70% higher than in whites. Native Americans, Hispanics, African Americans, and some Asian Americans and Pacific Islanders, including Japanese Americans, Samoans, and Native Hawaiians, are at particularly high risk for development of type 2 diabetes. Prevalence rates among American Indians are two to five times those of whites, with the Pima tribe of Arizona experiencing one of the highest rates in the world.

End Stage Renal Disease: In 1997, the incidence rates of ESRD were 218 per million population in whites, as compared to 873 in African Americans, and 586 in Native Americans and Alaska Natives.

Source: U.S. Department of Health and Human Services. NIH Strategic Research Plan to Reduce and Ultimately Eliminate Health Disparities, Fiscal Years 2002–2006. 2000. Available at: http://www.nih.gov/about/hd/strategicplan.pdf. Accessed August 5, 2006.

Box 6.2 Health Disparities Definitions

The term *health disparities* refers to differences in the incidence, prevalence, morbidity, mortality, and burden of diseases and other adverse health conditions that exist among specific population groups, usually racial and ethnic minority groups.

Racial and ethnic minority group means American Indians (including Alaska Natives, Eskimos, and Aleuts); Asian Americans; Native Hawaiians and other Pacific Islanders; blacks; or Hispanics. The term "Hispanic" refers to individuals whose origin is Mexican, Puerto Rican, Cuban, Central or South American, or any other Spanish-speaking country (see also Section 3.3.4.1 and Box 3.5).

A population is a *health disparity population* if there is a significant disparity in the overall rate of disease incidence, prevalence, morbidity, mortality, or survival rates in the population as compared to the health status of the general population. Nationally, health disparity population groups include but are not limited to African Americans, Hispanic Americans, American Indians/Alaska Natives, Native Hawaiians, and Pacific Islanders; medically underserved, low socioeconomic populations; and rural populations.

Box 6.3 Prevention

Prevention: Interventions at the individual, group, or community level to provide targeted audiences with the knowledge and skills to avert or minimize health risks.

Source: Abeles, R.P., and Heurtin-Roberts, S. Foreword. NIH Conference on Understanding and Reducing Health Disparities: Contributions form the Social Sciences. October 23-24, 2006. Abstract Book. Available at: http://obssr.od.nih.gov/HealthDisparities/images/Health%20Disparities%20Final.pdf. Accessed January 11, 2007.

---

and (4) reconsider the concept of the periodic medical checkup as an effective platform for prevention, early detection, and treatment.[2]

As a component of these efforts, the three organizations developed general prevention guidelines for all average-risk adults that focus on primary prevention through diet and exercise, monitoring body mass index (BMI) and blood pressure, and screening for diabetes and CVD by periodically checking plasma glucose and serum lipid levels.

They provided a schedule of these screening tests, which should be performed on individuals beginning at age 20 (see Table 6.1). At each regular healthcare visit, BMI should be calculated and blood pressure measured (unless blood pressure is < 120/80mm Hg, in which case it only needs to be measured once every 2 years). A test for blood glucose should be performed every 3 years starting at age 40, and a lipid profile is recommended every 5 years. The statement also contains recommendations for colorectal screening and prostate specific antigen testing and digital rectal exams for men over 50 years of age.

TABLE 6.1
Schedule of Screening Tests Recommended by the ACS, ADA, and AHA

Screening Test	Frequency
BMI	Each regular healthcare visit
Blood pressure	Each regular healthcare visit. Reduce to at least once every 2 years if BP is < 120/80 mm Hg
Lipid profile	Every 5 years
Blood glucose test	Every 3 years after age 40
Clinical breast exam (CBE) and mammography	CBE every 3 years until age 40; annually thereafter. Mammography annually starting at age 40
Pap test	Annually until age 30; every 1–3 years thereafter, depending on type of test and past results
Colorectal screening	Screening frequency depends on test preferred, starting at age 50
Prostate specific antigen test and digital rectal exam	Offer test and exam yearly, and assist informed decisions starting at age 50

Source: Eyre, H., Kahn, E.H., Robertson, R.M., et al. ACS/ADA/AHA Collaborative Writing Committee. Preventing cancer, cardiovascular disease, and diabetes: a common agenda for the American Cancer Society, the American Diabetes Association, and the American Heart Association. This article was published jointly in 2004 in *CA: A Cancer Journal for Clinicians* (online: July 13, 2004; print: July/August: July 14, 2004); *Diabetes Care* (online: June 25, 2004; print: June 25, 2004); *Circulation* (online: June 15, 2004; print: June 29, 2004); and *Stroke* (online: June 24, 2004; print: June 24, 2004) by the American Cancer Society, the American Diabetes Association, and the American Heart Association. Available at: http:/CAonline.AmCancerSoc.org. Accessed July 2, 2006.

ACS, ADA, and AHA also encourage primary care practitioners to review these general preventive guidelines with all average-risk adults:

- Achieve and maintain a healthy weight
- Exercise for at least 30 min on 5 or more days a week
- Eat at least five servings of vegetables and fruits daily
- Encourage tobacco cessation

Basically, these are the recommendations in the 2000 edition of the Dietary Guidelines for Americans (see Table 11.9).

6.2 DEPARTMENT OF HEALTH AND HUMAN SERVICES (HHS)

Racial and ethnic minority groups will comprise an increasingly larger portion of the U.S. population in coming years. While continuing the progress achieved in improving the overall health of the American people, the federal government supports programs and projects specifically aimed at reducing health disparities. Responsibility for these functions rests within several branches of the Department of Health and Human Services (HHS) — the Office of the Secretary, the National Institutes of Health (NIH), and the Centers for Disease Control and Prevention (CDC) (see Figure 6.1).

According to the General Accounting Office (GAO) (see Box 6.4), HHS is the primary federal entity involved in projects and research aimed at understanding and addressing disparities in healthcare, including the areas of diabetes, heart disease, and cancer. HHS also plays a major role

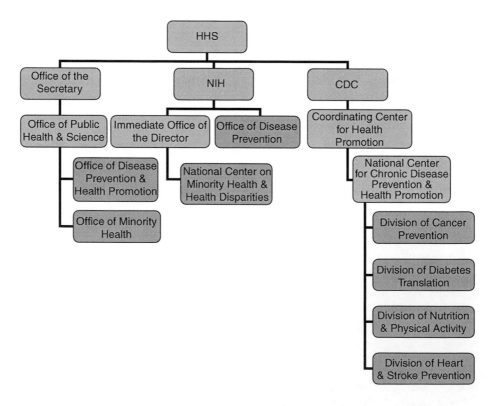

FIGURE 6.1 Agencies within HHS working to reduce health disparities. (From Maggie Meehan, M.A., R.D., M.P.H. Personal communication, 2006.)

Box 6.4 The General Accounting Office

The GAO is the audit, evaluation, and investigative arm of Congress. It exists to support Congress in meeting its constitutional responsibilities, and to help improve the federal government's performance and accountability. GAO examines the use of public funds, evaluates federal programs and policies, and provides analyses, recommendations, and other assistance to help Congress make informed oversight, policy, and funding decisions.

GAO documents are available through the GAO's Web site (www.gao.gov), which contains abstracts and full-text files of current reports and testimony, and an archive of older products. Each day a list of newly released GAO materials is posted under "Today's Reports," which contains links to the full-text document files. To be placed on the GAO e-mail list, go to www.gao.gov and select "Subscribe to e-mail alerts" under the "Order GAO Products" heading. The first copy of each printed report is free (but there is a charge for additional copies).

---

in financing healthcare for minority groups.[3] Also within HHS are located the Office of Minority Health (OMH) and the National Center on Minority Health and Health Disparities (NCMHD).

6.2.1 OFFICE OF THE SECRETARY

Two agencies under the direct purview of the Secretary are the Office of Disease Prevention and Health Promotion (ODPHP) and OMH.

6.2.1.1 Office of Disease Prevention and Health Promotion (ODPHP)

The mission of ODPHP is to work to strengthen the disease prevention and health promotion priorities of HHS within the collaborative framework of the HHS agencies. Health promotion programs under the aegis of the ODPHP include:

- *Steps to a HealthierUS* (Steps)[4] — Steps is the HHS's initiative to advance the HealthierUS goal of helping Americans live longer, better, and healthier lives. It will identify and promote programs that foster healthy behaviors and prevention. Priority areas for the Steps initiative are diabetes, obesity, asthma, heart disease, stroke, and cancer; also included are poor nutrition, physical inactivity, tobacco use, and youth risk taking (see Section 10.2.3.1).
- *Dietary Guidelines for Americans* 2005[5] — Published jointly with the USDA every 5 years since 1980, this publication is the statutorily mandated basis for many federal food assistance programs and for nutrition education activities (see Section 11.2.1).
- *Healthy People 2010*[6] — Released in 2001, Healthy People 2010 presents a comprehensive set of disease prevention and health promotion objectives developed to improve the health of all people in the U.S. during the first decade of the 21st century (see Section 10.2.2.3).
- *VERB™ It's What You Do*[7] — A national, multicultural, social marketing campaign that encourages young people ages 9 to 13 years ("tweens") to be physically active every day. The Youth Media Campaign focuses on motivating youth to increase physical activity in their lives, while helping parents, educators, and youth leaders appreciate the importance of physical activity to overall health (see Section 14.1.5.1.1).

6.2.2 OFFICE OF MINORITY HEALTH (OMH)

The OMH was established by HHS in 1986 to improve and protect the health of racial and ethnic minority populations through the development of health policies and programs that will eliminate health disparities. The Office advises the secretary of HHS and the Office of Public Health and Science (OPHS) on public health program activities affecting the racial and ethnic minority groups identified by the federal government.

6.2.3 NATIONAL INSTITUTES OF HEALTH (NIH)

The NIH is the primary federal agency for conducting and supporting medical research. NIH provides leadership and direction to programs designed to improve the health of the nation by conducting and supporting research in the causes, diagnosis, prevention, and cure of human diseases. Composed of 27 institutes and centers (see Figure 6.2), NIH provides leadership and financial support to researchers nationally and internationally. NIH's mission is to extend healthy life and reduce the burdens of illness and disability. Among its myriad goals, are protecting and improving health, and preventing disease. Of particular importance to nutrition in public health is the NIH Office of Disease Prevention (ODP), as well as the institutes listed in Table 6.2.

6.2.3.1 The National Center on Minority Health and Health Disparities (NCMHD)

The NCMHD was established by the passage of the Minority Health and Health Disparities Research and Education Act of 2000, P.L. 106–525. Its name makes its mission clear. The general purpose of the center is to conduct and support minority health disparities research, training, dissemination of information, and other programs with respect to minority health conditions and to other populations with health disparities.

6.2.3.2 Office of Disease Prevention (ODP)

The ODP is located within the office of the director of NIH. Its function is to coordinate research on disease prevention and health promotion across the 25 institutes and centers that comprise NIH. In particular, the ODP fosters, coordinates, and assesses research in prevention by collaborating with other federal agencies, academic institutions, the private sector, nongovernmental organizations and international organizations in the formulation of research initiatives and policies that promote public health.

The ODP advises the NIH on research related to disease prevention and health promotion and works with the NIH research institutes to initiate and develop requests for proposals (RFPs), requests for applications (RFAs), and program announcements (PAs) (see Section 16.2.1) to enhance program development.

6.2.4 CDC AND REACH

Racial and Ethnic Approaches to Community Health (REACH) is a cornerstone of the CDC's initiative to eliminate the disparities in health status experienced by ethnic minority populations (see also Section 7.2.3). It is designed to eliminate disparities in six priority areas, including cardiovascular disease and diabetes. In fiscal year 2005, Congress allocated $34.5 million for the REACH 2010 program, and $34.3 million in FY 2006. The program supports community coalitions in designing, implementing, and evaluating community-driven strategies to eliminate health disparities. Each coalition must include a community-based organization and three other organizations, at least one of which is either a local or state health department or a university or research organization. REACH 2010 grantees use local data to implement interventions that address one or more of the six priority areas and target one or more racial and ethnic groups. Sample community coalition activities include (1) continuing education on disease prevention for healthcare providers that emphasizes racial and ethnic differences among patients and 2) health education and health promotion programs that use lay health workers to reach community members.

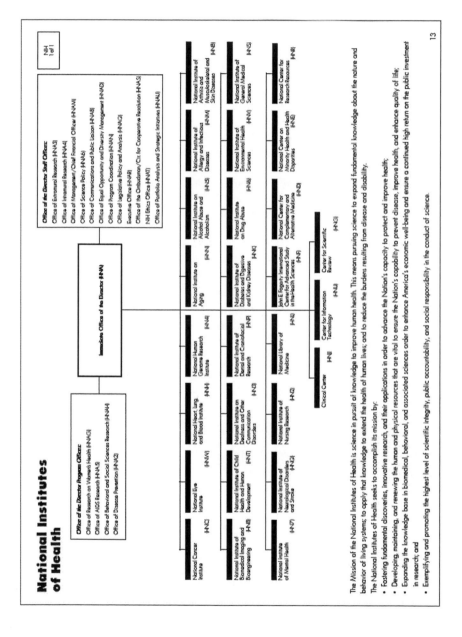

FIGURE 6.2 Organizational structure of NIH. (From http://www.pophealth.wisc.edu/ih/research/nihorg.pdf#search=%22organizational%20chart%20of%20the%20NIH%22.)

TABLE 6.2
Units of the National Institutes of Health with Nutrition

National Cancer Institute
National Heart, Lung, and Blood Institute
National Human Genome Research Institute
National Institute on Aging
National Institute on Alcohol Abuse and Alcoholism
National Institute of Allergy and Infectious Diseases
National Institute of Child Health and Human Development
National Institute of Dental and Craniofacial Research
National Institute of Diabetes and Digestive and Kidney Diseases
National Institute on Drug Abuse
National Institute of Environmental Health Sciences
National Institute of General Medical Sciences
National Institute of Mental Health
National Institute of Neurological Disorders and Stroke
National Library of Medicine
National Center for Complementary and Alternative Medicine
National Center on Minority Health and Health Disparities

Program priorities include expanding policy initiatives for environmental change, documenting the impact of cultural competency in coalitions, advancing the merits of community-based participatory research, and building program capacity to include research on social determinants of health. REACH 2010 will also help the CDC's Division of Adult and Community Health identify and disseminate effective community-based strategies to mobilize communities to improve the health of their residents and to reduce and eliminate seemingly intractable health disparities. The CDC will continue to expand this program by cultivating partnerships with national groups that can help support its mission.

Within the CDC are units that focus exclusively on (1) diabetes translation, (2) heart disease and stroke, (3) cancer prevention and control, and (4) nutrition and physical activity. These programs are described in the following sections.

6.2.4.1 Division of Diabetes Translation (DDT)

The CDC has had a diabetes division since 1977. In 1989, the name of the division was changed to the Division of Diabetes Translation (DDT), reflecting the division's mission to translate science into daily practice. The DDT is active in strengthening the public health surveillance systems for diabetes by working with those states using the diabetes-specific modules of the Behavioral Risk Factor Surveillance System (BRFSS) (see Section 5.1.3) to develop a nationwide, state-based surveillance system. It also conducts applied research that focuses on translating research findings into clinical and public health practice, such as the effectiveness of health practices to address risk factors for diabetes and demonstration of primary prevention of type 2 diabetes. The division provides funding for state-based Diabetes Prevention and Control Programs (DPCPs) throughout the U.S. Implementation of the National Diabetes Education Program (NDEP) is a joint initiative sponsored by the CDC and NIH, and provides public information about diabetes through various media strategies (see Section 6.4.6.1 and Section 11.3.2.2.1).

In 2004, CDC published *Diabetes: A National Plan for Action*.[8] Box 6.5 summarizes the plan's strategies for preventing diabetes as well as obesity and heart disease. Separate strategies are proposed for school personnel, healthcare providers, employers, community leaders, media spokespeople, researchers and professional educators, and government officials.

Box 6.5 Diabetes Prevention Strategies for School Personnel, HealthCare Providers, Employers, Community Leaders, Media Spokespeople, Researchers and Professional Educators, and Government Officials

Schools

The increase in type 2 diabetes among children makes schools essential partners in preventing the disease.

- Educate and share health promotion messages about sound nutrition and regular physical activity with teachers, school nurses, students, and parents.
- Educate children about the importance of balanced nutrition and regular exercise in preventing diabetes.
- Encourage children to develop plans for better nutrition and exercise and ways to measure their progress.
- Engage parents to increase their understanding of the importance of healthier diets and the benefits of exercise.
- Offer regular physical education/gym classes.
- Provide opportunities for unstructured activities for all ages at lunch and during breaks. For elementary school children, this might include actively participating in physical activities on the playground. For older students, sports equipment can be provided (e.g., basketballs, tennis rackets, etc.), with coaches encouraging participation in activities.
- Provide opportunities for nontraditional sports and alternatives to team sports for students who may not have the same physical talents as their peers.
- Provide after-school activities through the school or in partnership with other organizations, such as city parks and recreation leagues, religious organizations, community YMCAs, or boys and girls clubs.
- Provide tasty food options that are low in saturated fats and include fruits, vegetables, nuts, and whole grains for cafeteria and food cart choices.
- Provide healthy alternatives, such as milk, low-calorie beverages, or water in vending machines and in the cafeteria.
- Solicit help from school staff in setting examples for healthier eating and increased exercise.
- Foster the benefits of exercise through fun competitions and activities. For example, sponsor contests among teacher and student groups to register the most steps on their pedometers.
- Encourage all students to participate in exercise and support each other regardless of different abilities.
- Partner with State Diabetes Prevention and Control Programs run by the State Health Department.

Healthcare Providers

Healthcare providers play a key role in the prevention of type 2 diabetes. Medical providers are among the most important health messengers; patients are more likely to adopt new behaviors when instructed to do so by their health practitioners.

- Counsel patients with prediabetes about their risk of developing diabetes and develop a concrete plan for patients to help them decrease the likelihood of developing the disease.
- Refer high-risk individuals to appropriate resources for nutrition counseling and pre-diabetes education.
- Screen for overweight and obesity. Counsel patients who are overweight to lose weight. Set reasonable weight loss goals to avoid failure and frustration. Refer patients to local

resources or services that offer weight loss and physical activity programs and/or provide tools to help patients make lifestyle changes, activity logs, or meal plan guides.

- Provide information (e.g., handouts) on safe approaches to weight loss. Ready-to-use materials are available free of charge for providers through resources such as "Your Game Plan for Preventing Type 2 Diabetes: HealthCare Provider's Toolkit" (http://www.ndep.nih.gov/diabetes/pubs/GP_Toolkit.pdf).
- Encourage patients whose health permits to begin an exercise plan. Emphasize that even small steps can produce big rewards.
- Help patients set reasonable and realistic long-term and short-term exercise goals that can be measured over time so that they can see their successes.
- Build in accountability for patients. For example, after delivering the initial prevention messages and working with patients to set realistic goals, set up a reminder or follow-up system with patients who have been counseled to lose weight to assess progress and offer motivational messages.
- Acknowledge patients' efforts to adopt healthier behaviors, even if the initial changes reflect only part of the change needed.
- Encourage lifestyle changes for youth and counsel their parents on the importance of exercise and healthy eating to help prevent type 2 diabetes.
- Work with diabetes prevention and control programs run by the state health department.

Employers

Healthy employees are more productive and can be cost beneficial to companies. For example, a research study conducted on the return on investment (ROI) for worksite health promotion and disease prevention programs in nine companies, found significant ROI with the benefit to cost ratio ranging from $1.49 to $4.91 in benefits per dollar spent on the program.

- Be creative about developing exercise options. For example, think outside the "conference room box" by encouraging employees to hold discussions while walking with their colleagues rather than sitting in a conference room. The National Diabetes Education Program has developed tools to support providers in their efforts to encourage healthier lifestyle choices among their patients. These tools are available at http://www.ndep. nih.gov/resources/health.htm.
- Provide exercise space. For example, a conference room with a VCR player, a couple of low-impact aerobics tapes, and some low-cost mats made available at lunch time can serve as an exercise space for employees as well as a valuable networking activity that can improve morale and productivity.
- Provide healthy food options in cafeterias and vending machines.
- Encourage employees to adopt healthy behaviors. For example, offer contests with prizes to encourage exercise for employees.
- Consider providing health promotion or wellness programs and disease management programs for employees as part of their health benefits.
- Provide on-site education about diabetes prevention to employees.
- Utilize resources that are readily available at no cost to employers, such as Diabetes at Work (http://www.diabetesatwork.org/).
- Consider partnering with the local YMCA or community health club to offer discounted memberships to employees and their families.
- Partner with community organizations to develop and implement community health promotion and disease prevention initiatives.
- Request health insurers to provide appropriate information for employees to educate them on their health and diabetes prevention.
- Provide employees information about local parks and walking trails.

Communities

Local communities also play an important role in preventing or delaying type 2 diabetes by providing environments that promote healthier lifestyles through improved nutrition and increased physical activity. Civic and community organizations can partner with business groups, government agencies, and others to encourage healthier eating and increased physical activity for the community. Some actions communities can take to help prevent type 2 diabetes for their citizens.

- Promote environments that foster fitness, such as walking trails. Marking sidewalks with distance markers and messages can help encourage exercise.
- Encourage a community culture that promotes healthier eating habits. For example, community groups can sponsor "cook-offs" to create healthy culinary options among local chefs.
- Create community vegetable gardens.
- Organize community activities, such as community block parties with dancing and healthy food choices.

Media

The media serve as important partners in promoting diabetes prevention messages.

- Promote public awareness about the importance of diabetes prevention and the benefits of maintaining a healthy weight with regular physical activity and a healthy diet.
- Disseminate credible and accurate messages that encourage healthy habits and discourage risky behaviors. Media staff can help tailor messages to target specific audiences.
- Partner with medical professionals, federal, state, and local governments, and private sector community entities to help the public understand the importance of preventing diabetes. Publicize providers who are doing a particularly good job in facilitating behavior change or a hospital that has opened its doors to run a no-cost exercise program in a low-income area.
- Conduct or participate in research to study the effectiveness of media messages promoting healthy lifestyles.
- Use public access networks to broadcast local conferences or training videos on diabetes prevention.

Researchers and Professional Educators

Researchers and professional educators also play important roles in diabetes prevention.

- Continue research into the causes of type 1 and type 2 diabetes.
- Continue applied research into the prevention of diabetes and other relevant issues such as cost benefit analysis and evidence-based prevention strategies for combating the disease.
- Continue to conduct clinical trials like the DPP to prevent the onset of type 2 diabetes in individuals at high risk for developing the disease, such as minority populations.
- Continue to develop effective methods to translate research findings into clinical practice to prevent diabetes.
- Develop useful outcome measures for health promotion and diabetes prevention activities, services, and practices to assess progress in these areas, and provide information to inform program improvement.
- Develop and evaluate innovative methods to inform people about the importance of diabetes prevention and the link between the risk for diabetes and personal behaviors and choices, such as physical activity and dietary choices.
- Develop partnerships with community organizations to promote research and educational initiatives regarding diabetes prevention.

State and Local, Federal, and Tribal Governments

By taking action steps, the public sector plays an important role in (1) supporting healthy lifestyles among Americans that may prevent type-2 diabetes, (2) advancing research on how to prevent diabetes, and (3) supporting efforts to translate research into practice.

- Review and design policies that optimize strategies to address diabetes at all stages.
- Partner with communities and other entities to create environments that encourage healthy lifestyles and habits (for example, collaborate with communities to develop walking trails and parks where people can exercise safely) and implement initiatives.
- Disseminate information about the importance of healthy lifestyles to prevent diabetes. Tailor these messages to be meaningful to people of all ages, and cultural, socioeconomic, ethnic, and racial backgrounds.
- Support research on the effectiveness of different interventions to prevent diabetes.
- Conduct surveillance activities to measure progress toward achieving public health goals.
- Create an evidence base of effective strategies for preventing diabetes.
- Intensify prevention efforts among blacks, Hispanics, American Indians, and Alaska Natives, and other population groups who disproportionately suffer diabetes and its complications.
- Motivate government employees to adopt healthy lifestyles, thereby serving as a model to other employers.
- Foster interagency collaboration at federal, state, and tribal levels to promote healthy lifestyles in order to reduce the risks for diabetes.

Source: Adapted from U.S. Department of Health and Human Services. Diabetes: A National Plan for Action. Steps to a HealthierUS, 2004. Available at: http://aspe.hhs.gov/health/NDAP/NDAP04.pdf. Accessed August 5, 2006.

6.2.4.2 Division of Heart Disease and Stroke Prevention (DHDSP)

In 2006 the CDC formed the DHDSP,[9] whose mission is to provide public health leadership to improve cardiovascular health for all, reduce the burden of heart disease and stroke, and eliminate disparities associated with heart disease and stroke. The CDC released a public health action plan to prevent heart disease and stroke in 2003.[10]

6.2.4.3 Division of Cancer Prevention and Control (DCPC)

Through the DCPC, the CDC works with national cancer organizations, state health agencies, and other key groups to develop, implement, and promote effective strategies for preventing and controlling cancer.

6.2.4.4 Division of Nutrition and Physical Activity (DNPA)

The CDC's DNPA takes a public health approach to addressing the role of nutrition and physical activity in improving the public's health and preventing and controlling chronic diseases. The scope of the DNPA activities includes epidemiological and behavioral research, surveillance, training and education, intervention development, health promotion and leadership, policy and environmental change, communication and social marketing, and partnership development.[11]

The division maintains online interactive searchable databases. The Legislative Database makes available online (http://apps.nccd.cdc.gov/DNPALeg/) searches for state-level bills related to nutrition and physical activity topics. The DNPA state-based Physical Activity Program Directory site provides information about physical activity programs involving state departments of health.

6.3   OVERWEIGHT AND OBESITY

Estimates from the NHANES indicate that in 2003–2004, 17.1% of children and adolescents 2 to 19 years of age were overweight while 32.2% of adults were obese.[12] Although overweight and obesity occur in all population groups, prevalence varies by age, gender, race, ethnicity, and socioeconomic status (SES).

6.3.1   AGE

The prevalence of overweight and obesity increases with advancing age in both men and women, but starts to decline after the sixth decade of life. Analysis of data from the Behavioral Risk Factor Surveillance System (BRFSS) for 1994–1997 and from the National Health Interview Survey (NHIS) for 1993–1995 indicates that for the 50 states and District of Columbia, the prevalence of overweight decreases with increasing age among persons aged at least 55 years of age.[13]

6.3.2   GENDER, RACE, AND ETHNICITY

The prevalence of obesity varies by gender, race, and ethnicity. In 2003–2004, approximately one third of U.S. adults 20 years of age or older were overweight (BMI of 25 to 29.9), and another third were obese (BMI greater than or equal to 30). Overweight and obesity were more prevalent among minority women than among non-Hispanic white women. Non-Hispanic black women had the highest prevalence of obesity (53.9%), followed by Mexican American women (42.3%) and non-Hispanic whites (30.2%). Black men were more likely to be obese than their non-Hispanic white and Hispanic counterparts, although the prevalence of obesity among men differed little by race and ethnicity (31.1 to 34%).[14]

As indicated in Table 6.3, boys 2 to 19 years of age were more likely to be at risk of overweight or overweight than same-age girls. Considering the major racial and ethnic groups separately, overweight was estimated at 17.8% for non-Hispanic white boys and 14.8% of non-Hispanic white girls; 16.4 and 23.8% for non-Hispanic black boys and girls, respectively; and 22.0 and 16.2% for Mexican-origin boys and girls, respectively.

6.3.3   SOCIOECONOMIC STATUS

SES affects the prevalence of overweight and obesity in the population as a whole. Table 6.4 demonstrates an overall inverse relationship between poverty and obesity in adults (BMI greater than or equal to ≥ 30) and children (BMI ≥ 95th percentile on the sex- and age-specific 2000 CDC growth charts).

Women of lower SES are more likely to be obese than women with higher incomes. However, the likelihood that men will be overweight or obese is approximately equal regardless of SES group. Family income is not reliably associated with overweight prevalence among Mexican American and non-Hispanic black children and adolescents, although low-income non-Hispanic white adolescents are more likely to be overweight than those from higher-income families.

6.4   DIABETES

Diabetes is the fifth leading cause of death by disease in the U.S. Diabetes also contributes to higher rates of morbidity — people with diabetes are at higher risk for heart disease, blindness, kidney failure, extremity amputations, pregnancy complications, and deaths related to influenza and pneumonia.

6.4.1   EPIDEMIOLOGY

The prevalence of diabetes increases with age and is higher among certain racial and ethnic minority populations. The growth, aging, and increasing racial and ethnic diversity of the U.S. population portends a substantial increase in the segment of the population with diabetes.

TABLE 6.3

Prevalence of At-Risk of Overweight and Overweight in Children and Adolescents by Sex, Age, and Racial/Ethnic Groups for 2003–2004

	Male				Female			
	All (2–19 years)	2–5 years	6–11 years	12–19 years	All (2–19 years)	2–5 years	6–11 years	12–19 years
All (includes racial/ethnic groups not shown separately)								
At risk of overweight or overweight	34.8	27.3	36.5	36.8	32.4	25.2	38.0	31.7
Overweight	18.2	15.1	19.2	18.3	16.0	12.6	17.6	16.4
Non-Hispanic White								
At risk of overweight or overweight	35.4	26.6	35.6	38.7	31.5	23.5	38.2	30.4
Overweight	17.8	13.0	18.5	19.1	14.8	10.0	16.9	15.4
Non-Hispanic Black								
At risk of overweight or overweight	30.4	21.0	34.5	31.4	40.0	27.0	45.6	42.1
Overweight	16.4	9.7	17.5	18.5	23.8	16.3	26.5	25.4
Mexican American								
At risk of overweight or overweight	41.4	38.3	47.9	37.3	32.2	26.7	37.4	31.1
Overweight	22.0	23.2	25.3	18.3	16.2	15.1	19.4	14.1

Note: At risk of overweight: BMI for age at 85th percentile or higher. *Overweight*: BMI for age at 95th percentile of higher. Excludes pregnant females.

Source: Abstracted from Ogden, C.L., Carroll, M.D., Curtin, L.R., McDowell, M.A., Tabak, C.J., and Flegal, K.M. Prevalence of overweight and obesity in the United States, 1999–2004. *JAMA.* 295, 1549–1555, 2006. Available at: http://jama.ama-assn.org/cgi/content/full/295/13/1549. Accessed August 12, 2006.

Diabetes data are based on prevalence rates derived from the combined 1998, 1999, and 2000 files of the National Health Interview Survey (NHIS) (see Section 5.1.2). Combining 3 years' worth of the NHIS files created larger samples with which to estimate separate prevalence rates for each of 12 age groups by sex and by four race/ethnicity designations (see Box 6.6). The NHIS collects data on about 43,000 households of more than 106,000 people annually. Thus, the combined files for 1998–2000 created a sample of more than 320,000 individuals.

People with diabetes were identified using the survey question that asks whether the participant has been told by a doctor that he or she has diabetes (other than gestational diabetes). Responses to the question are coded as "yes," "no," "borderline," and "no response." People responding "yes" are coded as having diabetes. People responding "borderline" are not counted as having diabetes in this analysis.

Diabetes is becoming more and more common in the U.S. From 1980 through 2002, the number of Americans with diabetes more than doubled (from 5.8 million to 13.3 million);[15] it contributes to over 200,000 deaths a year. Type 2 diabetes affects 90%–95% of people with diabetes and is linked to obesity and physical inactivity. In fact, the increased prevalence of type 2 diabetes parallels the increased prevalence of obesity. More than 18% of adults older than age 65 have diabetes. Diabetes affects more women than men; its prevalence is 70% higher among African Americans

TABLE 6.4

Percentage of Overweight and Obese Adults and Overweight Children According to Poverty Status and Age, 1999–2002

	Adults				Children Overweight	
	Overweight		Obese			
Poverty Status	20–74 (age adjusted)	20 and over (age adjusted)	20–74 (age adjusted)	20 and over (age adjusted)	6–11	12–19
Poor	65.2	64.6	36	34.7	19.1	19.9
Near-poor	68.0	67.3	35.4	34.1	16.4	15.2
Non-poor	64.9	65.1	29.2	28.7	14.3	14.9

Note: Includes persons of all races and Hispanic origins. Data based on measured height and weight. Poverty status is based on family income and family size. Poor persons are defined as below the poverty threshold. Near-poor persons have incomes of 100% to less than 200% of the poverty threshold. Non-poor persons have incomes of 200% or greater than the poverty threshold. Persons with unknown poverty status are excluded.

Source: Adapted from Table 73: U.S. Department of Health and Human Services. National. *Health, United States, 2005. With Chartbook on Trends in the Health of Americans.* Hyattsville, MD: Center for Health Statistics, 2005. Available at: http://www.cdc.gov/nchs/data/hus/hus05.pdf. Accessed August 12, 2006.

than whites and nearly double the rate of Hispanics. The prevalence of diabetes among American Indians and Alaska Natives is more than twice that of the total population; the Pima of Arizona have the highest known prevalence of diabetes in the world. Diabetes can cause heart disease, stroke, blindness, and kidney failure, and can result in leg and foot amputations.

Box 6.6 Age and Race/Ethnicity Categories

The 12 age categories:
0–17
18–24
25–29
30–34
35–39
40–44
45–49
50–54
55–59
60–64
65–69
70 years

The four race/ethnicity categories:
Hispanic
Non-Hispanic white
Non-Hispanic black
Non-Hispanic other

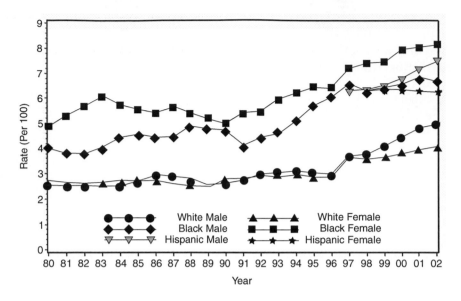

FIGURE 6.3 Age-Adjusted Prevalence of Diagnosed Diabetes per 100 Population by Race/Ethnicity and Sex, U.S., 1980–2002. (From Racial/Ethnic Disparities in Prevalence, Treatment, and Control of Hypertension — United States, 1999–2002. *MMWR*. 2005; 54(January 14): 7–9. Available at: http://www.cdc.gov/MMWR/preview/mmwrhtml/mm5401a3.htm. Accessed September 2, 2006.)

6.4.1.1 Prevalence

Currently, type 2 diabetes affects approximately 8% of adults.[16] Minority populations are affected disproportionately, as illustrated in Figure 6.3. According to data from the Third National Health and Nutrition Examination Survey (NHANES III, 1988 to1994) and NHANES (1999 to 2002), half of the adults in the U.S. who are diagnosed with diabetes are obese. Specifically, the prevalence of obesity among adults with diabetes was 45.7% (1988–1994) and 54.8% (1999–2002).[17]

If diabetes prevalence rates were to remain constant over time, controlling for age, sex, race, and ethnicity, then based on Census Bureau population projections, the number of people diagnosed with diabetes could increase to about 14.5 million by 2010 and to 17.4 million by 2020. It is likely that these figures are underestimates because the number of people with diabetes is based on self-reported data. These reports do not account for the considerable number of people with diabetes who do not report it or who are unaware they have the disease. About 5.9 million Americans are unaware they have diabetes.[18]

6.4.2 COST

In 2002, per capita medical expenditures totaled $13,243 for people with diabetes and $2,560 for people without diabetes. When adjusted for differences in age, sex, and race/ethnicity, people with diabetes had medical expenditures that were almost 2.5 times higher than expenditures than would be incurred by the same group in the absence of diabetes.

The direct and indirect costs of diabetes in 2002 were estimated at $92 billion and $40 billion, respectively, for a total of $132 billion. This estimate likely underestimates the true burden of diabetes because it omits intangibles such as pain and suffering, care provided by nonpaid (usually family) caregivers, and several areas of healthcare spending where people with diabetes probably use services at higher rates than people without diabetes (for example, dental care, optometry care, and the services of registered dietitians). In addition, this cost estimate excludes undiagnosed cases of diabetes. By 2010 and 2020 those totals are expected to reach $156 billion and $192 billion, respectively, based on the 2002 value of the dollar.[18]

TABLE 6.5
Diagnostic Thresholds for Diabetes and Lesser Degrees of Impaired Glucose Regulation

	TEST	
Category	Fasting Plasma Glucose	2-h 75-g Oral Glucose Tolerance Test
Normal	< 100 mg/dl (< 5.6 mmol/l)	< 140 mg/dl (< 7.8 mmol/l)
Impaired fasting glucose	100–125 mg/dl (5.6–6.9 mmol/l)	—
Impaired glucose tolerance	—	140–199 mg/dl (7.8–11.0 mmol/l)
Diabetes	≥ 126 mg/dl (≥ 7.0 mmol/1)	≥ 200 mg/dl (≥ 11.1 mmol/1)

Note: When both tests are performed, IFG or IGT should be diagnosed only if diabetes is not diagnosed by the other test. A diagnosis of diabetes needs to be confirmed on a separate day.

Source: From The Expert Committee on the Diagnosis and Classification of Diabetes Mellitus. Follow-up report on the diagnosis of diabetes mellitus. *Diabetes Care.* 26, 3160–3167, 2003. Available at: http://care. diabetesjournals.org/cgi/content/full/26/11/3160?ijkey=6bd479aa3ffe8753a6f9203c56a1b504c991198b & keytype 2=tf_ipsecsha. Accessed July 24, 2005.

6.4.3 PREDIABETES

Type 2 diabetes develops over a long period of time in adults, most of whom initially present with impaired glucose tolerance (IGT) and/or an impaired fasting glucose (IFG). IGT is defined as a plasma glucose concentration of 140 to 199 mg per deciliter (7.8 to 11.0 mmol per liter) 2 h after a 75-g oral glucose load. IFG is defined as a plasma glucose concentration of 100 to 125 mg per deciliter (5.6 to 6.9 mmol per liter) in the fasting state.[19] (See Table 6.5.)

Prediabetes in adults may be defined as the presence of IFG and/or IGT in individuals with a BMI greater than or equal to 25. Among Americans, 32% (31.0 million people) aged 40 to 74 years have IFG; 36.3% (or 37.3 million people) have prediabetes. IGT, an intermediate stage in the natural history of type 2 diabetes, predicts the risk of the development of diabetes and CVD.

Because strong evidence exists that appropriate changes in lifestyle can delay or prevent the progression from IGT to frank diabetes, emphasis has recently been placed on the early detection of glucose intolerance in overweight adults.[20] The immediate challenge is to implement programs and policies for diabetes prevention. The American Diabetes Association (ADA) recommends that all overweight people who are 45 years of age and older with prediabetes be considered candidates for diabetes prevention. People with prediabetes who are over 25 years with CVD risk factors, such as hypertension and dyslipidemia, are candidates for diabetes prevention, as well.[21]

6.4.4 METABOLIC SYNDROME

The metabolic syndrome is characterized by a cluster of risk factors in an individual. These factors include abdominal obesity (thought to be a better indicator of risk than BMI), hypertriglyceridemia, reduced high-density lipoprotein (HDL), hyperglycemia, and hypertension. Individuals who exhibit at least three of these medical conditions are defined as having metabolic syndrome.[22]

Table 6.6 presents the diagnostic criteria for these conditions. Of interest to those working with minority populations are the ethnic-group-specific (not country of residence-specific) waist circumference guidelines. These guidelines are suggested by the International Diabetes Federation for people from Europe, Central and Latin America, the Middle East, Asia, India, and Japan, regardless of their current residence.

TABLE 6.6
Clinical Identification of the Metabolic Syndrome

Indicator	United States Adult Treatment Panel III[a]	International Diabetes Federation[b]
Abdominal obesity, as measured by waist circumference. A high-risk waist line exceeds these measures	Women, 88 cm (35 in); men, 102 cm (40 in)	Europe: women, 80 cm (31.5 in), men, 94 cm (37 in); Central and Latin America, the Middle East, Asia, India: women, 80 cm (31.5 in), men, 90 cm (35.4 in); Japan: women, 90 cm (35.4 in), men, 85 cm (33.5 in); Other countries excluding North America): women, 80 cm (31.5 in), men, 94 cm (37 in)
Triglycerides	≥ 150 mg/dL (1.69 mmol/L)	≥ 150 mg/dL (1.69 mmol/L), or specific treatment for this lipid abnormality
HDL cholesterol		
Men	< 40 mg/dL (1.04 mmol/L)	< 40 mg/dL (1.04 mmol/L)
Women	< 50 mg/dL (1.29 mmol/L)	< 50 mg/dL (1.29 mmol/L), or specific treatment for this lipid abnormality
Blood pressure	≥ 130/85 mm Hg	≥ 130/85 mm Hg, or treatment of previously diagnosed hypertension
Fasting glucose	≥ 100 mg/dL (≥ 6.1 mmol/L)[c]	≥ 100 mg/dL (≥ 6.1 mmol/L), or previously diagnosed type 2 diabetes

[a] National Cholesterol Education Program. National Heart, Lung, and Blood Institute. Third Report of the National Cholesterol Education Program (NCEP) Expert Panel on Detection, Evaluation, and Treatment of High Blood Cholesterol in Adults (Adult Treatment Panel III) Final Report. NIH Publication No. 02-5215. National Institutes of Health. September 2002. Table II.6-1: Clinical identification of the metabolic syndrome, p. II-27. Available at: http://www.nhlbi.nih.gov/guidelines/cholesterol/atp3full.pdf. Accessed July 24, 2005.

[b] International Diabetes Federation (IDF). The IDF consensus worldwide definition of the metabolic syndrome. Available at: http://www.idf.org/webdata/docs/IDF_Metasyndrome_definition.pdf. Accessed August 4, 2006.

[c] In 2003, the American Diabetes Association changed the definition of impaired fasting glucose from 110 mg/dl to 100 mg/dl. Genuth, S., Alberti, K.G., Bennett, P., et al. Expert Committee on the Diagnosis and Classification of Diabetes Mellitus. Follow-up report on the diagnosis of diabetes mellitus. *Diabetes Care*. 26, 3160–3167, 2003.

Source: From National Heart, Lung, and Blood Institute. Table 3: Classification of blood pressure for adults in: Seventh Report of the Joint National Committee on Prevention, Detection, Evaluation, and Treatment of High Blood Pressure. U.S. Department of Health and Human Services. National Institutes of Health, August 2004. Available at: http://www.nhlbi.nih.gov/guidelines/hypertension/jnc7full.pdf. Accessed March 20, 2005.

Box 6.7 Age-Adjusted Incidence Rates

Age-adjusted rates are commonly used when comparing incidence rates, especially with chronic diseases such as heart disease and diabetes. Age adjustment is a statistical method used to allow health measures (such as rates of disease, death, or injuries) to be compared between communities with different age distributions. For example, populations with higher percentages of older residents will almost always have much higher crude incidence rates for major chronic conditions, compared to populations with younger populations. Age-adjusting incidence rates eliminates the bias of age in the composition of the populations being compared, thereby providing a much more reliable rate for comparison purposes.

People with the metabolic syndrome are at increased risk for developing diabetes and CVD as well as for increased mortality both from CVD and from all causes.[23] The NHANES III data indicate that consumption of fruits and vegetables is low among people with the metabolic syndrome. At the same time, adults with the syndrome have suboptimal concentrations of several antioxidants, which may partially explain their increased risk for diabetes and cardiovascular disease.[24]

Using 2000 census data, about 47 million U.S. residents (about one quarter of the population) have the metabolic syndrome.[25] The unadjusted prevalence of the syndrome in adults was 23.1% in NHANES III, and the age-adjusted prevalence was 24.1%.[26] Prevalence of the syndrome increased from 6.7% among survey participants aged 20–29 to 43.5% for participants aged 60–69 and 42.0% for those aged at least 70 years. Mexican Americans had the highest age-adjusted prevalence (31.9%). Among African Americans and Mexican Americans, women had a higher prevalence than men did.[27]

In a comparison of NHANES (1999–2000) data to NHANES III (1988–1994) data, the age-adjusted prevalence of the metabolic syndrome for women and men increased by 23.5% and 2.2%, respectively. Increases in high blood pressure, hypertriglyceridemia, and waist circumference accounted for much of the increase, particularly among women.[28] Continuing the comparisons between NHANES and NHANES III data, the unadjusted waist circumference in adults increased from 95.3 cm (age-adjusted, 96.0 cm) to 98.6 cm (age-adjusted, 98.9 cm) among men, and from 88.7 cm (age-adjusted, 88.9 cm) to 92.2 cm (age-adjusted, 92.1 cm) among women (see Box 6.7). These results demonstrate the rapid increase in obesity, especially abdominal obesity, among U.S. adults.[29]

6.4.5 End-Stage Renal Disease (ESRD)

ESRD is a complete or near-complete failure of the kidneys to excrete wastes, concentrate urine, and regulate electrolytes. The most common cause of ESRD in the U.S. is diabetes. ESRD occurs when the kidneys are no longer able to function at a level necessary for day-to-day life. It usually occurs as chronic renal failure progresses to the point where kidney function is less than 10% of baseline. At this point, kidney function is so diminished that without dialysis or kidney transplantation, complications are multiple and severe, and death will occur from accumulation of fluids and waste products in the body. Dialysis or kidney transplantation are the only treatments for ESRD. In the U.S., nearly 300,000 people are on long-term dialysis and more than 20,000 have a functioning transplanted kidney. Other treatments of chronic kidney failure may continue but are ineffective without dialysis or transplantation.

6.4.6 Treatment

The Diabetes Prevention Program (DPP) (see Box 6.8) has demonstrated that lifestyle modification is a cost-effective strategy to prevent type 2 diabetes in adults having impaired glucose tolerance. Lifestyle intervention in high-risk individuals provides greater health benefits at a lower cost than drug therapy and is thus the most fiscally responsible intervention choice for addressing the U.S. diabetes epidemic.[30] To that end, in 2005 the Joslin Diabetes Center released clinical nutrition guidelines for overweight and obese adults with type 2 diabetes, prediabetes, or at high risk for developing type 2 diabetes.[31] The nutrition and physical activity guidelines recommend approximately 40% of a person's daily calories come from carbohydrates; 20 to 30% from protein (unless the person has kidney disease); 30–35% from fat (mostly mono- and polyunsaturated fats), with at least 20–35 grams of fiber.

To initiate and continue weight reduction, a modest goal of one pound every one to two weeks is advised by reducing daily caloric intake by 250 to 500 cal. Total daily calories should not be less than 1,000 to 1,200 for women and 1,200 to 1,600 for men. A target of 60 to 90 min of modest intensity physical activity most days of the week, with a minimum of 150–175 min/week, is encouraged and should include cardiovascular, stretching, and resistance activities to maintain or increase lean body mass. Joslin's guidelines complement the 2005 *Dietary Guidelines for Americans.*

Box 6.8 The Diabetes Prevention Program (DPP)

DPP[1] is a large-scale, multisite randomized clinical trial designed to evaluate the safety and efficacy of interventions that may delay or prevent development of diabetes in people at increased risk for type 2 diabetes. Randomization of participants into the DPP over 2.7 years ended in June 1999. Nondiabetic persons (n = 3234) with elevated fasting and postload plasma glucose concentrations were randomly assigned to placebo, metformin (850 mg twice daily), or a lifestyle-modification program. The medication group received standard lifestyle recommendations in the form of written information and in an annual 20- to 30-min individual session that emphasized the importance of a healthy lifestyle. Participants were encouraged to follow the Food Guide Pyramid[2] and the equivalent of a National Cholesterol Education Program Step 1 diet,[3] to reduce their weight, and to increase their physical activity. The goals for the participants assigned to the intensive lifestyle intervention were to achieve and maintain a weight reduction of at least 7% of initial body weight through a healthy, low-calorie, low-fat diet and to engage in physical activity of moderate intensity, such as brisk walking, for at least 150 min per week. A 16-lesson curriculum covering diet, exercise, and behavior modification was designed to help the participants achieve these goals. The curriculum, taught by case managers on a one-to-one basis during the first 24 weeks after enrollment, was flexible, culturally sensitive, and individualized. Subsequent individual monthly sessions and group sessions with the case managers were designed to reinforce the behavioral changes.

The mean age of the participants was 51 years, and the mean body-mass index was 34.0. The population was 68% female and 45% were members of minority groups. The average follow-up was 2.8 years. The program was able to demonstrate that the most effective treatment was lifestyle intervention, followed by medication and placebo. The incidence of diabetes was 4.8, 7.8, and 11.0 cases per 100 persons in the lifestyle, drug, and placebo, groups, respectively. The lifestyle intervention reduced the incidence of diabetes by 58% (95% confidence interval, 48 to 66%) and the drug by 31% (95% confidence interval, 17 to 43%), as compared with placebo.

The lifestyle intervention manuals that were developed by the DPP Study Group are available on the DPP homepage at http://www.bsc.gwu.edu/dpp/index.htmlvdoc.

Sources:

[1] Knowler, W.C., Barrett-Connor, E., Fowler, S.E., Hamman, R.F., Lachin, J.M., Walker, E.A., and Nathan, D.M. Diabetes Prevention Program Research Group. Reduction in the incidence of type 2 diabetes with lifestyle intervention or metformin. *N Engl J Med*. 346, 393–403, 2002.

[2] The Food Guide Pyramid. Washington, D.C.: Department of Agriculture, Center for Nutrition Policy and Promotion, 1996. (Home and Garden Bulletin no. 252.)

[3] Step by step: eating to lower your high blood cholesterol. Bethesda, MD.: National Heart, Lung, and Blood 15.996 ptInstitute Information Center, 1987.

If successful, intensive efforts to reduce obesity in children who have impaired glucose tolerance through increased physical activity and better eating habits are likely to help to prevent their developing type 2 diabetes. Ongoing efforts to prevent and treat type 2 diabetes will require community and government involvement to reduce obesity and increase physical activity in both pediatric and adult populations. Women of childbearing age are also being targeted because exposure to obesity with or without diabetes *in utero* may be a major contributor to the increase in type 2 diabetes during childhood and adolescence. A number of government initiatives are underway.[32]

6.4.6.1 National Diabetes Education Program (NDEP)

HHS's NDEP was launched in 1997 to improve diabetes management and thus reduce the morbidity and mortality from diabetes and its complications among Americans with diabetes. NDEP is sponsored by NIDDK of the NIH and the CDC's DDT. The results of the Diabetes Prevention Program (DPP)[33] clinical trial (see Box 6.8) added a dramatic message to NDEP's outreach: among high-risk individuals: the onset of diabetes can be prevented or delayed. DPP showed that modest weight loss through regular physical activity and healthy eating could cut the risk of developing type 2 diabetes by more than half in people with prediabetes. Beginning in 2002, NDEP released messages and materials to translate the science of diabetes prevention into clinical practice and to raise awareness among high risk individuals. "Small Steps. Big Rewards. Prevent Type 2 Diabetes," the first national diabetes prevention campaign, targets Americans with prediabetes with tailored materials and messages for each high risk audience.[34]

6.5 DIABETES IN CHILDREN

The emerging public health problem of type 2 diabetes in youth reflects the increasing rates of childhood obesity discussed in Section 7.1.1. Type 2 diabetes has been described as a new epidemic in the American pediatric population. In 1992, type 2 diabetes was a rare occurrence in most pediatric centers, but by 1994, it represented up to 16% of new cases of diabetes diagnosed in urban areas, and by 1999 the incidence of new type 2 diagnoses in children ranged between 8% and 45%, depending on geographic location. This increased incidence has been observed primarily in African American, Mexican American, Native American, and Asian American children and youth.[35] Type 2 diabetes is now a common disease in American Indian children aged 10 or more years, which has increased dramatically over time, along with increasing weight. The Pima in Arizona are the group with the highest prevalence.[36]

6.5.1 DIAGNOSIS

According to the NDEP, only children at substantial risk for the presence or the development of type 2 diabetes should be tested. The primary factors that place youth at risk for type 2 diabetes in childhood include ancestry (African American, Alaska Native, American Indian, Asian and Pacific Islander American, and Hispanic American), obesity, and relatives with type 2 diabetes. Other risk factors include *Acanthosis nigricans*, hypertension, dyslipidemia, or polycystic ovarian syndrome (see Box 6.9).

Box 6.9 Testing Criteria and Diabetes Risk Factors for Early Identification of Type 2 Diabetes in Children

Overweight (BMI > 85th percentile for age and gender), plus any two of these risk factors: family history of type 2 diabetes in first- or second-degree relative; race/ethnicity of American Indian, African American, Hispanic/Latino, Asian American, or Pacific Islander; and/or signs of insulin resistance or conditions associated with insulin resistance, such as *Acanthosis nigricans* (the skin around the neck or in the armpits appears dark, thick, and feels velvety), hypertension, dyslipidemia, or polycystic ovarian syndrome. If a child is found to be at risk, then begin testing with a fasting plasma glucose at age 10 years or at onset of puberty, whichever occurs first; test every 2 years.

Source: Bobo, N., Evert, A., Gallivan, J., et al. Diabetes in Children Adolescents Work Group of the National Diabetes Education Program. An update on type 2 diabetes in youth from the National Diabetes Education Program. *Pediatrics.* 114, 259–263, 2004.

Box 6.10 The *We Can!* Parent Handbook

The *We Can!* parent handbook is available in hardcover at no cost, and also online. The balance of the materials for the program may be obtained online at: http://www.nhlbi.nih.gov/health/public/heart/obesity/wecan/.

Source: National Institutes of Health. *We Can! Families Finding the Balance. A Parent Handbook.* National Heart, Lung, and Blood Institute, National Institute of Diabetes and Digestive and Kidney Diseases, National Institute of Child Health and Human Development, National Cancer Institute. NIH Publication No. 05-5273. June 2005.

6.5.2 PREVALENCE

Very limited information about the epidemiology of type 2 diabetes in youth exists, although it is believed that the prevalence is increasing rapidly. Risk factors similar to those in adults with type 2 diabetes such as obesity and positive family history are thought to be important. However, there are no reliable epidemiologic studies of these risk factors in youth with type 2 diabetes using appropriate controls.

The prevalence of type 2 diabetes in children is difficult to determine because it can go undiagnosed for a long time, because children may have no or mild symptoms, and because blood tests are needed for diagnosis. The diagnostic criteria for type 2 diabetes in children have not been established, nor have they been established for differentiating between types of diabetes in children. For example, children with type 2 can develop ketoacidosis (common to type 1), whereas children with type 1 can be overweight (more likely with type 2). In addition, the overall prevalence of the disease may still be low.[37]

6.5.2.1 SEARCH for Diabetes in Youth

In response to the growing public health concern about type 2 diabetes in children, CDC and the National Institute of Diabetes and Digestive and Kidney Diseases (NIDDK) at NIH funded a 5-year, multicenter study — SEARCH for Diabetes in Youth (2000–2005) — to examine the current status of diabetes among children and adolescents in the U.S. The main objectives of the project

---

Box 6.11 Heart Disease and Stroke

Cardiovascular disease: Cardiovascular refers to the heart and blood vessels. ("Cardio" means heart; "vascular" means blood vessels.) Thus, cardiovascular disease refers to diseases of the heart and blood vessels.

Coronary Heart Disease (CHD): Disease of the heart caused by atherosclerotic narrowing of the coronary arteries likely to produce chest pain (angina pectoris) or heart attack.

Stroke (or cerebrovascular accident, CVA): An interruption of blood flow to the brain causing paralysis, slurred speech, and/or altered brain function. It may be caused by a blood clot blocking circulation or by bleeding into brain tissue causing tissue damage. A stroke can happen when a blood vessel carrying blood to the brain is blocked by a blood clot (*ischemic stroke*) or when a blood vessel breaks open due to trauma or an aneurysm ruptures, causing blood to leak into the brain (*hemorrhagic stroke*).

For the sake of brevity, these conditions are referred to as *heart disease* and *stroke*.

Source of definitions: American Heart Association. Cardiac Glossary. Available at: http://americanheart.org/presenter. jhtml?identifier=3038158#ablation. Accessed February 16, 2007.

are to assess the magnitude and burden of diagnosed diabetes through a multicenter registry system that covers more than 6% of the children and adolescents in the U.S., and to develop criteria to differentiate between the types of diabetes among young people in the U.S.[38] The prevalence of type 2 diabetes will be available from the CDC by the time this book is published.

In 2005 SEARCH was refunded for a second cycle (2006–2010).[39] Its funding may continue after 2010, as the longitudinal SEARCH elucidates the natural history of type 2 diabetes in children.

6.5.3 METABOLIC SYNDROME

In a sample of adolescents in the U.S. who were included in NHANES III (1988–1994), the prevalence of the metabolic syndrome was 6.8% among adolescents at risk of overweight (BMI 85th to < 95th percentile) and 28.7% among adolescents who were overweight (BMI ≥ 95th percentile), compared with 0.1% of those with a BMI < 85th percentile. Based on population-weighted estimates, in the mid-1990s, approximately 910,000 U.S. adolescents had the metabolic syndrome, approximately 4% of adolescents and nearly 30% of overweight adolescents in the U.S.[40]

When the effect of different degrees of overweight on the prevalence of the metabolic syndrome was studied in 430 overweight children and adolescents, its prevalence was found to be high and increased with increasing BMI. The syndrome reached 50% in the most overweight children and adolescents, a finding that has significant implications both for public health and clinical interventions.[41] Small studies suggest hypotheses for larger investigations, such as secondary analyses of NHANES data. For example, a study of metabolic syndrome in 163 predominantly white, ostensibly low-risk college students found that an unexpected 27% were overweight, 10% were dyslipidemic, and 6% were prediabetic.[42] These results need to be confirmed in studies with larger sample sizes in order to confidently recommend aggressive education among low risk as well as high risk groups, even in the absence of disease.

Because the implications of the metabolic syndrome for healthcare are substantial from a public health standpoint, identification of individuals with the metabolic syndrome may provide opportunities to intervene earlier in the development of shared disease pathways that predispose individuals to both diabetes and CVD.[43]

6.5.4 ETIOLOGY

Of the forms of diabetes that occur in children and youth, only type 2 diabetes is increasing in incidence. The other types of diabetes include: type 1, occurring in all races; atypical diabetes, seen as an autosomal dominantly transmitted disorder in African American populations; and maturity-onset diabetes of the young, seen rarely and only in Caucasians.[44]

Several risk factors have been identified as contributors to the development of type 2 diabetes and cardiovascular risk in youth. These factors include increased body and abdominal fat, insulin resistance, ethnicity (with greater risk in African American, Hispanic, and Native American children), and onset of puberty. There is no clear explanation of how these factors increase risk, although they appear to act in an additive fashion. The constellation of these risk factors may be especially problematic during the critical period of adolescent development, especially in individuals who may have compromised ß-cell function and an inability to compensate for severe insulin resistance.[45]

Another contributor to the increase in type 2 diabetes during childhood and adolescence may be exposure to diabetes or obesity *in utero*. Children who were large-for-gestational-age (birth weight > 90th percentile) and exposed to an intrauterine environment of either diabetes or maternal obesity are at increased risk of developing metabolic syndrome. Additionally, children exposed to maternal obesity alone are at increased risk of developing metabolic syndrome, suggesting that obese mothers who do not meet the clinical criteria for gestational diabetes may still have metabolic factors that affect fetal growth and postnatal outcomes.[46] Given the increased obesity prevalence, these findings have implications for perpetuating the cycle of obesity, insulin resistance, and its consequences in subsequent generations.

6.5.5 Epidemiology

Type 2 diabetes in youth is largely accounted for by minority populations and, as in adults, is associated with obesity. Overweight children and adolescents are now being diagnosed with IGT and type 2 diabetes. In addition, they evince early signs of the insulin resistance syndrome and cardiovascular risk. IGT and type 2 diabetes may not necessarily be new phenomena in children, but they are becoming more apparent as health screening measures improve. In addition, these risks may be affecting more absolute numbers of children concomitant with changing food patterns and increasing obesity rates.

Although no ethnic group is free of the problem, the disease disproportionately affects American Indian, African American, Mexican American, and Pacific Islander youth. True population-based prevalence data were not available as recently as 2004. However, extrapolating from NHANES III, for youth in the 12 to 19 year age group, 4.1 per 1000 had diabetes. However, depending upon the group, prevalence is estimated to be between 2 and 50 per 1000. In 15- to 19-year-old Pima Indians of Arizona, the prevalence of type 2 diabetes is 5%[47] (50 cases per 1000 population).

6.5.6 Prevention

Primary prevention of type 2 diabetes in children should ideally include a public health approach that targets the general population. Health professionals need to be involved in developing and implementing school- and community-based programs to promote improved dietary and physical activity behaviors for all children and their families. Programs that provide children and their families with the knowledge, attitudes, behavioral skills, and encouragement to consume a healthy diet and engage in regular physical activity may be effective in attenuating the expanding problem of obesity.

At the community level, schools, religious organizations, youth and family organizations, and government agencies should assume some responsibility for promoting a healthy lifestyle. School programs should promote healthy food choices and increased physical activity. Planning effective preventive efforts for populations at risk needs to involve members of the community (see Section 12.2.1).[48] The same public health programs that aim to increase physical activity, decrease sedentary behaviors, and decrease overweight and obesity count as their primary or secondary goals the decreased prevalence of type 2 diabetes in children and adults. SEARCH is expected to suggest future programs and interventions.[49,50]

6.5.6.1 *We Can!*

Ways to Enhance Children's Activity & Nutrition! (*We Can!*) was developed as a focused, collaborative, national public education outreach effort to help combat the persistent rise in overweight and obesity in the U.S. by creating synergy among public and private programs with related goals[51] (see Section 14.1.5.1.2). The program targets youth ages 8 to 13 and their parents and caregivers in home and community settings. Launched in 2005, *We Can!* features resources and activities for children, their parents, and caregivers and community-based programs that encourage healthy eating, increased physical activity, and reduced time engaged in sedentary activities. For example, a goal of the program is to help parents develop the skills to teach their children to:

- Eat a sufficient amount of a variety of fruits and vegetables every day
- Choose small portions at home and at restaurants
- Eat fewer high-fat and energy-dense foods that are low in nutrient value such as French fries, bacon, and doughnuts
- Substitute water or fat-free or low-fat milk for sweetened beverages such as sodas
- Engage in at least 60 min of moderate physical activity on most, preferably all, days of the week
- Reduce recreational screen time to no more than 2 h/d[52]

We Can! was developed by the Obesity Education Initiative at the National Heart, Lung, and Blood Institute (NHLBI). Because achieving and maintaining a healthy weight is a universal chronic disease prevention goal, the program is promoted by the NHLBI in collaboration with three other NIH Institutes: NIDDK, the National Cancer Institute (NCI), and the National Institute of Child Health and Human Development, as well as several national private sector organizations.

6.6 CARDIOVASCULAR DISEASE (CVD)

Almost one-fourth of the U.S. population has some form of CVD. Nationally, heart disease and stroke are the first and third leading causes of mortality, accounting for more than 40% of all deaths. About 950,000 Americans die of heart disease. Although this disease is often thought to affect men and older people primarily, it is also a major killer of women and people in the prime of life. Looking at only deaths due to CVD, however, understates the health effects of these two conditions. The economic effects of CVD on the U.S. healthcare system grows larger as the population ages.

6.6.1 HEART DISEASE

Heart disease is the nation's leading cause of death. Much of the burden of heart disease could be eliminated by reducing the prevalence rates of its major risk factors: high blood pressure, high blood cholesterol, tobacco use, diabetes, physical inactivity, and poor nutrition. Modest reductions in the rates of one or more of these risk factors can have a large public health impact. Heart disease can also be prevented or controlled through governmental policies (such as restricting access to tobacco) and through environmental changes (such as providing better access to healthy foods and opportunities for physical activity).[53]

- Heart disease, which killed more than 700,000 Americans in 2001, accounted for 29% of all deaths in the U.S.
- In 2001, the rate of death from heart disease was 31% higher among blacks than whites and 49% higher among men than women.
- In 2001, heart disease cost the nation $193.8 billion.
- About 66% of heart attack patients do not make a complete recovery.
- About 42% of people who experience a heart attack in a given year will die from it.

Heart disease is a leading cause of premature, permanent disability among working adults. Stroke alone accounts for the disability of more than 1 million Americans. Almost 6 million hospitalizations each year are due to CVD.

During the last two decades of the 20th century, the age-adjusted rate of deaths from coronary heart disease (CHD) declined sharply, falling from nearly 350 per 100,000 in 1980 to 196 in 2000; but the decrease fall shorts of reaching the *Healthy People 2010* target of 166 per 100,000 (Objective 12-1).

Among racial/ethnic groups, blacks showed the greatest disparity from the average in 2000, with a heart disease death rate of 243 deaths per 100,000. Geographically, CHD death rates have tended to be higher in the southern and southeastern states, particularly those along the Ohio and Mississippi river valleys and in the Appalachian region, as well as in New York, Oklahoma, Michigan, Rhode Island, and a portion of California.[54]

6.6.1.1 Prevention

On an individual level, adhering to the principles outlined in the Dietary Guidelines for Americans (see Section 11.12.1) or the general prevention guidelines presented at the beginning of this chapter (Section 6.1.1.1) would constitute health promotion and primary prevention of heart disease and stroke. See also Box 6.12 on recommendations to prevent heart disease and stroke.

Box 6.12 Recommendations to Prevent Heart Disease and Stroke

1. Develop policies for preventing heart disease and stroke at national, state, and local levels to assure effective public health action, including new knowledge on the efficacy and safety of therapies to reduce risk factors. Implement intervention programs in a timely manner and on a sufficient scale to permit rigorous evaluation and the rapid replication and dissemination of those most effective. Active intervention is needed continually to develop and support policies (both in and beyond the health sector) that are favorable to health, change those that are unfavorable, and foster policy innovations when gaps are identified. Policies that adversely affect health should be identified because they can be major barriers to the social, environmental, and behavioral changes needed to improve population-wide health.

2. Promote *cardiovascular health* and prevent heart disease and stroke through interventions in multiple settings, for all age groups, and for the whole population, especially high-risk groups. This recommendation defines the scope of a comprehensive public health strategy to prevent heart disease and stroke. Such a strategy must emphasize promotion of desirable social and environmental conditions and favorable population-wide and individual behavioral patterns to prevent major risk factors and assure full accessibility quality health services among people with risk factors or disease.

3. Strengthen public health agencies to assure that they develop and maintain sufficient capacities and competencies. Public health agencies at state and local levels should establish specific programs designed to promote cardiovascular health and prevent heart disease and stroke. Skills are required in the new priority areas of policy and environmental change, population-wide health promotion through behavioral change, and risk factor prevention. Public health agencies must also be able to manage and use health data systems to effectively monitor and evaluate interventions and prevention programs.

4. Define criteria and standards for population-wide health data sources. Expand these sources as needed to assure adequate long-term monitoring of population measures related to heart disease and stroke. Such measures include mortality, incidence, and prevalence rates; selected biomarkers of CVD risk; risk factors and behaviors; economic conditions; community and environmental characteristics; sociodemographic factors (e.g., age, race/ethnicity, sex, place of residence); and leading health indicators.

5. Upgrade and expand health data sources to allow systematic monitoring and evaluation of policy and program interventions. To learn what works best, all programs funded by public health agencies should allocate resources for evaluation upfront, and staff must be trained to develop and apply evaluation methods. The resulting data must be communicated effectively to other agencies and to policymakers.

6. Emphasize the critical roles of atherosclerosis and high blood pressure, which are the dominant conditions underlying heart disease and stroke, within a broad prevention research agenda. Prevention research on policy, environmental, and sociocultural determinants of risk factors is critical, as is rapid translation of this information into healthcare practice. Such research should focus especially on children and adolescents because atherosclerosis and high blood pressure can begin early in life. The *prevention research agenda* should be developed and updated collaboratively among interested parties, taking current and planned research programs into account.

7. Develop innovative ways to monitor and evaluate policies and programs, especially for policy and environmental change and populationwide health promotion. Public health agencies and their partners should conduct and promote research to improve surveillance

methods in multiple areas, settings, and populations. Marketing research can be used to evaluate public knowledge and awareness of key health messages and to update these messages over time. Methodological research can help assess the impact of new technologies and regulations on surveillance systems.

Source: U.S. Department of Health and Human Services. *A Public Health Action Plan to Prevent Heart Disease and Stroke.* Centers for Disease Control and Prevention. 2003. Available at: http://www.cdc.gov/dhdsp/library/action_plan/pdfs/action_plan_full.pdf. Accessed August 5, 2006.

6.6.1.1.1 The WISEWOMAN Program

The WISEWOMAN program is administered through CDC's DHDSP (see Section 6.2.4.2). The program provides low-income, under-insured, and uninsured women aged 40–64 with chronic disease risk factor screening, lifestyle intervention, and referral services in an effort to prevent cardiovascular disease. CDC funds 15 WISEWOMAN projects, which operate on the local level in states and tribal organizations. Projects provide standard preventive services including blood pressure and cholesterol testing, and programs to help women develop a healthier diet, increase physical activity, and stop using tobacco.

6.6.1.1.2 Community Prevention

Research conducted during the 1970s demonstrates that community interventions that change the environment are particularly effective in reducing heart disease throughout the entire community. For example, when a workplace adopts a no-smoking policy, all employees benefit, whether they smoke or not.

The first major community-based control program was conducted in North Karelia, Finland, which had a high CVD mortality rate. The North Karelia Project was launched in 1972 as a community-based program to influence diet and other lifestyles crucial in the prevention of CVD. The intervention employed comprehensive strategies. Broad community organization and the strong participation of community members were key elements. Evaluation has studied how the diet (particularly fat consumption) has changed and how these changes have led to a major reduction in population serum cholesterol and blood pressure levels. It has also shown a decline from 1971 to 1995 in ischemic heart disease mortality in a working-age population by 73% in North Karelia and by 65% throught Finland.

Although Finland is an industrialized country, North Karelia was rural, at a lower socioeconomic stratum, and with many social problems. The project was based on low-cost intervention activities, where individual participation and community organizations played a key role. Comprehensive interventions in the community were eventually supported by national activities — from expert guidelines and media activities to industry collaboration and policy.[55]

Similar changes have been implemented in the U.S. and other countries. In the U.S, NIH financed three major community-based intervention projects: the Stanford Five-City Project,[56] the Minnesota Heart Health Program,[57] and the Pawtucket Heart Health Program.[58] Other projects have been carried out in Israel,[59] Germany,[60] and Sweden.[61]

6.6.2 Hypertension

The World Health Organization estimates that high blood pressure causes one out of every eight deaths worldwide, making hypertension the third leading cause of death in the world.[62] Blood pressure categories for normal blood pressure, prehypertension, and stages 1 and 2 hypertension in adults are presented in Table 6.7.

Uncontrolled high blood pressure can lead to stroke, heart attack, heart or kidney failure by placing stress on a number of target organs. Elevated blood pressure is also associated with pregnancy complications, compromised sexual functioning, and may result in organ damage when

TABLE 6.7
Blood Pressure Categories in Adults

Category	Systolic Blood Pressure In millimeters of mercury	Diastolic Blood Pressure (mm Hg)
Normal blood pressure	< 120	< 80
Prehypertension	120–139	80–89
High blood pressure stage 1	140–159	90–99
High blood pressure stage 2	≥ 160	≥ 100

Source: Classification of blood pressure for adults in: National Heart, Lung, and Blood Institute. *Seventh Report of the Joint National Committee on Prevention, Detection, Evaluation, and Treatment of High Blood Pressure.* U.S. Department of Health and Human Services. National Institutes of Health, August 2004. Available at: http://www.nhlbi.nih.gov/guidelines/hypertension/jnc7full.pdf. Accessed March 20, 2005.

it occurs in children. Hypertension affects the heart, brain, kidneys, eyes, bones, sexual function, and pregnancy outcome, as presented in Box 6.13.

6.6.2.1 Prevalence

According to the NHLBI, between 1976–1980 and 1999–2000, the awareness of hypertension among Americans increased from 51 to 70%, the percentage of individuals with hypertension receiving treatment increased from 31 to 59%, and the percentage of patients with high blood pressure controlled to <140/90 mmHg increased from 10 to 34%. These changes have been associated with highly favorable trends in the morbidity and mortality attributed to hypertension.[63] Nevertheless, hypertension is found in almost one-third (32.3%) of U.S. adults, and another 28% are prehypertensive. As indicated in Figure 6.5, a disparity exists in the U.S. in the prevalence of hypertension.

The age-adjusted death rate for stroke declined during the 1980s and early 1990s (from 96.4 per 100,000 in 1980), plateaued in the early 1990s, then resumed a downward trend in the late 1990s, to reach a rate of 61 in 2000; however, the trend falls short of achieving the 2010 target of 48 per 100,000 (Objective 12-7). Of five racial/ethnic groups for whom data are available, the highest age-adjusted stroke death rate in 2000 was recorded for blacks (85 per 100,000) and the lowest for Hispanics (39 per 100,000). The age-adjusted death rates for females and males were about equal. Geographically, age-adjusted average annual stroke death rates are highest in the southeastern states, particularly in the so-called "stroke belt," a region comprising Georgia, South Carolina, eastern North Carolina, and adjacent parts of neighboring states. Rates are lowest in the Northeast and the noncoastal Southwest.[64]

6.6.2.2 Prevention

The prevention of high blood pressure is a major public health challenge in the U.S. Intervention on the individual, clinical level should target people with prehypertension. On the other hand, morbidity and mortality in the general population could be substantially reduced by decreasing the blood pressure level by even modest amounts. The National High Blood Pressure Education Program (NHBPEP) estimates that a 5 mm Hg reduction of systolic blood pressure in the population would result in a 14% overall reduction in mortality due to stroke, a 9% reduction in mortality due to CHD, and a 7% decrease in all-cause mortality.[65] Intervention should be aimed at modifying these causal factors of hypertension:[66]

Box 6.13 Hypertension and Its Sequelae

- *Heart:* High blood pressure places stress on a number of target organs, including the kidneys, eyes, and heart, causing them to deteriorate over time. About half of people who suffer their first heart attack have moderate hypertension (> 160/95 mm Hg). Depending on its severity high blood pressure increases the risk of a heart attack by up to five times, and precedes the development of congestive heart failure (CHF) in more than 90% of cases.[1]
- *Brain:* High blood pressure contributes to 75% of all strokes and heart attacks, and is particularly deadly in African Americans. Malignant hypertension, an emergency condition resulting from untreated primary hypertension, can be lethal. About two-thirds of people who suffer a first stroke have moderately elevated blood pressure ($\geq$ 160/95 mm Hg). Hypertensive people have up to 10 times the normal risk of stroke, depending on the severity of the blood pressure. Dementia and cognitive impairment occur more commonly in patients with hypertension. Hypertension is associated with vascular dementia and mixed dementia (the coexistence of Alzheimer's disease with vascular dementia).[2–4]
- *Kidney:* In patients with diabetes, both hyperglycemia and hypertension are independent risk factors for renal disease. High blood pressure is strongly associated with diabetic nephropathy. Blood pressure control is paramount in reducing CVD risk and the development of diabetic nephropathy: the target blood pressure is < 130/80 mm Hg in patients with type 2 diabetes.[5] Men with high blood pressure may also have a higher risk of kidney cancer.[6]
- *Eyes:* High blood pressure can lead to retinopathy.[7,8]
- *Bone loss:* Hypertension increases the excretion of calcium in urine that may lead to loss of bone mineral density, a significant risk factor for fractures.[9,10]
- *Sexual dysfunction:* Sexual dysfunction is more common and more severe in men with hypertension, particularly in smokers, than it is in the general population.[11]
- *Pregnancy and eclampsia:* Severe, sudden high blood pressure in pregnant women is one component of preeclampsia (commonly called *toxemia*) that can be serious for both mother and child. Preeclampsia occurs in up to 10% of pregnancies, usually in the third trimester of a first pregnancy, and resolves immediately after delivery. The condition may be caused by a failure of the placenta to embed properly in the uterus, which causes it to misconnect with the mother's blood vessels. As a result, the fetus does not receive a sufficient blood supply and the mother's own blood pressure increases to replace it. The reduced supply of blood to the placenta can cause low birth weight and eye or brain damage in the fetus. Severe cases of preeclampsia can cause kidney damage, convulsion, and coma in the mother and can be lethal to both mother and child. Women with existing hypertension are at risk for preeclampsia.[12]
- *Hypertension in children:* Early abnormalities, including enlarged heart and abnormalities in the kidney and eyes, may occur even in those children with mild hypertension. Children and adolescents with hypertension should be monitored and evaluated for possible early organ damage.[13,14]

Sources:

[1] American Heart Association. *Heart Disease and Stroke Statistics — 2005 Update*. Dallas, TX.: American Heart Association; 2004. Available at: http://www.americanheart.org/downloadable/heart/1105390918119HDSStats2005Update. pdf. Accessed July 24, 2005.

[2] Di Bari, M., Pahor, M., Franse, L.V., et al. Dementia and disability outcomes in large hypertension trials: lessons learned from the Systolic Hypertension in the Elderly Program (SHEP) trial. *Am J Epidemiol.* 153, 72–78, 2001.

[3] Feigin, V., Ratnasabapathy, Y., and Anderson, C. Does blood pressure lowering treatment prevents dementia or cognitive decline in patients with cardiovascular and cerebrovascular disease? *J Neurol Sci.* 229–230, 151–155, 2005. Epub 2005 January 7.

[4] Langa, K.M., Foster, N.L., and Larson, E.B. Mixed dementia: emerging concepts and therapeutic implications. *JAMA.* 292, 2901–2908, 2004.

[5] Lee, G.S. Retarding the progression of diabetic nephropathy in type 2 diabetes mellitus: focus on hypertension and proteinuria. *Ann Acad Med Singapore.* 34, 24–30, 2005. Available at: http://www.annals.edu.sg/pdf200502/GLee.pdf. Accessed March 21, 2005.

[6] Choi, M.Y., Jee, S.H., Sull, J.W., and Nam, C.M. The effect of hypertension on the risk for kidney cancer in Korean men. *Kidney Int.* 67(2), 647–52, February 2005.

[7] Wong, T.Y. and Mitchell, P. Hypertensive retinopathy. *N Engl J Med.* 351, 2310–2317, 2004.

[8] Porta, M., Grosso, A., and Veglio, F. Hypertensive retinopathy: there's more than meets the eye. *J Hypertens.* 23, 683–696, April 2005.

[9] Cappuccio, F.P., Kalaitzidis, R., Duneclift, S., and Eastwood, J.B. Unraveling the links between calcium excretion, salt intake, hypertension, kidney stones and bone metabolism. *J Nephrol.* 13, 169–77, 2000.

[10] Blackwood, A.M., Sagnella, G.A., Cook, D.G., and Cappuccio, F.P. Urinary calcium excretion, sodium intake and blood pressure in a multi-ethnic population: results of the Wandsworth Heart and Stroke Study. *J Hum Hypertension.* 15, 229–237, 2001. Available at: http://www.sin-italy.org/jnonline/Vol13n3/169.html. Accessed March 21, 2005.

[11] Giuliano, F.A., Leriche, A., Jaudinot, E.O., and de Gendre, A.S. Prevalence of erectile dysfunction among 7689 patients with diabetes or hypertension, or both. *Urology.* 64, 1196–1201, 2004.

[12] August, P., Helseth, G., Cook, E.F., and Sison, C. A prediction model for superimposed preeclampsia in women with chronic hypertension during pregnancy. *Am J Obstet Gynecol.* 191, 1666–1672, 2004.

[13] Sorof, J. and Daniels, S. Obesity hypertension in children: a problem of epidemic proportions. *Hypertension.* 40, 441–447, 2002. Available at: http://hyper.ahajournals.org/cgi/content/full/40/4/441. Accessed July 24, 2005.

[14] U.S. Department of Health and Human Services. National Institutes of Health. National Heart, Lung, and Blood Institute. The Fourth Report on the Diagnosis, Evaluation, and Treatment of High Blood Pressure in Children and Adolescents. NIH Publication No. 05-5267. Originally printed September 1996 (96-3790). Revised May 2005. Available at: http://www.nhlbi.nih.gov/health/prof/heart/hbp/hbp_ped.pdf. Accessed July 24, 2005.

- *Overweight.* At least 122 million Americans are overweight or obese.
- *High sodium intake.* The mean intakes for men and women in the U.S. are 4100 mg and 2750 mg per day, respectively, 75% of which comes from processed foods. It is recommended that the food industry, including manufacturers and restaurants, reduce sodium in the food supply by 50%. If implemented, this approach would reduce blood pressure in the population.
- *Low intake of fruits and vegetables.* Less than 25% of Americans consume at least 5 servings per day.

6.6.2.3 Population-Based Strategies

A population-based approach aimed at achieving a downward shift in the distribution of blood pressure in the general population is an important component for any comprehensive plan to prevent hypertension. A small decrement in the distribution of systolic blood pressure is likely to result in a substantial reduction in the burden of blood pressure-related illness. Public health approaches, such as lowering sodium content or caloric density in the food supply, and providing attractive, safe, and convenient opportunities for exercise are ideal population-based approaches for reduction of average blood pressure in the community. Enhancing access to appropriate facilities (parks, walking trails, bike paths) and to effective behavior change models is a useful strategy for increasing physical activity in the general population.[67]

Box 6.14 Gender, Racial, and Ethnic Variations in Cancer Incidence and Death Rates

Note: The numbers in parentheses are the rates per 100,000 persons. Incidence counts cover approximately 93% of the U.S. population. Death counts cover 100% of the U.S. population.

All cancers combined, men:

Incidence rates are highest among blacks (615.1), followed by whites (536.8), Hispanics (422.8), Asians/Pacific Islanders (324.3), and American Indians/Alaska Natives (267.2).
Death rates are highest among blacks (322.9), followed by whites (236.0), Hispanics (163.9), American Indians/Alaska Natives (145.3), and Asians/Pacific Islanders (138.8).

All cancers combined, women:

Incidence rates are highest among whites (408.9), followed by blacks (377.5), Hispanics (310.4), Asians/Pacific Islanders (264.5), and American Indians/Alaska Natives (215.4).
Death rates are highest among blacks (190.9), followed by whites (161.9), American Indians/Alaska Natives (114.5), Hispanics (107.4), and Asians/Pacific Islanders (96.6).

Among the five races and ethnicities presented:

American Indian/Alaska Native men have the lowest cancer incidence rates; however, Asian/Pacific Islander men have the lowest cancer death rates.
White women have the highest cancer incidence rates; however, black women have the highest cancer death rates.
American Indian/Alaska Native women have the lowest cancer incidence rates and the third-highest cancer death rates.

Source: U.S. Cancer Statistics Working Group. *United States Cancer Statistics: 1999–2002 Incidence and Mortality Web-based Report.* Atlanta: U.S. Department of Health and Human Services, Centers for Disease Control and Prevention and National Cancer Institute; 2005.

6.7 CANCER

Cancer is the leading cause of death among women 40 through 79 and among men 60 through 79. In 2002, 476,009 Americans younger than 85 died of cancer, whereas 450,637 died of heart disease. As cardiac deaths (the previous leading cause of death) fell sharply, cancer (the second leading cause) replaced heart disease in the hierarchy of mortality.[68] Box 6.14 details variations in cancer incidence and death rates by gender, race, and ethnicity. Figure 6.4 correlates cancer incidence by type of cancer and race/ethnicity.

The leading cause of cancer death in the U.S. overall for both men and women is lung cancer. The sites of the leading causes of cancer diagnosed in men and women are cancers of the prostate and breast, respectively.[69]

6.7.1 PREVENTION

Ample evidence demonstrates an association between cancer and body weight, weight gain, physical activity, consumption of fruits and vegetables, and alcohol.[70–75] Not only are most major cancers influenced by dietary patterns, but it is estimated that 30 to 40% of cancer cases worldwide are preventable by dietary means.[76]

Table I-19
AGE-ADJUSTED SEER INCIDENCE RATES AND TRENDS FOR THE TOP 15 CANCER SITES* BY RACE/ETHNICITY

Both Sexes

All Races	Rate[b] 2000-2003	APC[c] 1994-2003	White	Rate[b] 2000-2003	APC[c] 1994-2003	Black	Rate[b] 2000-2003	APC[c] 1994-2003
All Sites	471.3	-0.4	All Sites	478.4	-0.3	All Sites	504.4	-0.9*
Prostate[f]	74.8	0.5	Breast	72.4	-0.4	Prostate[f]	106.6	-0.9
Breast	70.4	-0.5	Prostate[f]	72.4	0.7	Breast	76.9	-1.3*
Lung and Bronchus	64.8	-1.2*	Lung and Bronchus	66.0	-1.1*	Lung and Bronchus	67.9	-0.4
Colon and Rectum	52.4	-1.0*	Colon and Rectum	52.0	-1.1*	Colon and Rectum	62.8	-0.8
Urinary Bladder	20.9	0.0	Urinary Bladder	22.8	0.2	Pancreas	14.9	-2.0*
Non-Hodgkin Lymphoma	19.1	-0.1	Melanoma of the Skin	21.1	2.1*	Non-Hodgkin Lymphoma	14.3	-0.1
Melanoma of the Skin	18.2	1.6*	Non-Hodgkin Lymphoma	19.9	-0.1	Kidney and Renal Pelvis	14.1	1.1
Corpus and Uterus, NOS[f]	12.6	-0.9*	Corpus and Uterus, NOS[f]	13.1	-1.0*	Stomach	12.8	-2.3*
Kidney and Renal Pelvis	12.6	1.9*	Kidney and Renal Pelvis	13.0	2.2*	Urinary Bladder	12.4	0.7
Leukemia	12.2	-0.9*	Leukemia	12.7	-0.9*	Corpus and Uterus, NOS[f]	11.3	1.2
Pancreas	11.3	-0.2	Pancreas	11.1	0.1	Oral Cavity and Pharynx	11.1	-2.9*
Oral Cavity and Pharynx	10.5	-1.5*	Oral Cavity and Pharynx	10.5	-1.3*	Myeloma	10.9	-1.5*
Thyroid	8.2	5.0*	Thyroid	8.6	5.4*	Leukemia	10.1	-0.5
Stomach	8.1	-1.5*	Ovary[h]	7.8	-1.0*	Liver & IBD[g]	7.2	3.5*
Ovary[h]	7.4	-1.0*	Stomach	7.1	-1.5*	Cervix Uteri[f]	6.4	-4.5*

Asian/Pacific Islander	Rate[b] 2000-2003	APC[c] 1994-2003	American Indian/Alaska Native	Rate[d] 1999-2002	APC[c] 1994-2002	Hispanic[e]	Rate[b] 2000-2003	APC[c] 1994-2003
All Sites	315.6	-0.6*	All Sites	325.8	-1.4	All Sites	353.1	-0.7
Breast	48.5	0.9	Colon and Rectum	46.5	-1.4	Prostate[f]	60.9	-0.2
Colon and Rectum	42.4	-0.7	Lung and Bronchus	43.1	-3.9*	Breast	48.1	-0.5
Prostate[f]	41.8	-0.7	Breast	40.0	-3.0	Colon and Rectum	39.0	-0.7
Lung and Bronchus	39.6	-0.8*	Prostate[f]	30.7	-3.4	Lung and Bronchus	32.6	-1.9*
Stomach	14.4	-3.2*	Stomach	16.2	4.7	Non-Hodgkin Lymphoma	16.1	-0.8*
Liver & IBD[g]	13.8	0.1	Kidney and Renal Pelvis	14.9	-2.0	Stomach	12.3	-1.9*
Non-Hodgkin Lymphoma	13.2	-0.1	Non-Hodgkin Lymphoma	12.4	3.3	Kidney and Renal Pelvis	12.1	2.7*
Urinary Bladder	9.3	0.6	Pancreas	10.8	1.5	Urinary Bladder	11.5	-0.2
Pancreas	8.9	-0.9	Liver & IBD[g]	9.9	-0.8	Pancreas	10.3	-1.1
Corpus and Uterus, NOS[f]	8.6	0.4	Corpus and Uterus, NOS[f]	8.4	-	Leukemia	9.5	-2.2*
Thyroid	8.4	2.3*	Oral Cavity and Pharynx	8.2	-8.4*	Liver & IBD[g]	9.5	1.3
Oral Cavity and Pharynx	7.9	-1.7	Urinary Bladder	7.2	-	Corpus and Uterus, NOS[f]	9.2	-0.5
Leukemia	7.3	-1.4*	Ovary[h]	7.1	-0.2	Cervix Uteri[f]	7.3	-3.7*
Kidney and Renal Pelvis	6.3	1.4	Leukemia	7.1	2.0	Thyroid	7.2	4.1*
Ovary[h]	5.3	0.2	Thyroid	6.4	1.3	Ovary[h]	6.2	-0.2

-   Statistic not shown. Rate based on less than 16 cases for the time interval. Trend based on less than 10 cases for at least one year within the time interval.
a   Top 15 cancer sites selected based on 2000-2003 age-adjusted rates for the race/ethnic group.
b   Incidence data used in calculating the age-adjusted rates are from the 17 SEER areas (San Francisco, Connecticut, Detroit, Hawaii, Iowa, New Mexico, Seattle, Utah, Atlanta, San Jose-Monterey, Los Angeles, Alaska Native Registry, Rural Georgia, California excluding SF/SJM/LA, Kentucky, Louisiana and New Jersey). Rates are age-adjusted to the 2000 US Std Population (19 age groups - Census P25-1130).
c   The APC is the Annual Percent Change over the time interval. Incidence data used in calculating the trends are from the 13 SEER areas (San Francisco, Connecticut, Detroit, Hawaii, Iowa, New Mexico, Seattle, Utah, Atlanta, San Jose-Monterey, Los Angeles, Alaska Native Registry and Rural Georgia). Trends are based on rates age-adjusted to the 2000 US Std Population (19 age groups - Census P25-1130).
d   Incidence data for American Indians/Alaska Natives include cases from Connecticut, Detroit, Iowa, New Mexico, Seattle, Utah, Atlanta, and the Alaska Native Registry for the time period 1994-2002.
e   Hispanic is not mutually exclusive from Whites, Blacks, Asian/Pacific Islanders, and American Indians/Alaska Natives. Incidence data for Hispanics are based on NHIA and exclude cases from Hawaii, Seattle, Alaska Native Registry and Kentucky.
f   The rates for sex-specific cancer sites are calculated using the population for both sexes combined.
g   IBD = Intrahepatic Bile Duct. ONS = Other Nervous System.
h   Ovary excludes borderline cases or histologies 8442, 8451, 8462, 8472, and 8473.
*   The APC is significantly different from zero (p<.05).

FIGURE 6.4 Cancer incidence by type and race/ethnicity. (From National Cancer Institute. Age-adjusted incidence rates and trends for the top 15 cancer sites by race/ethnicity. SEER [Surveillance Epidemiology and End Results]. Cancer Statistics Review 1975–2003. Available at: http://seer.cancer.gov/cgi-bin/csr/1975_2003/search.pl#results. Accessed August 30, 2006.)

6.7.1.1 Avoidance of Weight Gain

Avoidance of weight gain has a cancer-preventive effect with regard to cancers of the colon, breast (postmenopausal), endometrium, kidney (renal cell), and esophagus (adenocarcinoma). Physical activity has a preventive effect on cancers of the colon and the breast. Exercise and diet suggestions regarding prevention of these cancers include maintaining body weight in the lower part of the desirable range (BMI between 18.5 and 25), avoiding weight gain of more than 5 kg during adult life, and weight loss of 5 to 10% in already overweight or obese individuals. Moderate physical activity — such as brisk walking or cycling for at least 30 min several days a week — reduces the risk of other chronic diseases, such as coronary heart disease and diabetes, and is therefore encouraged.

Programs to encourage individuals to avoid weight gain often overlap with other health concerns, such as diabetes and heart disease. These programs are cited in numerous place throughout this text and include Steps to a HealthierUS, VERB It's What You Do, NDEP, Sisters Together, and *We Can!*

6.7.1.2 Alcohol

Alcohol increases the risk of mouth, pharyngeal, laryngeal, and esophageal cancers, the risks for which are also increased by smoking. Consumption of alcohol is not recommended, but for those

Characteristic**	Hypertension prevalence		Awareness of condition		Under current treatment		Condition controlled	
	%	(95% CI††)	%	(95% CI)	%	(95% CI)	%	(95% CI)
Sex								
Men	27.8	(24.9–29.7)	59.4	(55.8–63.1)	45.2	(40.9–49.6)	27.5	(23.7–31.3)
Women	29.0	(27.3–30.8)	69.3	(61.7–77.0)	56.1	(29.2–63.1)	35.5	(28.4–42.7)
Race/Ethnicity								
White, Non-hispanic	27.4	(25.3–29.5)	62.9	(57.3–68.5)	48.6	(44.1–53.1)	29.8	(25.7–34.0)
Black, Non-hispanic	40.5	(38.2–42.8)	70.3	(64.9–75.8)	55.4	(51.2–59.6)	29.8	(25.2–34.5)
Mexican American	25.1	(23.1–27.1)	49.8	(40.4–59.2)	34.9	(27.5–42.3)	17.3	(10.7–23.8)§§
Age group (yrs)								
20–39	6.7	(5.3–8.2)	48.7	(38.8–58.7)	28.1	(20.1–36.1)	17.6	(11.6–23.7)
40–59	29.1	(25.9–32.4)	73.5	(69.1–77.9)	61.2	(57.1–65.2)	40.5	(36.4–44.5)
>60	65.2	(62.4–68.0)	72.4	(70.0–74.7)	65.6	(61.9–69.3)	31.4	(28.7–34.2)
Total¶¶	**28.6**	**(26.8–30.4)**	**63.4**	**(59.4–67.4)**	**45.3**	**(45.3–52.8)**	**29.3**	**(26.0–32.7)**

* Had a blood pressure measurement ≥140 mm Hg systolic or ≥ 90 mm Hg diastolic or took antihypertensive medication.
† Told by a health-care professional that blood pressure was high.
§ Took antihypertensive medication.
§ Hypertension levels < 140 mm Hg systolic and > 90 mm Hg diastolic.
** All characteristic estimates (excluding age group) are age adjusted.
†† Confidence interval.
§§ Estimate should be used with caution; relative standard error is 20%–29%.
¶¶ Total population estimates (including sex and age group) include only non-Hispanic whites, Non-Hispanic blacks, and Mexican Americans.

FIGURE 6.5 Disparities in Hypertension. (From Racial/Ethnic Disparities in Prevalence, Treatment, and Control of Hypertension — United States, 1999–2002. *MMWR*. 2005; *54*(January 14): 7–9. Available at: http://www.cdc.gov/MMWR/preview/mmwrhtml/mm5401a3.htm. Accessed September 2, 2006.)

who do drink alcohol, intake should be restricted to less than 5% of total energy for men and less than 2.5% of total energy for women, or fewer than two drinks per day for men and one for women. Excessive consumption of alcohol is discouraged.

6.7.1.2.1 Strengthening Families Program (SFP)

The Strengthening Families Program (SFP), which focuses on high-risk families, is an evidence-based family skills training program found to significantly reduce problem behaviors, delinquency, and alcohol and drug abuse in children and to improve social competencies and school performance.

A National Institute on Drug Abuse (NIDA) research grant in the early 1980s, found the program to be effective, corroborated by more than 15 subsequent independent replications. Both culturally adapted versions and the core version of SFP have been found effective with African American, Hispanic, Asian, Pacific Islander, and American Indian families.[77]

6.7.1.3 Fruits and Vegetables

Consumption of fruits and vegetables lowers the risk of gastrointestinal cancers (mouth and pharynx, esophagus, stomach, and colorectal). Vegetables may have a protective effect against ovarian cancer, cruciferous vegetables may have a protective effect against cancer of the stomach and lung, and fruits may have an effect on bladder cancer.

Recommendations include consuming vegetables and fruits that provide 7% or more of total energy, or 15 to 30 oz (5 or more servings) per day of a variety of vegetables and fruits (see Section 14.1.5.3.3). Increases from 250 to 400 g/d of fruits and vegetables may result in a 23% reduction in overall cancer incidence; diets high in vegetables and fruits (more than 400 g/day) could prevent at least 20% of all cancer incidence.[78] These recommendations are incorporated into the 2005 *Dietary Guidelines for Americans.*[79]

6.7.1.3.1 Body & Soul

Developed for African American churches, Body & Soul encourages church members to eat a healthy diet rich in fruits and vegetables every day for better health.

Body & Soul was developed in partnership with NCI, ACS, and CDC. The four pillars of the program are

- Pastoral leadership
- Educational activities
- A church environment that supports healthy eating
- Peer counseling[80]

6.8 CONCLUSION

Reducing health disparities — such as the incidence rates of CVD, diabetes, and cancer — is one of the two overarching goals of HealthyPeople 2010. although socioeconomic status is often the most significant determinant of health status, disparities reveal themselves in comparing population subgroups to the general population. Thus, particular minorities within the population are at greater risk for developing diet-related chronic diseases than the population at large.

Numerous programs at the federal, state, and local levels exist to assess these disparities and try to effect change. It is important that these programs target the correct audiences with effective materials sensitive to cultural differences among groups. Reducing disparities has potentially enormous economic and societal ramifications in light of our rapidly changing demographics and escalating healthcare costs.

6.9 ACRONYMS

ACS	American Cancer Society
ADA	American Diabetes Association (also American Dietetic Association)
AHA	American Heart Association
BMI	Body mass index
BRFSS	Behavioral Risk Factor Surveillance System
CDC	Centers for Disease Control and Prevention
CHD	Coronary heart disease
CHF	Congestive heart failure
cm	Centimeter
CVD	Cardiovascular disease
DCPC	Division of Cancer Prevention and Control
DDT	Division of Diabetes Translation
DHPSP	Division of Heart Disease and Stroke Prevention
DNPA	Division of Nutrition and Physical Activity
DPCP	Diabetes Prevention and Control Program
DPP	Diabetes Prevention Program
ESRD	End-stage renal disease
FAS	Fetal alcohol syndrome
GAO	Government Accounting Office
HDL	High density lipoprotein
HHS	Department of Health and Human Services
IFG	Impaired fasting glucose
IGT	Impaired glucose tolerance
mmol	Millimole
NCCDPHP	National Center for Chronic Disease Prevention and Health Promotion
NCI	National Cancer Institute
NCMHD	National Center on Minority Health and Health Disparities
NDEP	National Diabetes Education Program
NIDA	National Institute on Drug Abuse
NIDDK	National Institute of Diabetes and Digestive and Kidney Diseases
NIH	National Institutes of Health
NHANES	National Health and Nutrition Examination Survey (1999 to 2002)
NHANES III	Third National Health and Nutrition Examination Survey (1988 to1994)
NHBPEP	National High Blood Pressure Education Program
NHIS	National Health Interview Survey
NHLBI	National Heart, Lung, and Blood Institute
ODP	Office of Disease Prevention
ODPHP	Office of Disease Prevention and Health Promotion
OMH	Office of Minority Health
OPHS	Office of Public Health and Science
PA	Program announcement
PL or P.L.	Public law
REACH	Racial and Ethnic Approaches to Community Health
RFA	Request for Applications
RFP	Request for Proposal
SES	Socioeconomic status
SFP	Strengthening Families Program
We Can!	Ways to Enhance Children's Activity & Nutrition!
YRBSS	Youth Risk Behavior Surveillance System

REFERENCES

1. Eyre, H., Kahn, R., and Robertson, R.M., The ACS/ADA/AHA Collaborative Writing Committee. Preventing cancer, cardiovascular disease, and diabetes: a common agenda for the American Cancer Society, the American Diabetes Association, and the American Heart Association. *CA Cancer J Clin.* 54, 190–207, 2004. Available at: http://caonline.amcancersoc.org/cgi/content/full/54/4/190. Accessed March 6, 2005.

2. Kahn, E.H. and Robertson, R.M., ACS/ADA/AHA Collaborative Writing Committee. Preventing cancer, cardiovascular disease, and diabetes: a common agenda for the American Cancer Society, the American Diabetes Association, and the American Heart Association. This article was published jointly in 2004 in *CA: A Cancer Journal for Clinicians* (online: July 13, 2004; print: July/August: July 14, 2004); *Diabetes Care* (online: June 25, 2004; print: June 25, 2004); *Circulation* (online: June 15, 2004; print: June 29, 2004); and *Stroke* (online: June 24, 2004; print: June 24, 2004) by the American Cancer Society, the American Diabetes Association, and the American Heart Association. Available at: http:/CAonline.AmCancerSoc.org. Accessed July 2, 2006.

3. U.S. General Accounting Office. HealthCare: Approaches to Address Racial and Ethnic Disparities. GAO-03-862R. 2003. Available at: http://www.gao.gov/new.items/d03862r.pdf. Accessed August 5, 2005.

4. Steps to a Healthier U.S. homepage: www.healthierus.gov/steps/.

5. Dietary Guidelines 2005 homepage: http://www.healthierus.gov/dietaryguidelines/.

6. Healthy People 2010 homepage: http://www.healthypeople.gov/.

7. VERB™ homepage: http://www.cdc.gov/youthcampaign/index.htm.

8. U.S. Department of Health and Human Services. *Diabetes: A National Plan for Action. Steps* to a Healthier U.S., 2004. Available at: http://aspe.hhs.gov/health/NDAP/NDAP04.pdf. Accessed August 5, 2006.

9. CDC. Division of Heart Disease and Stroke Prevention (DHDSP) homepage. Available at: http://www.cdc.gov/DHDSP/index.htm. Accessed August 5, 2006.

10. U.S. Department of Health and Human Services. *A Public Health Action Plan to Prevent Heart Disease and Stroke.* Centers for Disease Control and Prevention. 2003. Available at: http://www.cdc.gov/d hdsp/library/action_plan/pdfs/action_plan_full.pdf. Accessed August 5, 2006.

11. CDC. Division of Nutrition and Physical Activity homepage. Available at: http://www.cdc.gov/nccdphp/dnpa/index.htm. Accessed August 5, 2006.

12. Ogden, C.L., Carroll, M.D., Curtin, L.R., McDowell, M.A., Tabak, C.J., and Flegal, K.M. Prevalence of overweight and obesity in the United States, 1999–2004. *JAMA.* 295, 1549–1555, 2006. Available at: http://jama.ama-assn.org/cgi/content/full/295/13/1549. Accessed August 12, 2006.

13. Kamimoto, L.A., Easton, A.N., Maurice, E., Husten, C.G., and Macera, C.A. Surveillance for five health risks among older adults — United States, 1993–1997. *MMWR.* 48(SS08), 89–130, 1999. Available at: http://www.cdc.gov/mmwr/preview/mmwrhtml/ss4808a5.htm. Accessed August 12, 2006.

14. Ogden, C.L., Carroll, M.D., Curtin, L.R., McDowell, M.A., Tabak, C.J., and Flegal, K.M. Prevalence of overweight and obesity in the United States, 1999–2004. *JAMA.* 295, 1549–1555, 2006.

15. Centers for Disease Control and Prevention, National Center for Health Statistics, Division of Health Interview Statistics, data from the National Health Interview Survey. U.S. Bureau of the Census, census of the population and population estimates. Data computed by the CDC's Division of Diabetes Translation, National Center for Chronic Disease Prevention and Health Promotion.

16. Knowler, W.C., Barrett-Connor, E., Fowler, S.E., Hamman, R.F., Lachin, J.M., Walker, E.A., Nathan, D.M. Diabetes prevention program research group. reduction in the incidence of type 2 diabetes with lifestyle intervention or metformin. *N Engl J Med.* 346, 393–403, 2002.

17. Prevalence of Overweight and Obesity Among Adults With Diagnosed Diabetes — United States, 1988–1994 and 1999–2002. *MMWR.* 53, 1066–1068, 2004.

18. Hogan, P., Dall, T., and Nikolov, P. American Diabetes Association. Economic costs of diabetes in the U.S. in 2002. *Diabetes Care.* 26, 917–932, 2003. Available at: http://care.diabetesjournals.org/cgi/content/full/26/3/917. Accessed July 25, 2005.

19. The expert committee on the diagnosis and classification of diabetes mellitus: follow-up report on the diagnosis of diabetes mellitus. *Diabetes Care.* 26, 3160–3167, 2003.

20. Sinha, R., Fisch, G., Teague, B., Tamborlane, W.V., Banyas, B., Allen, K., Savoye, M., Rieger, V., Taksali, S., Barbetta, G., Sherwin, R.S., Caprio, S. Prevalence of impaired glucose tolerance among children and adolescents with marked obesity. *N Engl J Med.* 346, 802–810, 2002.

21. The expert committee on the diagnosis and classification of diabetes mellitus: follow-up report on the diagnosis of diabetes mellitus. *Diabetes Care.* 26, 3160–3167, 2003.

22. U.S. Department of Health and Human Services. Public Health Service. National Institutes of Health. National Heart, Blood, and Lung Institute. *Third Report of the National Cholesterol Education Program Expert Panel on Detection. Evaluation, and Treatment of High Blood Cholesterol in Adults (Adult Treatment Panel III): Final Report.* NIH Publication No. 02-5215, September 2002. Available at: http://www.nhlbi.nih.gov/guidelines/cholesterol/atp3full.pdf. Accessed February 1, 2005.

23. Ford, E.S., Giles, W.H., and Dietz, W.H. Prevalence of the metabolic syndrome among U.S. adults: findings from the Third National Health and Nutrition Examination Survey. *JAMA.* 287, 356–359, 2002.

24. Ford, E.S., Mokdad, A.H., Giles, W.H., and Brown, D.W. The metabolic syndrome and antioxidant concentrations: findings from the Third National Health and Nutrition Examination Survey. *Diabetes.* 52, 2346–2352, 2003.

25. Ford, E.S., Giles, W.H., and Dietz, W.H. Prevalence of the metabolic syndrome among U.S. adults: findings from the Third National Health and Nutrition Examination Survey. *JAMA.* 287, 356–359, 2002.

26. Ford, E.S., Giles, W.H., and Mokdad, A.H. Increasing prevalence of the metabolic syndrome among U.S. adults. *Diabetes Care.* 27, 2444–2449, 2004.

27. Ford, E.S., Giles, W.H., and Dietz, W.H. Prevalence of the metabolic syndrome among U.S. adults: findings from the Third National Health and Nutrition Examination Survey. *JAMA.* 287, 356–359, 2002.

28. Ford, E.S., Giles, W.H., and Mokdad, A.H. Increasing prevalence of the metabolic syndrome among U.S. adults. *Diabetes Care.* 27, 2444–2449, 2004.

29. Ford, E.S., Mokdad, A.H., and Giles, W.H. Trends in waist circumference among U.S. adults. *Obes Res.* 11, 1223–1231, 2003.

30. Herman, W.H., Hoerger, T.J., Brandle, M., Hicks, K., Sorensen, S., Zhang, P., Hamman, R.F., Ackermann, R.T., Engelgau, M.M., and Ratner, R.E. Diabetes Prevention Program Research Group: the cost-effectiveness of lifestyle modification or metformin in preventing type 2 diabetes in adults with impaired glucose tolerance. *Ann Intern Med.* 142, 323–332, 2005.

31. Joslin Diabetes Center. *The Joslin Clinical Nutrition Guideline For Overweight and Obese Adults With Type 2 Diabetes, Prediabetes or at High Risk for Developing Type 2 Diabetes.* Joslin Diabetes Center, Publications Department. Available at: https://diabetesmanagement.joslin.org/Guidelines/Nutrition_ClinGuide.pdf. Accessed April 12, 2005.

32. SEARCH for Diabetes in Youth homepage. Available at: http://www.searchfordiabetes.org/index.cfm. Accessed July 25, 2005.

33. Knowler, W.C., Barrett-Connor, E., Fowler, S.E. et al. Reduction in the incidence of type 2 diabetes with lifestyle intervention or metformin. *N Engl J Med.* 346, 393–403, 2002.

34. U.S. Department of health and Human Services. Small Steps. Big Rewards: prevent type 2 Diabetes. National Diabetes Education Program. Available at: http://www.ndep.nih.gov/campaigns/SmallSteps/SmallSteps_index.htm. Accessed August 6, 2006.

35. Kaufman, F.R. Type 2 diabetes mellitus in children and youth: a new epidemic. *J Pediatr Endocrinol Metab.* 15(S), 737–744, 2002.

36. Dabelea, D., Hanson, R.L., Bennett, P.H., Roumain, J., Knowler, W.C., and Pettitt. D.J. Increasing prevalence of Type II diabetes in American Indian children. *Diabetologia.* 41, 904–910, 1998.

37. American Diabetes Association. Type 2 diabetes in children and adolescents. *Pediatrics.* 105, 671–680, 2000.

38. The SEARCH Writing Group. SEARCH for Diabetes in Youth: a multi-center study of the prevalence, incidence and classification of diabetes mellitus in youth. *Controlled Clin Trials.* 25, 458–471, 2004.

39. SEARCH for diabetes in youth. Protocol phase 2. February 2006. Available at: http://www.searchfordiabetes.org/documents/SEARCH_Protocol_Complete_Document_Phase_2.pdf. Accessed August 6, 2006.

40. Cook, S., Weitzman, M., Auinger, P., Nguyen, M., Dietz, W.H. Prevalence of a metabolic syndrome phenotype in adolescents: findings from the third National Health and Nutrition Examination Survey, 1988–1994. *Arch Pediatr Adolesc Med.* 157, 821–827, 2003.

41. Weiss, R., Dziura, J., Burgert, T.S., et al. Obesity and the metabolic syndrome in children and adolescents. *N Engl J Med.* 350, 2362–2374, 2004.

42. Huang, T.T., Kempf, A.M., Strother, M.L., Li, C., Lee, R.E., Harris, K.J., and Kaur, H. Overweight and components of the metabolic syndrome in college students. *Diabetes Care.* 27, 3000–3001, 2004.

43. McNeill, A.M., Rosamond, W.D., Girman, C.J., Golden, S.H., Schmidt, M.I., East, H.E., Ballantyne, C.M., and Heiss, G. The metabolic syndrome and 11-year risk of incident cardiovascular disease in the atherosclerosis risk in communities study. *Diabetes Care.* 28, 385–390, 2005.

44. Rosenbloom, A.L., Joe, J.R., Young, R.S., and Winter, W.E. Emerging epidemic of type 2 diabetes in youth. *Diabetes Care.* 22, 345–354, 1999. Available at: http://care.diabetesjournals.org/cgi/reprint/22/2/345. Accessed March 19, 2005.

45. Goran, M.I., Ball, G.D.C., and Cruz, M.L. Obesity and risk of type 2 diabetes and cardiovascular disease in children and adolescents. *J Clin Endocrin Metab.* 88, 1417–1427, 2003.

46. Boney, C.M., Verma, A., Tucker, R., and Vohr, B.R. Metabolic syndrome in childhood: association with birth weight, maternal obesity, and gestational diabetes mellitus. *Pediatrics.* 115, e290–e296, 2005. Available at: http://pediatrics.aappublications.org/cgi/content/full/115/3/e290. Accessed July 25, 2005.

47. Bobo, N., Evert, A., Gallivan, J., et al. Diabetes in Children Adolescents Work Group of the National Diabetes Education Program. an update on type 2 diabetes in youth from the National Diabetes Education Program: *Pediatrics.* 114, 259–263, 2004. Available at: http://pediatrics.aappublications. org/cgi/content/full/114/1/259. Accessed July 24, 2005.

48. American Diabetes Association. Type 2 diabetes in children and adolescents. American Diabetes Association. Consensus Statement. *Diabetes Care.* 23, 381–389, 2000. Available at: http://care.diabetesjournals.org/cgi/reprint/23/3/381. Accessed July 25, 2005.

49. The SEARCH Writing Group. SEARCH for diabetes in youth: a multi-center study of the prevalence, incidence and classification of diabetes mellitus in youth. *Controlled Clin Trials.* 25, 458–471, 2004.

50. SEARCH homepage. www.searchfordiabetes.org/. Accessed August 4, 2006.

51. U.S. Department of Health and Human Services. National Heart, Lung, and Blood Institute. Obesity Education Initiative. Healthy Weight Community Outreach Initiative Strategy Development Workshop Report. February 17–18, 2004. January 2005. Available at: http://www.nhlbi.nih. gov/health/prof/heart/obesity/hwcoi/hwcoi_full.pdf. Accessed July 24, 2005.

52. U.S. Department of Health and Human Services. National Institutes of Health. *Ways to Enhance Children's Activity and Nutrition. We Can!* homepage. Available at: http://www.nhlbi.nih.gov/ health/public/heart/obesity/wecan_mats/toolkit.pdf. Accessed July 25, 2005.

53. Centers for Disease Control and Prevention. The Burden of Chronic Diseases and Their Risk Factors: National and State Perspectives 2004. Available at: http://www.cdc.gov/nccdphp/burdenbook2004. February 2004. Accessed March 16, 2005.

54. U.S. Department of Health and Human Services. Public Health Service. Progress Review: Heart Disease and Stroke. April, 2003. Available at: http://www.healthypeople.gov/data/2010prog/focus12/. Accessed March 20, 2005.

55. Pekka, P., Pirjo, P., and Ulla, U., Influencing public nutrition for non-communicable disease prevention: from community intervention to national programme — experiences from Finland. *Public Health Nutr.* 5(S), 245–251, 2002.

56. Farquhar, J.W., et al. Effect of community-wide education on cardiovascular disease risk factors: the Stanford Five-City Project. *JAMA.* 264, 359–365, 1990.

57. Luepker, R.V., et al. Community education for cardiovascular disease prevention: risk factor changes in the Minnesota Heart Health Program. *Am J Public Health.* 84, 1383–1393, 1994.

58. Carleton, R.A., et al. The Pawtucket Heart Health Program: community-wide education effects assessed by changes in cardiovascular disease risk. *Am J Public Health.* 85, 777–785, 1995.

59. Abrahamson, J.K., et al. Evaluation of a community program for the control of cardiovascular risk factors: the CHAD program in Jerusalem. *Israel J Med Sci,* 17, 201–212, 1981.

60. GCP Study Group. The German Cardiovascular Prevention (GCP) study: design and methods. *Eur Heart J.* 10, 629–646, 1988.

61. Brännström, I., et al. Changing social patterns of risk factors for cardiovascular disease in a Swedish community intervention programme. *Int J Epidemiol.* 22, 1026–1037, 1993.

62. The World Health Report 2002. *Reducing Risks, Promoting Healthy Life.* Geneva, Switzerland: World Health Organization, 2002.

63. National Heart, Lung, and Blood Institute. Seventh Report of the Joint National Committee on Prevention, Detection, Evaluation, and Treatment of High Blood Pressure. U.S. Department of Health and Human Services. National Institutes of Health, August 2004. Available at: http://www.nhlbi.nih. gov/guidelines/hypertension/jnc7full.pdf. Accessed March 20, 2005.

64. U.S. Department of Health and Human Services. Public Health Service. Progress Review: Heart Disease and Stroke. April, 2003. Available at: http://www.healthypeople.gov/data/2010prog/focus12/. Accessed March 20, 2005.

65. Whelton, P.K., He, J., Appel, L.J., et al., National High Blood Pressure Education Program Coordinating Committee. Primary prevention of hypertension: clinical and public health advisory from The National High Blood Pressure Education Program. *JAMA.* 288, 1882–1888, 2002.

66. Chobanian, A.V., Bakris, G.L., Black, H.R., et al. The National High Blood Pressure Education Program Coordinating Committee. The Seventh Report of the Joint National Committee on Prevention, Detection, Evaluation, and Treatment of High Blood Pressure (JNC 7). Joint National Committee on Prevention, Detection, Evaluation, and Treatment of High Blood Pressure. National Heart, Lung, and Blood Institute; National Institutes of Health. U.S. Department of Health and Human Services, 2003. Available at: http://www.nhlbi.nih.gov/guidelines/hypertension/. Accessed March 21, 2005.

67. Jemal, A., Murray, T., Ward, E., et al. Cancer statistics, 2005. *CA Cancer J Clin.* 55, 10–30, 2005. Available at: http://caonline.amcancersoc.org/cgi/content/full/55/1/10. Accessed February 1, 2005.

68. U.S. Cancer Statistics Working Group. *United States Cancer Statistics: 2001 Incidence and Mortality.* Atlanta: Department of Health and Human Services, Centers for Disease Control and Prevention and National Cancer Institute, 2004. Available at: http://www.cdc.gov/cancer/npcr/uscs/pdf/USCS.pdf. Accessed February 1, 2005.

69. Diet, Nutrition and the Prevention of Chronic Diseases. WHO Technical Report. 2003. Available at: http://www.6omdagen.dk/dokumentation/WHO_FAO_2003.pdf. Accessed January 28, 2005.

70. International Association of Research on Cancer. *IARC Handbooks of Cancer Prevention: Vol. 6. Body Weight and Physical Activities.* Lyon, France: IARC Press, 2002.

71. International Association of Research on Cancer. *IARC Handbooks of Cancer Prevention: Vol. 8. Fruits and Vegetables.* Lyon, France: IARC Press, 2003.

72. International Association of Research on Cancer. *IARC Handbooks of Cancer Prevention: Vol. 9. Cruciferous Vegetables.* Lyon, France: IARC Press, 2004.

73. U.S. Department of Health and Human Services. National Institutes of Health. National Institute on Alcohol Abuse and Alcoholism. State of the Science Report of the Effects of Moderate Drinking 2003. Available at: http://www.niaaa.nih.gov/publications/ModerateDrinking-03.htm. Accessed January 30, 2005.

74. U.S. Department of Health and Human Services. National Institutes of Health National Cancer Institute. PDQ Cancer Information Summaries: Prevention. http://cancer.gov/cancerinfo/pdq/prevention. Accessed January 30, 2005.

75. World Cancer Research Fund and American Institute for Cancer Research. *Food, Nutrition and the Prevention of Cancer: A Global Perspective.* Washington, D.C.: American Institute for Cancer Research, 1997. [The 2007 edition was forthcoming when this book went to press.]

76. Strengthening Families Program. Available at: www.strengtheningfamiliesprogram.org/index.html. Accessed August 30, 2006.

77. World Cancer Research Fund and American Institute for Cancer Research. *Food, Nutrition and the Prevention of Cancer: A Global Perspective.* Washington, D.C.: American Institute for Cancer Research, 1997.

78. U.S. Department of Health and Human Services, U.S. Department of Agriculture. *Dietary Guidelines for Americans 2005.* HHS Publication number HHS-ODPHP-2005-01-DGA-A. USDA Publication number: Home and Garden Bulletin No. 232. Available at: http://www.health.gov/dietaryguidelines/dga2005/document/pdf/DGA2005.pdf. Accessed January 30, 2005.

79. Body and Soul: A Celebration of Health Eating and Living. Available at: www.bodyandsoul.nih.gov/index.html. Accessed August 30, 2006.

7 Weight Control: Challenges and Solutions

Watermelon — it's a good fruit. You eat, you drink, you wash your face.

Enrico Caruso (1873–1921)

In 2001, then U.S. Surgeon General Satcher described overweight and obesity as having reached "nationwide epidemic proportions," noting that approximately 300,000 deaths a year in the U.S. are currently associated with these conditions. Health risks associated with obesity include type 2 diabetes, heart disease, stroke, hypertension, sleep apnea, psychological disorders such as depression, some cancers, and premature death. Dr. Satcher called for the prevention and treatment of overweight and obesity and their associated health problems by:

- Promoting the recognition of overweight and obesity as major public health problems
- Helping people balance healthful eating with regular physical activity to achieve and maintain a healthy or healthier body weight
- Identifying effective and culturally appropriate interventions to prevent and treat overweight and obesity
- Encouraging environmental changes that help prevent overweight and obesity
- Developing and enhancing public–private partnerships to help implement these goals[1]

Rising rates of overweight and obesity — as indicated by national surveys — impact not only individual health, but also national healthcare costs, levels of work productivity, and social interactions. Advertising, increased snacking and portion sizes, the "built environment," and lack of physical activity have all been implicated in our escalating national weight. Solutions range from the individual diet to federally implemented education campaigns.

7.1 DEFINING OVERWEIGHT AND OBESITY

The body mass index or BMI is weight in kilograms divided by height in meters squared. BMI is highly correlated with body fat. The National Institutes of Health (NIH) defines a healthy weight in adults as a BMI of 18.5 to 24.9 kg/m^2, overweight as a BMI of 25 to 29.9 kg/m^2, obesity as a BMI equal to or greater than 30 kg/m^2, and extreme obesity as a BMI of at least 40 kg/m^2.[2] (See Figure 7.1.)

7.2 PREVALENCE

Data indicate that the prevalence of obesity has significantly increased among the U.S. population since the 1960s. Recent studies in the U.S. have found high levels of obesity among adults, high levels of overweight among children, and an increase of overweight in preschool-aged children.

Estimates of rates of overweight and obesity in the U.S. differ, based on whether heights and weights are self-reported or are measured by trained personnel. Self-reported weights tend to be lower than weights measured by survey personnel. Therefore, surveys that rely on measured weights produce higher calculated BMIs than surveys using self-reported weights. However, surveys that rely on measured weights and heights may be limited by the fact that some people, such as the extremely obese, are less likely to submit to examinations.[3] Nevertheless, national examination surveys that use measured weight and height data provide the best opportunity to track BMI trends.

BMI	19	20	21	22	23	24	25	26	27	28	29	30	31	32	33	34	35
Height (inches)								Body Weight (pounds)									
58	91	96	100	105	110	115	119	124	129	134	138	143	148	153	158	162	167
59	94	99	104	109	114	119	124	128	133	138	143	148	153	158	163	168	173
60	97	102	107	112	118	123	128	133	138	143	148	153	158	163	168	174	179
61	100	106	111	116	122	127	132	137	143	148	153	158	164	169	174	180	185
62	104	109	115	120	126	131	136	142	147	153	158	164	169	175	180	186	191
63	107	113	118	124	130	135	141	146	152	158	163	169	175	180	186	191	197
64	110	116	122	128	134	140	145	151	157	163	169	174	180	186	192	197	204
65	114	120	126	132	138	144	150	156	162	168	174	180	186	192	198	204	210
66	118	124	130	136	142	148	155	161	167	173	179	186	192	198	204	210	216
67	121	127	134	140	146	153	159	166	172	178	185	191	198	204	211	217	223
68	125	131	138	144	151	158	164	171	177	184	190	197	203	210	216	223	230
69	128	135	142	149	155	162	169	176	182	189	196	203	209	216	223	230	236
70	132	139	146	153	160	167	174	181	188	195	202	209	216	222	229	236	243
71	136	143	150	157	165	172	179	186	193	200	208	215	222	229	236	243	250
72	140	147	154	162	169	177	184	191	199	206	213	221	228	235	242	250	258
73	144	151	159	166	174	182	189	197	204	212	219	227	235	242	250	257	265
74	148	155	163	171	179	186	194	202	210	218	225	233	241	249	256	264	272
75	152	160	168	176	184	192	200	208	216	224	232	240	248	256	264	272	279
76	156	164	172	180	189	197	205	213	221	230	238	246	254	263	271	279	287

BMI	36	37	38	39	40	41	42	43	44	45	46	47	48	49	50	51	52	53	54
58	172	177	181	186	191	196	201	205	210	215	220	224	229	234	239	244	248	253	258
59	178	183	188	193	198	203	208	212	217	222	227	232	237	242	247	252	257	262	267
60	184	189	194	199	204	209	215	220	225	230	235	240	245	250	255	261	266	271	276
61	190	195	201	206	211	217	222	227	232	238	243	248	254	259	264	269	275	280	285
62	196	202	207	213	218	224	229	235	240	246	251	256	262	267	273	278	284	289	295
63	203	208	214	220	225	231	237	242	248	254	259	265	270	278	282	287	293	299	304
64	209	215	221	227	232	238	244	250	256	262	267	273	279	285	291	296	302	308	314
65	216	222	228	234	240	246	252	258	264	270	276	282	288	294	300	306	312	318	324
66	223	229	235	241	247	253	260	266	272	278	284	291	297	303	309	315	322	328	334
67	230	236	242	249	255	261	268	274	280	287	293	299	306	312	319	325	331	338	344
68	236	243	249	256	262	269	276	282	289	295	302	308	315	322	328	335	341	348	354
69	243	250	257	263	270	277	284	291	297	304	311	318	324	331	338	345	351	358	365
70	250	257	264	271	278	285	292	299	306	313	320	327	334	341	348	355	362	369	376
71	257	265	272	279	286	293	301	308	315	322	329	338	343	351	358	365	372	379	386
72	265	272	279	287	294	302	309	316	324	331	338	346	353	361	368	375	383	390	397
73	272	280	288	295	302	310	318	325	333	340	348	355	363	371	378	386	393	401	408
74	280	287	295	303	311	319	326	334	342	350	358	365	373	381	389	396	404	412	420
75	287	295	303	311	319	327	335	343	351	359	367	375	383	391	399	407	415	423	431
76	295	304	312	320	328	336	344	353	361	369	377	385	394	402	410	418	426	435	443

FIGURE 7.1 BMI chart. The table shown has already done the math and metric conversions. To use the table, find the appropriate height in the left-hand column. Move across the row to the given weight. The number at the top of the column is the BMI for that height and weight. (From U.S. Department of Health and Human Services. *The Practical Guide. Identification, Evaluation, and Treatment of Overweight and Obesity in Adults.* National Heart, Lung, and Blood Institute. NIH Publication Number 00-4084. October 2000. Available at: http://www.nhlbi.nih.gov/guidelines/obesity/prctgd_c.pdf. Accessed August 24, 2006.)

7.3 SURVEYS

7.3.1 NATIONAL HEALTH AND NUTRITION EXAMINATION SURVEY (NHANES)

The CDC's NHANES III, conducted from 1988 through 1994, was designed to obtain nationally representative information on the health and nutritional status of the U.S. population. Approximately 31,000 civilian, noninstitutionalized individuals aged 2 months and older received direct physical examinations, including measurements of height and weight. Based on these data, it is estimated that 22.5% of the adult population is obese. Please refer to Chapter 5 for a more detailed description of NHANES origins and methodology.

NHANES IV entered the field in 1999. Again, heights and weights were among the measurements obtained from 4115 adults and 4018 children in 1999–2000, and from 4390 adults and 4258 children in 2001–2002. In 1999–2002, of adults aged at least 20 years, 65.1% were overweight or obese, 30.4% were obese, and 4.9% were extremely obese. Among children aged 6 through 19 years, 31.0% were either at risk for overweight or overweight and 16.0% were overweight.

Between 1999–2000 and 2001–2002, there were no significant changes among adults in prevalence of overweight or obesity (64.5 vs. 65.7%), obesity (30.5 vs. 30.6%), or extreme obesity (4.7 vs. 5.1%), or among children aged 6 through 19 years in prevalence of at risk for overweight or overweight (29.9 vs. 31.5%) or overweight (15.0 vs. 16.5%). However, although there was no change, these results do not indicate that the prevalence of obesity among adults and overweight among children is decreasing.

7.3.2 BEHAVIORAL RISK FACTOR SURVEILLANCE SYSTEM (BRFSS)

The BRFSS is a cross-sectional telephone survey conducted monthly by state health departments with assistance from CDC (see Chapter 5). Self-reported data in BRFSS from 1991 to 1994 showed a prevalence of obesity of 12 to 14.4%. Thus, the NHANES figures are more than 50% higher than the BRFSS estimates.[4]

In 2002, self-reported data collected through the BRFSS indicated a prevalence of overweight among U.S. adults of 37% and a prevalence of obesity of 22.2%. Mississippi had the highest rate of obesity (24.3%) and Colorado had the lowest (13.8%). Trends in state-specific obesity for the year 2002 appear in Table 7.1. The most recent available state-specific and national prevalence data may be found on the BRFSS interactive Web site at www.cdc.gov/brfss/index.htm.

TABLE 7.1
Overweight and Obesity Prevalence Rate, by State (2002)

State	Overweight BMI = 25.0 to 29.9 kg/m²	Obese BMI = 30.0 kg/m²	Overweight + Obese BMI = 25 kg/m²
Alabama	36.8	23.9	60.7
Alaska	38.2	21	59.2
Arizona	36.8	19.2	56
Arkansas	36.6	23.3	59.9
California	37.4	19.9	57.3
Colorado	33.8	14.2	48
Connecticut	36.3	17.4	53.7
Delaware	39.2	16.6	55.8
District of Columbia	31.7	21.5	53.2
Florida	35.2	18.7	53.9
Georgia	37.9	21.5	59.4
Hawaii	34.5	15.7	50.2
Idaho	36.8	18.9	55.7
Illinois	37.2	21.7	58.9
Indiana	36.5	21.8	58.3
Iowa	38.5	21.5	60
Kansas	37.9	20.8	58.7
Kentucky	38	23	61
Louisiana	36.5	23.6	60.1
Maine	36.3	20	56.3

(Continued)

TABLE 7.1 (Continued)
Overweight and Obesity Prevalence Rate, by State (2002)

State	Overweight BMI = 25.0 to 29.9 kg/m²	Obese BMI = 30.0 kg/m²	Overweight + Obese BMI = 25 kg/m²
Maryland	36.5	20.2	56.7
Massachusetts	36.1	16.8	52.9
Michigan	38.7	22.4	61.1
Minnesota	37.6	17.4	55
Mississippi	36.7	25	61.7
Missouri	34.4	22.1	56.5
Montana	37.2	15.9	53.1
Nebraska	37.4	21.1	58.5
Nevada	35.3	17.9	53.2
New Hampshire	36.5	18.1	54.6
New Jersey	38.3	18.5	56.8
New Mexico	36.2	19.3	55.5
New York	39.2	17.7	56.9
North Carolina	37.4	21.8	59.2
North Dakota	40	20.4	60.4
Ohio	35.7	21.5	57.2
Oklahoma	36.6	19.7	56.3
Oregon	36.1	21.5	57.6
Pennsylvania	36.4	21.2	57.6
Puerto Rico	39.3	21.7	61
Rhode Island	36.6	17.1	53.7
South Carolina	36.9	22	58.9
South Dakota	38.9	19.8	58.7
Tennessee	36.5	22.9	59.4
Texas	36.7	23.1	59.8
Utah	35	19.1	54.1
Vermont	34.6	18.2	52.8
Virginia	38	18.2	56.2
Washington	36.3	18.8	55.1
West Virginia	36.5	23.2	59.7
Wisconsin	37.8	20	57.8
Wyoming	37.2	18	55.2

Source: From CDC. Behavioral Risk Factor Surveillance System. Prevalence Data. Risk Factors and Calculated Variables — 2002. Available at BRFSS homepage: www.cdc.gov/brfss/index.htm. Accessed March 5, 2005.

7.3.3 RACIAL AND ETHNIC APPROACHES TO COMMUNITY HEALTH (REACH) 2010

In 2001, the CDC began to conduct annual Risk Factor Surveys in minority communities to monitor the health of black, Hispanic, Asians/Pacific Islanders (A/PI), and American Indians/Alaska Natives. These surveys are part of the REACH 2010 project, which was launched in 1999 and is the CDC's cornerstone initiative aimed at eliminating disparities in health status experienced by ethnic minority populations in key health indicators.[5] For a more complete discussion of health disparities, please refer to Chapter 6.

Data from the REACH 2010 Risk Factor Survey reveal that residents in minority communities bear greater risks for disease compared with the general population. REACH 2010 indicates that the median prevalence of obesity ranged from a low of 2.9% for men and 3.6% for women in A/PI communities to a high of 39.2% for men and 38.0% for women in American Indian communities. The prevalence of obesity was substantially higher among both men and women in American Indian communities and among women in black communities compared with national 2001 BRFSS data. Overall, more than one third of American Indian men and women and of black women was obese in the surveyed communities, whereas approximately one fifth of adults were obese in the national BRFSS survey. Obesity was rare in A/PI communities (see Table 7.2).

7.4 CHILDREN

The 2000 Centers for Disease Control and Prevention (CDC) growth charts represent the revised version of the 1977 National Center for Health Statistics (NCHS) growth charts. Most of the data used to construct these charts come from the National Health and Nutrition Examination Survey (NHANES), which has periodically collected height and weight and other health information on the American population since the early 1960s. In 2000, the CDC introduced charts representing BMI-for-age for children and youth, ages 2–19 years (see Figure 7.2 and Figure 7.3). The BMI-for-age charts are used to assess underweight, risk for overweight, and overweight. According to the CDC, a child with a BMI-for-age that is at the 85th to 95th percentile indicates "risk for overweight," whereas a child with a BMI-for-age that is equal to or greater than the 95th percentile is considered to be "overweight." As of 2006, CDC did not have a definition for obesity for children and adolescents.

CDC's BMI Table for Overweight Children and Adolescents is available on the agency's Web site (www.cdc.gov/nchs/data/hus/tables/2002/02hus071.pdf) as are numerous clinical growth charts (www.cdc.gov/nchs/about/major/nhanes/growthcharts/clinical_charts.htm).

When the CDC released the 2000 growth charts, they included nutritional status indicators for *overweight* (defined as a BMI greater than or equal to the 95th percentile of BMI-for-age) and *at risk for overweight* (defined as greater than or equal to the 85th and less than the 95th percentile of BMI-for-age.) *The term obese did not appear.*

In contrast to CDC's definitions of unhealthy weight in children, the American Obesity Association (AOA) uses the 85th percentile of BMI-for-age as the reference point for overweight and the 95th percentile of BMI-for-age as the reference point for obesity. Their rationale is that the 95th percentile for BMI-for-age in children corresponds to an adult BMI of 30 kg/m^2, which is the reference point for obesity. The 85th percentile for BMI-for-age in children corresponds to an adult BMI of 25 kg/m^2, which is the marker for overweight.

Suggest reasons why CDC and AOA use different vocabulary to describe the same phenomena.

7.4.1 Prevalence among Children

In the 1960s, less than 5% of children 6–19 years of age were overweight, as indicated in Table 7.3. As of 2002, about 10% of 2–5-year-olds and 15% of 6–19-year-olds were overweight. Taking into consideration those deemed at risk of being overweight, the current percentages double to 20% for preschoolers ages 2–5 and 30% for children to 19 years of age. Among children of color, the rates are even higher, with 40% of Mexican American and African American youth ages 6–19 years considered overweight or at risk of being overweight.[6]

Longitudinal data suggest an overweight future for overweight children. In the PedNSS study discussed in the following section, data on 380,518 low-income children from birth to age 59 months born between 1985 and 1990 indicate that overweight during infancy persists through the preschool years.[7] In another study, data on 2610 children ages 2–17 years of age in 1973 who were followed to ages 18–37 years in 1996 (the mean follow-up was 17.6 years) indicate that childhood levels of both BMI and triceps skinfold thickness (TSF) were associated with adult levels of BMI and adiposity. The magnitude of these longitudinal associations increased with childhood age, and the BMI levels of even the youngest children were moderately associated with adult adiposity.

TABLE 7.2
Percentage of Adults Who Were Obese in REACH 2010 Communities, 2001–2002, Compared with National BRFSS 2000–2001 Data by Race/Ethnicity and Sex in U.S.

Reach 2010 Community	REACH 2010 Racial/Ethnic Populations*								Comparison Populations from BRFSS	
	Black		Hispanic		Asian/Pacific Islander		American Indian[†]		MMSA/State[§]/Nation	
	%	(95%, CI[¶])	%	(95%, CI)	%	(95%, CI)	%	(95%, CI)	%	(95%, CI)
Men										
Boston, MA	19.9	(14.5–26.6)							18.2	(17.1–19.4)
Charlotte, NC	27.1	(21.4–33.7)							22.7	(18.6–26.9)
Los Angeles County, CA	24.8	(19.3–31.2)							21.3	(18.4–24.1)
Fulton County, GA	25.3	(16.6–36.5)							20.5	(17.6–23.3)
Nashville, TN	23.6	(16.8–32.2)							22.4	(17.9–26.8)
Charleston and Georgetown Counties, SC	28.9	(23.0–35.6)							22.7	(20.1–25.2)**
Orleans Parish, LA	31.3	(25.1–38.2)							24.6	(21.4–27.7)
Alabama	32.3	(27.0–38.1)							24.1	(21.1–27.0)**
San Diego, CA	28.0	(20.0–37.8)							19.8	(14.0–25.6)
Southwest Chicago, IL	27.6	(20.9–35.3)	16.1	(9.7–25.5)					20.1	(18.0–22.1)
Lawndale, Chicago, IL	27.5	(18.3–39.0)	25.0	(18.5–33.0)					20.1	(18.0–22.1)
Detroit, MI	26.8	(19.8–35.2)	23.0	(15.0–33.4)					24.7	(21.6–27.8)
Bronx, New York City, NY	20.0	(13.6–28.4)	24.2	(18.0–31.8)					15.2	(12.8–17.5)
Lawrence, MA			24.2	(19.3–29.8)					18.2	(17.1–19.4)
Lower Rio Grande Valley, South Texas			38.4	(34.0–43.0)					24.5	(22.5–26.4)**
Seattle and King County, WA	17.1	(7.4–34.8)	9.7	(3.1–26.2)	3.7	(0.9–13.6)			18.0	(15.7–20.2)
Santa Clara County, CA					2.1	(1.1–3.8)			20.6	(18.2–23.0)**
Lowell, MA					5.3	(2.7–10.0)			18.2	(17.1–19.4)
Los Angeles and Orange Counties, CA					1.1	(0.6–2.1)			21.3	(18.4–24.1)
Oklahoma							32.6	(27.0–38.8)	24.5	(22.0–27.0)**
Jackson and Swain Counties, NC							45.7	(41.4–50.1)	22.6	(20.1–25.1)**
Median	27.0		24.2		2.9		39.2		21.3‡	
Low	17.1		9.7		1.1		32.6		15.1‡	
High	32.3		38.4		5.3		45.7		25.7‡	

Women

Boston, MA	41.0 (35.2–47.1)				16.4 (15.5–17.4)
Charlotte, NC	37.7 (33.7–42.0)				24.0 (19.8–28.1)
Los Angeles County, CA	36.2 (31.5–41.1)				20.1 (17.3–22.8)
Fulton County, CA	35.2 (28.7–42.3)				19.9 (17.6–22.2)
Nashville, TN	38.0 (31.8–44.6)				21.4 (18.0–24.7)
Charleston and Georgetown Counties, SC	40.7 (36.1–45.5)				22.2 (19.8–24.5)**
Orleans Parish, LA	39.2 (33.9–44.7)				24.0 (21.6–26.4)
Alabama	40.6 (36.7–44.6)				24.8 (22.4–27.1)**
San Diego, CA	27.1 (21.2–34.0)				20.3 (15.1–25.4)
Southwest Chicago, IL	39.4 (34.8–44.3)	36.6 (27.1–47.3)			21.7 (19.9–23.6)
Lawndale, Chicago, IL	44.9 (36.8–53.3)	24.5 (17.7–32.9)			21.7 (19.9–23.6)
Detroit, MI	40.2 (34.9–45.7)	28.1 (20.6–37.2)			23.6 (21.0–26.1)
Bronx, New York City, NY	29.9 (24.7–35.7)	27.1 (22.9–31.7)			19.9 (17.5–22.4)
Lawrence, MA		21.2 (17.9–24.9)			16.4 (15.5–17.4)
Lower Rio Grande Valley, South Texas		39.2 (35.4–43.2)			24.7 (22.9–26.4)**
Seattle and King County, WA	28.3 (16.6–44.0)	10.1 (4.2–22.1)	5.2 (2.0–12.6)		14.5 (12.7–16.3)
Santa Clara County, CA			1.7 (1.0–2.9)		23.1 (21.0–25.4)**
Lowell, MA			4.3 (3.1–5.8)		16.4 (15.5–17.4)
Los Angeles and Orange Counties, CA			2.9 (1.6–5.2)		20.1 (17.3–22.8)
Oklahoma				32.6 (27.7–37.9)	20.8 (18.8–22.8)**
Jackson and Swain Counties, NC				42.3 (38.6–46.2)	23.2 (21.0–25.4)**
Median	38.0	27.1	3.6	37.5	20.9‡
Low	27.1	10.1	1.7	32.6	14.8‡
High	44.9	39.2	5.2	42.3	28.2‡

* Body mass index ≥ 30 kg/m², calculated from self-reported height and weight.

† The REACH 2010 project now includes 42 minority communities across the United States. Although the Alaska Native community was one of the REACH 2010 intervention communities, they did not participate in the Risk Factor Survey for the period covered and therefore were excluded from this report.

§ Metropolitan/micropolitan statistical area, 2000–2001.

¶ Confidence interval.

** Data from 2001 state BRFSS.

‡ Data from 2001 BRFSS from 53 states/territories and the District of Columbia.

Source: From Liao, Y., Tucker, P., Okoro, C.A., Giles, W. H., Mokdad, A.H. Harris, V.B. REACH 2010 Surveillance for Health Status in Minority Communities — United States, 2001–2002. Table 5. *MMWR Surveill Summ.* 53: 1–36, 2004. Available at: www.cdc.gov/mmwr/preview/mmwrhtml/ss5306a1.htm#tab5. Accessed July 25, 2006.

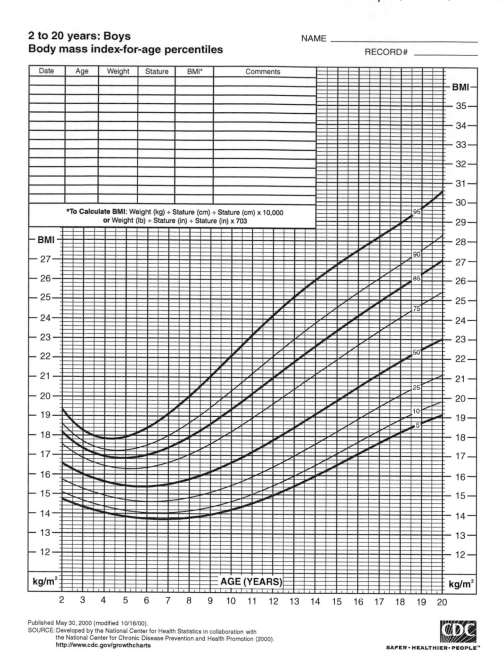

FIGURE 7.2 BMI-for-age for boys. Published May 30, 2000; modified October 16, 2000. (From Developed by the National Center for Health Statistics in collaboration with the National Center for Chronic Disease Prevention and Health Promotion, 2000. Available at: http://www.cdc.gov/growthcharts.)

Overweight 2–5-year-olds were more than 4 times as likely to become overweight adults as were children with a BMI below the 50th percentile.[8] In sum, many overweight children will become overweight adults.

7.4.2 THE PEDIATRIC NUTRITION SURVEILLANCE SYSTEM (PEDNSS)

As described in Chapter 5, PedNSS[9] is a cross-sectional survey of health records of low-income children enrolled in the Special Supplemental Nutrition Program for Women, Infants, and Children

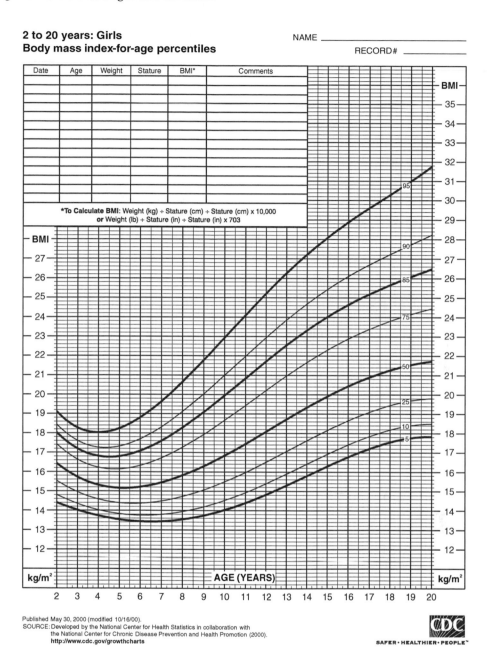

2 to 20 years: Girls
Body mass index-for-age percentiles

NAME _____

RECORD# _____

Published May 30, 2000 (modified 10/16/00).
SOURCE: Developed by the National Center for Health Statistics in collaboration with
the National Center for Chronic Disease Prevention and Health Promotion (2000).
http://www.cdc.gov/growthcharts

FIGURE 7.3 BMI-for-age for girls. Published May 30, 2000, modified October 16, 2000. (Developed by the National Center for Health Statistics in collaboration with the National Center for Chronic Disease Prevention and Health Promotion, 2000. Available at: http://www.cdc.gov/growthcharts.)

(WIC) and other childcare agencies. An analysis of PedNSS data for 2–4-year old children indicates increases in overweight between 1989 and 2000.

Overweight was defined as weight-for-height ≥ 95th percentile. Although the expected prevalence of overweight among children is 10%, in 1989 11 states reported a prevalence of overweight greater than 10% in the 2–4-year old population. By 2000, 28 states reported a prevalence of overweight greater than the expected 10%. From 1989 to 2000, the overall prevalence of overweight increased from 10.8 to 13.68% in the low-income preschool population. As indicated in

TABLE 7.3
Prevalence of Overweight in Children and Teens in the U.S.: NHANES, 1963–2002

	NHANES I 1963–1970	NHANES I 1971–1974	NHANES II 1976–1980	NHANES III 1988–1994	NHANES IV 1999–2002
Boys, 6–11 years	4.0%	4.3%	6.6%	11.6%	15.8%
Girls, 6–11 years	4.5%	3.6%	6.4%	11.0%	14.7%
Male teens, 12–19 years	4.6%	6.1%	5.0%	10.5%	16.1%
Female teens, 12–19 years	4.7%	6.2%	5.3%	9.7%	15.4%

Note: Overweight = Greater than or equal to the 95th percentile for BMI, by age and sex.

Source: From Ogden, C.L., Flegal, K.M., Carroll, M.D., Johnson, C.L. *JAMA.* 288: 1728–1732, 2002; Hedley, A.A., Ogden, C.L., Johnson, C.L., Carroll, M.D., Curtin, L.R., Flegal, K.M. *JAMA.* 291: 2847–2850, 2004.

Table 7.4, Puerto Rico and the Inter-Tribal Council of Arizona reported the highest prevalences of overweight, at 22 and 21.2%, respectively. Puerto Rico realized the greatest increase in overweight, averaging just over half of 1% (0.55) per year. The prevalence of overweight in low-income preschool children in Washington, D.C., decreased slightly, although the amount (0.05%) is statistically significant. Nevertheless, this trend analyses documents significant increases in overweight in 30 states (p < 0.01).

Of the overweight 3 year olds, 62.5% were still overweight a year later, whereas only 4.1% of the nonoverweight 3-year-olds became overweight a year later, indicating that overweight during infancy persists through the preschool years. Tracking of overweight appears to become stronger as children get older, suggesting that preschoolers' height and weight status should be monitored as a strategy for preventing obesity in adolescence and adulthood.[10] These findings urge the expansion of prevention and intervention efforts in the U.S. to reverse the rising trend of overweight.

TABLE 7.4
Selected Area Prevalences of Overweight in Low-Income Preschool Children

State	Percent Overweight 1989	2000	Change per Year
Utah	4.7	7.3	0.24
Hawaii	5.8	10.4	0.42
Idaho	6.4	10.3	0.35
Georgia	6.8	10.9	0.37
New Mexico	6.8	8.8	0.18
New York	13.3	16.4	0.28
District of Columbia	13.5	12.9	−0.05
California	14.3	16.8	0.23
Puerto Rico	16.0	22.0	0.55
Inter-Tribal Council of Arizona	19.0	21.2	0.20

Source: From Sherry, B., Mei, Z., Scanlon, K.S., Mokdad, A.H., Grummer-Strawn, L.M. Trends in state-specific prevalence of overweight and underweight in 2- through 4-year-old children from low-income families from 1989 through 2000. *Arch Pediatr Adolesc Med.* 158: 1116–1124, 2004.

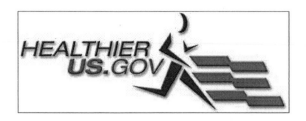

FIGURE 7.4 HealthierUS logo. (From HealthierUS homepage: http://www.healthierus.gov. Accessed January 11, 2007.)

7.5 THE IMPACT ON PUBLIC HEALTH

A combination of poor diet and sedentary lifestyle not only undermine quality of life, life expectancy, and productivity, they also contribute to about 20% of the two million annual deaths in the U.S.

Specific diseases and conditions, such as cardiovascular disease, hypertension, and diabetes are linked to diet. Overweight in adults increases blood pressure and cholesterol levels, and increases the risk of developing type 2 diabetes and its sequelae. Overweight people are at greater risk of becoming obese. Lack of physical activity is also associated with a number of conditions, including diabetes, overweight and obesity, cardiovascular disease, and certain cancers. About 30% of women and 25% of men get little or no exercise.

Overweight children and teenagers are also at greater risk for developing type 2 diabetes and risk factors for heart disease at an earlier age. Several decades may pass for the effects of the present childhood obesity epidemic to manifest themselves as health problems in adults.

7.6 THE COSTS OF OVERWEIGHT AND OBESITY

Escalating rates of obesity in the U.S. have resulted in higher direct and indirect economic costs. Direct medical costs include prevention, diagnosis, and treatment related to obesity. Indirect costs are further subdivided into morbidity and mortality costs. Morbidity costs represent lost income from reduced productivity, restricted physical activity, absenteeism, and bed days. Mortality costs encompass lost future income due to premature death.[11]

Using the 1996 and 1997 National Health Interview Surveys (NHIS) and the 1998 Medical Expenditure Panel Survey (MEPS), Finkelstein et al. computed per capita and total medical spending attributable to both overweight (BMI of 25.0–29.9 kg/m²) and obesity (BMI ≥ 30.0 kg/m²). Annual obesity-attributable medical spending ranged from $26.8 billion (MEPS data) to $47.5 billion (NHIS data), with 5.3% of medical spending for the U.S. adult population attributable to obesity. The public sector finances nearly half of the overweight- and obesity-attributable medical spending. The authors note that annual medical spending for overweight and obesity combined exceeds that attributable to smoking.[12] Thompson and Wolf's review of the literature, with its finding that 5.5–7.0% of health spending in the U.S. is attributable to obesity essentially corroborates Finkelstein et al.'s figure of 5.3%.[13]

Obesity-attributable healthcare costs are not confined to a single point in time but persist long after an acute event such as myocardial infarction.[14] In a hypothetical population of 1 million persons, hypertension would be the most prevalent of obesity-related diseases and type 2 diabetes, the most costly.[15] These costs do not occur in isolation. Bungum et al.'s cross-sectional study of normal and overweight/obese city workers found that BMI not only predicted healthcare costs, but job absenteeism as well.[16] Oster's analysis suggests that although healthcare comprises 41% of the total costs related to obesity, other economic costs account for the remaining 59%.[15]

Wolf and Colditz observe that "indirect costs have a greater effect at the individual and societal levels because they reflect the value of lost health and vitality caused by morbidity."[17] In a later study, Wolf notes that roughly 27% of the labor force in the U.S. has a BMI $\geq$ 29 kg/m^2. She cites numerous studies that evaluated decreased productivity (days missed due to illness), increased restricted activity, and impact on long-term disability due to obesity and concludes, "the evidence is quite strong that obesity impacts productivity and potentially all indirect morbidity outcomes."[18]

Using the 1988 NHIS data, Wolf and Colditz determined that increases in indices of functional impairment and morbidity due to obesity such as restricted-activity, bed, and work-loss days resulted 52.9 million days of lost productivity, costing employers $4 billion in 1990.[17] People having a BMI > 30 kg/m^2 had on average 2.87 more bed days per year than those with a BMI < 23 kg/m^2.[17]

7.7 THE GLOBAL PICTURE

The obesity epidemic is not confined to the U.S. — it is increasing worldwide. Developing countries are facing a double burden of disease. Paradoxically, the prevalence of both overweight and obesity are rising among adults while high rates of undernutrition persist among children.[19] Some evidence indicates that this increase has occurred more rapidly in developing countries such as Brazil, where obesity is increasing more quickly among lower socioeconomic groups. In most parts of Latin America, obesity is the second most important risk factor for mortality and disease.[20] In many developing countries the prevalence of obesity is greater than that of undernutrition.[21] It is estimated that by 2020, two thirds of the global burden of disease will be attributable to nutrition-related noncommunicable diseases (NR-NCD), most of them strongly associated with diet.

Indigenous cuisine and traditional food habits are being supplanted by a Westernized, energy-dense diet with its unhealthy concentration on soft drinks and meat consumption. A sharp decline in the cost of vegetable oils and sugar has put them in direct competition with cereals as the least expensive food ingredients worldwide. This in turn has reduced the proportion of the diet derived from grain and grain products and greatly increased world average energy consumption of sugar and oil, although this increase is not evenly distributed throughout the world's population. Taken together, this transition towards foods of animal origin, increased fats, and refined foods, along with the more sedentary lifestyle that accompanies urbanization, contribute to the current global epidemics of obesity, diabetes, and cardiovascular disease.

The pace of change for both diet and physical activity has accelerated to varying degrees in different regions of the world. The shift of countries and large populations into the stage of development characterized by high prevalence of these NR–NCDs is known as the *nutrition transition*.[22,23,24]

7.8 THE NUTRITION TRANSITION AND ITS REPERCUSSIONS

In 2001, representatives from Africa, the Mideast, Europe, and the Americas met in Bellagio, Italy, to discuss the health implications of the nutrition transition. The Bellagio Declaration, which summarizes the findings of this meeting, states that although the control and prevention of undernutrition remains a challenge in many developing countries, NR–NCDs have become the main causes of disability and death.[25]

The World Health Organization (WHO) and many national governments also recognize that the patterns of disease throughout the developing world are changing rapidly. Changes in food systems and patterns of work and leisure, and therefore in diets and physical activity, are causing overweight, obesity, diabetes, high blood pressure, cardiovascular disease (including stroke), and increasingly cancer, even in the poorest countries. Malnutrition early in life, followed by inappropriate diets and physical inactivity in childhood and adult life, increases vulnerability to chronic diseases.

In many developing countries, NR–NCDs prematurely disable and kill a large proportion of economically productive people, a preventable loss of precious human capital. This includes countries where HIV/AIDS is a dominant problem. Four out of five deaths from NR-NCDs occur in middle- and low-income countries. The incidence of new cases of diabetes is larger in India than in any other country, and when combined with China comprises the majority of new cases of diabetes in the world.[26]

Low-income communities appear to be especially vulnerable to nutrition-related chronic diseases, once thought to be diseases only of affluence. The Bellagio Declaration concluded that immediate action to prevent and control nutrition-related chronic diseases is not only a public health imperative but also a political, economic, and social necessity. Successful programs integrate strategies to promote healthful diets and regular physical activity throughout life into all relevant policies and programs, including those designed to combat undernutrition. In addition, they must be multidisciplinary and include government, industry, the health professions, the media and civil society, and international agencies as partners. Community empowerment and action are crucial to overcome the environmental, social, and economic constraints to improvement in dietary quality and reduction of a sedentary lifestyle.

Successful programs in a few developed countries such as Finland and Norway have demonstrated that chronic diseases are preventable. Programs in developing countries include massive community participation in physical activity encouraged by *Agita São Paulo* in Brazil, protection of the traditional low-fat/high-vegetable diet in South Korea through strong support from home economics and dietetic professionals and infrastructure, selective price policies promoting consumption of soy products in China, and development of food-based dietary guidelines in several countries based on local disease patterns and available foods. School-based programs to promote healthy diets and physical activity provide additional opportunities for early prevention, aimed at protecting health over the life span. Examples include Brazil's national school food program that provides fresh, unprocessed food to school children and Thailand's national physical activity program.[25,26]

7.9 ENVIRONMENTAL DETERMINANTS OF OVERWEIGHT AND OBESITY

While it is true that overweight and obesity result from an energy imbalance caused by consuming too many calories relative to one's energy needs, body weight more realistically depends on a complex amalgam of genetics, metabolism, behavior, culture, economics, and socioeconomic status. A public health perspective is most concerned with the environmental factors that influence individual choices that lead to overweight. There is a growing awareness that we have inadvertently created what has been described as an *obesogenic* environment that discourages physical activity while encouraging overeating.[27] Table 7.5 lists some of the environmental causes of obesity. Unfortunately, increasingly obesogenic environments, reinforced by many of the cultural changes associated with globalization, make the adoption of healthy lifestyles, especially by children and adolescents, more and more difficult.

7.9.1 THE BUILT ENVIRONMENT

Aspects of the environment that can potentially affect health include physical and social factors, such as housing, urban development, land use, transportation, industry, and agriculture. Environmental health refers to assessing and controlling these factors that comprise the "built environment," a component of environmental health.[28]

The built environment encompasses all buildings and spaces created or modified by people. It includes homes, schools, workplaces, parks and recreation areas, greenways, business areas, and transportation systems. It extends overhead in the form of electric transmission lines, underground

TABLE 7.5
Environmental Causes of Obesity

Location	Environmental Factors
Home	*Food access and availability*
	Increase in ready-made foods for meal preparation
	Limited time to cook
	Opportunities for physical activity
	Increased competition from attractive passive entertainment activities, such as television, video/DVD, video/computer games, Internet
	Increase in the use of modern appliances (e.g., microwaves, dishwashers, washing machines, vacuum cleaners)
Work	*Food access and availability*
	Employee lunchrooms and cafeterias that do not make nutritious food available
	Vending machines that are not stocked with nutritious snacks
	Opportunities for physical activity
	Increase in sedentary occupational lifestyles due to technology, increase in computerization
Public places	*Food access and availability*
	Food courts in shopping malls
	Opportunities for physical activity
	Increase in the use of elevators, escalators, and even automatic doors
Urban residence	*Food access and availability*
	Paucity of supermarkets in low-income neighborhoods
	Opportunities for physical activity
	Limited open areas for physical activity
	Policies that connect energy intake and expenditure to the built environment
	Fear of crime in urban areas
Suburban residence	*Policies that connect energy intake and expenditure to the built environment*
	Increase number of neighborhoods that depend on private automobiles mobility
	Rise in car ownership
	Increase in driving shorter distances
Community	*Food access and availability*
	Unreasonably large portions of food served in restaurants
	Food outlets with low availability of low-calorie and/or nutritionally-dense food items
	Fund-raising events that promote high-calorie foods, such as cookie and candy sales
	Opportunities for physical activity
	Few opportunities for physical activity in communities
School	*Food access and availability*
	School breakfast and lunch program meals that do not meet national standards
	Using food as a reward
	Availability of high-calorie low nutrition competitive foods in school vending machines and on a la carte lines
	Opportunities for physical activity
	Low level of required physical education
	Policies that connect energy intake and expenditure to the built environment
	Crowded lunchrooms, short lunch period, long lunch lines
	Limited safe walking routes to school

Source: Compiled from various sources, primarily "The Surgeon General's Call to Action to Prevent and Decrease Overweight and Obesity, 2001."

Box 7.1 Health and Community Design

In their 2003 book, *Health and Community Design: The Impact of the Built Environment on Physical Activity*, L.D. Frank, P.O. Engelke, and T.L. Schmid maintain that the American iconization of the automobile has had dire consequences for the built environment, curtailing our physical and aesthetic existence.

The authors carefully explore the history and development of community design, the changing nature of physical activity in daily life, and the devastating impact of the one upon the other. In the beginning, cities grew "organically" — unplanned and as the need arose. Streets were winding and close together as befitted the primary mode of transportation: walking. Although large, rich civilizations such as the Roman Empire planned cities, their grid pattern continued to accommodate the pedestrian. More recently, as violent epidemics of typhus and cholera ripped through crowded slums, the close proximity of people to people, of homes to commerce was seen as antithetical to the public health. A belief in the benefits of space, light, and trees in combination with the advent of the automobile gave birth to the modern suburban development and changed the nature of our cities.

The authors posit the concepts of *proximity* (nearness of homes, businesses, shops, and schools to each other) and *connectivity* (ease of moving between homes, businesses, shops, and schools) in the context of the basic activities of walking and biking. They argue that reductions in proximity (for example, by zoning for single use and placing residences far from commerce) as well as decreases in connectivity (by thinking of roadways as deadly, high-speed, car-centric arteries leading to isolated residential dead ends) have made it unappealing if not impossible for inhabitants to engage in walking or biking for transport, thus eliminating much needed physical activity and contributing to obesity.

---

in the form of waste disposal sites and subway trains, and across the country in the form of highways. It includes land-use planning and policies that impact our communities in urban, rural, and suburban areas. The built environment influences obesity through food access and availability, opportunities for physical activity, and policies that support physical activity. Urban communities, particularly those of lower socioeconomic status, typically have limited access to safe outdoor activities or to healthy food choices, whereas residents of suburban neighborhoods suffer from a heavy reliance on automobiles. (See Box 7.1 Health and Community Design and Box 7.2 Public–Private Partnership to Examine How Surroundings Encourage Active Lifestyles.)

Because it may take years to achieve the long-term population goals of reducing the prevalence of obesity, environmental modifications offer the best opportunity for the prevention and treatment of obesity. The most effective environmental strategies include interventions that address energy intake and energy expenditure in different levels and settings throughout the built environment. (See Box 7.3.)

Box 7.2 Public–Private Partnership to Examine How Surroundings Encourage Active Lifestyles

In 2004, NIH's National Institute of Environmental Health Sciences (NIEHS) partnered with the Robert Wood Johnson Foundation's (RJWF) Active Living by Design Program to examine how better community design encourages people to be more physically active in their daily lives. The RWJF has provided each of 25 community partnerships across the U.S. with $200,000 grants to increase "active living" (a way of life that integrates physical activity into daily routines). In addition to the grant, each partnership receives technical assistance to address community design, land use, transportation, architecture, trails, parks, and other issues that influence healthier lifestyles. The communities will develop partnerships to collaborate among a variety of organizations in public health and other disciplines, such as city planning, transportation, architecture, recreation, crime prevention, traffic safety and education, as well as key groups concentrating on land use, public transit, nonmotorized travel, public spaces, parks, trails, and architectural practices that advance physical activity. Each grantee is expected to establish innovative approaches to increase physical activity through community design and communications strategies.

The NIEH is funding the $2.8 million 5-year evaluation component of the project, assessing the impact on physical activity, obesity and other health indicators of local design and transportation changes. The evaluators will identify how the built environment contributes to obesity and how environmental changes can combat the problem. Results from these 25 communities (the experimental group) will be compared against communities that haven't improved their surroundings to encourage physical activity (the control group). If the evaluators determine that simple changes in the built environment and in individual behavior can enhance physical activity and reduce obesity for residents, then local municipalities throughout the country can adopt some of the effective strategies that were developed. Information about this project is available online at: http://www.activelivingbydesign.org/index.php?id=6.

Box 7.3 Sample Physical Activity Programs Developed by DHHS

Hearts N' Parks was piloted during the summer of 1999 in 33 sites in 12 North Carolina communities involving more than 2000 participants. It is a community-based initiative supported by the National Heart, Lung, and Blood Institute (NHLBI) of the National Institutes of Health and the National Recreation and Park Association (NRPA). This innovative program aims to reduce the growing trend of obesity and the risk of coronary heart disease in the U.S. by encouraging Americans of all ages to aim for a healthy weight, follow a heart-healthy eating plan, and engage in regular physical activity. Hearts N' Parks demonstrates the impact that community park and recreation programs can have on helping people improve and maintain their health. Nearly 75% of Americans live within a 2-mi walking distance of a public park. These facilities are widely accessible to individuals from culturally and socioeconomically diverse populations, as well as to individuals with disabilities. Hearts N' Parks activities can be incorporated into a variety of programs including nutrition and fitness activities, stress reduction or family life programs, and so on. Activities can be adapted for children, youth, adults, and seniors. Recreation and park departments and other community organizations receive staff training and resources to integrate heart-healthy activities into existing activities or to develop new activities. Program materials available to local initiatives include consumer-oriented literature to communicate heart-healthy messages related to weight management, physical activity, high blood pressure, cholesterol, and heart disease; materials targeted to specific populations, such as African Americans and Hispanics; and evaluation materials to measure the program's impact.

KidsWalk-to-School is a community-based program developed by the CDC to increase opportunities for daily physical activity by encouraging children to walk to and from school in groups accompanied by adults. Similarly, the *Walking School Bus* provides children with a safe and healthy mode of transportation to school. The designated adult supervisor "picks up" each student, house by house, on foot. The group walks to school together along a set route, all the while enjoying fresh air, exercise, and friendly conversation.

Source: National Recreation and Park Association. About Hearts 'n Parks. Available at: http://www.nhlbi.nih.gov/ health/ prof/heart/obesity/hrt_n_pk/hnp_ab.htm. Accessed July 26, 2006; CDC. Nutrition and Physical Activity Program. KidsWalk-to-School homepage. Available at: http://www.cdc.gov/nccdphp/dnpa/kidswalk/index.htm. Accessed July 26, 2006.

The Institute of Medicine[29] suggests these intermediate environmental goals:

- *Food access and availability.* Increase the access to and affordability of fruits and vegetables for low-income populations.
- *Opportunities for physical activity.* Increase the following: (1) availability of outlets that sell healthful foods located within walking distance of the communities they serve, (2) the number of children who can safely walk and bike to school, (3) the play and physical activity opportunities in the neighborhood, and (4) the availability and use of community recreational facilities.
- *Policies that connect energy intake and expenditure to the built environment.* Change institutional and environmental policies to support energy balance.

7.9.2 THE ECONOMIC ENVIRONMENT

In addition to an individual's socioeconomic status, the economic environment as it impacts food choices includes but is not limited to federal and state policies regulating agriculture and advertising.

7.10 U.S. AGRICULTURAL POLICIES

The Institute for Agriculture and Trade Policy argues that an often overlooked but significant contributor to obesity in the U.S. is our government's farm policy. Over the past five decades, while the price of fruits and vegetables has continued to rise, government support has consistently kept the price of a few commodities such as corn and soybeans low, encouraging their use as ingredients in numerous food products (see Box 7.4 U.S. Food Consumption Trends). Not coincidently, these commodities fall into the dietary categories of added fats and sugars linked to obesity. Low-cost, processed foods high in added fats and sugars are often more available and more affordable than healthier choices.[30]

Farmers, as well as the public health sector, have been negatively affected by policies that favor the production of low-value bulk crops over those of higher value. While farmers struggle to stay

---

Box 7.4 U.S. Food Consumption Trends

- As a country, we spend over half of every food dollar on ready-to-eat food, most of which is high in added fats and sugars.
- Processed grocery foods, frozen foods, and baked goods represented over 40% of supermarket sales in 2000, whereas produce claimed only 9%.
- On any given day, about a quarter of U.S. adults eat in a fast food restaurant, contributing to the $110 billion we spend at such outlets each year.
- U.S. consumption of high fructose corn syrup, which is used as a sweetener, increased from virtually no consumption in 1970 to 43.4 lb per year in 2003. On a daily basis, that translates to 1.9 oz or 12.8 teaspoons, delivering 205 cal.
- Annual per capita average U.S. consumption of added fats and oils increased from 53.4 lb in 1970 to 74.5 lb in 2000.
- The average American consumes over 50 gal of carbonated soft drinks a year.
- Nearly one third of our calories come from foods with little or no redeeming nutritional value, i.e., junk food.

Source: Schoonover, H. and Muller, M. Food without thought: how U.S. farm policy contributes to obesity. Institute for Agriculture and Trade Policy: Environment and Agriculture Program. March 2006. Available at: http://www.iatp.org/iatp/publications.cfm?accountID=421&refID= 80627. Accessed July 26, 2006.

in business by growing low value grains and oilseeds, U.S. consumers are becoming ever more dependent on imports of high-value crops. Governmental inertia supports the status quo, yet consumers have begun to seek other routes to healthier foods such as direct purchasing from farmers. Schools and workplaces are also establishing policies to supply cafeterias with fresh, local food, and food councils and farm-to-table networks are becoming more commonplace (see Chapter 10).[30]

7.11 ADVERTISING

Food manufacturers spent $7 billion on food advertising in 1997, over 75% of which went to television commercials. As indicated in Table 7.6, food product categories with the highest advertising intensity tend to be highly-processed and expensively-packaged foods that are over-consumed in the U.S. relative to federal dietary recommendations.[31]

7.11.1 TELEVISION ADVERTISING TARGETING CHILDREN

An examination of data on 13,000 children who participated in the National Health Examination Survey (NHES, a precursor to NHANES) found that among 12- to 17-year olds, the prevalence of obesity increased by 2% for each additional hour of television viewed.[32] The authors suggest that 29% of the cases of obesity could be prevented by reducing television viewing to less than 1 h per week.[33] Similarly, an analysis of NHANES III (1988–1994) data indicates that among 8- and 16-year-old youth, those who watched the most television had higher BMIs than those who watched less. The prevalence of obesity is lowest among children watching one or fewer hours of television a day, and highest among those watching four or more hours of television a day.[34]

TABLE 7.6
Advertising Expenditures by Food Manufacturers, 1997

Product Category	$ Millions	Percentage Share
Prepared, convenience foods: Soups, cereals, jams, jellies, peanut butter, health and dietary foods, infant foods, pasta products and dinners, all other prepared dinners and entrees, and miscellaneous prepared foods	1,563	22.1
Confectionery and snacks: Candy, gum, mints, cookies, crackers, nuts, chips, and other salty snacks	1,095	15.5
Alcoholic beverages	1,082	15.3
Soft drinks and bottled water	702	9.9
Cooking products and seasoning: Sugars, syrups, artificial sweeteners, shortening, cooking oils, margarine, baking mixes, crusts, flour and other baking ingredients, seasoning, spices, extracts, gelatins, puddings, condiments, pickles, relishes, sauces, gravies, dips, salad dressings, mayonnaise, and other miscellaneous ingredients	675	9.5
Beverages: Coffee, tea, cocoa, fruit juices and fruit drinks, and vegetable juices	625	8.8
Dairy products and substitutes	505	7.1
Bakery goods	408	5.8
Meat, poultry, and fish	210	3.0
Fruits, vegetables, grains, and beans	159	2.2
General promotions	50	0.7
Total	7,074	100.0

Source: From Gallo, A. Food advertising in the United States. Chap. 9 in Frazao E., ed. *America's Eating Habits: Changes and Consequences.* Agriculture Information Bulletin No. (AIB750). 1999. Available at: http://www.ers.usda.gov/publications/aib750/aib750i.pdf#search=%22advertising%20expenditures%20by%20food%20manufacturer%20%22. Accessed August 24, 2006.

Although increased television viewing is associated with increased BMI in children[35] and altering this behavior affects weight gain,[36,37] there is no incontrovertible evidence that watching television commercials in particular causes pediatric obesity.[38] Nevertheless, children are the target of intense and aggressive food marketing and advertising efforts. Television advertising and in-school marketing are two of the most prevalent forms of marketing to children. Food is the most frequently advertised product category on children's television, accounting for more than one-half of all ads — most of which are for foods that are high in sugar or fat. Low income children are exposed to the most advertising because they watch more television than their more affluent counterparts.[39]

A review of the research on the role of media in childhood obesity indicates that television food ads influence the food choices children make.[40] The amount of time children spend watching television has been shown to be a significant predictor of how often they request products in the grocery store. As many as three-quarters of these requests were for products seen in television ads. In addition, preschoolers preferred specific foods that appeared in a video they were shown as compared to children in a control group who had not seen the video.[41] Despite these findings, exactly how media contributes to childhood obesity has not been conclusively documented. The likely main mechanism may be through children's exposure to billions of dollars worth of food advertising and marketing.[42]

7.12 SOCIOECONOMIC STATUS AND ETHNICITY

Socioeconomic status (SES) categorizes individuals based on economic or social factors or according to occupational prestige and power. Occupation and income are frequently used as indicators of SES.[43] Traditionally it was held that there exists an inverse relationship between obesity and SES in developed countries, particularly among women, and a positive relationship between obesity and SES in developing countries.[44] That is, obesity increases as income level decreases. Nevertheless, coincident with the increase in obesity in the U.S. over the past three decades, epidemiologists have observed the relationship between BMI and SES has weakened. Analysis of data from NHANES I-III (1971–1994) and NHANES (1999–2000) indicates that high-SES groups are manifesting a significant "catch-up" in the prevalence of obesity.[45] Additionally, the view that there is a positive relationship of obesity to SES in societies in developing countries has recently been disputed.[46] In Brazil, for example, obesity is increasing faster among the groups with lower incomes.[47] (See Section 7.4.1 The nutrition transition and its repercussions.)

Among children, NHANES III (1988–1994) data indicate that low-income adolescents were at a higher risk for obesity, and high-income adolescents were at a lower risk. This association became significant only among adolescents at age 12 and again became insignificant at age 17. SES was not significantly related to obesity among children who were less than 10 years of age.[48] Ethnicity was also shown to be a significant risk factor for overweight and obesity. Compared to white youth, black and Mexican American children and adolescents were at a higher risk for obesity and overweight. However, when income and urban–rural residence were adjusted for, ethnicity became insignificant. These findings may suggest that the SES differences across ethnic groups are a more likely explanation for the difference in obesity prevalence than ethnicity.

The Growth and Health Study (NGHS), a large-scale multisite National Heart, Lung, and Blood Institute (NHLBI)-funded study, sought to determine whether SES as measured by education and income is inversely associated with obesity in 9- to 10-year-old black and white girls and their parents. The prevalence of obesity in the girls and their parents was examined in relation to SES and selected environmental factors. Less obesity was observed at higher levels of household income and parental education in white girls, but not in black girls. Among the mothers of the study participants who were seen, lower prevalence of obesity was observed with higher levels of income and education for white mothers, but no consistent patterns were seen in black mothers. A lower prevalence of obesity was seen at higher levels of SES in white girls, whereas no clear relationship was detected in black girls. These findings raise new questions regarding the correlates of obesity in black girls.[49]

7.13 FOOD INSECURITY, ENERGY DENSITY, AND WEIGHT

Food insecurity, as defined in 1989 by the Expert Panel of the American Institute of Nutrition, means "the limited or uncertain availability of nutritionally adequate and safe foods or limited or uncertain ability to acquire acceptable foods in socially acceptable ways."[50,51] Food insecurity is associated with lower food expenditures, low fruit and vegetable consumption, and lower-quality diets.[52] Frequency of consumption of fruit, salad, carrots, and vegetables declined significantly as food insecurity increased.[51] Some U.S. policymakers have doubted the existence of food insecurity because of the prevalence of overweight in lower income groups.[50] Excess body weight and inadequate food supply do seem paradoxical. Yet, mildly and moderately food insecure women were 41% and 52% overweight, respectively, compared to food-secure women.[50,51,53]

Fresh fruits and vegetable are perceived as luxury items and are not always easily accessible. Householders with diminishing incomes first consume less expensive foods to save money and maintain energy intakes, but at a lower cost.[52] An important strategy used by low-income consumers is to stretch the food budget by consuming energy-dense foods (see Box 7.5). These foods are less expensive than foods that are not energy-dense, allowing for a higher energy consumption at a lower cost. In other words, there is an inverse relation between energy density (kilocalories per gram) and energy cost (dollar per kilocalories).[52] Although cost is the most significant predictor of dietary choice,[54] there has been little emphasis on the low economic cost of becoming obese.[52] The Thrifty Food Plan, developed by the USDA to aid low-income house-holders in shopping for food, becomes more expensive when healthier, lower-fat options are included. (See Box 7.6.)

Cost constraints reduce the proportion of energy contributed by fruits, vegetables, meat, and dairy and increase the proportion of energy contributed by cereals, added fats, and sweets. The low cost of energy-dense foods may in turn promote overconsumption. Income disparities affect diet quality more than total energy intake does.[52] Nutrient intake was found to be lower for the food insecure for all nutrients except vitamin A and fat.[51]

Box 7.5 Energy Density: Volume vs. Calories

All foods have a certain number of calories within a given amount (volume). Some foods, such as desserts, candies, and processed foods, are high in energy density. This means that a small volume of that food has a large number of calories. For example, just a half-cup of mixed nuts delivers more than 400 cal.

Alternatively, some foods, such as vegetables and fruit, have a low energy density. These foods provide a larger portion size with a fewer number of calories. For example, in a half-cup serving, raw broccoli contains just 15 cal, and a half-cup of cubed cantaloupe has 28 cal.

Two factors play an important role in what makes food less energy-dense and more filling: water and fiber.

- *Water.* Many fruits and vegetables are high in water, which provides volume but not calories. Grapefruit, for example, is about 90% water and has just 39 cal in a half-cup serving. Carrots are about 88% water and have only 52 cal in 1 cup.
- *Fiber.* High-fiber foods, such as vegetables, fruits, and whole grains, not only provide volume, but also take longer to digest, leading to a sense of satiety for a longer period of time.

Source: MayoClinic.com. Energy density and weight loss: feel full on fewer calories. Available at: www.mayoclinic.com/ health/weight-loss/NU00195. Accessed July 27, 2006.

Box 7.6 The Thrifty Food Plan

The standard Thrifty Food Plan (TFP) market basket is a low-cost meal plan developed by the USDA that demonstrates how people on a modest budget can meet minimum USDA food pyramid guidelines. The TFP contains 2 weeks of meal plans with grocery shopping lists that are the basis for market basket studies. Although the TFP meets the food pyramid guidelines, it does not include many of the healthier recommended choices, such as low-fat and fat-free dairy products, lean meat, and whole grains. Comparing the cost of a standard market basket of foods to a healthier basket with low-fat meat and dairy, and whole grains reveals that the healthier basket was 16 to 22% more expensive due to higher costs of whole grains, lean beef, and skinless poultry.

Source: Jetter, K.M. and Cassady, D.L. The availability and cost of healthier food items. University of California. Agricultural Issues Center. AIC Issues Brief No. 29, March 2005.

7.14 THE FOOD ENVIRONMENT

What foods are available to an individual whether at home,[55] at school, at work, or in one's neighborhood comprises the food environment. Availability of food is affected by both accessibility and affordability.

7.14.1 FOOD AWAY FROM HOME

Americans are eating more meals away from home,[55] and eating frequently in restaurants is one of the behaviors associated with obesity.[56,57,58,59]

- The share of total food expenditure that Americans spend on dining out has risen from 28% in 1962 to 47% in 2003.
- The per capita number of fast-food restaurants doubled between 1972 through 1997, whereas the per capita number of full-service restaurants rose by 35%.
- Between 1977–1978 and 1994–1996, consumption of food away from home (FAFH) increased from 18% to 32% of total calories.
- Compared to home-cooked foods, foods eaten away from home are more calorie-dense.[60] FAFH meals and snacks contain more calories per eating occasion. FAFH is higher in total fat and saturated fat on a per-calorie basis than at-home food.[61] (Parenthetically, FAFH contains less dietary fiber, calcium, and iron on a per-calorie basis. For adults but not children, food prepared away from home is more sodium and cholesterol dense.[62])

7.14.2 PORTION SIZES

The size of food portions have increased over time and exceed federal standards as defined by the USDA in MyPyramid and the FDA for food labels. (See DHHS, NIH, Portion Distortion available at: http://hp2010.nhlbihin.net/portion/.) Larger portions contain more calories and simultaneously encourage people to eat more.[63]

In 1916, Coca Cola came in 6.5 oz bottles. By the 1950s, 10-oz and 12-oz "king-sized" bottles were available; however, the 6.5 oz size still accounted for 80% of sales. Currently, soft drinks marketed for individual consumption come in 20-oz and 32-oz bottles. The 20-oz size has replaced the 12-oz in vending machines and at convenience stores. This size inflation is pervasive (see Table 7.7 Size Inflation). An analysis of 66 restaurants showed a 12% increase in menu offerings described as "king size" or "queen size" between 1988 and 1993.[64]

TABLE 7.7
Size Inflation

| Food | Common Portion Size | |
	1960	2000
Bagel	2–3 oz	4–6 oz
Muffin	2–3 oz	5–7 oz
Coca-Cola, bottle	6.5 fl oz	20 fl oz
Chocolate bar	1 oz	1.5-8 oz
Potato chips, bag	1 oz	2–4 oz
McDonald's hamburger	1.5 oz	1.5-8 oz
McDonald's soda	7 fl oz	12–42 fl oz
McDonald's French fries	2.4 oz	2.4–7.1 oz
Pasta entrée	1.5 cups	3 cups
Beer, can	12 fl oz	12–24 fl oz

Source: From Young, L. *The Portion Teller.* New York: Morgan Road Books, 2005, p. 9.

Analysis of nationally representative data from the Nationwide Food Consumption Survey (1977–1978) and the Continuing Survey of Food Intake by Individuals (CSFII, 1989–1991, 1994–1996, and 1998) indicates that for each survey year, average portion size consumed from specific food items (salty snacks, desserts, soft drinks, fruit drinks, french fries, hamburgers, cheeseburgers, pizza, and Mexican food) increased both inside and outside the home for all categories, except pizza. For example, a typical hamburger grew from 5.7 oz in the 1970s to an average of 7 oz — 97 calories more — by the mid-1990s. A serving of french fries increased from 3.1 to 3.6 oz, adding 68 calories. A typical serving of soft drink climbed 6.8 fluid ounces, or about 50 calories, to 19.9 oz. The large portion-size increases were observed for food consumed at home as well as FAFH, a shift that indicates marked changes in eating behavior in general. For some foods, such as french fries, hamburgers, and Mexican foods, people reported eating the biggest portions at home, not at restaurants. For instance, the analysis found that the average home-cooked hamburger now weighs about 8 oz, vs. 5.5 oz in full-service restaurants and 7 oz at fast-food outlets.[65]

7.14.3 SNACKS

A comparison of food consumption data from the CSFII of 1977–1978 and 1994–1996 indicates that reported daily consumption increased by 268 calories for men and 143 calories for women. *Most of the increase is in energy consumed as snacks.*[66]

7.14.4 SCHOOL FOOD

In the latter half of the 20th century, the federal government developed and expanded a set of measures to combat the problems of domestic hunger and malnutrition. Congress passed the National School Lunch Act in 1946 (now known as the Richard B. Russell National School Lunch Act) as a measure of national security, to safeguard the health and well-being of the nation's children, and to encourage the domestic consumption of nutritious agricultural commodities. The bill made permanent the school lunch program, under which all students receive low-cost lunches and low-income students receive them at no cost. The School Breakfast Program began as a pilot program in 1966 and was expanded into a permanent program in 1975.

School breakfasts must provide, on average over each school week, at least one fourth of the daily Recommended Dietary Allowances (RDA) for protein, iron, calcium, and vitamins A and C.

Lunches must provide, on average over each school week, at least one third of the daily RDA of these nutrients. The choice of foods served and how they are prepared and presented are made by local schools. Since its inception in 1946, Congress has improved the child school nutrition program to better serve children and families and adjust to changes in nutrition recommendations and guidelines, families, workplaces, schools, and communities.

The Healthy Meals for Children Act (Public Law 104–149 §1, May 29, 1996, 110 Stat. 1379.) effective in 1997, established that to be eligible for federal reimbursement by the United States. Department of Agriculture (USDA), schools must serve breakfasts and lunches consistent with the applicable recommendations of the most recent Dietary Guidelines for Americans (see Chapter 10). Through Team Nutrition, USDA provides schools with technical training and assistance to help school service personnel prepare meals that meet federal guidelines. Team Nutrition also offers nutrition education to help children understand the link between diet and health.

The Child Nutrition and WIC Reauthorization Act of 2004 (Public Law 108–265.) requires each local education authority to establish a School Wellness Policy for participating schools. The policy must include goals for nutrition education, physical activity, and other school-based activities designed to promote health and prevent obesity (see Chapter 10).

Although many overweight low-income children participate in the School Breakfast and Lunch Programs, a review commissioned by the USDA found no published research to demonstrate that participation in food assistance programs causes overweight in children.[67]

7.14.5 Competitive Food

Most schools allow food to be sold outside of the official food service. These "competitive foods" have been criticized as providing many children with unneeded calories (from fat and sugar), supplanting the more nutritionally-dense foods available through the federal food programs.

Although they have long been a source of concern to nutritionists, supporters contend that competitive foods, particularly those sold through vending machines, generate significant revenues

---

Box 7.7 Competitive Foods

Competitive foods include all foods and beverages sold in schools during the lunch hour except for meals provided through the federal school meal programs. Current federal regulations restrict only a subset of competitive foods, foods of minimal nutritional value (FMNV), from being sold during mealtimes in food service areas. FMNV means: (1) in the case of artificially sweetened foods, a food which provides less than 5% of the Reference Daily intakes (RDI) for each of eight specified nutrients per serving, and (2) in the case of all other foods, a food which provides less than 5% of the RDI of each of 8 specified nutrients per serving. The eight nutrients to be assessed for this purpose are protein, vitamin A, vitamin C, niacin, riboflavin, thiamine, calcium, and iron. The categories of FMNV include: soda water, water ices, chewing gum, certain candies, hard candy, jellies and gums, marshmallow candies, fondant, licorice, spun candy, and candy coated popcorn. Competitive foods are sold in a variety of locations on a many school campuses nationwide. The types of competitive foods available often differ by location where they are sold, with healthy foods more often sold in a la carte lines in the cafeteria and less healthy foods more often sold through vending machines, school stores, canteens, and snack bars.

Source: Federal Regulation 7 CFR § 210.11 Competitive Food Services; United States General Accounting Office. School Meal Programs. Competitive Foods Are Available in Many Schools; Actions Taken to Restrict Them Differ by State and Locality. Report to Congressional Requesters. GAO-04-673. April 2004. Available at: http://www.gao.gov/new.items/d04673.pdf. Accessed March 14, 2005.

that fund special activities or items not covered in a school's budget. Beverage companies, which offer bonuses to schools for signing contracts that permit exclusive use of their particular brand, have been a major source of funds for school districts. The schools receive cash and other incentives, and the beverage company receives the right to sell sodas in vending machines and to advertise on scoreboards, in hallways, on book covers, and other places. Such "pouring rights" have been available on college campuses since the early 1990s and have more recently appeared in schools for children of all ages.[68] Approximately 60% of all U.S. middle and high schools sell soft drinks in vending machines. In 2002, an estimated 240 U.S. school districts had entered into exclusive pouring rights contracts with soft drink companies. These contracts reward schools for selling more soda to students, and some even directly link the school's revenues to the amount of soda sold.[69]

Preliminary small-scale studies suggest that the presence of competitive foods in schools is related to a decrease in fruit and vegetable consumption and an increase in calories obtained from fat. A small study examining the behaviors of 598 7th-grade students found that, on average, students in schools with a la carte programs consumed fewer fruits and vegetables and obtained more of their daily calories from total fat and saturated fat than students in schools without a la carte programs.[70]

In another study, changes in food and beverage consumption were examined over time for 2 student cohorts of a total of 594 middle school students. In year 1, 4th graders in the experimental group had access only to the school lunch program but gained snack bar access in year 2 when they transitioned to the 5th grade. Compared to the control group, average consumption of fruits, regular vegetables and milk decreased, and average consumption of high-fat vegetables and sweetened beverages increased for students moving from fourth to fifth grade. These middle school students who gained access to school snack bars consumed fewer healthy foods compared with the previous school year when they were in elementary school and had access only to lunch meals served at school. Snack bar access may have played a role in some of the observed changes.[71]

In accordance with P.L. 108-265, school districts establish their own policies regarding competitive foods. Several large school districts have enacted policies to restrict competitive foods beyond federal regulations. The New York City Department of Education, which administers the largest school district in the U.S., eliminated candy, soda, and other snack foods from all vending machines in 2003. Vending machines on school grounds are limited to selling water, low-fat snacks, and 100% fruit juices. The following year, the Los Angeles Board of Education, the second largest school district in the U.S., banned soda, fried chips, candy, and other snack foods from school vending machines and school stores. In recent years, several individual schools across the U.S. have taken actions to restrict competitive foods in schools beyond federal, state, and school board regulations. These actions include removing all food from vending machines except water and juice, removing soda and candy from vending machines and replacing them with juices and cereal bars, removing all vending machines selling soda and snack food, and removing sodas and other foods with minimal nutritional value (FMNV) from vending machines.

7.15 OBESITY PREVENTION

Ideally, the treatment of obesity should parallel its prevention: "increasing physical activity, improving diet, then sustaining these lifestyle changes can reduce both body weight and risk of diabetes."[72] (See Box 7.8.) This is, of course, easier said than done.

Several recent studies have found only a small fraction of the U.S. population adheres to a healthy lifestyle. Reeves and Rafferty defined four healthy lifestyle characteristics (HLCs) — nonsmoking, healthy weight, fruit and vegetable consumption, and regular physical activity — that together serve as a single healthy lifestyle indicator. Using data from the 2000 BRFSS, they

---

Box 7.8 WHO Recommendations for Developing Strategies to Reduce Obesity

- Strategies should be comprehensive and address all major dietary and physical activity risks for chronic diseases together, alongside other risks (such as tobacco use) from a multisectoral perspective.
- Each country should select what will constitute the optimal mix of actions that are in accord with national capabilities, laws, and economic realities.
- Governments have a central steering role in developing strategies, ensuring that actions are implemented and monitoring their impact over the long term.
- Ministries of health have a crucial convening role — bringing together other ministries needed for effective policy design and implementation.
- Governments need to work together with the private sector, health professional bodies, consumer groups, academics, the research community, and other nongovernmental bodies if sustained progress is to occur.
- A life-course perspective on chronic disease prevention and control is critical. This starts with maternal and child health, nutrition, and care practices, and carries through to school and workplace environments and access to preventive health and primary care, as well as community-based care for the elderly and disabled people.
- Strategies should explicitly address equality and diminish disparities; they should focus on the needs of the poorest communities and population groups. This requires a strong role for government.
- Strategies should be gender sensitive, as women generally make decisions about household nutrition.

Source: Diet, Nutrition and the Prevention of Chronic Diseases: report of a Joint WHO/FAO Expert Consultation. Geneva, January 28–February 1, 2002. WHO technical report series 916. Geneva, Switzerland: WHO, 2003. Available at: http://www.who.int/nut/documents/trs_916.pdf. Accessed July 24, 2005.

---

determined that only 3.0% of U.S. adults practiced all four health behaviors.[73] A subsequent study by Ford et al., using the same 4 HLCs examined data from NHANES III. They found that only 6.8% of the population engaged in all four healthy lifestyle factors and concluded, "There is a long road to travel" before a preponderance of Americans adopt a healthy lifestyle.[74]

7.15.1 Dieting

With nearly a third of adults trying to lose weight at any one time, Americans seek the one perfect diet. Of these, the low-carbohydrate, high-fat diet popularized by Dr. Atkins had a stunning run of popularity. Why? The basic philosophy of the diet — that fat calories don't matter and that carbohydrates are bad — contradicts the tenets of the less glamorous, hard-working, high-carbohydrate diet where weight loss can only occur if caloric expenditure exceeds intake.[75,78] True, the fantasy low-carbohydrate, high-fat diet of steak and bacon results in fairly rapid, early weight loss; however, by 12 months there is no appreciable difference in results.[75,] In its favor, the low-carbohydrate diet raises HDL and lowers triglyceride levels but does so at the expense of the rest of the lipoprotein profile.[79] Through the alchemy of ketosis, the low-carbohydrate advocates claim excess fat melts away. Unfortunately, the long-term effects of ketosis — such as possible kidney and liver damage — are not resolved. Similar discord arises in discussions of insulin resistance.[75]

No weight-loss diet is easy to adhere to. There are many well-accepted methods to reduce initial body weight by 7–10%, but long-term maintenance of that lost weight is more problematic.

Box 7.9 Strategies for Successful Weight Loss Maintenance

Successful weight loss maintainers enrolled in the National Weight Control Registry (NWCR) consistently report four strategies they use to maintain their weight loss.

- Consuming a low-calorie, low-fat diet. It is estimated that registry members eat about 1800 calories per day, with about one-quarter of calories from fat. Registry members report consuming 2.5 meals per week in restaurants and 0.74 meals per week in fast food establishments, much less frequently than the national average.
- Regularly engaging in high levels of physical activity for 1 h/d. Three-quarters of the respondents walk briskly everyday; other activities engaged in most frequently includes weight lifting, cycling, and aerobics.
- Weighing themselves frequently. Almost half of the respondents weigh themselves everyday. This frequent monitoring of weight would allow these individuals to catch small weight gains and hopefully initiate corrective behavior changes.
- Consuming breakfast daily.

Source: Wing, R.R. and Phelan, S. Long-term weight loss maintenance. *Am J Clin Nutr.* 82(Suppl.), 222S–225S, 2005. Available at: http://www.ajcn.org/cgi/content/full/82/1/222S. Accessed August 24, 2006.

On average, among treatment-seeking populations, approximately one-third of lost weight is regained by 1 year; by 5 years most or all previously lost weight is regained.[78] An ongoing registry using a convenience sample of long-term weight maintainers is providing valuable information about behaviors endorsed by those with long-term success. As reported by the National Weight Control Registry (http://www.nwcr.ws/), 90% of people who are successful at maintaining their weight loss consume a diet with 20–30% of energy from fat, restrict total energy intake, and participate in regular physical activity.[76] In essence, people who are successful at losing weight and who maintain their lower weight status are always dieting,[80] or so it seems to their overweight counterparts. (See Box 7.9.)

7.15.2 PROPOSED OBESITY PREVENTION POLICIES

7.15.2.1 Regulating Advertising to Children

Although television watching may contribute to childhood obesity, use of the media may also provide opportunities to positively affect the problem. Leading policy options include reducing or regulating food ads targeted to children, expanding public education campaigns to promote healthy eating and exercise, incorporating messages about healthy eating into TV storylines, and supporting interventions to reduce the time children spend with media.

The American Public Health Association (APHA) has a long history of supporting legislation to limit television advertising aimed at children. For example, in 1977 it supported regulation of sugared snacks advertisements to children. Currently, the APHA supports congressional action to eliminate television food advertising aimed at young children[81] or at least to limit the amount of advertising permitted on children's television to no more than five to six commercial minutes per hour. At present, the FTC allows 10.5 min of commercials to be broadcast per hour of children's television shows aired on weekends, and 12 min/h on weekdays. Additional policies supported by APHA include banning advertising in schools; developing school policies that promote a healthful eating environment, including a ban on the sale of soft drinks and other high-calorie, low nutrition foods during the school day; convening a national conference to develop recommendations to address the issue of advertising food to children; allocating NIH funds to study the effects of food advertising and marketing on health behaviors of children and adolescents; and developing school-based media literacy curricula for children and adolescents.

According to the American Psychological Association (APA), children under the age of eight are unable to critically comprehend televised advertising messages and are prone to accept advertiser messages as truthful, accurate, and unbiased, which can lead to unhealthy eating habits. As sugared cereals, candies, sweets, sodas, and snack foods are the most common products marketed to children, advertising of unhealthy food products to young children may be a variable in the current epidemic of pediatric overweight. Research on children's commercial recall and product preferences confirms that advertising does typically get young consumers to buy products. A series of studies on product choices demonstrates that children not only recall content from the ads to which they have been exposed but also exhibit preferences for a product with as little as a single commercial exposure, a preference that is strengthened with repeated exposures. These product preferences can affect children's product purchase requests, putting pressure on parents' purchasing decisions and insti-gating parent–child conflicts when parents deny requests. The accumulation of evidence on adver-tising to children is compelling enough to warrant regulatory action by the government. APA recommends that restrictions be placed on advertising to children too young to recognize its persuasive intent, a policy that would bring the U.S. alongside Australia, Canada, Sweden, and Great Britain, which have already adopted regulations prohibiting advertising on programs whose audiences are young children.[82]

As expected, the advertising industry opposes any such regulation, citing its long history of self-regulation. The private organization Children's Advertising Review Unit (CARU) has developed self-regulating guides for advertisers to follow when advertising to children[83] First Amendment free speech protection is also frequently invoked (see Box 7.10). Industry spokespersons claim that advertising's role in preventing obesity is in adhering to the marketing principles outlined in CARU's guidelines for advertising directed to children under 12 years of age. They also tout activities such as their ad campaigns for obesity prevention[84] and disease prevention[85] that aim to promote an active lifestyle and other behaviors that will result in reducing the risk of developing type 2 diabetes, CVD, and cancer.

Box 7.10 First Amendment, U.S. Constitution

Congress shall make no law respecting an establishment of religion, or prohibiting the free exercise thereof; or abridging the freedom of speech, or of the press; or the right of the people peaceably to assemble, and to petition the Government for a redress of grievances. First Amendment rights are the foundation of democracy in the U.S. They help to create an open society in which people have the ability to share and discuss differing opinions and beliefs. The First Amendment was written precisely to protect controversial and/or offensive speech and ideas (other speech and ideas would not have to be protected). It covers spoken and written words, as well as pictures, art, and other forms of expression of ideas and opinions, such as armbands and insignia. *It is a restriction on the power of government* rather than on individuals or private businesses. There are times when the government can regulate the time, place, and manner of speech, but — generally — it cannot censor the *content* of protected expression. Most advertising is considered commercial speech. Commercial speech does receive First Amendment protection, although the government may restrict commercial speech that is false, misleading, or promotes a product, service, or conduct that is illegal. For example, broadcast media (television, radio) has been highly regulated through licenses granted by the Federal Trade Commission.

7.15.2.2 Labeling and Taxation

To promote nutrition and activity, the Center for Science in the Public Interest (CSPI) suggests policy options such as requiring nutrition labeling on menus and menu boards at chain restaurants[86] and levying taxes on foods of low nutritional value (such as soft drinks and some snack foods) and using the revenues to fund health promotion programs.[87]

The Food and Drug Administration's (FDA) Obesity Working Group proposed an action plan to cover critical dimensions of the obesity problem from FDA's perspective and authorities. In addition to encouraging restaurants to provide nutritional information to consumers, policy recommendations include modifying the food label to display calorie count more prominently and to use meaningful serving sizes, stepping-up enforcement actions concerning accuracy of food labels, initiating a consumer education campaign focusing on the "Calories Count" message, and revising FDA guidance for developing drugs to treat obesity.[88] (See Box 7.11.)

Box 7.11 Recommendations of the FDA Working Group on Obesity

Food Labeling: The report recommends that FDA take the following actions:

- Publish an advance notice of proposed rulemaking (ANPRM) to seek comment on how to give more prominence to calories on the food label (e.g., increasing the font size for calories, including a percent daily value column for total calories, and eliminating the listing for calories from fat).
- Publish an ANPRM to seek comment on authorizing health claims on certain foods that meet FDA's definition of "reduced" or "low" calorie. An example of a health claim for a "reduced" or "low" calorie food might be: "Diets low in calories may reduce the risk of obesity, which is associated with type 2 diabetes, heart disease, and certain cancers."
- Publish an ANPRM to seek comment on whether to require additional columns on the NFP to list quantitative amounts and percent daily value of an entire package on those products/package sizes that can reasonably be consumed at one eating occasion (or declare the whole package as single serving).
- Publish an ANPRM to seek comment on which, if any, reference amounts customarily consumed of food categories appear to have changed the most over the past decade and require updating.
- File petitions the agency has received that ask FDA to define terms such as "low," "reduced," and "free" carbohydrate; provide guidance for the use of the term "net" in relation to carbohydrate content of food.
- Encourage manufacturers to use dietary guidance statements, an example of which would be, "To manage your weight, balance the calories you eat with your physical activity."
- Encourage manufacturers to take advantage of the flexibility in current regulations on serving sizes to label as a single-serving those food packages where the entire contents of the package can reasonably be consumed as a single serving.
- Encourage manufacturers to use appropriate comparative labeling statements that make it easier for consumers to make healthy substitutions.

Enforcement: Accurate information in the NFP is crucial for consumers to monitor their intake of calories and nutrients. In particular, meaningful serving sizes can help consumers understand how many calories they consume. The report recommends that FDA take the following actions:

- Consider enforcement activities against those manufacturers that declare inaccurate serving sizes.
- Highlight in the Food Labeling Compliance Program enforcement against inaccurate declarations of serving sizes.
- Continue to work with the Federal Trade Commission to target dietary supplement products with false or misleading weight-loss claims.

Education: The OWG report recommends that FDA focus its education strategy on influencing behavior, as well as imparting knowledge, in the context of healthy eating choices for consumers and with the basic message that "Calories Count." The report specifically recommends that FDA, as part of a larger DHHS effort, take the following actions:

- Establish relationships with private and public sector groups to give consumers a better understanding of the food label and how to use the label to help them make healthier and wiser food choices.
- Pursue relationships with youth-oriented organizations, such as the Girl Scouts of the U.S. and the 4-H program, to provide educational programs that emphasize caloric balance and proper diet for weight management.

Restaurants/Industry: American consumers now spend approximately 46% of their food budget on food consumed outside of the home, and these foods account for a significant portion of total calories consumed, especially from quick-service restaurants. The report specifically recommends the following actions:

- Urge the restaurant industry to launch a nationwide, voluntary, and point-of-sale nutrition information campaign for consumers.
- Encourage consumers routinely to request nutrition information when eating out.
- Develop a series of options for providing voluntary, standardized, simple, and understand-able nutrition information, including calorie information, at the point-of-sale to consumers in restaurants.
- Explore the concept of third-party certification of weight-loss diet plans and related products.

Therapeutics: FDA recognizes that obese and extremely obese individuals are likely to need medical intervention to reduce weight and mitigate associated diseases and other adverse health effects. The report recommends that FDA take the following actions:

- Convene a meeting of a standing FDA advisory committee to address challenges, as well as gaps in knowledge, about existing drug therapies for obesity.
- Continue discussions with pharmaceutical and medical device sponsors about new obe-sity medical products.
- Revise the 1996 "Guidance for the Clinical Evaluation of Weight-Control Drugs" draft guidance on developing obesity drugs and reissue it for comment.

Research: One of the mandates of the OWG was to identify applied and basic research needs that include the development of healthier foods as well as a better understanding of consumer behavior and motivation. The report recommends that FDA take the following actions:

- Support and collaborate, as appropriate, on obesity-related research with others, including NIH.
- Collaborate with the U.S. Department of Agriculture/Agricultural Research Service on a USDA-sponsored national obesity prevention conference (in October 2004).
- Pursue five other areas of obesity research: (1) information to facilitate consumers' weight management decisions, (2) the relationship between overweight/obesity and food consumption patterns, (3) incentives for product reformulation, (4) the potential for FDA-regulated products unintentionally to contribute to or result in obesity, and (5) the extension of basic research findings to the regulatory environment.

Source: U.S. Food and Drug Administration. *Backgrounder.* Report of the Working Group on Obesity. March 12, 2004. Available at: www.fda.gov/oc/initiatives/obesity/backgrounder.html. Accessed July 27, 2006.

7.15.2.3 School-Based Programs

Schools play a critical role in promoting student health, preventing childhood obesity, and combating problems associated with poor nutrition and physical inactivity. To formalize and encourage this role, P.L. 108–265 required each school district participating in the National School Lunch and/or Breakfast Program to establish a local wellness policy by the start of the 2006 school year (see Box 7.12). This legislation supports the HealthierUS initiative (see Section 7.6.3.1) that encourages Americans to be physically active, eat a nutritious diet, get preventive screening, and make healthy choices. The legislation places the responsibility of developing a wellness policy at the local level so that the individual needs of each district can be addressed.

Box 7.12 Commponents of a Local Wellness Policy

As required by law, a local wellness policy, at a minimum, must include:

- *Goals for nutrition education, physical activity and other school-based activities* that are designed to promote student wellness in a manner that the local educational agency determines is appropriate.
- *Nutrition guidelines* selected by the local educational agency for all foods available on each school campus under the local educational agency during the school day with the objectives of promoting student health and reducing childhood obesity.
- *Guidelines for reimbursable school meals,* which are no less restrictive than regulations and guidance issued by the Secretary of Agriculture pursuant to Subsections (a) and (b) of Section 10 of the Child Nutrition Act (42 U.S.C. 1779) and Section 9(f)(1) and 17(a) of the Richard B. Russell National School Lunch Act (42 U.S.C. 1758(f)(1), 1766(a)0, as those regulations and guidance apply to schools. This requirement implies that districts must ensure that reimbursable school meals meet the program requirements and nutrition standards set forth under the 7 CFR Part 210 and Part 220.
- *A plan for measuring implementation of the local wellness policy,* including designation of one or more persons within the local educational agency or at each school, as appropriate, charged with operational responsibility for ensuring that each school fulfills

the district's local wellness policy.
- *Community involvement*, including parents, students, and representatives of the school food authority, the school board, school administrators, and the public in the development of the school wellness policy.

Source: From USDA, Food and Nutrition Service. Healthy schools: local wellness policy requirements. Available at: www.fns.usda.gov/tn/Healthy/wellness_policyrequirements.html. Accessed July 27, 2006.

Significant online support for developing school wellness policies is available from USDA's Team Nutrition and the National Alliance for Nutrition and Activity (NANA: www.nanacoalition. org). The Team Nutrition Web site http://www.fns.usda.gov/tn/Healthy/wellnesspolicy.html provides local wellness policy requirements, information on creating a policy, examples of extant policies, implementation tools and resources, and sources of funding for supporting policy implementation. NANA's site makes available resources about general nutrition, school meals, meal times and scheduling, nutrition standards for foods and beverages sold individually, fruit and vegetable promotion in schools, fundraising activities, snacks, rewards, celebrations, promoting physical activity, physical education, food marketing, and monitoring and policy review.

7.15.2.4 Private, Nonprofit Organizations

In 2005, the American Heart Association and the William J. Clinton Foundation teamed up to form the Alliance for a Healthier Generation (http://www.healthiergeneration.org/engine/renderpage.asp? pid=s034.), to combat the spread of childhood obesity and associated morbidities such as heart disease and diabetes. Alliance programs focus on healthy schools, industry, physical activity in children, and healthcare. In 2006, the Alliance announced an initiative to collaborate with schools to help them create environments that foster healthy lifestyles and ultimately prevent overweight and obesity among students. The program was made possible by an $8 million grant from the Robert Wood Johnson Foundation (RWJF http://www.rwjf.org/).

RJWF is self-described as the nation's largest philanthropy devoted exclusively to improving the health and healthcare of all Americans. In addition to its support of the Alliance for a Healthier Generation, the foundation has initiated Healthy Eating Research, a national program to support research that identifies, analyzes, and evaluates environmental and policy approaches to increasing healthy eating among children.

7.15.2.5 Federal Programs

7.15.2.5.1 HealthierUS

In 2002, the HealthierUS initiative was undertaken "to help Americans live longer, better, and healthier lives." The four focus areas of this national campaign are initiatives addressing physical fitness and nutrition, as well as prevention (screenings and tests for blood pressure and cholesterol) and healthy choices (washing one's hands regularly, wearing a safety belt, and avoiding risky behaviors such as using tobacco or drugs and abusing alcohol).[89] A portal to the program is available online at www.healthierus.gov/. Personal responsibility for the choices Americans make, plus social responsibility to ensure that policymakers support programs that foster healthy behaviors and prevent disease, lie at the heart of this campaign. Policymakers, the health community, and the public are being encouraged to establish programs and policies that support behavior changes, encourage healthier lifestyle choices, and reduce disparities in healthcare. (See also Box 7.13.)

Box 7.13 Materials Developed by the Federal Government Designed to Facilitate Implementation of Obesity Prevention Programs and Policies

- *Making It Happen — School Nutrition Success Stories*, a joint product of HHS, USDA, and ED provides case studies of 32 schools and school districts that have implemented innovative strategies to improve the nutritional quality of foods and beverages offered and sold on school campuses. The most consistent theme emerging from these vignettes is that students will buy and consume healthful foods and beverages — and schools can make money from healthful options.
- *The Health Education Curriculum Analysis Tool* is a user-friendly checklist designed by CDC to help schools select or develop curricula based on the extent to which they have characteristics that research has identified as being critical for leading to positive effects on youth health behaviors. The companion Physical Education Curriculum Analysis Tool will help school districts develop state-of-the-art physical education curriculum based on insights gained from research and best practice.
- *Media Smart Youth: Food, Fitness, and Fun* is a curriculum with supporting materials developed by the National Institute of Child Health and Human Development for youth ages 11–13 years. It is designed to create awareness of the role that media play in shaping values concerning physical activity and nutrition, while building skills to encourage critical thinking, healthy lifestyle choices, and informed decision making, now and in their future.
- The *School Health Index (SHI) Self-Assessment and Planning Guide* was developed by CDC in partnership with school administrators and staff and non-governmental agencies in order to enable schools to identify strengths and weaknesses in their health and safety policies and programs; help schools develop an action plan for improving student health, which can be incorporated into the School Improvement Plan; and engage stakeholders (teachers, parents, students, the community) in promoting health-enhancing behaviors and better health. The 2005 edition of the SHI covers safety, physical activity, nutrition, and tobacco use (additional health topics will be added in future editions). CDC has developed guidelines for schools to address each of these risk behaviors, which are typically established during childhood and adolescence.
- *Fruit and Vegetables Galore*, developed in 2003 by USDA in collaboration with HHS, provides strategies for school foodservice professionals on planning, purchasing, preparing, presenting, and promoting fruits and vegetables in school food programs. The program also includes suggestions for working with teachers by providing them with teaching tools and by supporting their educational efforts (making daily meal offerings competitive with other commercial options available to students) and motivating students to choose a more healthful diet.

Source: U.S. Department of Agriculture. Team Nutrition. *Making It Happen! School Nutrition Success Stories.* March 2005. Available at: http://www.fns.usda.gov/tn/Resources/makingithappen.html. Accessed July 18, 2005; U.S. Department of Agriculture. Food and Nutrition Service. *Fruits & Vegetables Galore — Helping Kids Eat More.* FNS-365. February 2004. Available in four parts at: http://www.fns.usda.gov/tn/Resources/eye_prize.pdf; http://www.fns.usda. gov/tn/Resources/ quality_intro.pdf; http://www.fns.usda.gov/tn/Resources/tricks_trade.pdf; http://www.fns.usda.gov/ tn/Resources/meal_ appeal.pdf. Accessed July 21, 2005.

Steps to a HealthierUS (Steps)[90] was launched by the U.S. Department of Health and Human Services (DHHS) in 2003 to advance the government's *HealthierUS* agenda. The *Steps* initiative aims to identify and promote programs that encourage small behavior changes through the combined efforts of all DHHS agencies, including the CDC, FDA, and NIH. *Steps* encourages

- Health promotion programs to motivate and support responsible health choices.
- Community initiatives to promote and enable healthy choices.
- Healthcare and insurance systems that put prevention first by reducing risk factors and complications of chronic disease.
- State and federal policies that invest in the promise of prevention for all Americans.
- Cooperation among policymakers, local health agencies, and the public to invest in disease prevention instead of spending our resources to treat diseases after they occur.

A centerpiece of *Steps* is a 5-year (2003–2008) cooperative agreement program through which states, cities, and tribal entities receive funds to implement chronic disease prevention efforts focused on reducing the burden of diabetes, overweight and obesity, and asthma and addressing three related risk behaviors: physical inactivity, poor nutrition, and tobacco use. In 2003, *Steps* allocated $13.6 million to fund 12 grantees representing 24 communities (7 large cities, 1 tribe, and 4 states that coordinate grants to 16 small cities and rural communities).

In 2004, almost $36 million was granted to increase funding to the existing communities and to fund an additional 10 grantees representing 16 communities (5 large cities, 2 tribes, and 3 states that coordinate grants to 9 small cities and rural communities). These 40 funded communities are implementing community action plans to reduce health disparities and promote quality healthcare and prevention services. They are expected to serve as models for other communities, and include programs in schools, healthcare, and workplace settings that offer organized community interventions such as walking programs, health education trainings, and media campaigns; environmental interventions such as smoking cessation programs and increasing healthy food choices in schools; and educational interventions such as enhancing coordinated school health programs.

Steps programs target rural communities, low-income populations, Hispanics and Latinos, American Indians and Alaska Natives, African Americans, immigrants, youth, senior citizens, uninsured and underinsured people, and other populations at high risk. Partners include departments of education and health, school districts, healthcare providers, national and local health organizations, faith-based agencies, private sector organizations, and academic institutions.[91]

The HealthierUS initiative sets the overall framework for the work of the USDA's Center for Nutrition Policy and Promotion (CNPP). In concert with the DHHS, CNPP is responsible for the revisions made to the *Dietary Guidelines for Americans* as well as the USDA's food guidance system, MyPyramid (www.mypyramid.gov). CNPP's work emphasizes the importance of nutrition combined with physical activity, prevention, and making healthier choices. The overall goal for the revision of the U.S. government's food guidance system in 2005 was to develop individualized tools to assist Americans in developing healthier lifestyles and improve overall health.

7.15.2.5.2   CDC Initiatives

The CDC has extensive experience in population-based prevention efforts through schools and worksites, the communications and marketing fields, and the nation's public health system. About 15 CDC divisions and programs currently conduct overweight and obesity-related public health activities. (Visit the CDC's obesity response Web site at: www.cdc.gov/doc.do/id/0900f3ec803207fd.)

7.15.2.5.3   Nutrition and Physical Activity Program to Prevent Obesity and Other Chronic Diseases

This program is designed to help states prevent obesity and other chronic diseases by addressing two closely related factors: poor nutrition and inadequate physical activity. The program supports states in developing and implementing science-based nutrition and physical activity interventions. The program's major goals are balancing caloric intake and expenditure, increasing physical activity, improving nutrition through increased consumption of fruits and vegetables, reducing television time, and increasing breastfeeding. In 2004–2005, 23 states were funded at $300,000 to $450,000 for "capacity-building," and 5 additional states were funded at $800,000 to $1.5 million for basic implementation. Health departments in the states that are in the capacity-building stage gather data, build partnerships, and create statewide health plans in order to lay the critical foundation before implementing nutrition and physical activity interventions. States in the basic implementation stage are in the process of developing new interventions, evaluating existing ones, and/or supporting additional state and local efforts to prevent obesity and other chronic diseases.[92] The CDC has developed a resource guide for nutrition and physical activity interventions to prevent and control obesity and other chronic diseases. Topics covered in the guide include obesity prevention and control (including caloric intake and expenditure), increased physical activity, improved nutrition (including increased breastfeeding and increased consumption of fruits and vegetables), and reduced television time.[93]

7.15.2.5.4   Other Programs Sponsored by the CDC

- The 5-A-Day for Better Health Program is a national effort to achieve the *Healthy People 2010* objective for increasing the per capita consumption to five or more servings of fruits and vegetables daily. www.5aday.gov/homepage/index_content.html
- Active Community Environment (ACES) promotes walking, bicycling, and the development of accessible recreation facilities. The site contains a working paper that discusses how land use and transportation systems impact health. www.cdc.gov/nccdphp/dnpa/aces.html
- *KidsWalk-to-School* (see Box 7.3) is a community-based program that aims to increase opportunities for daily physical activity by encouraging children to walk to and from school in groups accompanied by adults. An online guide is available that contains strategies to encourage individuals and organizations to work together to identify and create safe walking routes to school. www.cdc.gov/nccdphp/dnpa/kidswalk/
- Verb™ (see Chapter 14, Section 14.1.5.1.1. VERB™ It's What You Do) is a national, multicultural, social marketing youth marketing campaign designed to encourage young people ages 9–13 years ("tweens") to be physically active everyday. Verb™ combines paid advertising, marketing strategies, and partnership efforts to reach children and their adults/influencers (parents, educators, and youth leaders). www.cdc.gov/youthcampaign/

7.15.2.5.5   NIH Initiatives

To help families adopt healthier lifestyles, in 2005 the NHLBI of NIH launched a national public education program targeting parents and caregivers of children ages 8 to 13. *Ways to Enhance Children's Activity & Nutrition!* (*We Can!*) (see Chapter 14, Section 14.1.5.1.2 *We Can!*) provides resources to encourage healthy eating, increase physical activity, and reduce sedentary time. The program offers a parents' handbook in Spanish and English as well as a curriculum for parents and curricula for children tested at community-based sites. Online resources (www.nhlbi.nih.gov/health/ public/heart/obesity/wecan/) provide parents, caregivers, communities, national partners, and media strategies for maintaining a healthy weight for families. *We Can!* helps parents teach their children to:

- Eat a sufficient amount of a variety of vegetables and fruits each day
- Choose small portions at home and at restaurants
- Eat fewer high-fat foods and energy-dense foods that are low in nutrient value such as french fries, bacon, and doughnuts
- Substitute water or fat-free (skim) or low-fat (1%) milk for sweetened beverages such as sodas
- Engage in at least 60 min of moderate physical activity on most, preferably all, days of the week
- Reduce recreational screen time to no more than 2 h/d

7.15.2.6 Workplace Wellness Programs

Employee wellness programs that account for both individual and environmental influences can improve the health status of the workforce and quantifiably reduce healthcare costs. One evaluation found an average reduction of $3.35 in healthcare costs for each dollar spent on health promotion programs. In addition, absenteeism rates and associated costs are also reduced.[94,95]

Successful workplace health promotion programs share a set of common characteristics including attention to the need of the individual to identify his or her own health issues and health-related goals, variable needs for social support, interdependent health practices (for example, smoking and alcohol use), and lack of time. Success is further mediated by both management support (where employees sense the commitment of their employers to their well-being) and a supportive climate (for example, by placing reasonable demands on time and energy and enabling employees to "participate in the governance of their own work.")[96]

In the U.S., total employment in March 2006 was 143.6 million, with 63% of the population age 16 and over holding jobs.[97] One investigation of workplaces concluded that a health and fitness plan could improve the health of 53% of a workplace's employees;[98] thus, employee health programs have the potential to reach at least or 76 million people (143.6 million × 53%) nationwide.

Objective 7–5 of *HealthyPeople 2010* is to "increase the proportion of worksites that offer a comprehensive employee health promotion program to their employees." Objective 22–13 aims to "increase the proportion of worksites offering employer-sponsored physical activity and fitness programs."[99] Legislative efforts are being made nationwide to induce behavioral change through the workplace; businesses receiving a tax credit and reduced healthcare costs would have a stake in sustaining a wellness program.

At present, Illinois and Virginia make grants to employers to help them provide health promotion or wellness services, including aerobic exercise and physical fitness. New Jersey has established a state council on physical fitness whose responsibilities include assisting businesses in establishing fitness programs for employees. In 2002, a California task force was established to promote fitness in schools and workplaces by generating media interest and providing an informational Web site. Although a Colorado bill encourages citizens to value their health and workplaces to provide a supportive environment, it does not offer a tax credit or other incentives. The Massachusetts Department of Public Health, Mississippi's State Board of Health, and the West Virginia county boards are all mandated to provide health programs, including physical fitness, to public employees.[100]

A state-based tax credit to businesses is not the only approach, nor likely the only solution, to increasing physical activity. Wellness Councils of America (WELCOA) has developed guidelines to build and sustain a wellness at work program. Their Web site (http://www.welcoa.org) offers benchmarks to success, links to key resources, and recognition awards for successful programs.

7.16 CONCLUSION

Over the last 40 years, the rates of overweight and obesity in the U.S. have increased across all population categories to the point where they are now described as epidemic. In 2001, in response to this alarming trend, the Surgeon General published a call to action to prevent and decrease overweight and obesity. Just as overweight and obesity have no single, identifiable cause, they have no single solution. Action must be taken on all fronts, from the individual making informed health choices, to the federal government introducing and supporting effective policies. The built, economic, work, and food environments each play a role in inducing and reducing obesity. Although it is imperative that immediate action be taken to halt the rising rates of overweight and obesity and their attendant morbidities, the impact of any undertaking will likely take several decades to become evident.

7.17 ACRONYMS

ACES	Active Community Environment
AOA	American Obesity Association
APA	American Psychological Association
APHA	American Public Health Association
BMI	Body Mass Index
BRFSS	Behavioral Risk Factor Surveillance System
CARU	Children's Advertising Review Unit
CDC	Centers for Disease Control and Prevention
CNPP	Center for Nutrition Policy and Promotion
CSFII	Continuing Survey of Food Intake by Individuals
CSPI	Center for Science in the Public Interest
DHHS	Department of Health and Human Services
FAFH	Food eaten away from home
FDA	United States Food and Drug Administration
HDL	High density lipoprotein
HLC	Healthy lifestyle characteristics
MEPS	Medical Expenditure Panel Survey
NANA	National Alliance for Nutrition and Activity
NGHS	Growth and Health Study
NHANES	National Health and Nutrition Examination Survey
NHES	National Health Examination Survey
NHIS	National Health Interview Surveys
NHLBI	National Heart, Lung, and Blood Institute
NIH	National Institutes of Health
NR-NCD	Nutrition-related noncommunicable diseases
PedNSS	Pediatric Nutrition Surveillance System
RDA	Recommended Dietary Allowance
REACH 2010	Racial and Ethnic Approaches to Community Health 2010
SES	Socioeconomic status
USDA	United States Department of Agriculture
We Can!	Ways to Enhance Children's Activity and Nutrition!
WHO	World Health Organization
WIC	Special Supplemental Nutrition Program for Women, Infants, and Children

REFERENCES

1. U.S. Department of Health and Human Services. The Surgeon General's call to action to prevent and decrease overweight and obesity. Rockville, MD: U.S. Department of Health and Human Services, Public Health Service, Office of the Surgeon General, 2001. Available at: http://www.surgeongeneral. gov/ library. Accessed March 6, 2005.
2. National Institutes of Health (NIH), National Heart, Lung, and Blood Institute (NHLBI). Clinical guidelines on the identification, evaluation, and treatment of overweight and obesity in adults. HHS, Public Health Service (PHS), 1998. Available at: http://www.nhlbi.nih.gov/guidelines/obesity/ob_ gdlns. pdf. Accessed March 7, 2005.
3. Baskin, M.L., Ard, J., Frankllin, F., and Allison, D.B. Prevalence of obesity in the United States. *Obes Rev.* 6, 5–7, 2005.

4. Flegal, K.M., Carroll, M.D., Kuczmarski, R.J., and Johnson, C.L. Overweight and obesity in the United States: prevalence and trends, 1960–1994. *Int J Obes Relat Metab Disord.* 22, 39–47, 1998.

5. Liao, Y., Tucker, P., Okoro, C.A., Giles, W.H., Mokdad, A.H., and Harris, V.B. REACH 2010 Surveillance for Health Status in Minority Communities — United States, 2001–2002. *MMWR Surveill Summ.* 53, 1–36, 2004. Available at: www.cdc.gov/mmwr/preview/mmwrhtml/ss5306a1.htm. Accessed March 7, 2005.

6. CDC. Table 71. Overweight children and adolescents 6–19 years of age, according to sex, age, race, and Hispanic origin: United States, selected years 1963–1965 through 1999–2000. Available at: http://www.cdc.gov/nchs/data/hus/tables/2002/02hus071.pdf. Accessed July 24, 2006.

7. Mei, Z., Grummer-Strawn, L.M., and Scanlon, K.S. Does overweight in infancy persist through the preschool years? An analysis of CDC Pediatric Nutrition Surveillance System data. *Sozial-und Praventivmedizin.* 48, 161–167, 2003.

8. Freedman, D.S., Khan, L.K., Serdula, M.K., Dietz, W.H., Srinivasan, S.R., and Berenson, G.S. The relation of childhood BMI to adult adiposity: the Bogalusa Heart Study. *Pediatrics.* 115, 22–27, 2005.

9. Sherry, B., Mei, Z., Scanlon, K.S., Mokdad, A.H., and Grummer-Strawn, L.M. Trends in state-specific prevalence of overweight and underweight in 2- through 4-year-old children from low-income families from 1989 through 2000. *Arch Pediatr Adolesc Med.* 158, 1116–1124, 2004. Available at: http://archpedi.ama-assn.org/cgi/content/full/158/12/1116. Accessed March 5, 2005.

10. Mei, Z., Grummer-Strawn, L.M., and Scanlon, K.S. Does overweight in infancy persist through the preschool years? An analysis of CDC Pediatric Nutrition Surveillance System data. *Sozial-und Praventivmedizin.* 48, 161–167, 2003.

11. CDC. Overweight and obesity economic consequences. http://www.cdc.gov/nccdphp/dnpa/obesity/economic_consequences.htm. Accessed July 25, 2006.

12. Finkelstein, E.A., Fiebelkorn, I.C., and Wang, G. National medical spending attributable to overweight and obesity: how much, and who's paying?. *Health Affairs.* W3, 219–226, 2003.

13. Thompson, D. and Wolf, A.M. The medical-care cost burden of obesity. The International Association for the Study of Obesity. *Obes Rev.* 2, 189–197, 2001.

14. Eisenstein, E.L., Shaw, L.K., Nelson, C.L., Anstron, K.J., Hakim, Z., and Mark, D.B. Obesity and long-term clinical and economic outcomes in coronary artery disease patients. *Obes Res.* 10(2), 83–91, 2002.

15. Oster, G., Edelsberg, J., O'Sullivan, A.K., and Thompson, D. The clinical and economic burden of obesity in a managed care setting. *Am J Managed Care.* 6(6), 681–689, 2000.

16. Bungum, T., Satterwhite, M., Jackson, A.W., and Morrow, J.R. The relationship of body mass index, medical costs, and job absenteeism. *Am J Health Behav.* 27(4), 456–462, 2003.

17. Wolf, A.M. and Colditz, G.A. Social and economic effects of body weight in the United States. *Am J Clin Nutr.* 63(S), 466S–469S, 1996.

18. Wolf, A.M. Economic outcomes of the obese patient. *Obes Res.* 10(S1), 58S–62S, 2002.

19. Doak, C. Large-scale interventions and programmes addressing nutrition-related chronic diseases and obesity: examples from 14 countries. *Public Health Nutr.* 5(S1A), 275–277, 2002.

20. World Health Organization. *Obesity: Preventing and Managing the Global Epidemic.* Geneva: WHO, 2000. WHO Technical Report Series, No. 894.

21. Popkin, B.M. and Du, S. Dynamics of the nutrition transition toward the animal foods sector in China and its implications: a worried perspective. *J. Nutr.* 133, 3898S–3906S, 2003.

22. Caballero, B. and Popkin, B.M. Eds. *The Nutrition Transition: Diet and Disease in the Developing World.* London: Academic Press, 2002.

23. Popkin, B.M. The nutrition transition and obesity in the developing world. *J Nutr.* 131(S), 871S–873S, 2001.

24. Drewnowski, A. Nutrition transition and global dietary trends. *Nutrition.* 16(7–8), 486–487, 2000.

25. Bellagio Declaration. Nutrition and health transition in the developing world: the time to act. *Pub Health Nutr.* 5(1A), L279–L280, 2002. Available at www.cpc.unc.edu/projects/nutrans/bellagio/papers.html. Accessed July 26, 2006.

26. Popkin, B.M. An overview on the nutrition transition and its health implications: the Bellagio meeting. *Pub Health Nutr.* 5(1A), 93–103, 2002. Available at: www.cpc.unc.edu/projects/nutrans/bellagio/papers.html. Accessed July 26, 2006.

27. Swinburn, B., Egger, G., and Raza, F. Dissecting obesogenic environments: the development and application of a framework for identifying and prioritizing environmental interventions for obesity. *Prev Med.* 29(6 Pt. 1), 563–570, 1999.

28. Srinivasan, S., O'Fallon, L.R., and Dearry, A. Creating healthy communities, healthy homes, healthy people: initiating a research agenda on the built environment and public health. *Am J Public Health.* 93, 1446–1450, 2003.

29. Koplan, J.P., Liverman, C.T., and Kraak, V.I. Preventing childhood obesity: health in the balance: executive summary. *J Am Diet Assoc.* 105, 131–138, 2005. Reprinted from Koplan, J.P., Liverman, C.T., Kraak, V.I., Eds. and the Committee on Prevention of Obesity in Children and Youth. *Preventing Childhood Obesity: Health in the Balance.* Washington, D.C.: The National Academies Press, 2005. Available at: www.nap.edu/catalog/11015.html. Accessed July 26, 2006.

30. Schoonover, H. and Muller, M. Food without thought: how U.S. farm policy contributes to obesity. Institute for Agriculture and Trade Policy: Environment and Agriculture Program. March 2006. Available at: http://www.iatp.org/iatp/publications.cfm?accountID=421&refID=80627. Accessed July 26, 2006.

31. Gallo, A.E. Food Advertising in the United States. Chap. 9 in Frazao E., Ed. *America's Eating Habits: Changes and Consequences.* Agriculture Information Bulletin No. 750. May 1999. Available at: http://www.ers.usda.gov/publications/aib750/. Accessed July 26, 2006.

32. Dietz, W, and Gortmaker, S. Do we fatten our children at the TV set? Obesity and television viewing in children and adolescents. *Pediatrics.* 75, 807–812, 1985.

33. Dietz, W. and Gortmaker, S. TV or not TV: fat is the question. *Pediatrics.* 91, 499–500, 1993.

34. Crespo, C.J., Smit, E., Troiano, R.P., Bartlett, S.J., Macera, C.A., and Andersen, R.E. Television watching, energy intake, and obesity in U.S. children: results from the third National Health and Nutrition Examination Survey, 1988–1994. *Arch Pediatr Adolesc Med.* 155, 360–365, 2001.

35. Proctor, M.H., Moore, L.L., Gao, D., Cupples, L.A., Bradlee, M.L., Hood, M.Y., and Ellison, R.C. Television viewing and change in body fat from preschool to early adolescence: the Framingham Children's Study. *Int J Obes Relat Metab Disord.* 27, 827–833, 2003.

36. Robinson, T.N. Reducing children's television viewing to prevent obesity: a randomized controlled trial. *JAMA.* 282, 1561–1567, 1999.

37. Gortmaker, S.L., Peterson, K., Wiecha, J., et al. Reducing obesity via a school-based interdisciplinary intervention among youth: Planet Health. *Arch Pediatr Adolesc Med.* 153, 409–418, 1999.

38. Robinson, T.N. Does television cause childhood obesity? *JAMA.* 279, 959–960, 1998.

39. Koplan, J.P., Liverman, C.T., Kraak, V.I., Eds. *Preventing Childhood Obesity: Health in the Balance.* Washington, DC: The National Academies Press, 2005. Available at: http://www.nap.edu/. Accessed March 9, 2005.

40. Kaiser Family Foundation. The role of media in childhood. Issue Brief. Report No. 7030. February 2004. Available at: http://www.kff.org/. Accessed March 9, 2005.

41. Borzekowski, D.L.G. and Robinson, T.N. The 30-second effect: an experiment revealing the impact of television commercials on food preferences of preschoolers. *J Am Diet Assoc.* 101, 42–46, 2001.

42. Kaiser Family Foundation. The role of media in childhood. Issue Brief. Report No. 7030. February 2004. Available at: http://www.kff.org/. Accessed March 9, 2005.

43. Liberatos, P., Link, B.G., and Kelsey, J.L. The measurement of social class in epidemiology. *Epidemiol Rev.* 10, 87–121, 1988.

44. Sobal, J. and Stunkard, A.J. Socioeconomic status and obesity: a review of the literature. *Psychol Bull.* 105, 260–275, 1989.

45. Zhang, Q. and Wang, Y. Trends in the association between obesity and socioeconomic status in U.S. adults: 1971 to 2000. *Obes Res.* 12, 1622–1632, 2004.

46. Monteiro, C.A., Moura, E.C., Conde, W.L., Wolney, L., and Popkin, B.M. Socioeconomic status and obesity in adult populations of developing countries: a review. *Bull World Health Org.* 82, 940–946, 2004. Available at: http://www.scielosp.org/pdf/bwho/v82n12/v82n12a11.pdf. Accessed March 13, 2005.

47. Monteiro, C.A., Conde, W.L., and Popkin, B.M. Is obesity replacing undernutrition? Evidence from different social classes in Brazil. *Public Health Nutr.* 5, 105–112, 2002.

48. Wang, Y. Cross-national comparison of childhood obesity: the epidemic and the relationship between obesity and socioeconomic status. *Int J Epidemiol.* 30, 1129–1136, 2001.

49. Kimm, S.Y., Obarzanek, E., Barton, B.A., Aston, C.E., Similo, S.L., Morrison, J.A., Sabry, Z.I., Schreiber, G.B., and McMahon, R.P. Race, socioeconomic status, and obesity in 9- to 10-year-old girls: the NHLBI Growth and Health Study. *Ann Epidemiol.* 6, 266–275, 1996.

50. Townsend, M.S., Peerson, J., Love, B., Achterberg, C., and Murphy, S.P. Food insecurity is positively related to overweight in women. *J Nutr.* 131, 1738–1745, 2001.

51. Kendall, A., Olson, C.M., and Frongillo, E.A. Relationship of hunger and food insecurity to food availability and consumption. *J Am Diet Assoc.* 96, 1019–1024, 1996.

52. Drewnowski, A. and Specter, S.E. Poverty and obesity: the role of energy density and energy costs. *Am J Clin Nutr.* 79, 6–15, 2004.

53. Kendall, A. and Kennedy, E. Position of the American Dietetic Association: domestic food and nutrition security. *J Am Diet Assoc.* 98(9), 337–342, 1998.

54. Morland, K., Wing, S., Roux, A.D., and Poole, C. Neighborhood characteristics associated with the location of food stores and food service places. *Am J Prev Med.* 22(1), 23–29, 2002.

55. Chou, S.-Y., Grossman, M., and Saffer, H. An economic analysis of adult obesity: results from the behavioral risk factor surveillance system. *J Health Econ.* 23, 565–587, 2004.

56. McCrory, M.A., Fuss, P.J., Hays, N.P., Vinken, A.G., Greenberg, A.S., and Roberts, S.B. Overeating in America: association between restaurant food consumption and body fatness in healthy adult men and women ages 19–80. *Obes Res.* 7, 564–571, 1999.

57. Binkley, J.K., Eales, J., and Jekanowski, M. The relation between dietary change and rising U.S. obesity. *Int J Obes Relat Metab Disord.* 24, 1032–1039, 2000.

58. French, S.A., Harnack, L., and Jeffery, R.W. Fast food restaurant use among women in the Pound of Prevention Study: dietary, behavioral and demographic correlates. *Int J Obes Relat Metab Disord.* 24, 1353–1359, 2000.

59. Clemens, L.H.E., Slawson, D.L., and Klesges, R.C. The effect of eating out on quality of diet in premenopausal women. *J Am Diet Assoc.* 99, 442–444, 1999.

60. Variyam, J.N. The price is right: economics and the rise in obesity. *Amber Waves.* 3, 2005 [serial online]. Available at: Accessed March 8, 2005.

61. Guthrie, J.F., Lin, B.H., and Frazao, E. Role of food prepared away from home in the American diet, 1977–1978 versus 1994–1996: changes and consequences. *J Nutr Educ Behav.* 34, 140–150, 2002.

62. Guthrie, J.F., Lin, B.H., and Frazao, E. Role of food prepared away from home in the American diet, 1977–1978 versus 1994–1996: changes and consequences. *J Nutr Educ Behav.* 34, 140–150, 2002.

63. Young, L.R. and Nestle, M. The contribution of expanding portions sizes to the U.S. obesity epidemic. *Am J Pub Health.* 92, 246–249, 2002.

64. French, S.A., Story, M., and Jeffery, R.W. Environmental influences on eating and physical activity. *Annu Rev Public Health.* 22, 309–335, 2001.

65. Nielsen, S.J. and Popkin, B.M. Patterns and trends in food portion sizes, 1977–1998. *JAMA.* 289, 450–453, 2003.

66. Cutler, D.M., Glaeser, E.L. and Shapiro, J.M. Why have Americans become more obese? *J Econ Perspect.* 17, 93–118, 2003.

67. U.S. Department of Agriculture, Food and Nutrition Service, Office of Analysis, Nutrition and Evaluation. *Obesity, Poverty, and Participation in Food Assistance Programs.* Report No. FSP-04-PO, 2004. Available at: http://www.fns.usda.gov/oane/MENU/Published/NutritionEducation/Files/ObesityPoverty.pdf. Accessed March 14, 2005.

68. Nestle, M. Soft drink "pouring rights": Marketing empty calories to children. *Public Health Rep.* 115, 308–319, 2000.

69. Fried, E.J. and Nestle, M. The growing political movement against soft drinks in schools. *JAMA.* 288, 2181, 2002.

70. Kubik, M.Y., Lytle, L.A., Hannan, P.J., Perry, C.L., and Story, M. The association of the school food environment with dietary behaviors of young adolescents. *Am J Public Health.* 93, 1168–1173, 2003.

71. Cullen, K.W. and Zakeri, I. Fruits, vegetables, milk, and sweetened beverages consumption and access to à la carte/snack bar meals at school. *Am J Public Health.* 94, 463–467, 2004.

72. Mokdad, A.H., Ford, E.S., Bowman, B.A., Dietz, W.H., Vinicor, F., Bales, V.S., and Marks, J.S. Prevalence of obesity, diabetes, and obesity-related health risk factors, 2001. *JAMA.* 289, 76–79, 2003.

73. Reeves, M.J. and Rafferty, A.P. Healthy lifestyle characteristics among adults in the United States. *Arch Intern Med.* 165, 854–857, 2005.

74. Ford, E.S., De Proost Ford, M.A., Will, J.C., Galuska, D.A., and Ballew, C. Achieving a healthy lifestyle among United States adults: a long way to go. *Ethn Dis.* 11, 224–231, 2001.

75. Blackburn, G.L., Phillips, J.C.C., and Morreale, S. Physician's guide to popular low-carbohydrate weight-loss diets. *Cleve Clin J Med.* 68, 761–774, 2001.

76. Kennedy, E.T., Bowman, S.A., Spence, J.T., Freedman, M., and King, J. Popular diets: correlation to health, nutrition, and obesity. *J Am Diet Assoc.* 101, 411–420, 2001.

77. St. Jeor, S.T., Howard, B.V., Prewitt, T.E., Bouee, V., Bazzarre, T., and Eckel, R. AHA science advisory. Dietary protein and weight reduction: a statement for healthcare professionals from the Nutrition Committee of the Council on Nutrition, Physical Activity, and Metabolism of the American Heart Association. *Circulation.* 104, 1869–1878, 2001.

78. Tapper-Gardzina, Y., Cotunga, N., and Vickery, C. Should you recommend a low-carb, high-protein diet?. *Nurse Pract.* 27, 52–59, 2002.

79. Foster, G.D., Wyatt, H.R., Hill, J.G., et al. A randomized trial of low-carbohydrate diet for obesity. *N Engl J Med.* 348(21), 2082–2090.

80. Shick, S.M., Wing, R.R., Klem, M.L., McGuire, M.T., and Hill, J.O., and Seagle, H. Persons successful at long-term weight loss and maintenance continue to consume a low-energy, low-fat diet. *J Am Diet Assoc.* 98, 408–413, 1998.

81. Story, M. Food marketing and advertising directed at children and adolescents. American Public Health Association policy statement, 2003.

82. Wilcox, B., Cantor, J., Dowrick, P., Kunkel, D., Linn, S., and Palmer, E. Report of the APA Task Force on Advertising to Children: Summary of findings and conclusions. February 2004. Available at: http://www.apa.org/releases/childrenads.html. Accessed March 10, 2005.

83. Children's Advertising Review Unit. Self-Regulatory Guidelines for Children's Advertising. Available at: http://www.caru.org/index.asp. Accessed March 11, 2005.

84. Ad Council. Campaign for Obesity Prevention. Available at: http://www.adcouncil.org/campaigns/healthy_lifestyles/. Accessed March 13, 2005.

85. Ad Council. Campaign for Disease Prevention. Available at: http://www.adcouncil.org/campaigns/disease_prevention/. Accessed March 13, 2005.

86. Center for Science in the Public Interest. *Anyone's Guess — The Need for Nutrition Labeling at Fast-Food and Other Chain Restaurants.* Washington, D.C.: Center for Science in the Public Interest, November 2003. Available at: http://www.cspinet.org/restaurantreport.pdf. Accessed June 16, 2005.

87. Jacobson, M. and Brownell, K. Small taxes on soft drinks and snack foods to promote health. *Am J Public Health.* 90, 854–857, 2000. Available at: http://www.cspinet.org/reports/jacobson.pdf. Accessed June 16, 2005.

88. Food and Drug Administration. Working Group on Obesity. Calories Count. March 12, 2004. Available at: http://www.cfsan.fda.gov/~dms/owg-toc.html. Accessed June 15, 2005.

89. Bush, G.W. *Healthier U.S.: The President's Health and Fitness Initiative.* June 2002. Available at: http://www.whitehouse.gov/infocus/fitness/fitness-policy-book.pdf. Accessed June 15, 2005.

90. Steps to a Healthier U.S. Prevention: a Blueprint for Action. Department of Health and Human Services, April 2004. Available at: http://aspe.hhs.gov/health/blueprint/. Accessed June 15, 2005.

91. Department of Health and Human Services. Partners Invited To Participate in Steps to a Healthier U.S. *Federal Register.* 68, 2003, pp. 60393–60394. Available at: www.healthierus.gov/steps/rfa/2004OrgsRFA/FR04232004.htm. Accessed June 15, 2005.

92. Division of Nutrition and Physical Activity. CDC's State-Based Nutrition and Physical Activity Program to Prevent Obesity and Other Chronic Diseases. National Center for Disease Prevention and Health Promotion. Available at www.cdc.gov/nccdphp/dnpa/obesity/state_programs/index.htm. Accessed June 15, 2005.

93. Nutrition, Physical Activity, and Obesity Prevention Program. Resource Guide for Nutrition and Physical Activity Interventions to Prevent Obesity and Other Chronic Diseases. Department of Health and Human Services. Centers for Disease Control and Prevention, 2003. Available at: www.cdc.gov/nccdphp/dnpa/obesityprevention.htm. Accessed June 15, 2005.

94. Pennsylvania HealthCare Cost Containment Council. Employee health promotion programs can help contain costs. Available at: http://www.phc4.org/reports/fyi/fyi4.htm. Accessed March 19, 2006.

95. The Florida Department of Health. The facts about employee wellness. Available at: http://www.doh.state.fl.us/Family/heart/PDF/FactsEmployeeWellness.pdf. Accessed March 19, 2006.

96. Shain, M. and Kramer, D.M. Health promotion in the workplace: framing the concept; reviewing the evidence. *Occup Environ Med.* 61, 643–648, 2004.

97. Employment Situation Summary. The employment situation: March 2006. Bureau of Labor Statistics. U.S. Department of Labor. Available at: http://www.bls.gov/news.release/empsit.nr0.htm. Accessed April 24, 2006.

98. Chang, S.F. Worksite health promotion — the effects of an employee fitness program. *J Nurs Res.* 11(3), 227–229, 2003.
99. Healthy People 2010. Available at: http://www.healthypeople.gov/Publications/. Accessed March 19, 2006.
100. National Conference of State Legislatures. State legislation and statutes database: health promotion. Available at: http://www.ncsl.org/programs/health/pp/healthpromo.cfm. Accessed May 2, 2006.

8 Special Populations

8.1 INTRODUCTION

This chapter examines three populations that are (or should be) of special interest to public health nutritionists: lactating mothers, people with HIV/AIDS, and inmates in correctional facilities. We focus on these groups for diverse reasons.

- The incidence and duration of breastfeeding took a turn for the worse in the middle of the last century; public health has a mandate to reverse this trend.
- With the advent of highly active antiretroviral therapy (the combination of several antiretroviral medications, which slows the rate at which HIV multiplies in the body), the population that is HIV seropositive is living longer, turning HIV into a chronic disease that requires constant dietary vigilance.
- Inmates with chronic diseases who have not learned self-management techniques while they are incarcerated will reenter society less likely to take care of themselves than if their heart disease, high blood pressure, and diabetes were under control.

8.2 LACTATING MOTHERS AND BREASTFED INFANTS

The American Dietetic Association (ADA, 2005),[1] American Academy of Pediatrics (AAP, 2005),[2] the World Health Organization (WHO, 2001),[3] and the U.S. Department of Health and Human Services (HHS, Healthy People 2010, released in 2001)[4] all recommend increases in the proportion of mothers who breastfeed their babies. In particular, *Healthy People 2010* and the AAP call for a 75% breastfeeding initiation rate, a 50% continuation rate to 6 months, and a 25% rate at 1 year.

According to the Ross Mothers' Survey (see Section 8.2.3.1) conducted in 1988, almost two-thirds of new mothers breastfed in the early postpartum period, less than one third breastfed at 6 months, and only 16% breastfed at 1 year. For the past 25 years, breastfeeding rates among WIC participants have lagged behind those of non-WIC mothers.[5] Unarguably, a goal of public health nutrition must be to help increase the initiation and duration of breastfeeding, with special attention to the 50% of U.S. infants who participate in WIC.[6] To increase the initiation and duration of breastfeeding, public health measures should target the populations with the lowest breastfeeding rates and invest in institutional changes that will support this behavioral outcome.

8.2.1 BREASTFEEDING TRENDS

Despite its benefits, rates of breastfeeding in the U.S. declined dramatically during the mid-20th century. According to the ADA,[7] almost all infants were breastfed in colonial America, but by the 1880s, mothers began to supplement breastfeeding with raw cow's milk and to wean their infants before they were 3 months old. Infants fed raw cow's milk had higher mortality rates than their breastfed counterparts. The decline continued during the period when milk substitutes (evaporated cow's milk and infant formula) became widely available. These human milk substitutes were aggressively marketed as being both more convenient for the mother and more nutritious for her infant than human milk.

In 1936–1940, rates of breastfeeding initiation were about 77%. Breastfeeding initiation gradually declined to a low of 25% in 1971 and then rose to 62% in 1982. Through the 1980s, breastfeeding initiation again declined to 52% in 1989, then increased through the 1990s and reached 70% in 2003.

The number of breastfeeding mothers and trends in breastfeeding varied widely across socio-economic and cultural categories. Among the groups experiencing the most precipitous declines in breastfeeding levels from the late 1950s to the late 1970s were black women, women with less than 12 years of education, and women who never worked outside the home.[8]

Significant differences in rates of breastfeeding have persisted among racial groups over time. In the 1950s, black and Hispanic mothers were more likely to breastfeed their babies than white mothers. But during the decline in breastfeeding prevalence in the early 1970s, rates of breastfeeding dropped most dramatically for blacks and have not fully recovered. In contrast, breastfeeding rates among white and Hispanic mothers rose sharply beginning in the 1970s, and reached or exceeded 1950s levels by the late 1980s.[9]

8.2.2 BENEFITS OF BREASTFEEDING

The physiological benefits of breastfeeding to mother and child are well-documented, yet other apparent benefits have not yet received unqualified support. In addition to these physiologic advantages, breastfeeding boasts several nonphysiological benefits that have major implications for public health.

8.2.2.1 Physiologic

The documented health benefits of breastfeeding for new mothers are decreased postpartum bleeding and more rapid uterine involution. For the infant, human milk feeding has been shown to decrease the incidence and/or severity of a wide range of infectious diseases, including bacterial meningitis, bacteremia, gastroenteritis, respiratory tract infection, necrotizing enterocolitis, otitis media, urinary tract infection, and late-onset sepsis in preterm infants.

Three childhood diseases that commonly afflict children under 2 years of age include otitis media, gastroenteritis, and necrotizing enterocolitis.

- *Otitis media* is an inflammation of the ear and is the most frequently reported diagnosis for children under the age of 2 years.
- *Gastroenteritis* refers to vomiting or diarrhea as a discrete illness for a 24-h period.
- Necrotizing enterocolitis (NEC) is the most common gastrointestinal tract disease in the neonatal intensive care unit, the leading cause of emergency surgical treatment in newborns, and a major cause of neonatal death. Over 90% of NEC cases affect premature infants. Incidence approaches 12% of all low birth weight (LBW) premature infants. The onset of NEC is usually within the first 10 d of life. Its incidence in exclusively breastfed LBW infants is 1%, compared with an incidence of 7% in formula-fed LBW infants.

In addition to the known benefits of breastfeeding, there is preliminary evidence of its associations with decreased rates of sudden infant death syndrome (SIDS) in the first year of life, and with reductions in types 1 and 2 diabetes, lymphoma, leukemia, Hodgkin's disease, overweight and obesity, hypercholesterolemia, and asthma in older children and adults. Breastfeeding has also been associated with slightly enhanced tests of cognitive development.

8.2.2.2 Nonphysiologic

Economic, family, and environmental benefits result from breastfeeding. These benefits include the potential for decreased environmental burden from reduced disposal of formula cans and bottles, decreased energy costs associated with the manufacture and transport of artificial feeding products, decreased medical bills due to the decreased incidence of the conditions outlined in Section 8.2.2.1, and decreased employee absenteeism to care for sick children. An unknown proportion of the medical care savings would be offset by increased costs associated with lactation. These extra expenses would include consultations by physicians and others, and equipment associated with breastfeeding, such as breast pumps. All of these should be covered, in part, by third-party reimbursement.

8.2.2.2.1 Decreased Employee Absenteeism and Decreased Healthcare Costs

Breastfeeding results in decreased national healthcare costs and decreased employee absenteeism to care for infants who are ill. Based on epidemiological studies that relate breastfeeding to the risk of otitis media, gastroenteritis, and NEC, and estimates of treatment costs, the USDA estimated that an increase in breastfeeding rates from the 1988 levels to the year 2010 targets of 75% at discharge and 50% at 6 months would save a minimum of $3.6 billion annually. The majority of these savings are attributable to preventing premature deaths due to NEC. Because this analysis represents savings from treating only 3 childhood illnesses, the $3.6 billion figure is probably an underestimation.[10]

The annual cost of treating U.S. children less than 5 years of age for otitis media is estimated at $5 billion per year.[11] Breastfeeding reduces the incidence of otitis media; in the first year of life, infants who breastfed exclusively for at least 4 months have half as many episodes of acute otitis media as formula-fed infants.

As for the individual family, the cost savings in 1999 for breastfed infants when compared with formula-fed babies were estimated to be between $331 and $475 per child in a single year, based on less frequent episodes of otitis media, diarrhea, and lower respiratory tract infections.[12]

8.2.2.2.2 Decreased Environmental Burden

Breastfeeding contributes to the health of the environment in numerous ways. Human milk is a renewable natural resource manufactured at the cost of only 450[13] to 500[14] kcal/d per infant during the first few months postpartum. Human milk is delivered at no cost at all or very inexpensively in terms of breast pumping and milk storage for later use. Unlike artificial feeding, bottle, breastfeeding consumes no energy associated with transportation, shipping, and disposing of containers.[15]

8.2.3 BREASTFEEDING SURVEILLANCE

A number of surveys and surveillance systems measure breastfeeding in the U.S., each of which faces its own challenges and problems.

8.2.3.1 Ross Mother's Survey

Although flawed, the oldest data about breastfeeding in the U.S. comes from the Ross Mother's Survey (RMS). Ross Products, a division of Abbott Laboratories, a U.S. marketer of pediatric nutritionals, started conducting periodic surveys in 1955 to examine infant feeding patterns during the 1st year of life. It remains the only source of long-term infant-feeding trends available.[16]

8.2.3.2 National Immunization Survey

The National Immunization Survey (NIS) is sponsored by the National Immunization Program (NIP) and conducted jointly by NIP and the National Center for Health Statistics (NCHS), Centers for Disease Control and Prevention. The NIS is a random-digit dialing telephone survey of households with children 9 to 36 months of age.[17] Since 2003, breastfeeding questions have been added to the survey in order to assess the population's breastfeeding practices. The 2005 survey included these questions:

- Was [child's name] ever breastfed or fed breast milk?
- How long was [child's name] breastfed or fed breast milk?
- How old was [child's name] when [he/she] was fed something other than breast milk. This includes formula, juice, solid foods, cow's milk, water, sugar water, anything else.

A study of the validity and reliability (see Figure 8.1) of maternal recall of breastfeeding history revealed that maternal recall is a valid and reliable estimate of breastfeeding initiation and duration, especially when the duration of breastfeeding is recalled after a short period of time (through 3 years). However, validity and reliability of maternal recall for the age at introduction of food and fluids other than breast milk are less satisfactory.[18]

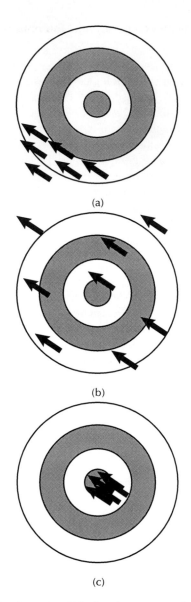

FIGURE 8.1 Validity and reliability. A test is valid when it measures what it is meant to measure. How valid a test is depends on its purpose — for example, a ruler may be a valid measuring device for length but is not valid for measuring volume. A test is reliable if it yields consistent results. A test can be both reliable and valid, one or the other, or neither. However, reliability is a prerequisite for measurement validity. To visualize the relationship between reliability and validity, consider the center of a target as the factor being measured. For each factor (for example, blood pressure), the researcher aims at the target. When the center of the target is hit, the factor is both valid and reliable. The following targets depict three possible situations: (a) The target is hit consistently, but the center is missed. This illustrates consistent and systematic measurement, but of the wrong value for all individuals being measured. Thus, while this measure is reliable, it is not valid. (b) Hits are randomly spread across the target. While the center of the target is seldom hit, on average, the researcher is getting the correct answer for the group, although it is often not the right answer for individuals. The measure provides only a valid group estimate; information about the individual cannot be inferred. This case illustrates that reliability is directly related to the variability of the measure. (c) The center of the target is consistently hit, indicating that the measure is both reliable and valid. (Adapted from Georgetown University. Department of Psychology. Research Methods & Statistics Resources. Available at: http://www.georgetown._edu/departments/ psychology/researchmethods/researchanddesign/validityandreliability.htm. Accessed August 20, 2006.)

8.2.3.3 Sociodemographic Factors of Lactating Mothers

Understanding the sociodemographic characteristics of women who do and do not breastfeed is important for many activities, including designing and implementing breastfeeding promotion campaigns. Before developing lactation programs, healthcare planners must know the age, income, and other demographic characteristics of the target population they hope to reach. When health educators are preparing lactation-related educational materials or activities, they need to know the demographic profile of the target audience, so that appropriate programs or efforts are made available.

The 2005 NIS provides overall population estimates for the initiation, duration, and exclusivity of breastfeeding. It also provides geographically-specific breastfeeding rates, as indicated in Table 8.1.

When household income is used as a proxy for SES, the highest income women have the highest prevalences of having ever breastfed, having breastfed exclusively for 3 or 6 months, and having breastfed partially up to 1 year. The lowest breastfeeding rates are evident in women with 1 or more of these characteristics: unmarried, under the age of 20 years, income below the poverty threshold, less than a high school education, and a WIC recipient. Understandably, these findings prompted WIC to concentrate on promoting breastfeeding. The WIC initiatives to increase the initiation and duration of breastfeeding are discussed in Section 8.2.4.6.3.

Asians, Native Hawaiians, and Latinas are the most likely to breastfeed exclusively for at least 3 months, whereas blacks and American Indians/Alaska Natives are the least likely.

8.2.3.4 Geographic Considerations

The 2005 NIS of breastfeeding practices reveals that 21 states achieved the national Healthy People 2010 objective of 75% of mothers initiating breastfeeding. The objective of having 50% of mothers breastfeeding their children at six months of age was achieved by 11 states. There were 5 states — California, Hawaii, Oregon, Vermont, and Washington — that achieved the objective of having 25% of infants still breastfeeding at 12 months of age.

Consistent with previous research, the NIS breastfeeding data reveal that non-Hispanic black and low SES groups have the lowest breastfeeding rates. The AAP recommends that an infant be breastfed without supplemental foods or liquids for the first 6 months of life, known as "exclusive breastfeeding." NIS data indicate that by 2005, only Oregon had achieved the AAP's breastfeeding goals (see Box 8.1).

8.2.4 OVERCOMING BARRIERS TO BREASTFEEDING

A number of factors act as barriers to breastfeeding initiation and continuation. The major deterrents to breastfeeding include aggressive formula product marketing, lack of social support, lack of role models, lack of proper guidance from healthcare providers, lack of timely and postpartum follow-up care, disruptive hospital maternity care practices, and an increasing number of women in the workforce. An examination of these factors appears in the next two sections. The discussion is based on the CDC's *Guide to Breastfeeding Interventions*, released in 2005.

8.2.4.1 Social Support

According to the CDC,[19] social networks influence women's decision-making processes. Networks can be either barriers or points of encouragement for breastfeeding. New mothers' preferred resource for concerns about child rearing is other mothers (such as advice from a friend). Perceived social support has also been found to predict success in breastfeeding.

Peer support represents a cost-effective, individually-tailored, and culturally competent (see Chapter 9) way to promote and support breastfeeding for women of varying socioeconomic backgrounds, especially when peer mothers have the same or similar sociocultural background as those

TABLE 8.1
Breastfeeding Rates by Sociodemographic Factors, 2005 (Percent ± Half 95% Confidence Interval)

Sociodemographic Factors	Number in Sample	Breastfeeding for Any Time	Breastfeeding at 6 Months	Breastfeeding at 12 Months	Exclusive Breastfeeding at 3 Months	Exclusive Breastfeeding at 6 Months
U.S., nationally	27,423	72.9 ± 0.9	39.1 ± 0.9	20.1 ± 0.8	38.7 ± 1.0	13.9 ± 0.7
Infant's Race/Ethnicity						
American Indian or Alaska	904	67.3 ± 5.5	33.7 ± 5.1	16.7 ± 4.0	30.7 ± 5.1	11.3 ± 2.9
Asian or Pacific islander	1,724	81.4 ± 2.9	47.5 ± 3.9	24.5 ± 3.2	43.1 ± 3.9	18.1 ± 2.9
Asian	1,432	81.9 ± 3.1	47.1 ± 4.2	24.2 ± 3.4	43.2 ± 4.2	18.5 ± 3.2
Native Hawaiian and other	365	78.5 ± 6.9	51.2 ± 8.8	28.0 ± 8.4	43.0 ± 8.8	17.5 ± 7.5
Black or African American[a]	4,921	59.6 ± 2.3	27.1 ± 2.1	13.5 ± 1.7	29.7 ± 2.2	10.0 ± 1.4
White	21,409	75.7 ± 1.0	41.5 ± 1.1	21.5 ± 0.9	40.9 ± 1.1	14.6 ± 0.8
Hispanic or Latino	5,832	79.0 ± 1.7	42.0 ± 2.1	22.0 ± 1.8	43.9 ± 2.2	14.1 ± 1.5
Not Hispanic or Latino	21,591	70.7 ± 1.0	38.0 ± 1.0	19.3 ± 0.8	36.8 ± 1.0	13.8 ± 0.7
Black or African American[b]	4,062	55.4 ± 2.5	24.8 ± 2.2	11.9 ± 1.8	26.8 ± 2.3	9.2 ± 1.5
White	16,749	74.1 ± 1.1	41.1 ± 1.2	21.0 ± 1.0	39.3 ± 1.2	14.7 ± 0.8
Does the Infant Receive WIC[c]						
Received WIC	12,296	65.8 ± 1.4	30.3 ± 1.4	15.7 ± 1.1	31.7 ± 1.4	10.5 ± 0.9
No, but WIC but eligible	1,358	77.6 ± 3.4	48.6 ± 4.2	28.5 ± 3.7	49.1 ± 4.2	20.4 ± 3.4
No, and WIC and ineligible	12,457	81.9 ± 1.1	49.2 ± 1.4	24.5 ± 1.2	46.4 ± 1.4	17.3 ± 1.0
Maternal Age (at Child's Birth)						
Less than 20 years	589	50.0 ± 6.5	14.8 ± 4.4	5.4 ± 2.3	17.5 ± 4.7	6.7 ± 3.0
20–29 years	10,689	68.4 ± 1.4	31.7 ± 1.4	15.8 ± 1.2	32.8 ± 1.5	10.1 ± 0.9
30 or more years	16,145	77.7 ± 1.1	46.2 ± 1.3	24.2 ± 1.1	44.6 ± 1.3	17.3 ± 1.0
Maternal Education						
Less than high school	3,110	63.6 ± 2.6	32.2 ± 2.7	17.9 ± 2.3	33.6 ± 2.7	12.3 ± 1.9
High school	6,755	64.8 ± 1.8	29.3 ± 1.7	14.9 ± 1.4	30.6 ± 1.8	10.2 ± 1.2
Some college	4,618	76.8 ± 1.9	39.3 ± 2.3	19.5 ± 2.0	39.5 ± 2.3	13.3 ± 1.5
College graduate	12,940	84.5 ± 0.9	52.5 ± 1.3	26.6 ± 1.2	49.3 ± 1.3	18.6 ± 1.0
Maternal Marital Status						
Married	20,258	78.4 ± 0.9	45.2 ± 1.1	23.7 ± 1.0	43.7 ± 1.1	16.1 ± 0.8
Unmarried[d]	7,165	60.3 ± 1.9	25.0 ± 1.7	11.6 ± 1.3	27.2 ± 1.8	8.8 ± 1.1

TABLE 8.1 (Continued)
Breastfeeding Rates by Sociodemographic Factors, 2005 (Percent ± Half 95% Confidence Interval)

Sociodemographic Factors	Number in Sample	Breastfeeding for Any Time	Breastfeeding at 6 Months	Breastfeeding at 12 Months	Exclusive Breastfeeding at 3 Months	Exclusive Breastfeeding at 6 Months
Poverty (% of Federal Poverty Threshold)						
< 100%	4,610	63.5 ± 2.3	29.7 ± 2.2	16.7 ± 1.9	31.7 ± 2.3	10.7 ± 1.4
100% to< 185%	4,512	70.8 ± 2.1	35.4 ± 2.3	18.7 ± 1.9	36.7 ± 2.4	13.0 ± 1.8
185% to < 350%	6,159	73.6 ± 1.9	41.0 ± 2.0	20.3 ± 1.6	38.9 ± 2.0	14.2 ± 1.4
350% or more	8,987	82.4 ± 1.2	48.3 ± 1.6	23.5 ± 1.4	46.0 ± 1.6	17.0 ± 1.2

Note: Exclusive breastfeeding is defined in this 2005 study as *only* breast milk — no solids, no water, and no other liquids. This new definition is a diversion from the 2003 NIS data, which had defined exclusive breastfeeding as "only breast milk and water – no solids or other liquids."

[a] Black/African American and white rates are for all mothers who indicate they are Black/African American or white, including those who report they are Hispanic or Latina and those who indicate they are not Hispanic or Latina.
[b] Most frequently, we report breastfeeding prevalence for three main groups: Black/African American non-Hispanic, white non-Hispanic, and Hispanic.
[c] WIC = Special Supplemental Nutrition Program for Women, Infants, and Children.
[d] Unmarried includes never married, widowed, separated, divorced.

Source: Adapted from the 2005 National Immunization Survey, Centers for Disease Control and Prevention, Department of Health and Human Services. Available at: http://www.cdc.gov/breastfeeding/data/NIS_data/2005/sociodemographic. htm. Accessed August 12, 2006.

whom they support. The goal of peer support is to encourage and support pregnant women and those who currently breastfeed. Peer support, provided by mothers who are currently breastfeeding or who have done so in the past, includes individual counseling and mother-to-mother support groups. Peer mothers provide support and counseling to help women address their barriers to breastfeeding and assist them in preventing and managing breastfeeding problems. Peer support includes psychoemotional support, encouragement, education about breastfeeding, and help with solving problems. Women who provide peer support undergo specific training and may work in an informal group or one-on-one through telephone calls or visits in the home, clinic, or hospital.

8.2.4.1.1 WIC Peer Counseling

In 2004, WIC launched a national initiative to institutionalize peer counseling as a core service. Many WIC state agencies already provide successful peer counseling programs, whereas the rest are implementing new programs as part of this national effort. After receiving extensive training, peer counselors work primarily from home to provide telephone support to pregnant and breast-feeding mothers. In many programs, peer counselors also provide clinic-based counseling, make home visits during the early postpartum period, lead prenatal breastfeeding classes and postpartum support groups, and provide one-to-one support in the hospital setting (see Section 8.2.6.4.3).

Box 8.1 State Rankings in Breastfeeding Incidence

To see how any state has ranked in breastfeeding incidence from 2003 to the present, click on "geographic-specific breastfeeding rates" at CDC's breastfeeding Web site: http://www.cdc.gov/breastfeeding.

8.2.4.2 Education

In the U.S., most new mothers do not have direct, personal knowledge of breastfeeding, and many find it hard to rely on family members for consistent, accurate information and guidance about infant feeding. Further, although many women have a general understanding of the benefits of breastfeeding, they lack exposure to sources of information regarding how breastfeeding is actually carried out. The CDC found that *prenatal breastfeeding education is the most effective single intervention for increasing breastfeeding initiation and short-term duration.*

The goal of educating mothers is to influence their attitudes toward breastfeeding as well as to increase their breastfeeding knowledge and skills. Breastfeeding education occurs most often during the prenatal and intrapartum periods and should be taught by someone with expertise or training in lactation management. This instruction typically occurs within an informally structured small group setting but may be given one-to-one. This education primarily includes information and resources. The target audience is usually pregnant or breastfeeding women but may also include fathers and others who support the breastfeeding mother.

8.2.4.2.1 Intrapartum Education

Intrapartum breastfeeding education is time sensitive. This type of education is often less formal than education provided during pregnancy, is generally conducted individually, and almost always occurs within a hospital setting. Intrapartum education usually focuses on immediate issues, such as fostering appropriate latch and positioning, adequate milk removal, stability of the infant, and comfort of the mother. It also provides an opportunity to reassure and support a concerned mother or family member, provides mothers and family members with referral information for further postpartum support, and allows the reiteration of signs of success or potential problems in the first few days after hospital discharge. All hospitals that routinely handle births should have staff with adequate training and knowledge to address and facilitate routine, standard breastfeeding education in the intrapartum period for all breastfeeding mothers and infants.

The professional member of the healthcare team for complex breastfeeding problems and lactation management is generally the international board certified lactation consultant (IBCLC). Other health professionals with expertise in breastfeeding support include dietitians, physicians, and nurses who specialize in lactation. Starting in 2008, the International Board of Certified Lactation Examiners will offer a complementary credential to individuals trained to provide basic lactation support.[20]

8.2.4.3 Maternity Care Practices

Breastfeeding is a time-sensitive relationship. Experiences with breastfeeding in the first hours and days of life influence an infant's later feeding. Because of its inextricable relationship with the birth experience, breastfeeding must be supported throughout the maternity hospital stay, not delayed until the infant goes home. The hospital stay, although short, is a critical period for the establishment of breastfeeding. Many of the experiences of mothers and newborns in the hospital and the practices in place there affect how likely breastfeeding is to be established.

Prenatal education on breastfeeding can affect a mother's decision to even consider it as a feeding option. Medications and procedures administered to the mother during labor affect the infant's behavior at the time of birth, which in turn affects the infant's ability to suckle in an organized and effective manner at the breast. Infants who are put to the breast within the first few hours after birth continue breastfeeding longer than those whose first breastfeeding is delayed. Mothers who room-in with their infants will have more opportunities to practice breastfeeding because of the infant's proximity.

Maternity care practices supportive of breastfeeding include developing a written policy on breast-feeding, providing all staff (e.g., nurses, physicians, radiology staff, pharmacy staff, food service and housekeeping staff) with education and training, encouraging early breastfeeding initiation, supporting cue-based feeding, restricting supplements and pacifiers for breastfed infants, and providing for post-discharge follow-up. Both the use of medications during labor and cesarean birth have been shown to have a negative effect on breastfeeding, while providing continuous support during labor and maintaining skin-to-skin contact between mother and baby after birth has a positive effect on breastfeeding.

8.2.4.3.1 Baby-Friendly Hospital Initiative Ten Steps Program

The Baby-Friendly Hospital Initiative (BFHI) is a global United Nations International Children's Emergency Fund/World Health Organization (UNICEF/WHO)-sponsored effort to promote breastfeeding. The initiative is based on ten policy or procedure statements that were jointly developed and published in 1989 by UNICEF and WHO in consultation with international experts. In 1990, the Ten Steps were accepted as the central theme of the Innocenti Declaration and, later that year, endorsed at the World Summit on Children. In 1992, UNICEF and WHO launched a major international campaign to encourage all hospitals with maternity services to accept the Ten Steps as basic maternity and newborn infant care policies and procedures (see Box 8.2).

Box 8.2 The Innocenti Declaration on the Protection, Promotion, and Support of Breastfeeding and the WHO/UNICEF International Code of Marketing of Breastmilk Substitutes

The Innocenti Declaration on the protection, promotion, and support of breastfeeding was developed and adopted by participants at the WHO/UNICEF policymakers' meeting on "Breastfeeding in the 1990s: A Global Initiative" cosponsored by the U.S. Agency for International Development (USAID) and the Swedish International Development Authority, held in 1990 at the *Spedale degli Innocenti*, located in Florence, Italy. The Declarations states:

As a global goal for optimal maternal and child health and nutrition, all women should be enabled to practise exclusive breastfeeding and all infants should be fed exclusively on breast milk from birth to 4–6 months of age. Thereafter, children should continue to be breastfed, while receiving appropriate and adequate complementary foods, for up to two years of age or beyond. This child-feeding ideal is to be achieved by creating an appropriate environment of awareness and support so that women can breastfeed in this manner.

The Declaration set four extremely ambitious operational targets to be met. By 1995, all governments should:

- Appoint a national breastfeeding coordinator and establish a multisectoral national breastfeeding committee composed of representatives from relevant government departments, nongovernmental organizations, and health professional associations.
- Ensure that every facility providing maternity services fully practices all ten of the Ten Steps to Successful Breastfeeding set out in the joint WHO/UNICEF statement "Protecting, promoting and supporting breastfeeding; the special role of maternity services."
- Take action to enforce the principles and aim of all Articles of the International Code of Marketing of Breastmilk Substitutes and subsequent relevant World Health Assembly resolutions. [This goal is regarded as the minimum starting point for effective action.]
- Enact imaginative legislation protecting the breastfeeding rights of working women and establish means for its enforcement.

On the broadest possible scale, international advisory commissions should:

- Establish action strategies for protecting, promoting, and supporting breastfeeding, including global monitoring and evaluation of their strategies.
- Support national situation analyses and surveys, and the development of national goals and targets for action.
- Encourage and support national authorities in planning, implementing, monitoring, and evaluating their breastfeeding policies.

Countries have made significant progress in reaching these goals, although they have not been fully achieved. There are 80 countries having some form of national authority, about 19,000 hospitals have been certified and designated as baby-friendly in 150 countries, more than 80 countries have laws or regulations implementing the International Code of Marketing of Breastmilk Substitutes either fully or in part, and 59 countries have ratified at least one of three maternity protection conventions to support employed mothers.

The WHO/UNICEF International Code of Marketing of Breastmilk Substitutes was adopted in 1981 by Resolution WHA34.22 of the World Health Assembly (WHA) to promote infant health by protecting and supporting breastfeeding. The Code bans all *promotion* of bottle feeding and establishes requirements for labeling and information on infant feeding products. Any activity that undermines breastfeeding violates the aim and spirit of the Code. The Code pertains to all products that are marketed in a manner suggesting they should replace breast-feeding, even if the product is not suitable for that purpose. The products include but are not limited to infant formula, follow-up formula, baby foods, juices (for infants under 4 months of age), and infant feeding paraphernalia such as bottles, nipples, bottles with collapsible liners, and so on. When the Code was adopted by the WHA it was recognized that it may require clarification or even revision. Accordingly, Resolutions have been adopted every two years since 1982. The subsequent Resolutions have equal status to the International Code and close many of the loopholes capitalized on by the baby food industry.

The International Code and its resolutions do not ban breast milk substitutes, but they set out how companies are permitted to market them. These stipulations are regarded as the minimum requirement for effective action to promote breastfeeding. In particular, baby food companies may not engage in the following:

- Promote their products in hospitals, shops, or to the general public.
- Give free samples to mothers or free or subsidized supplies to hospitals or maternity wards.
- Give gifts to health workers or mothers.
- Promote their products to health workers: any information provided by companies must contain only scientific and factual matters.
- Promote foods or drinks for babies.
- Give misleading information.

Source: Innocenti Declaration On the Protection, Promotion, and Support of Breastfeeding. Available at: http://www.unicef.org/programme/breastfeeding/innocenti.htm. Accessed August 16, 2006.

1990–2005 — Celebrating the Innocenti Declaration on the Protection, Promotion, and Support of Breastfeeding. Past Achievements, Present Challenges and the Way Forward for Infant and Young Child Feeding. UNICEF. Florence, Italy: UNICEF Innocenti Research Centre, 2005. Available at: http://www.unicef.org/brazil/1990_2005_gb.pdf.sed_. Accessed August 16, 2006.

Official designation as Baby-Friendly requires a careful assessment completed by a trained external team to confirm that the institution is truly carrying out all Ten Steps and conforming to the International Code of Marketing of Breastmilk Substitutes. A maternity facility can be designated baby-friendly when it does not accept free or low-cost breast milk substitutes, feeding bottles, or nipples, and has implemented these ten specific steps to support successful breastfeeding:

1. Have a written breastfeeding policy that is routinely communicated to all healthcare staff.
2. Train all healthcare staff in skills necessary to implement this policy.
3. Inform all pregnant women about the benefits and management of breastfeeding.
4. Help mothers initiate breastfeeding within a half-hour of birth.
5. Show mothers how to breastfeed and how to maintain lactation even if they should be separated from their infants.

6. Give newborn infants no food or drink other than breast milk, unless medically indicated.
7. Practice rooming-in — allow mothers and infants to remain together — 24 hours a day.
8. Encourage breastfeeding on demand.
9. Give no artificial teats or pacifiers to breastfeeding infants.
10. Foster the establishment of breastfeeding support groups and refer mothers to them on discharge from the hospital or clinic.

The Ten Steps have been implemented in over 19,000 maternity care facilities worldwide as part of the BFHI. The BFHI is considered one of the most successful international efforts ever undertaken to protect, promote, and support breastfeeding. Although it does not ensure that mothers will aspire to or achieve the widely accepted goal of approximately 6 months of exclusive breastfeeding, it helps mothers to initiate exclusive nursing, an essential step in the right direction.[21]

8.2.4.3.2   Baby-Friendly Hospital Initiative in the U.S.

Boston Medical Center (BMC) reported that breastfeeding initiation rates rose from 58% in 1995 before implementation of their program to 87% in 1999 after the policies were in place, including an increase in breastfeeding initiation among U.S.-born African American mothers from 34 to 74%.[22]

The BFHI is implemented in less than 60 facilities in the U.S.[23] (see Box 8.3). In the attempt to increase the number of maternity centers that meet all the standards required to achieve BFHI certification, the proposed HeLP America Act of 2005 contains a section (§105) that would provide hospitals up to $20,000 to offset the cost associated with achieving the Baby-Friendly designation.

Box 8.3 U.S. Baby-Friendly Hospitals (through July 2006)

Alice Peck Day Memorial Hospital, Lebanon, NH
Aurora Lakeland Medical Center, Elkhorn, WI
Boston Medical Center, Boston, MA
Cape Canaveral Hospital, Cocoa Beach, FL
Central Maine Medical Center, Lewiston, MA
Community Hospital Anderson, Anderson, IN
Community Hospital of Anaconda, Anaconda, MO
Community Hospital of the Monterey Peninsula, Monterey, CA
Corona Regional Medical Center, Corona, CA
Elmbrook Memorial Hospital, Brookfield, WI
Evergreen Hospital Medical Center, Kirkland, WA
Glendale Memorial Hospital and Health Center, Glendale, CA
Goleta Valley Cottage Hospital, Santa Barbara, CA
Hartford Hospital, Hartford, CT
Inland Midwife Services–The Birth Center, Redlands, CA
Kaiser Permanente Medical Center, Honolulu, HI
Kaiser Permanente Medical Center, Hayward, CA
Kaiser Permanente Riverside Medical Center, Riverside, CA
Kaiser Sunnyside Medical Center, Clackamas, OR
Kootenai Medical Center, Coeur d'Alene, ID
Lisa Ross Birth & Women's Center, Knoxville, TN
Madison Birth Center, Middleton, WI
Mercy Hospital Anderson, Cincinnati, OH
Mercy Hospital Fairfield, Fairfield, OH
Meriter Hospital, Madison, WI

Methodist Hospital, Indianapolis, IN
Methodist Hospital, Omaha, NE
Middlesex Hospital, Middletown, CT
Miles Memorial Hospital, Damariscotta, ME
Morton Plant Hospital, Clearwater, FL
Newport Hospital, Newport, RI
Northeastern Vermont Regional Hospital, St. Johnsbury, VT
Okanogan–Douglas District Hospital, Brewster, WA
PeaceHealth Nurse Midwifery Birth Center, Eugene, OR
Pekin Hospital, Pekin, IL
Providence Medford Medical Center, Medford, OR
Reading Birth and Women's Center, Reading, PA
Robert E. Bush Naval Hospital, Twentynine Palms, CA
Rochester General Hospital, Rochester, NY
Scripps Memorial Hospital Encinitas, Encinitas, CA
St. Elizabeth Medical Center, Edgewood, KY
St. Francis Hospital, Milwaukee, WI
St. John's Hospital, Springfield, IL
St. Joseph Hospital, Nashua, NH
St. Mary Medical Center, Walla Walla, WA
South County Hospital, Wakefield, RI
Tacoma General Hospital, Tacoma, WA
Three Rivers Community Hospital, Grants Pass, OR
UCSD Medical Center, San Diego, CA
US Army MEDDAC, Heidelberg, Germany
Ventura County Medical Center, Ventura, CA
Weed Army Community Hospital, Fort Irwin, CA
Women's Health and Birth Center, Santa Rosa, CA
Women's Wellness and Maternity Center, Madisonville, TN

Source: BHFI USA. Available at: http://www.babyfriendlyusa.org/eng/03.html. Accessed August 14, 2006.

8.2.4.3.3 *Pursuing Baby-Friendly Status*

As described by the BMC breastfeeding committee,[24] becoming Baby-Friendly entails strategic planning, implementing, and maintaining change throughout an entire institution, staff education at all levels, cooperation between many departments, the support of senior staff members, and expense. Persuading a large institution to pay for infant formula, which most U.S. hospitals receive for free from infant formula manufacturers, was cited as an especially difficult barrier to overcome.[25]

8.2.4.3.3.1 *Paying for Infant Formula that Could Be Free*

To comply fully with the Baby-Friendly Hospital Initiative, an institution must pay fair market price for all formula and infant feeding supplies that it uses; it cannot accept free or heavily

---

Box 8.4 Research Question

Does a change in state law to explicitly permit public breastfeeding help to increase the rate of breastfeeding by removing or reducing an existing barrier? Suggestion: Compare the changes over time in prevalence of breastfeeding in states with and without breastfeeding legislation.

discounted formula and supplies. Hospitals have problems achieving this step to being designated Baby-Friendly. When a hospital is already receiving free formula, it seems illogical to persuade administrators to reverse a trend and pay for a product that is usually free. The BMC researchers caution that any facility interested in pursing the Baby-Friendly designation must consider the ramifications of this added expense. Nevertheless, they encourage facilities to apply for the certificate of intent and begin work, even if it is not immediately clear how the formula will be paid for.

Each of the Ten Steps takes the hospital along an important course, is never wasted effort, and increases the number of breastfeeding mothers (thereby reducing formula costs). Demonstrating a willingness to invest time and energy for the benefit of patients and the institution as a whole is valuable when requesting support for formula payment. Hospital administrators, who may make the final decision regarding formula payment, will be more willing to listen to breastfeeding advocates if they have already accomplished significant goals within the institution and have collected supporting data. The authors conclude that although for BMC not accepting free formula was the most difficult barrier to overcome on the path to Baby-Friendly designation, it was not insurmountable.

8.2.4.4 Workplace Accommodations

As indicated in the CDC's *Guide to Breastfeeding Interventions* (2005),[26] mothers are the fastest-growing segment of the U.S. labor force. Approximately 70% of employed mothers with children younger than 3 years work full time. About one-third of them return to work within 3 months after birth and two-thirds return within 6 months. Working outside the home is related to a shorter duration of breastfeeding and intentions to work full time are significantly associated with lower rates of breastfeeding initiation and shorter duration. Low-income women are more likely than their higher-income counterparts to return to work earlier and to hold jobs that compromise their ability to continue breastfeeding. Given the substantial presence of new mothers in the workforce, there is a need to establish lactation support in the workplace. Support for breastfeeding in the workplace includes these employee benefits and services:

- Flexible work schedules to provide time for milk expression.
- Access to a private location for milk expression.
- Access to a nearby clean and safe water source and sink for washing hands and rinsing out any breast-pump equipment.
- Access to high-quality breast pumps and hygienic storage options for the mother to store her breast milk.

Legislation to protect breastfeeding mothers when they return to work has been enacted in ten states: California, Connecticut, Georgia, Hawaii, Illinois, Minnesota, Rhode Island, Tennessee, Texas, and Washington. In 1993, the World Alliance for Breastfeeding Action (WABA) launched the Mother-Friendly Workplace Initiative (MFWI) to take baby friendliness outside the hospital and into women's working environments. The initiative aims to help women continue breastfeeding after returning to work.[27] States such as Texas and California used the WABA model to create their own Mother Friendly Workplaces. With the passage of Assembly Bill 1025 in 2001, the State of California became one of the first states to reduce a major barrier to breastfeeding by enacting legislation requiring employers to provide unpaid break time and a private space to express breast milk during the workday.

The *proposed* HeLP America Act of 2005 (S. 1074) section "Healthy Workplace for New Moms" would require employers with 50 or more employees to make reasonable efforts, in break time and space, to allow mothers to express milk or to breastfeed. It also establishes a federal taskforce to identify ways by which to improve the ability of new mothers to breastfeed when they return to work.

8.2.4.5 State Legislation

In recent years, the practice of breastfeeding has expanded. As a consequence of this trend, 38 states and Puerto Rico have enacted legislation associated with breastfeeding. The laws vary considerably in their scope and in their coverage. Initially, legislation concerned itself with issues about breast-feeding in public, clarifying that mothers have a right to breastfeed their babies wherever they go. Since then, other issues have arisen, such as exempting breastfeeding mothers from jury duty or protecting breastfeeding mothers when they return to work, as discussed in the previous section. Maine and Michigan have enacted laws that require courts in family law cases (divorce or separation) to consider breastfeeding in making custody and visitation or parenting time decisions. Maryland became the first state to provide an exemption from the sales tax laws for breastfeeding accessories, such as pumps, shields, and other paraphernalia used by breastfeeding mothers.

State laws may be generally classified into six broad categories: permitting a mother to breastfeed in any public or private location where the mother is legally entitled to be; exempting breastfeeding from public indecency laws; laws related to breastfeeding in the workplace; exempting breast-feeding mothers from jury duty; and laws implementing or encouraging the development of breastfeeding awareness programs.[28]

8.2.4.6 Federal Policies and Initiatives to Support Breastfeeding

More than three-quarters of the states have enacted laws that pertain to breastfeeding. However, there exist only two types of federal laws regarding breastfeeding, although many laws have been proposed.

8.2.4.6.1 Proposed Federal Legislation and Policy

There were 2 bills dealing with breastfeeding introduced in 2003 during the 108th Congress and 4 during the 109th Congress (see Box 8.5). None has emerged from Committee consideration at this time (September 2006). Three of the bills (S 418, HR 2790, and HR 2122) would amend the Civil Rights Act of 1964 to protect breastfeeding by new mothers. The practical effect of these amendments on the Civil Rights Act would be to include breastfeeding and the expression of milk within the definitions of "because of sex" and "on the basis of sex" for the purposes of the discrimination prohibitions of the Act. In addition, HR 2790 would provide for a performance standard for breast pumps and would provide tax incentives to encourage employers to permit breastfeeding.

Box 8.5 Breastfeeding: Proposed Federal Legislation

- S 418: 108th Congress (1st Session). Pregnancy Discrimination Act Amendments of 2003. "To amend the Civil Rights Act of 1964 to protect breastfeeding by new mothers."
- HR 2790: 108th Congress (1st session). Breastfeeding Promotion Act."To amend the Civil Rights Act of 1964 to protect breastfeeding by new mothers; to provide for a performance standard for breast pumps; and to provide tax incentives to encourage breastfeeding."
- HR 2122: 109th Congress (1st session). Pregnancy Discrimination Act Amendments of 2005. "To amend the Civil Rights Act of 1964 to protect breastfeeding by new mothers; to provide for a performance standard for breast pumps; and to provide tax incentives to encourage breastfeeding."
- S 1074: 109th Congress (2nd session). HeLP America Act. "Healthy Lifestyles and Prevention America Act or the `HeLP America Act." Title II will assist businesses and communities in offering a range of opportunities for people to start leading healthier lives. Initiatives include creating a more "mom-friendly" breastfeeding environment in the workplace.
- S 403 (Resolution): 109th Congress (2nd session). "Recognizing the benefits of breast-feeding and for other purposes."

HR 5951: 109th Congress (2nd session). Healthy Lifestyles and Prevention America Act or the HelP America Act. "To improve the health of Americans and reduce healthcare costs by reorienting the nation's healthcare system toward prevention, wellness, and self-care."

8.2.4.6.2   Current Federal Laws and Policy

Current laws regarding breastfeeding relate to women who breastfeed on federal property and with breastfeeding promotion through WIC. A woman may breastfeed at any location in a federal building or on federal property, if she and her child are otherwise authorized to be present at the location. These statutes are more symbolic than utilitarian. They demonstrate to the nation the intent of Congress, expecting that state governments will follow suit. Indeed, as indicated in Box 8.6, 32 states have enacted laws that specifically sanction breastfeeding in public places.

Box 8.6 State Breastfeeding Statutes

More than three-quarters of the states (39%) have enacted legislation related to breastfeeding.

- *Thirty-two states allow mothers to breastfeed in any public or private location.* California, Colorado, Connecticut, Delaware, Florida, Georgia, Hawaii, Illinois, Indiana, Iowa, Kentucky, Louisiana, Maine, Maryland, Minnesota, Missouri, Montana, Nevada, New Hampshire, New Jersey, New Mexico, New York, North Carolina, Oklahoma, Ohio, Oregon, Rhode Island, South Dakota, Utah, Texas, Vermont, and Virginia.
- *Fifteen states exempt breastfeeding from public indecency laws.* Alaska, Florida, Illinois, Michigan, Montana, Nevada, New Hampshire, North Carolina, Oklahoma, Rhode Island, South Dakota, Utah, Virginia, Washington, and Wisconsin.
- *Ten states have laws related to breastfeeding in the workplace.* California, Connecticut, Georgia, Hawaii, Illinois, Minnesota, Rhode Island, Tennessee, Texas, and Washington.
- *Ten states exempt breastfeeding mothers from jury duty.* California, Idaho, Illinois, Iowa, Kansas, Minnesota, Nebraska, Oklahoma, Oregon, and Virginia.
- *Four states have implemented or encouraged the development of a breastfeeding awareness education campaign.* California, Illinois, Missouri, and Vermont.

Eight states have unique laws related to breastfeeding, such as:

- California and Texas have laws related to the procurement, processing, distribution, or use of human milk.
- Louisiana prohibits any child care facility from discriminating against breastfed babies.
- Maine and Michigan have laws regarding divorcing and favored parents. Maine's law is intended to protect the health and well-being of a nursing infant of separated or divorcing parents. The law adds the situation of whether the mother is breastfeeding an infant under one year of age to the list of factors that a judge must consider in deciding parental rights and responsibilities. Michigan's law concerns child custody. Among the factors to be considered for "parenting time" is whether the child is a nursing child less than six months of age, or less than one year of age if the child receives substantial nutrition through nursing.
- Maryland exempts from the sales and use tax the sale of tangible personal property that is manufactured for the purpose of initiating, supporting or sustaining breastfeeding.
- Rhode Island requires the Department of Health to prepare a consumer mercury alert notice, explaining the danger of eating mercury-contaminated fish to women who are pregnant or breastfeeding their children.
- Illinois law gives a woman denied the right to breastfeed in a public or private location, other than a private residence or place of worship, the right to bring an action to enjoin

future denials of the right to breastfeed; if she prevails in her suit, she shall be awarded reasonable attorney's fees and reasonable litigation expenses.

- New York corrections law requires that when a woman is committed to a correctional institution and gives birth or is nursing a child in her care under one year of age, the child may accompany/remain with her in the institution.

Note: Effective through April 2006.

Source: Weimer, D.R. Summary of State Breastfeeding Laws and Related Issues. Congressional Research Service. The Library of Congress. January 12, 2005. Order Code RL31633. Available at: http://maloney.house.gov/documents/olddocs/breastfeeding/050505CRSReport.pdf. Accessed August 13, 2006; National Conference of State Legislatures. 50 State Summary of Breastfeeding Laws (Updated April 20, 2006). Available at: http://www.ncsl.org/programs/health/breast50.htm. Accessed August 14, 2006.

Of more practical significance are the federal laws regarding breastfeeding in the WIC program because half of the babies born in the U.S. participate in WIC.

8.2.4.6.3 WIC

WIC operates under the broad goal of improving the health of women, infants, and children by providing supplemental foods, nutrition and breastfeeding education, and access to health services. Since the program began in 1974, WIC program staff have counseled and encouraged women, both before and after delivery, regarding breastfeeding and infant care. Although these services continue to be a major program focus, breastfeeding promotion and support has been strengthened over the years.

Program and funding changes enabled WIC state agencies to provide breastfeeding aids, such as breast pumps and breast pads, offer an enhanced food package to women who breastfeed exclusively, and designate a staff person to coordinate breastfeeding promotion activities at the state level. Beginning in 1989, Congress began designating a specific portion of each state's WIC budget allocation to be used exclusively for the promotion and support of breastfeeding among its participants.

The Child Nutrition and WIC Reauthorization Act of 2004 earmarks up to $20 million per year for special nutrition education such as breastfeeding peer counseling and related activities to help achieve the breastfeeding goals, increasing the proportion of mothers who breastfeed their babies to 75% in the early postpartum period and to 50% at 6 months. In FY 2004, $14.9 million was appropriated for this additional WIC breastfeeding support and $14.8 million was appropriated in FY 2005 and FY 2006. State agencies use these funds to implement or expand peer counseling programs in accordance with the USDA Food and Nutrition Service Model for a Successful Peer Counseling Program (see Box 8.7, Box 8.8, and Box 8.9). An extensive collection of breastfeeding support materials is also available at the WIC Program's Web site http://www.nal.usda.gov/wicworks/Learning_Center/Breastfeeding_campaigns.html.

Box 8.7 U.S. Department of Agriculture Food and Nutrition Service Model for a Successful Peer Counseling Program

A "peer counselor" is a paraprofessional, recruited and hired from the target population, who is available to WIC clients outside usual clinic hours and outside the WIC clinic environment.

Adequate Program Support from State and Local Management

- Designated breastfeeding peer counseling program managers and/or coordinators at State and/or local level
- Defined job parameters and job descriptions for peer counselors

- Adequate compensation and reimbursement of peer counselors
- Training of appropriate WIC State/local peer counseling management and clinic staff (including use of "Using Loving Support to Manage Peer Counseling Programs" and "Peer Counseling: Making a Difference for WIC Families" training curriculum and PowerPoint presentations)
- Establishment of standardized breastfeeding peer counseling program policies and procedures at the State and local level as part of Agency nutrition education plan
- Adequate supervision and monitoring of peer counselors
- Establishment of community partnerships to enhance the effectiveness of a WIC peer counseling program

Adequate Program Support of Peer Counselors

- Adequate training and continuing education of peer counselors
- Timely access to breastfeeding coordinators and other lactation experts for assistance with problems outside of peer counselor scope of practice
- Regular, systematic contact with supervisor
- Participation in clinic staff meetings and breastfeeding in-service opportunities as part of the WIC team
- Opportunities to meet regularly with other peer counselors

Source: USDA, WIC Learning Center. *Loving Support Model for a Successful Peer Counseling Program.* Available at: http://www.nal.usda.gov/wicworks/Learning_Center/FNS_model.pdf#search=%22USDA%20Model%20successful%20peer%20counseling%22. Accessed August 31, 2006.

Box 8.8 Legislative History of Breastfeeding Promotion Requirements in WIC

- 1972 — P.L. 92–443. Congress authorized a 2-year pilot project to serve pregnant and lactating women, infants, and children up to age 4. In addition to meeting the income guidelines, participants were required to be at nutritional risk.
- 1975 — P.L. 94–105. WIC officially became a permanent national health and nutrition program. Congress explicitly used the term "breastfeeding" in the legislation. Breastfeeding women were defined as women who breastfed their infants up to 1 year of age. Nonbreastfeeding postpartum women could participate up to 6 months postpartum. Eligibility for children was extended to age five.
- 1989 — P.L. 101–147. Further increased emphases on breastfeeding promotion WIC by requiring the following:
  - That the USDA define the term "breastfeeding," as well as develop standards to ensure adequate breastfeeding promotion and support at the state and local levels
  - Authorization of the use of WIC nutrition services and administrative (NSA) funds to purchase breastfeeding aids such as breastpumps that directly support the initiation and continuation of breastfeeding
  - The addition of an expert in breastfeeding promotion and support to the National Advisory Council on Maternal, Infant and Fetal Nutrition
  - That WIC state agencies spend annually, at a minimum, their share of $8 million specifically targeted for breastfeeding promotion and support
  - Each state agency to make (a) a yearly evaluation of their breastfeeding promotion and support activities [this mandate was rescinded in 1996], (b) provide nutrition education and breastfeeding materials in languages other than English as appropriate, (c) include in their state plan a plan to provide nutrition education and breastfeeding promotion and

a plan to coordinate operations with local agency programs for breastfeeding promotion, and (d) designate a breastfeeding coordinator to provide training on breastfeeding promotion and support to local agency staff responsible for breastfeeding

- 1992 — P.L. 102–342. Required the Secretary of Agriculture to establish a national breastfeeding promotion program to promote breastfeeding as the best method of infant nutrition, foster wider public acceptance of breastfeeding in the U.S., and assist in the distribution of breastfeeding equipment to breastfeeding women. To do so, the secretary may develop or assist others to develop appropriate materials. Authorized the USDA to enter into cooperative agreements with federal, state, local, or other entities to carry out a breastfeeding promotion program and further authorized USDA to solicit and accept donations from outside sources for establishing a breastfeeding promotion program.
- 1994 — P.L. 103–448. Revised the formula for determining the amount of funds to be expended for WIC breastfeeding promotion and support; required WIC State agencies to spend $21 per pregnant and breastfeeding woman in support of breastfeeding promotion; required each WIC state agency to collect data on the incidence and duration of breastfeeding among participants and report this information to Congress every 2 years.
- 1996 — P.L. 104–193. Eliminated the state agency requirement for annually evaluating breastfeeding promotion and support activities.
- 1998 — P.L. 105–336. Authorized WIC state agencies to use food funds for the purchase or rental of breast pumps.

Box 8.9 WIC Breastfeeding Promotion Activities Carried Out at the State Level

Each state agency designates a breastfeeding promotion coordinator to coordinate breastfeeding promotion efforts identified in the state plan. The state plan must include the state agency's nutrition education goals and action plans, including a description of the methods that will be used to promote breastfeeding. Breastfeeding women are certified at intervals of approximately 6 months, ending with the breastfed infant's first birthday.

Nutrition education. State agencies perform the following activities in carrying out nutrition education responsibilities:

1. Provide training on the promotion and management of breastfeeding to staff at local agencies who will provide information and assistance on this subject to participants. All pregnant participants shall be encouraged to breastfeed unless contraindicated for health reasons.
2. Identify or develop resources and educational materials for use in local agencies, including breastfeeding promotion and instruction materials; taking reasonable steps to include materials in languages other than English in areas where a significant number of or proportion of the populations needs the information in a language other than English.
3. Establish standards for breastfeeding promotion and support which include, at a minimum, (a) a policy that creates a positive clinic environment that endorses breastfeeding as the preferred method of infant feeding, (b) a requirement that each local agency designate a staff person to coordinate breastfeeding promotion and support activities, (c) a requirement that each local agency incorporate task-appropriate breastfeeding promotion and support training into orientation programs for new staff involved in direct contact with WIC clients, and (d) a plan to ensure that women have access to breastfeeding promotion and support activities during the prenatal and postpartum periods.

Source: U.S. Department of Agriculture. Breastfeeding Promotion in WIC: Current Federal Requirements. Food and Nutrition Service. Available at: http://www.fns.usda.gov/wic/breastfeeding/bfrequirements.HTM. Accessed August 14, 2006.

Box 8.10 Research Activity

Use THOMAS to identify federal breastfeeding legislation that has been introduced in Congress in the past 5 years and to determine breastfeeding support legislation that has been enacted in the past 5 years.

Box 8.11 Nutrition Education Priorities for People Living with HIV Disease and AIDS

Information and guidance should be provided on the following topics:

- Consumption of a healthy diet
- Maintaining or increasing lean body mass
- Achieving and maintaining normal growth in children
- Management of metabolic complications related to HIV and antiretroviral therapy
- Management of medication–food interactions
- Management of gastrointestinal side effects of medications
- Cultural and ethnic beliefs related to food and diet
- Exercise
- Management of nausea and diarrhea
- Substance abuse and nutrition
- Nutrition during acute illnesses
- Food safety
- Nutrition during pregnancy
- Access to food, including infant formula
- Breastfeeding and HIV transmission
- Use of herbal and nutritional supplements
- Community sources of food and nutrition support

Source: Adapted from Nerad, J., Romeyn, M., Silverman, E., et al. General nutrition management in patients infected with human immunodeficiency virus. *Clin Infect Dis.* 36(Suppl. 2), S52–S62, 2003.

Box 8.12 Update

Search THOMAS for an update on the most recent reauthorization of the CARE Act. Where in the act has nutrition been included?

As discussed in Section 13.5, in 2006 WIC food packages were redesigned to promote the benefits of breastfeeding. Mother–infant pairs who rely on breastfeeding as the primary feeding method are provided with greater amounts and a wider variety of foods than before. The WIC food package for mothers who primarily breastfeed includes more milk, eggs, cheese, and whole grains than the packages for women who formula-feed. The packages for older infants who are given no formula contain twice the amount of baby food fruits and vegetables than the packages for their formula-fed counterparts.

8.2.4.6.4 Federal Breastfeeding Policy

In the short span of 16 years (1989 to 2005) the federal government produced sweeping legislation and policy statements regarding the promotion of breastfeeding.

- *1989–1992*: WIC breastfeeding initiatives are ramped-up through enactment of PL 101–147 and PL 102–342. The breastfeeding promotion requirements are summarized in Box 8.8.
- *2000:* Publication of *Blueprint for Action on Breastfeeding* by the Surgeon General of the U.S. presents a plan for breastfeeding based on education, training, awareness, support, and research. The *Blueprint* offers action steps for the healthcare system, families, the community, employers, and researchers. Its recommendations include training on breastfeeding counseling for healthcare professionals who provide maternal and childcare; ensuring that women who return to work after childbirth can continue breastfeeding; the creation of social support and information resources; and supporting research.
- *2001*: The U.S. Breastfeeding Committee publishes *Breastfeeding in the U.S.: A National Agenda* that calls for (1) access to comprehensive, current, and culturally appropriate lactation care and services for all women, children, and families; (2) recognition of breastfeeding as the normal and preferred method of feeding infants and young children; (3) all federal, state, and local laws relating to child welfare and family law to recognize and support the importance and practice of breastfeeding; and increase protection, promotion, and support for breastfeeding mothers in the workforce[29] (see Table 8.2).

TABLE 8.2
Strategic Plan for Breastfeeding in the United States

Goal 1	Assure access to comprehensive, current, and culturally appropriate lactation care and services for all women, children, and families
Objectives	Identify and disseminate evidence-based best practices and polices throughout the healthcare system
	Educate all healthcare providers and payers regarding appropriate breastfeeding and lactation support
	Ensure that all women have access to appropriate breastfeeding support within the family and/or community
	Ensure the routine collection and coordination of breastfeeding data by federal, state, and local government and other organizations, and foster additional research of breastfeeding
Goal 2	Ensure that breastfeeding is recognized as the normal and preferred method of feeding infants and young children
Objectives	Develop a positive and desirable image of breastfeeding for the American public
	Reduce the barriers to breastfeeding posed by the marketing of breast milk substitutes
Goal 3	Ensure that all federal, state, and local laws relating to child welfare and family law recognize and support the importance and practice of breastfeeding
Objective	Ensure that all lawmakers and government officials at federal, state, and local levels are aware of the importance of protecting, promoting, and supporting breastfeeding
Goal 4	Increase protection, promotion, and support for breastfeeding mothers in the workforce
	The rights of women in the workplace will be recognized in public and private sectors
Objectives	Ensure that all mothers are able to seamlessly integrate breastfeeding and employment

Source: United States Breastfeeding Committee. *Breastfeeding in the United States: A National Agenda.* Rockville, MD: U.S. Department of Health and Human Services, Health Services and Research Administration, Maternal and Child Health Bureau, 2001. Available at: http://www.usbreastfeeding.org/USBC-Strategic-Plan-2001.pdf. Accessed August 11, 2006.

- *2001*: *Healthy People 2010* outlines the measurable objectives regarding changes sought in the initiation and duration of breastfeeding. The targets are for 75% of new mothers to be breastfeeding when discharged from the hospital; 50% breastfeeding by the time the baby is 6 months of age; and 25% breastfeeding when the child is 12 months of age.
- *2005*: Publication of *The Guide to Breastfeeding Interventions* by the CDC, which describes successful breastfeeding interventions: maternity care practices, workplace support, peer support, educating mothers, professional support, and media and social marketing. Professional education, public acceptance, and hotlines and other information resources were found to be only marginally successful.

8.3 HIV/AIDS

Since the first cases of acquired immunodeficiency syndrome (AIDS) were reported in 1981, infection with human immunodeficiency virus (HIV) has grown to pandemic proportions, resulting in an estimated 65 million infections and 25 million deaths. During 2005 alone, an estimated 2.8 million persons died from AIDS, 4.1 million were newly infected with HIV, and 38.6 million were living with HIV. At the end of 2003, an estimated 1,039,000 to 1,185,000 persons in the U.S. were living with HIV/AIDS, with blacks and Hispanics together accounting for 69% of all reported cases.

By killing or damaging cells of the body's immune system, HIV progressively destroys the body's ability to fight infections and certain cancers. People living with HIV progress to the diagnosis of AIDS when they develop life-threatening diseases called opportunistic infections. These infections are caused by viruses or bacteria that make people with healthy immune systems sick.

Effective treatment of HIV infection with antiretroviral therapy (ART) is now available and 55% of persons in the U.S. in need of ART received it in 2005. HIV/AIDS drug therapies are prolonging the lives of people with HIV/AIDS who have access to medical treatment, effectively rendering HIV a chronic disease. In the U.S., ART has prolonged life by an estimated 13 years.[30] Better treatments have also led to an increase in the number of persons who are living with HIV/AIDS. Between 2000 and 2004, the estimated number of persons in the U.S. living with AIDS increased from 320,000 to 415,000 — an increase of 30%. Nonetheless, comprehensive programs are needed to reach all persons who require treatment and to prevent transmission of new infections.[31]

Good nutrition is essential to the management of HIV infection. People living with HIV/AIDS (PLWH/A) have special dietary requirements that must be managed in order to delay weight loss, wasting, and malnutrition. Nutritious food profoundly affects the immune system, may delay disease progression, increases tolerance of medical treatments, and can have a major impact on the quality of life.

8.3.1 Nutrition and HIV/AIDS[32]

Nutritional status is strongly predictive of survival and functional status among PLWH/A. Nutritional problems may occur at any stage of disease and can contribute to impaired immune response, accelerate disease progression, increase the frequency and severity of opportunistic infections, and impede the effectiveness of medications. Many nutritional disturbances are preventable and manageable.

Access to food, nutritional assessments, and nutrition interventions such as counseling and therapy can have a positive impact on morbidity, mortality, and quality of life. Nutritional interventions can also decrease or delay hospitalizations, emergency room visits, and costly and invasive treatments. The primary care setting offers an important opportunity to help prevent and mitigate nutrition-related complications. Yet, nutritional services are not always integrated into the primary care framework. Care teams sometimes do not include anyone with expertise in nutrition in HIV/AIDS. As a result, many nutrition-related problems go undiagnosed and untreated. The medical and physiological sources of nutritional problems associated with HIV/AIDS may be grouped into three general categories: inadequate intake, poor absorption, and altered metabolism.

8.3.2 Nutritional Problems and HIV/AIDS

Preventing, diagnosing, and treating nutritional disturbances require providers to navigate a complex and cyclical web of cause and effect. The systems that regulate nutrient intake and absorption are affected by — and, in turn, affect — HIV disease itself, opportunistic infections associated with the disease, and the effects of drugs used to fight HIV and HIV-induced illnesses. Inadequate nutrition makes it hard for PLWH/A to preserve their already weakened immune systems, increasing the risk of opportunistic infections and reducing the effectiveness of treatment. Infections can further compromise nutritional status and the strength of the immune system. Finally, HIV medications involve numerous food–drug interactions, so successful treatment adherence requires specific timing of medication doses and complicated dietary regimens.

8.3.2.1 Inadequate Intake

Many factors affect whether PLWH/A can ingest enough calories and nutrients to maintain health. Reduced nutrient intake can lead to weight loss as well as protein, vitamin, and mineral deficiencies. It generally results from loss of appetite caused by nausea, vomiting, altered sense of taste, fatigue, opportunistic infections in the gastrointestinal (GI) tract, or depression caused by receiving a diagnosis that is positive for HIV.

8.3.2.2 Altered Absorption

Malabsorption is a common manifestation of HIV infection, which may be secondary to lactose intolerance or GI infections. Even early on, HIV disease can directly damage the GI tract and interfere with nutrient absorption, resulting in depleted levels of micronutrients, particularly the carotenoids, B-vitamins, vitamin C, selenium, and zinc. As HIV disease progresses, opportunistic infections, including intestinal parasites and candidiasis, can further impair intestinal absorption. Malabsorption may also appear as a side effect of medication.

8.3.2.3 Altered Nutrient Metabolism

Metabolic abnormalities alter the way the body uses, stores, and excretes nutrients and may result in an increased need for calories and protein. Metabolic problems include impaired regulation of glucose and lipid abnormalities that may arise from immune dysfunction, medication side effects, opportunistic infections, hormonal alterations, or the direct effects of HIV itself.

8.3.2.4 AIDS Wasting and Lipodystrophy

Although the efficacy of antiretroviral therapy has reduced the incidence of some HIV-related nutritional problems, new nutrition-related challenges have emerged in their place. In some cases, the problems are complications of medical progress — either the direct result of treatment advances or simply a function of prolonged survival. Among the most important nutritional disturbances are AIDS wasting syndrome and lipodystrophy.

AIDS wasting syndrome (AWS) is characterized by involuntary weight loss of more than 10% of body weight along with either chronic diarrhea or weakness and fever. AWS incidence fell after the introduction of highly active antiretroviral therapy (HAART). However, weight loss and muscle wasting remain significant concerns, even in people with access to treatment. For example, lesser degrees of weight loss, such as dropping 5% of body weight within 6 months, although not included in the technical definition of AWS, is associated with increased morbidity and mortality. Unlike starvation-induced weight loss, HIV-associated wasting results in loss primarily of lean body mass (LBM), which increases the likelihood of opportunistic infections and is an independent predictor of increased morbidity and mortality, even if total body weight is preserved.

People on antiretroviral therapy who develop AWS may not exhibit the symptoms characteristic of the pre-HAART era. Monitoring of weight and physical appearance may be insufficient measurements for assessing the development of AWS, particularly in people with lipodystrophy, which may camouflage depletion of LBM. Therefore, routine monitoring of changes in weight, body mass, and body composition is essential.

Lipodystrophy is characterized by two types of changes in body fat distribution, which may occur alone or in combination: (1) the loss of fat in certain areas, particularly in the cheeks, temples, buttocks, arms, and legs and (2) isolated fat deposits, most commonly at the back of the neck and shoulders and around the abdomen. These changes to body shape can interfere with daily activities, such as exercising, sleeping, and even breathing. Lipodystrophy has been associated with increased risk for high blood pressure and dyslipidemia (abnormal cholesterol or triglyceride levels). The cause of lipodystrophy is not known, but may be related to HAART because the syndrome was identified only after the use of HAART became widespread.

8.3.3 Nutritional Care and HIV/AIDS

As nutritional changes can occur early in HIV infection, nutrition intervention should begin soon after diagnosis. Nutrition screening and a complete baseline nutrition assessment should be part of every care plan, as should ongoing reassessment. The key components of nutritional care risk are screening, comprehensive baseline evaluation or assessment, and ongoing monitoring and treatment — including self-care training, nutrition education, and various interventions.

8.3.3.1 Screening and Referral

Screening for nutritional status is a critical part of early intervention to identify and treat nutrition problems. At a minimum, it should include patient history, basic body measurements, and laboratory tests. Ideally, nutrition screening is conducted by a registered dietitian (RD) with experience in HIV/AIDS, but all HIV/AIDS providers should be able to identify nutrition-related problems and know when and how to refer clients for further evaluation and treatment.

Various forms are available to guide providers in assessing risk in their HIV-positive clients. This includes the tools contained in *HealthCare and HIV: Nutritional Guide for Providers and Clients,* developed by the AIDS Education and Training Centers (AETC) Program of the Ryan White CARE Act (see Section 8.3.3), available at http://www.aids-etc.org/aidsetc?page=et-30-20-01.

Referrals to a RD should be automatic when one or more risk factors are identified during the screening, as outlined in Nutrition Referral Criteria for Adults with HIV/AIDS, located at http://www.hivaidsdpg.org. Risk levels are defined as follows:

1. *High risk*, for example, greater than 10% unintentional weight loss over 4 to 6 months, severely dysfunctional psychosocial situation, and two or more medical co-morbidities should be evaluated by an RD within one week.
2. *Moderate risk,* for example, possible lipodystrophy; chronic diarrhea, and chronic nausea and vomiting should be evaluated by an RD within one month.
3. *Low risk*, for example, no manifestations of nutrition-related problems, should be seen by an RD as needed.

Additional criteria signaling the need for referral to an RD include oral and GI symptoms, metabolic complications, barriers to nutrition, impaired functional status, and unusual eating behaviors.

8.3.3.2 Medical Nutrition Therapy

According to the HIV/AIDS dietetic practice group of the ADA, the major goals of medical nutrition therapy for persons living with HIV are to:

- Optimize nutrition status, immunity, and overall well-being
- Prevent the development of specific nutrient deficiencies
- Prevent loss of weight and LBM
- Reduce risk for onset or complications of co-morbidities such as diabetes, cardiovascular, kidney, and liver diseases
- Maximize effectiveness of medical and pharmacological treatments
- Minimize healthcare cost[33]

8.3.3.3 The Ryan White Comprehensive AIDS Resources Emergency (CARE) Act

The Ryan White Comprehensive AIDS Resources Emergency (CARE) Act is federal-level legislation that addresses the unmet health needs of PLWH/A by funding primary healthcare and support services. It is the largest discretionary investment solely devoted to the care of PLWH/A in the U.S., reaching more than 500,000 people a year in all 50 states, the District of Columbia, Puerto Rico, and the U.S. territories. The program is administered through the HIV/AIDS Bureau of the Health Resources and Services Administration (HRSA) within HHS. It is named after Ryan White, an Indiana teenager infected with the illness after a blood transfusion, who died shortly before the act was originally passed in 1990.

The legislation, which must be reauthorized every 5 years, was extended in 1996 (by P.L. 104–146) and in 2000 (P.L. 106–345). It was due for reauthorization in September 2005, but by September 2006 it had not yet received Congressional action. Nevertheless, the program was funded for about $2 billion in 2005 and again in 2006. The President's FY2007 budget request for the CARE Act is about the same. A separate act of Congress appropriates the money on a yearly basis.

As indicated in Table 8.3, the CARE Act includes six parts: emergency relief (Title I); HIV care (Title II); early intervention (Title III); women, infants, children and youth (Title IV); AIDS Education Training Centers (AETC); and dental reimbursements. Roughly 55% of the budget is allocated for HIV care, 30% for emergency relief, and 15% for the remaining programs. In testimony

---

TABLE 8.3
FY 2006 Appropriations for the Ryan White CARE Act[a]

Program	FY 2006 Appropriations
Part A: (Title I) — Emergency Relief	$611,581,200
Part B: (Title II) — HIV Care	$1,134,595,500
(STATE)	(330,972,000)
(ADAP)	(789,546,000)
Part C: (Title III) — Early Intervention	$196,054,400
Part D: (Title IV) — Women, Infants, Children & Youth	$72, 695,900
Part E: AIDS Ed Training Centers (AETC)	$34,700.000
Part F: Dental Reimbursements	$13,086,000
Total: Ryan White CARE Act	$2,062,713,000

[a] *Journal of Correctional HealthCare* homepage. Available at: http://www.ncchc.org/pubs/journal.html. Accessed August 10, 2006.

before Congressional committee staff members, ADA recommended the following provisions be included in the 2005 reauthorization of the Ryan White CARE Act:[34]

- Titles I and II: Medical Nutrition Therapy (MNT) should be required and specifically listed as a core service in all titles, but especially Titles I and II.
- HIV/AIDS Education and Training Centers should specifically include nutrition faculty and dietetics professionals among those eligible for training.
- Title I: HIV Service Planning Councils should include representation by food and nutrition professionals.

8.3.3.4 Community-Based Programs

The Association of Nutrition Services Agencies (ANSA) collaborates with other national organizations having nutrition and/or HIV/AIDS as a core issue to help ensure the long-term sustainability of their members' programs and to move the entire field of nutrition services forward with a unified voice. ANSA advocates for (1) Ryan White CARE Act reauthorization, (2) new funding for non-HIV/AIDS critically ill populations, and (3) building a national coalition — the National Nutrition Collaborative — comprised of national organizations with hunger and nutrition as core issues.

8.3.3.4.1 Food Assistance

Three types of food assistance are available to PLWH/A: groceries, congregate meals, and home-delivered meals (see Box 8.13).

- *Pantry bags (groceries) and food vouchers* allow PLWH/A with limited financial resources access to nutritious food. In conjunction with nutrition services, PLWH/A are able to increase their levels of independence by preparing meals and making their own food choices.
- *Congregate meals* are served in community locations fostering access to healthcare, prevention, and supportive services, while meeting the nutritional needs of PLWH/A. Many participants who use the congregate meal programs are indigent, homeless, or in marginal housing which lack kitchen facilities and food preparation equipment.
- *Home-delivered meals* help to maintain or improve the health and well-being of home restricted individuals by providing calorie- and protein-rich, therapeutically tailored meals, and snacks. For PLWH/A who lack the ability to shop for and prepare food, home-delivered meals fulfill a critical need, often allowing them to leave the hospital sooner and remain in the community longer.

Box 8.13 Model Community-based Comprehensive Care Program

Harlem United Community AIDS Center is a Ryan White-funded community-based organization providing a continuum of care for over 2,300 clients per year, most of whom are socially and economically disenfranchised people living with HIV/AIDS, whose diagnoses are often complicated by addiction, mental illness, and homelessness. Harlem United's clients are integrated into a healthy and healing community that offers access to a full range of medical, social, and supportive services. Harlem United's "one-stop shop" for services allows the center to treat the whole person — mind, body, and spirit — in a compassionate and supportive environment. The staff of over 150 full-time employees works in partnership with Harlem United's clients at each stage of care: HIV testing; treatment and education; primary medical care; substance use counseling; mental health services; pastoral counseling; and an array of expressive therapies. Harlem United has become a national model of comprehensive care in a community-based setting. The Food and Nutrition Services component of Harlem United provides comprehensive nutritional services that include nutrition education in a group setting and individual level nutrition counseling, as well as a hot, balanced evening meal. Metrocards are provided to individuals to get home after program services as well as to return the next evening.

Source: Harlem United Community AIDS Center. Available at: http://www.harlemunited.org/index.html. Accessed August 17, 2006.

8.4 PRISON INMATES

Bernard P. Harrison, J.D., and B. Jaye Anno, Ph.D., introduced the concepts of national standards and voluntary accreditation as means to upgrade healthcare in correctional facilities. Their work marked the beginning of the field known as correctional health. In the early 1970s, Harrison and Anno brought to the nation's attention the tremendous inadequacy of healthcare for the incarcerated, spearheading efforts to survey and research the state of healthcare in correctional healthcare facilities. They demonstrated the gravity of health problems of inmates, the risk that these problems posed to the health of the public beyond jails and prisons, and the inadequacy of care that was being provided to inmates. Along with key organizations and constituencies, they increased awareness of the problem and sought to improve standards for health services in prisons. Attributed to their work was a subsequent fourfold increase in the detection of previously undiagnosed and untreated illnesses among inmates and a Supreme Court ruling, (*Estelle v. Gamble*) requiring states to ensure that an inmate's basic needs are met, including healthcare.

In 1981 Anno and Harrison founded the National Commission on Correctional HealthCare (NCCHC), a nonprofit organization dedicated to improving healthcare in the nation's jails, prisons, and juvenile detention and confinement facilities. The organization has created a certification program for correctional health personnel, sets standards for health services in correctional facilities, and provides a voluntary accreditation program for facilities that meet NCCHC standards.[35]

8.4.1 Constitutional Right to Healthcare

One of the most contested aspects of imprisonment is access to healthcare. The U.S. is unique among Western countries in that it has no general governmental oversight of prisons and jails. Therefore, it is left to the courts to develop the minimum standards for treatment of prisoners.

That an inmate has the right to adequate healthcare was determined by the Supreme Court decision in *Estelle v. Gamble*, 429 U.S. 97 (1976). The Court ruled that "deliberate indifference" to a prisoner's health was "cruel and unusual punishment," which is prohibited by the Eighth Amendment to the Constitution. *In this case*, the Court interpreted the Eighth Amendment protections to require that healthcare for convicted felons must meet a standard equal to that in the community. Although the 8th Amendment is the usual focus of a discussion of prisoners' rights, any official actions rising to a violation of a prisoner's civil liberties may impact their 14th Amendment right to equal protection under the law, as well as their right to due process.

Beginning in the early 1970s a series of cases was decided in the federal courts that served to further clarify the scope and extent of inmates' Eighth Amendment rights to medical treatment. As a result of these decisions, prisoners are the only Americans with a constitutional right to healthcare.

8.4.2 Correctional Health in Public Health

Health conditions overrepresented in incarcerated populations include substance abuse; HIV and other infectious diseases; perpetration of and victimization by violence; mental illness; chronic disease; and reproductive health problems.[36] Whereas the vast majority of individuals affected by these conditions develop them prior to incarceration, the period of incarceration provides a window of opportunity to serve the broad public health interest by providing testing, treatment, counseling, health education, and health promotion to an otherwise disenfranchised population prior to their ultimate release back into the community.[37]

Prisons and jails offer a unique opportunity to establish better disease control in the community by providing improved healthcare and disease prevention to inmates before they are released. In 1998, over 11 million men and women were released from prison into the community, many thousands with undiagnosed or untreated chronic diseases. Not only would it be cost effective to treat several of these diseases while the individuals are incarcerated, but in quite a few instances it would save money in the long run.[38,39] Periods of incarceration offer opportunities to public health and criminal justice agencies to provide a range of health interventions needed by this underserved population. Timely discharge planning is essential, as are linkages with community-based organizations and agencies that can provide medical care, health education, and necessary supportive services.[40]

The vast majority of the prison population is arrested in and returned to urban, low-income communities. These men, women, and adolescents have high rates of health problems,[40] predominantly mental health, substance abuse, and communicable diseases.[41] The prison population has had little prior access to primary healthcare or health interventions, and many are returning to their communities without critical preventive health information and skills, appropriate medical services, and other necessary support.[42]

Correctional systems can have a direct effect on the health of urban populations by offering healthcare and health promotion in jails and prisons, by linking inmates to community services after release, and by assisting in the process of community reintegration.

8.4.3 JAILS AND PRISONS

Jails are locally-operated correctional facilities that confine persons before or after adjudication. Inmates sentenced to jail usually have a sentence of a year or less, although jails also incarcerate persons in a wide variety of other categories. Prisons, on the other hand, are federal or state facilities that house felons who must serve a sentence longer than 1 year.

8.4.3.1 Federal Detention

The Federal Bureau of Prisons was responsible for the custody and care of approximately 180,000 federal offenders in 2004, over 80% of whom were confined in bureau-operated correctional institutions and detention centers. The rest are confined in privately-operated prisons, detention centers, community corrections centers, and juvenile facilities, as well as facilities operated by state or local governments. The federal prison system is a nationwide system of prisons and detention facilities for the incarceration of inmates who have been sentenced to imprisonment for federal crimes and the detention of individuals awaiting trial or sentencing in federal court; the system is also responsible for incarcerating the District of Columbia's sentenced felon inmate population. The bureau places most inmates in community corrections centers (halfway houses) prior to their release from custody to help them adjust to life in the community after their release.[43] At year end 2004, the federal system was 40% over-capacity.

8.4.3.2 State Detention

In addition to the federal system, each state has its own department of corrections (New York has both a New York State and a New York City Department of Corrections). The Federal Bureau of Prisons operated the largest prison system at year end 2004, followed by Texas (168,000), California (167,000), Florida (86,000), and New York (64,000 plus 14,500 in the city system).

The states with the highest incarceration rates in 2004 were Louisiana (8.16 sentenced prisoners per 1,000 state residents), Texas (6.94), Mississippi (6.69), Oklahoma (6.49), and Georgia (5.74).

The states with the lowest incarceration rates were Maine (1.48 sentenced inmates per 1,000 state residents), Minnesota (1.71), Rhode Island (1.75), New Hampshire (1.87), and North Dakota (1.95). At year end 2004, 24 state prison systems were operating at or above their highest capacity.

8.4.4 Demographic Trends in Correctional Populations

State and federal prison authorities had in custody 1.4 million inmates at year end 2004 (1.2 million in state custody and almost 171,000 in federal custody). Local jails held more than 700,000 persons awaiting trial or serving a sentence at mid-year 2004.

If incarceration rates remain unchanged, 6.6% of U.S. residents born in 2001 will go to prison at some time during their lifetime.[44]

8.4.4.1 Race and Ethnicity

Cities have more poor people, more people of color, and higher crime rates than suburban and rural areas; thus, urban populations are overrepresented in the nation's jails and prisons. As a result, U.S. incarceration policies and programs have a disproportionate impact on urban black and Latino communities.[45]

At year end 2004, there were 3.218 black male prison inmates per 1000 black males in the U.S., compared to 1.220 Hispanic male inmates per 1000 Hispanic males and 0.463 white male inmates per 1000 white males. About 8.4% of all black male U.S. residents between 25 and 29 years old were in a state or federal prison in 2004, compared to 2.5% of Hispanic males in the same age group and 1.2% of white males. Among male and female prisoners combined, 41% were black, 34% were white, 19% Hispanic, with the rest of other races or two or more races.[46]

8.4.4.2 Women

Although the number of incarcerated women is substantially less than the number of incarcerated men, women make up the fastest growing segment of the U.S. incarcerated population, increasing an average of 5% each year between 1995 and 2003. In mid-year 2003,[47] the female inmate population reached just over 100,000.

8.4.4.3 The Aging Inmate Population

The past decade has seen a dramatic increase in the number of incarcerated elderly, due to mandatory minimum sentencing, longer sentences, and tighter parole policies. Corrections officials recognize that the cost of maintaining older prisoners is nearly triple that of other inmates, primarily due to the expense of healthcare. Poor living conditions in prison, inadequate medical treatment, and prior lifestyles (which accelerate aging and medical conditions) make older prisoners a unique population with special prerelease needs. Solutions to the aging inmate challenges that have been suggested by the Administration on Aging include the establishment of private medical prisons, early release of nonviolent, low-risk older offenders, and the exploration of alternatives to incarceration.[48]

8.4.5 Food Service in the Prison Systems

8.4.5.1 In the Federal System

The meals provided through the federal system meet Recommended Dietary Allowances (RDA). Special meals are available to accommodate inmates' religious and medical dietary requirements. Meal preparation is accomplished primarily by inmate workers (about 12% of the population) under the supervision of Bureau staff. Inmates assigned to a food service department have the opportunity to acquire skills and abilities that may assist them in obtaining employment upon release.

Recently, court battles have been waged by inmates for the right to receive kosher or halaal meals in prison, claiming that denial of such a request violates their First Amendment rights to free exercise of religion. In response, federal prisons have adopted a policy whereby inmates requesting a religious diet will be provided with a "common fare religious diet program," consisting of foods that largely require no preparation, contain no pork or pork derivatives, do not mix meat or dairy products in the service of food items, and are served with utensils that have not come in contact with pork or pork derivatives. To the extent practicable, this diet contains approximately three hot entrees a week and meets or exceeds the RDA. Inmates requesting a religious diet must submit an application to the prison chaplain, who is responsible for approving such requests. An inmate shall ordinarily begin eating from the common fare menu within two days after food service receives the chaplain's authorization.[49]

8.4.5.2 In the State Systems

In state facilities, the daily energy allowance for inmates is determined by the state legislatures and varies across states. In Illinois, for example, the daily minimum energy allotment is 2,700 kcal/day, whereas Wyoming and Montana require, respectively, 1,800 and 3,500 kcal/day.[50] In 38 states, recipes are reviewed regularly by dietitians, though the basis for identifying and using recipes in 26 states comes from the military. Correctional food service is subcontracted out to private contractors in Kansas and New Mexico.[50]

In some cases, federal standards for religious meals have been adopted by states, in whole or in part. Pork-free meals are available in state prisons in 20 states, vegetarian meals in 11 states, meatless meals in 7 states, kosher foods in 6 states, and lacto-ovo meals in 3 states.[51]

On average nationwide, state departments of correction spent $2.62 per capita to feed inmates each day. Pennsylvania ($5.69) and Washington ($5.68) reported the largest amounts, followed by Maine ($5.03), Hawaii ($4.87), and Iowa ($4.81). North Carolina indicated the lowest cost ($0.52), followed by Alabama ($0.72), Mississippi ($0.81), and Louisiana ($0.96). Reports of low food costs often reflected prisoner-operated farm and food processing operations. For example, facilities in Mississippi grew a wide variety of fruits, vegetables, and grains, and even raised livestock for other prisons in the state, whereas prison enterprises in North Carolina operated a cannery, a meat processing plant, warehouses, and trucks to deliver food and equipment to correctional facilities statewide.[52]

Food service in correctional facilities is big business. In 2006 the Aramark company provided services to more than 475 correctional facilities.

8.4.5.2.1 Scenario
Input from inmates has helped bring about positive changes in some correctional facilities. The South Dakota Women's Penitentiary in Pierre, SD, developed a wellness program to educate their inmates on the importance of a healthy weight, proper nutrition, and daily exercise. This program evolved in response to inmate complaints about obesity and the high-fat, high-energy meals being served. The reduced calorie meal plan is based on modifying the regular cycle menu; for example, chicken should be baked instead of fried. To be eligible for the low-energy meals, the inmates must commit to the program for at least one month. Nutrition analysis of food is posted so that the women may keep track of their intakes. The commissary began stocking more healthful snack options as well.[51]

8.4.5.3 Dietary Needs of Juvenile Offenders

For facilities with youthful offenders, the menus for children are the same as for adults, except the children receive more milk. Some facilities with large juvenile populations are approved by the Child Nutrition Program. When necessary, the physician or other medical personnel will order therapeutic diets (renal, hepatic, diabetic, low-sodium, low cholesterol, low-fat, low-energy, high-energy, high protein, cardiovascular, medical-soft, dental-soft, low-lactose, pregnancy, bland, pureed, and liquid diets), derived from the facility's regular cycle menu. In some cases, such as in Kentucky, the specialized meals are available only at correctional hospital facilities.[53]

8.4.5.4 Nutrition-Related Chronic Diseases in Inmates

An estimated 80,000 inmates have diabetes and more than 280,000 have hypertension, with prevalence rates of about 5% and 18%, respectively.[54] The current estimated prevalence of diabetes and hypertension in correctional institutions is somewhat lower than the overall U.S. prevalence of these conditions, perhaps because the incarcerated population is younger than the general population. The prevalence of diabetes and its related co-morbidities and complications, however, will continue to increase in the prison population as current sentencing guidelines continue to increase the number of aging prisoners *and* as the incidence of diabetes in young people continues to increase.

Prevalence rates for several diseases vary by age, race, and sex. For example, the prevalences of diabetes and hypertension are considerably higher for inmates 50 years or older than for younger prisoners. Diabetes is more common among black and Hispanic inmates than among white inmates, similar to patterns in the general population.[55]

8.4.5.4.1 Managing Nutrition-Related Chronic Diseases

People with diabetes, high blood pressure, and high blood cholesterol in correctional facilities should receive care that meets national standards. Correctional institutions have unique circumstances that need to be considered so that all standards of care may be achieved. Correctional institutions should have written policies and procedures for the management of diabetes, hypertension, and elevated cholesterol, and for training medical and correctional staff in diabetes care practices. These policies must take into consideration issues such as security needs, transfer from one facility to another, and access to medical personnel and equipment, so that all appropriate levels of care are provided.

In terms of diabetes, policies should encourage or at least allow patients to self-manage their disease. Ultimately, diabetes management is dependent upon having access to needed medical personnel and equipment. Ongoing diabetes therapy is important in order to reduce the risk of later complications, including cardiovascular events, vision loss, renal failure, and amputation. Early identification and intervention for people with diabetes is also likely to reduce short-term risks for acute complications requiring transfer out of the facility, thus improving security. [56]

Inmates with diabetes, hypertension, and/or hypercholesterolemia who have special dietary needs may benefit from simple solutions such as a reduced fat, reduced sodium salad bar that would relieve food service of the burden of preparing individual trays and would allow otherwise healthy prisoners to live outside of special units.[57]

NCCHC has adopted clinical guidelines[58] to help correctional healthcare professionals effectively manage diet-related chronic diseases commonly found in jails, prisons, and juvenile confinement facilities. Guidelines are available for diabetes (2001), high blood pressure (2003), and high blood cholesterol (2005). The guidelines are adapted for the correctional environment from nationally accepted clinical guidelines prepared by the ADA and the National Heart, Lung, and Blood Institute of the National Institutes of Health. The guidelines are written to specifically help correctional healthcare providers improve patient care outcomes. They encourage total disease management, which requires clear indicators of the degree of control of the patient's disease and, frequently, the more subtle distinction as to whether the condition is stable, improving, or deteriorating. Table 8.4 presents indicators for management of diabetes, hypertension, and dyslipidemia in the inmate population.

TABLE 8.4
Indicators of Disease Control and Clinical Status

	Disease			
Control	**Diabetes**	**Hypertension + Diabetes**	**Cardiac/Hypertension**	**Dyslipidemia**
Good	HbA$_{1c}$ is within acceptable range (< 7%)	Systolic < 130 mm/Hg Diastolic < 80 mm/Hg	Systolic < 140 mm/Hg Diastolic < 90 mm/Hg	LDL-C at goal
Fair	HbA$_{1c}$ is 7%	Systolic 130–150 mm/Hg Diastolic 80–95 mm/Hg	Systolic 140–160 mm/Hg Diastolic 90–100 mm/Hg	LDL-C 130–159 mg/dL
Poor	HbA$_{1c}$ is 8%	Systolic > 150 mm/Hg Diastolic > 95 mm/Hg	Systolic > 160 mm/Hg Diastolic > 100 mm/Hg	LDL-C ≥ 160 mg/dL
	Status			
Improved	Reduction in HbA$_{1c}$ or the average of finger-stick levels, or for type 2 diabetes there has been intentional weight loss of 5% or more through diet and exercise; or HbA$_{1c}$ is within acceptable range.	BP is lower than at the previous visit	BP is lower than at the previous visit	LDL-C has decreased or reached goal level since previous visit
Unchanged	When the HbA$_{1c}$ or the average of finger-stick levels are the same as previously recorded and for type 2 diabetes weight is relatively unchanged.	No change in BP, weight, and/or lab values since last visit	No change in BP, weight, and/or lab values since last visit	LDL-C has not changed since previous visit
Poorer	When the HbA$_{1c}$ or the average of finger stick levels is increased, or for type 2 diabetes there has been a weight gain of 5% or more.	Increase in BP, weight, and/or lab values; or nonadherence to treatment plan; or development of more acute symptoms since previous visit	Increase in BP, weight, and/or lab values; or nonadherence to treatment plan; or development of more acute symptoms since previous visit	LDL-C has increased since previous visit

Source: Definitions of Disease Control and Status (2004): http://www.ncchc.org/clinical_guidelines/2004_defs_of_ control.pdf.

8.4.5.5 The Dietitian's Role

Corrections dietitians in the U.S. represent a minority in the field of nutrition and dietetics and food service management. The roles of the correctional dietitian vary, depending on the agency and facility, but this list represents an overview of the tasks that are performed:[59]

- Promote the use of standardized menus and diets.
- Ensure compliance with standards and policies.
- Ensure nutritional adequacy of menus via computerized nutritional analysis.

Box 8.14 Ethical Issue

Modifying Food Service to Control Behavior

The American Correctional Association standards preclude the use of food as a disciplinary measure (ACA Standard 3–4301, Ref. 2–4252/Adult Correctional Facilities). Inmates and staff, except those on special medical or religious diets, are expected to eat the same meals, and food should not be withheld as a disciplinary sanction. Though compliance to these standards is voluntary, they are viewed as valid and acceptable standards of operation within the industry.

Nevertheless, occasionally an inmate will be served a food product known as the "Loaf" (or variously, Special Management Meal, Behavioral Loaf, Nutri-Loaf, or Prison Loaf), which is designed to be nutritionally complete. Three loaves per day meet the basic nutritional needs of an adult inmate (2,400–3,900 calories with a distribution of approximately 10–15% protein, 50–79% carbohydrate and 5–38% fat). The loaf is often served in a disposable container with no eating utensils and is accompanied by a beverage. This meal is a nutritionally complete, *albeit* tasteless alternative to the regular food service. The individual governing agency, warden, or jail administrator decides whether to use the loaf as either a reprimand for severe, deviant, antisocial behavior by the inmate or as a protective measure so that the inmate is less likely to injure himself.

As it is not a special diet in the medical sense, Anno asserts that the food loaf should not be devised or prescribed by health professionals.

There are no reliable statistics regarding how many facilities use the loaf. An informal survey indicated that it was used by half of the 19 facilities that responded for typically 1 to 3 d (but as many as 30). Respondents indicated that the loaf was used for discipline or behavior modification. In the majority of cases, administrative and/or medical personnel approved its use with strict monitoring procedures. Two respondents were sued; both cases were resolved in favor of the prison authority.

Discuss the ethical issues faced by a nutrition professional who is asked to develop a recipe for a food loaf to be used as a reprimand in her detention facility.

Sources:

Wakeen, B. and Montgomery, J.W. The "loaf" — part II. *ACFS Insider.* Summer 2003, pp. 19–20. Available at: http://www.acfsa.org/cfppgm/pdfs/diet103.pdf. Accessed August 9, 2006.

Anno, B.J. Correctional HealthCare: Guidelines for the Management of an Adequate Delivery System, 2001 edition. National Commission on Correctional HealthCare, 2001.

- Review and approve menus annually and/or semiannually and make recommendations as needed.
- Write menus.
- Write medical diets or provide guidance for diets as requested. Typical therapeutic diets include the following types: low fat, diabetic, vegetarian, lactose-free, mechanical soft, religious (such as kosher and Muslim), allergy, and gluten-free.
- Set policy. Although there is general consensus that the DRIs and RDAs should be met, each system establishes its own standards regarding nutrients and energy provided in meals (see also Box 8.14).

8.4.5.6 Dietary Guidelines

Since publication of the sixth edition of the Dietary Guidelines for Americans, corrections dietitians have been faced with the challenge of modifying corrections menus in order to meet the new meal pattern recommendations within the constraints of a limited budget.[60] In many ways, corrections dietitians face challenges similar to those faced by the school lunch programs.

- How are state and federal correction facilities modifying menus to meet these guidelines?
- How can sodium be reduced to 2300 mg when large caloric levels and processed foods are served, and when 2300 mg of sodium is considered a therapeutic level of sodium in many correctional facilities?
- What modifications are being made both to menus and by manufacturers to accommodate the fat, cholesterol, and saturated fat restrictions?
- Is meeting the DRIs and RDAs sufficient to be in compliance with agency standards?
- To help meet the dietary guidelines, will facilities accept menu modifications that include reducing overall calories, increasing meatless meals, and/or incorporating soy products into recipes to offset fat and cholesterol, offering skim milk, omitting and/or limiting nonnutritional items, such as sugar and coffee, and cooking without added salt?[60]

8.4.6 REENTRY

Prisons and jails offer a unique opportunity to establish better disease control in the community by providing improved healthcare and disease prevention to inmates before they are released. Unarguably, tens of thousands of inmates are being released into the community every year with undiagnosed or untreated communicable disease, chronic disease, and mental illness. Thus, in 1997, Congress instructed the U.S. Department of Justice (DOJ) to investigate the health status of soon-to-be-released inmates. At question was the extent that changes in correctional healthcare might be able to improve the public health of communities at large. NCCHC studied the problem and in 2002 released to Congress *The Health Status of Soon-to-Be-Released Inmates*.[61] The following key findings regarding chronic diseases are from the report.

In addition to disproportionately high rates of infectious disease and mental illness, the incarcerated population is afflicted with high rates of nutrition-related chronic diseases, such as dental problems, diabetes, hypertension, and heart disease. Because inmates are a relatively young population the estimated prevalence rates for diabetes and hypertension among inmates are still high when compared to the total U.S. population considering the two diseases are much more likely to afflict older individuals. Although prisons and jails are channels to the community, corrections and public health maintain related, yet often uncoordinated, systems. In addition to the public health benefits, coordinating health treatment approaches could also result in financial savings to taxpayers. Only 29 of the 41 systems indicated that inmates with chronic disease were given a supply of medication when released. Although many may view such care as outside the responsibility of publicly-funded correctional agencies, inadequate access to care and follow-up services creates a cost burden (in dollars and in the potential development of resistance to treatment) for public health institutions once inmates are released.

It is suggested that federal, state, and local reentry programs provide a three-phase, comprehensive assistance and support services approach from the (a) prerelease phase, with education, mental health, and substance abuse treatment, job training, and risk assessment, to the (b) transition phase prior to and immediately following offender release, and the (c) postrelease, sustained, long-term mentoring, counseling, and support phase. In New York City,[62] for example, case managers with the New York City Link program are responsible for creating a community-services plan for inmates at the city's jail (Rikers Island), filing benefit applications on inmates' behalf and providing housing referrals. The

Medication Grant Program (MGP) is the primary mechanism to connect individuals with mental illnesses to benefits such as Medicaid, food stamps, and cash assistance after release. The program assists inmates in the application process and to secure MGP cards upon their release. Under the program, a Medicaid application can be submitted up to 45 days before or within seven days after release.

8.4.6.1 Scenario

Faced with explosive growth in its prison population and a legal mandate to improve medical care for incarcerated offenders, the state of Texas implemented a novel correctional managed healthcare program in 1994. The organizational structure of the program is based on a series of contractual relationships between the state prison system and two of the state's academic medical centers, which provide all medical, dental, and psychiatric care for the state's inmates. The health delivery system is composed of several levels of care, including primary ambulatory care clinics in each prison unit, infirmaries at strategic locations throughout the state, several regional medical facilities, and a dedicated prison hospital with a full range of services. Specialized treatment programs have been established at various units for patients with such chronic conditions as hypertension and diabetes mellitus.

Ten years after the managed care program was established, researchers reported significant positive health outcomes and millions of dollars saved. Significant changes in diet-related chronic conditions were reported from 1995 to 2003. The mean blood glucose level for patients with type 1 diabetes mellitus decreased from 230 mg/dL to 188 mg/dL, the mean LDL-C level among patients with hyperlipidemia decreased from 174 mg/dL to 132 mg/dL, and the proportion of inmates with essential hypertension (blood pressure $\geq$ 140/90 mm/Hg) decreased from 83% to 51%.[63]

8.4.7 RESOURCES AND PROFESSIONAL AFFILIATIONS

In a short span of time, the correctional health field has established itself as a significant subspecialty within public health. Physicians who work in corrections may belong to the Society of Correctional Physicians. Similarly, there are two correctional health associations for nutrition professionals. Dietitians in Corrections is a subgroup of the American Correctional Food Service Association (ACFSA).[64] Corrections is a subunit of Consultant Dietitians in HealthCare Facilities,[65] a practice group of the ADA. The subunit sponsors a corrections electronic mailing list, and in 2004, its members published *Correctional Foodservice and Nutrition Manual*, second edition.

The NCCHC, a nonprofit organization dedicated to improving healthcare in the nation's jails, prisons, and juvenile detention and confinement facilities, has created a certification program for correctional health personnel, sets standards for health services in correctional facilities, and provides a voluntary accreditation program for facilities that meet NCCHC standards.[66] The NCCHC *Journal of Correctional HealthCare* is the only national, peer-reviewed journal to address correctional healthcare topics. This quarterly publication features original research, case studies, best practices, and literature reviews in the areas of health services administration, personnel and staffing, ethical issues, clinical and support services, medical records, continuous quality improvement, risk management and medical–legal issues. As NCCHC develops clinical guidelines and position statements, these also are also published in the journal.

Other associations for professional correctional health personnel include:

- Academy of Correctional Health Professionals, http://www.correctionalhealth.org/
- American Correctional Health Services Association, achsa@mindspring.com
- Corrections Connection Online Healthcare Network, www.corrections.com/healthnet
- Institute for Criminal Justice Healthcare, http://www.icjh.org/

8.5 CONCLUSION

This chapter has examined three distinctly different populations: breastfeeding mothers and infants, persons living with HIV/AIDS, and those who have been incarcerated. Combined, they comprise a substantial (though sometimes overlapping) portion of our population. Increasing the number of women who breastfeed and the duration of breastfeeding among all economic and ethnic strata of our society will significantly impact general population health and healthcare costs in the future. Similarly, improving nutrition and thus the health of PWLH/A and the incarcerated have ramifications beyond the health status of any one individual. It is particularly important to focus on special populations such as these as they are often those least likely to have access to or be able to afford healthcare, nutrition education, or healthy foods.

8.6 ACRONYMS

AAP	American Academy of Pediatrics
ACA	American Correctional Association
ACFSA	American Correctional Food Service Association
ADA	American Dietetic Association
AETC	AIDS Education and Training Center
AIDS	Autoimmune deficiency syndrome
ART	Antiretroviral treatment. Highly active antiretroviral therapy
AWS	AIDS wasting syndrome
BFHI	Baby-Friendly Hospital Initiative
BMC	Boston Medical Center
CARE Act or RWCA	Ryan White Comprehensive AIDS Resources Emergency Act
CDC	Centers for Disease Control and Prevention
dL	Deciliter
DOJ	U.S. Department of Justice
DRI	Dietary Reference Intake
GI	Gastrointestinal tract
HAART	Highly active antiretroviral therapy
HeLP America	Healthy Lifestyles and Prevention America Act of 2005
HHS	Department of Health and Human Services
HIV	Human immunodeficiency virus
IBCLC	International Board Certified Lactation Consultant
LBM	Lean body mass
LBW	Low birth weight
LDL-C	Low density lipoprotein cholesterol
MFWI	Mother-Friendly Workplace Initiative
mm Hg	Millimeters of mercury
MNT	Medical Nutrition Therapy
NCCHC	National Commission on Correctional HealthCare
NCHS	National Center for Health Statistics
NEC	Necrotizing enterocolitis
NIP	National Immunization Program
NIS	National Immunization Survey
PLWH/A	Persons living with HIV/AIDS
RD	Registered dietitian
RDA	Recommended Dietary Allowance
RMS	Ross Mother's Survey
SES	Socioeconomic status
SIDS	Sudden Infant Death Syndrome
UNICEF	United Nations International Children's Emergency Fund
USDA	U.S. Department of Agriculture
WHO	World Health Organization
WIC Program	Special Supplemental Nutrition Program for Women, Infants, and Children

REFERENCES

1. American Dietetic Association. Position of the American Dietetic Association. Promoting and supporting breastfeeding. *J Am Diet Assoc.* 105, 81–818, 2005.
2. Gartner, L.M., Morton, J., Lawrence, R.A., et al. American Academy of Pediatrics Section on Breastfeeding. Breastfeeding and the use of human milk. *Pediatrics.* 115, 496–506, 2005. Available at: http://pediatrics.aappublications.org/cgi/content/full/115/2/496. Accessed August 20, 2006.
3. World Health Organization. The optimal duration of exclusive breastfeeding. Report of an expert consultation. Department of Child and Adolescent Health and Development. Geneva, Switzerland: WHO, 2001. Available at: http://www.who.int/child-adolescent-health/publications/NUTRITION/WHO_FCH_CAH_01.24.htm. Accessed August 20, 3006.
4. U.S. Department of Health and Human Services. *Healthy People 2010: Conference Edition—Volumes I and II.* Washington, D.C.: U.S. Department of Health and Human Services, Public Health Service, Office of the Assistant Secretary for Health. 47–48, 2000. Available at: http://www.healthypeople.gov/Document. Accessed August 20, 2006.
5. Ryan, A.S. and Zhou, W. Lower breastfeeding rates persist among the Special Supplemental Nutrition Program for Women, Infants, and Children participants, 1978–2003. *Pediatrics.* 117, 1136–1146, 2006.
6. U.S. Department of Agriculture, Food and Nutrition Service, Office of Analysis, Nutrition and Evaluation, WIC Participant and Program Characteristics 2004, WIC-04-PC. Bartlett, S., Bobronnikov, E., Pacheco, N. et al. Project Officer, Lesnett F. Alexandria, VA: March 2006. Available at: http://www.fns.usda.gov/oane/MENU/Published/WIC/FILES/pc2004.pdf. Accessed August 20, 2006.
7. American Dietetic Association. Position of the American Dietetic Association. Promoting and supporting breastfeeding. *J Am Diet Assn.* 105, 2005.
8. Hirschman, C. and Hendershot, G.E. Trends in breast feeding among American mothers. *Vital Health Stat.* Series 23, Data from the National Survey of Family Growth. November 1979, pp. 1–39.
9. U.S. Department of Agriculture, Food and Nutrition Service, Office of Analysis, Nutrition and Evaluation, Breastfeeding Intervention Design Study-Final Evaluation Design and Analysis Plan. McLaughlin, J.E., Burstein, N.R., Tao, F., Fox, M.K. Project Officer, McKinney, P. Alexandria, VA: 2004. Available at: http://www.fns.usda.gov/oane. Accessed August 20, 2006.
10. Weimer, J.P. The economic benefits of breastfeeding: a review and analysis. Food and Rural Economics Division, Economic Research Service, U.S. Department of Agriculture. Food Assistance and Nutrition Research Report No. 13. Available at: http://www.ers.usda.gov/publications/fanrr13/fanrr13.pdf. Accessed August 14, 2006.
11. Bondy, J., Berman, S., Glazner, J., and Lezotte, D. Direct expenditures related to otitis media diagnoses: extrapolations from a pediatric Medicaid cohort. *Pediatrics.* 105, e72, 2000. Available at: http://www.pediatrics.org/cgi/content/full/105/6/e72. Accessed August 14, 2006.
12. Ball, T.M. and Wright, A.L. Healthcare costs of formula-feeding in the first year of life. *Pediatrics.* 103(4 Pt. 2), 870–876, 1999. Available at: http://pediatrics.aappublications.org/cgi/content/full/103/4/S1/870. Accessed August 20, 2006.
13. Butte, N.F. and King, J.C. Energy requirements during pregnancy and lactation. *Public Health Nutr.* 8, 1010–1027, 2005.
14. Picciano, M.F. Pregnancy and lactation: physiological adjustments, nutritional requirements and the role of dietary supplements. *J Nutr.* 133, 1997S–2002S, 2003.
15. American Dietetic Association. Position of the American Dietetic Association. Promoting and supporting breastfeeding. *J Am Diet Assn.* 105, 81–818, 2005.
16. Ryan, A.S. The truth about the Ross Mothers Survey. *Pediatrics.* 113, 626–267, 2004. Available at: http://pediatrics.aappublications.org/cgi/content/full/113/3/626. Accessed August 13, 2006.
17. Zell, E.R., Ezzati-Rice, T.M., Battaglia, M.P., and Wright, R.A. National Immunization Survey: the methodology of a vaccination surveillance system. *Public Health Rep.* 115, 65–77, 2000. Available at: http://www.pubmedcentral.nih.gov/articlerender.fcgi?tool=pubmed&pubmedid=10968587. Accessed August 19, 2006.
18. Li, R., Scanlon, K.S., and Serdula, M.K. The validity and reliability of maternal recall of breastfeeding practice. *Nutr Rev.* 63, 103–110, 2005.

19. Shealy, K.R., Li, R., Benton-Davis, S., and Grummer-Strawn, L.M. *The CDC Guide to Breastfeeding Interventions.* Atlanta: U.S. Department of Health and Human Services, Centers for Disease Control and Prevention, 2005. Available at: http://www.cdc.gov/breastfeeding/pdf/breastfeeding_interventions. pdf. Accessed August 14, 2006.

20. International Board of Lactation Consultant Examiners homepage. Available at: http://www.iblce.org/. Accessed August 15, 2006.

21. Naylor, A.J. Baby-Friendly Hospital Initiative. Protecting, promoting, and supporting breastfeeding in the twenty-first century. *Pediatr Clin North Am.* 48, 475–483, 2001.

22. Philipp, B.L., Merewood, A., Miller, L.W. et al. Baby-Friendly Hospital Initiative improves breast-feeding initiation rates in a U.S. hospital setting. *Pediatrics.* 108, 677–681, 2001. Available at: http://pediatrics.aappublications.org/cgi/content/full/108/3/677. Accessed August 14, 2006.

23. Shealy, K.R., Li, R., Benton-Davis, S., and Grummer-Strawn, L.M. *The CDC Guide to Breastfeeding Interventions.* Atlanta: U.S. Department of Health and Human Services, Centers for Disease Control and Prevention, 2005. Available at: http://www.cdc.gov/breastfeeding/pdf/breastfeeding_interventions. pdf. Accessed August 14, 2006.

24. Philipp, B.L., Merewood, A., Miller, L.W., et al. Baby-friendly hospital initiative improves breast-feeding initiation rates in a U.S. hospital setting. *Pediatrics.* 108, 677–681, 2001. Available at: http://pediatrics.aappublications.org/cgi/content/full/108/3/677. Accessed August 14, 2006.

25. Merewood, A. and Philipp, B.L. Becoming baby-friendly: overcoming the issue of accepting free formula. *J Hum Lact.* 16, 279–282, 2000. Available at: http://jhl.sagepub.com/cgi/reprint/16/4/279?ijkey=9b7d9047e78f6f4738952b807c661633dbab6e5e&keytype2=tf_ipsecsha. Accessed August 20, 2006.

26. Shealy, K.R., Li, R., Benton-Davis, S., and Grummer-Strawn, L.M. *The CDC Guide to Breastfeeding Interventions.* Atlanta: U.S. Department of Health and Human Services, Centers for Disease Control and Prevention, 2005. Available at: http://www.cdc.gov/breastfeeding/pdf/breastfeeding_ interventions.pdf. Accessed August 14, 2006.

27. World Alliance for Breastfeeding Action (WABA) homepage. Available at: http://www.waba.org. my/wwaba.htm. Accessed August 14, 2006.

28. Weimer, D.R. Summary of State Breastfeeding Laws and Related Issues. Congressional Research Service. The Library of Congress. January 12, 2005. Order Code RL31633. Available at: http://maloney. house.gov/documents/olddocs/breastfeeding/050505CRSReport.pdf. Accessed August 13, 2006.

29. U.S. Breastfeeding Committee. *Breastfeeding in the United States: A National Agenda.* Rockville, MD: U.S. Department of Health and Human Services, Health Services and Research Administration, Maternal and Child Health Bureau, 2001. Available at: http://www.usbreastfeeding.org/USBC-strategic-plan-2001.pdf. Accessed August 11, 2006.

30. Walensky, R.P., Paltiel, A.D., Losina, E., et al. The survival benefits of AIDS treatment in the United States. *J Infect Dis.* 194, 11–19, 2006.

31. The Global HIV/AIDS Pandemic, 2006. Available at: http://www.cdc.gov/mmwr/preview/mmwrhtml/mm5531a1.htm?s_cid=mm5531a1_e. MMWR. 2006;55:841–844 Accessed August 17, 2006.

32. This section is based on: Providing HIV/AIDS Care in a Changing Environment. HRSA Care Action. August 2004. Available at: http://hab.hrsa.gov/publications/aug04. Accessed August 16, 2006.

33. Need for HIV Medical Nutrition Therapy. Available at: http://www.hivaidsdpg.org. Accessed August 17, 2006.

34. Watts, M.L. American Dietetic Association White Paper: Ryan White CARE Act Reauthorization. Presentation to the professional staff members of the Senate Health, Education, Labor and Pensions Committee and House Energy and Commerce Committee. January 19, 2006. Available at: http://www.eatright.org/ada/files/written_january_19_2006_feedback_session_ryan_white.doc. Accessed August 16, 2006.

35. Institute of Medicine Press Release. Innovators in field of correctional healthcare receive Institute of Medicine's 2003 Lienhard Award. 2003. Available at: http://www.iom.edu/?id=16009. Accessed August 10, 2006.

36. Freudenberg, N. Jails, prisons, and the health of urban populations: a review of the impact of the correctional system on community health. *J Urban Health.* 78, 214–235, 2001.

37. American Public Health Association. Correctional HealthCare Standards and Accreditation. 2004. Available at: http://www.apha.org/legislative/policy/policysearch/index.cfm?fuseaction=view&id=1291. Accessed August 9, 2006.

38. Anno, B.J. *Correctional HealthCare: Guidelines for the Management of an Adequate Delivery System,* 2001 edition. Chicago, IL: National Commission on Correctional Health, 2001. Available at http://www.nicic.org/pubs/2001/chc-files/fulldocument.pdf. Accessed September 23, 2004.

39. National Commission on Correctional HealthCare: *The Health Status of Soon-to-Be Released Inmates: A Report to Congress.* Vol. 1. Chicago, IL, NCCHC, 2002.

40. Hammett, T.M., Gaiter, J.L., and Crawford, C. Reaching seriously at-risk populations: health interventions in criminal justice settings. *Health Educ Behav.* 25, 99–120, 1998.

41. Watson, R., Stimpson, A., and Hostick, T. Prison healthcare: a review of the literature. *Int J Nurs Stud.* 41, 119–128, 2004.

42. Hammett, T.M., Gaiter, J.L., and Crawford, C. Reaching seriously at-risk populations: health interventions in criminal justice settings. *Health Educ Behav.* 25, 99–120, 1998.

43. Federal Bureau of Prisons web site. Available at: http://www.bop.gov/. Accessed August 9, 2006.

44. U.S. Department of Justice. Bureau of Justice Statistics. Prevalence of Imprisonment in the U.S. Population, 1974–2001. Available at: http://www.ojp.usdoj.gov/bjs/abstract/piusp01.htm. Accessed August 9, 2006.

45. Freudenberg, N. Jails, prisons, and the health of urban populations: a review of the impact of the correctional system on community health. *J Urban Health.* 78, 214–235, 2001.

46. U.S. Department of Justice. Bureau of Justice Statistics. Corrections Statistics. Available at: http://www.ojp.usdoj.gov/bjs/welcome.html. Accessed August 9, 2006.

47. National Commission on Correctional HealthCare. Position Statement. Women's healthcare in correctional settings. 2005. Available at: http://www.ncchc.org/resources/statements/womenshealth 2005. html. Accessed August 9, 2006.

48. U.S. Department of Health and Human Services. Older adults in prisons. Administration on Aging. Available at: http://www.aoa.gov/prof/notes/docs/older_adults_in_prisons.pdf. Accessed August 9, 2006.

49. Ogden, A. and Rebein, P. Do prison inmates have a right to vegetarian meals? *Vegetarian J.* March 2001. Available at: http://www.findarticles.com/p/articles/mi_m0FDE/is_2_20/ai_72607721. Accessed August 10, 2006.

50. Stein, K. Foodservice in correctional facilities. *J Am Diet Assoc.* 100, 508–509, 2000.

51. Vitucci, N. Facility implements weight loss and nutrition education plan. *CorrectCare.* 9, 1999.

52. James, J.S. State Prison Expenditures, 2001. U.S. Department of Justice. Office of Justice Programs. Bureau of Justice Statistics. Special Report. June 2004. Available at http://www.ojp.usdoj.gov/bjs/pub/ascii/spe01.txt. Accessed September 22, 2004.

53. Karen, S. Foodservice in correctional facilities. *J Am Diet Assoc.* 100, 508–509, 2000.

54. Hornung, C.A., Greifinger, R.B., and Gadre, S. A projection model of the prevalence of selected chronic diseases in the inmate population. In *The Health Status of Soon-To-Be-Released Inmates,* Vol. II. A Report to Congress. Chicago, IL: National Commission on Correctional HealthCare, 2002. Available at: http://www.ncchc.org/stbr/volume2/Report3_hornung.pdf. Accessed August 10, 2006.

55. Raimer, B.G. and Stobo, J.D. Healthcare delivery in the Texas prison system: the role of academic medicine. *JAMA.* 292, 485–489, 2004.

56. Lorber, D.L., Chavez, S., Dorman, J., et al.; American Diabetes Association. Diabetes Management in Correctional Institutions. *Diabetes Care.* 27(S1):S114–S121, 2004. Available at: http://care.diabetesjournals.org/cgi/content/full/27/suppl_1/s114. Accessed September 22, 2004.

57. Stoller, N. Improving Access to HealthCare for California's Women Prisoners. Executive Summary. A working paper for the California Program on Access to Care. October 2000. Available at www.ucop.edu/cprc. Accessed September 23, 2004.

58. National Commission on Correctional HealthCare. Clinical Guidelines. Available at: http://www.ncchc.org/resources/clinicalguides.html. Accessed August 10, 2006.

59. Wakeen, B. and Macqueen, S. Building global relationships — corrections "Down Under." *ACFSA Insider.* Fall 2005, pp. 15–17.

60. Wakeen, B. Meeting dietary goals based upon the Dietary Guidelines. *ACFSA Insider.* Summer 2005, pp. 14–15. Available at: http://www.acfsa.org/cfppgm/pdfs/Dietitians_Summer_2005.pdf. Accessed August 10, 2006.
61. National Commission on Correctional HealthCare. *The Health Status of Soon-to-be-Released Inmates, A Report to Congress*, 2 volumes. Chicago, IL: The National Commission on Correctional HealthCare, 2001. Available at: http://www.ncchc.org/pubs/pubs_stbr.html. Accessed August 17, 2006.
62. Best Practices: Access to Benefits for Prisoners with Mental Illnesses. A Brazelon Center Issue Brief. Available at: http://www.bazelon.org/issues/criminalization/publications. Accessed August 17, 2006.
63. Raimer, B.G. and Stobo, J.D. Healthcare delivery in the Texas prison system: the role of academic medicine. *JAMA.* 292, 485–489, 2004.
64. Dietitians in Corrections homepage. Available at: http://www.acfsa.org/cfppgm/frmdiet.htm. Accessed August 10, 2006.
65. Consultant Dietitians in Healthcare Facilities web site. Available at: http://www.cdhcf.org/index2.html. Accessed August 10, 2006.
66. Institute of Medicine Press Release. Innovators in field of correctional healthcare receive Institute of Medicine's 2003 Lienhard Award. 2003. Available at: http://www.iom.edu/?id=16009. Accessed August 10, 2006.

9 Cultural Competence

Whenever I meet people I always approach them from the standpoint of the most basic things we have in common. We each have a physical structure, a mind, and emotions. We are all born in the same way, and we all die.

His Holiness, the 14th Dalai Lama (1935–)

Cultural competence is vital for public health policymakers and health program planners who are operating in an increasingly multi- and cross-cultural society. This chapter explores some of the issues pertaining to cultural competence. We examine the steps required to improve the quality of food and nutrition services for minority, immigrant, and ethnically diverse communities by promoting cultural and language competence, and look at the foodways of the major ethnic groups in the U.S.

9.1 WHAT IS CULTURAL COMPETENCE?

The National Institutes of Health (NIH) has defined cultural competence as the healthcare provider's ability to deliver culturally appropriate and specifically tailored care to populations with diverse values, beliefs, and behaviors.

The definition that is quoted most frequently is that of Cross, who speaks in terms of cultural competence of institutions as well as of individuals. According to Cross,[1] cultural and linguistic competence is a set of compatible behaviors, attitudes, and policies that work together in a system, agency, or among professionals that enables effective functioning in cross-cultural situations. Cultural competence is a developmental process that evolves over an extended period. Both individuals and organizations are at various levels of awareness, knowledge, and skills along the cultural competence continuum.

The term "cultural competence" is not universally accepted. Experts speak of cultural awareness, cultural diversity, cultural sensitivity, and other concepts. Many professionals who work in this area have developed their own definitions and explanations (see Box 9.1).

9.2 WHY IS CULTURAL COMPETENCE IMPORTANT?

Racial, ethnic, cultural, and linguistic differences within the U.S. population present a unique challenge for those who promote the public's health. Major disparities exist in the health status, incidence of illness, and access to healthcare among different population groups. This is particularly true for minority populations, such as African Americans, Latino/Hispanic Americans, and

---

Box 9.1 Cultural Competence

Culture refers to patterns of human behavior that include the language, thoughts, communications, actions, customs, beliefs, values, and institutions of racial, ethnic, religious, or social groups. *Competence* implies having the capacity to function effectively as an individual and an organization within the context of the cultural beliefs, behaviors, and needs presented by consumers and their communities.

Native Americans, Alaska Natives, and Pacific Islanders, who face a disproportionate burden of disease compared to the nonminority U.S. population (see also, Chapter 6). Minority groups will comprise almost half of the U.S. population by 2050. Hypertension, cardiovascular diseases, stroke, diabetes, and anemia are some of the diet-related diseases disproportionately affecting minorities.

The National Center for Cultural Competence (NCCC) has identified reasons for incorporating cultural competence into organizational policy.[2]

- To respond to current and projected demographic changes in the U.S.
- To eliminate disparities in the health status of people of diverse racial, ethnic, and cultural backgrounds
- To improve the quality of services and health outcomes
- To meet legislative, regulatory, and accreditation mandates
- To gain a competitive edge in the marketplace, and to decrease the likelihood of liability/malpractice claims

Although many assume that cultural competence will have a positive effect on clinical outcomes, research on the effects of cultural competence is still at an early stage.[3,4]

9.3 CURRENT AND PROJECTED DEMOGRAPHIC CHANGES IN THE U.S.

The make-up of the American population is changing as a result of immigration patterns and significant increases among racially, ethnically, culturally, and linguistically diverse populations already residing in the U.S. Healthcare organizations and programs, and federal, state, and local governments must implement systemic change in order to meet the health needs of this diverse population.

In 2006 the U.S. population reached 300 million. By 2050, the population is projected to grow to over 403 million people; ethnic and racial minorities will comprise more than 90% of those 130 million additional Americans.

More legal immigrants (7.6 million) came to the U.S. between 1991 and 1999 than in any other decade except 1901 to 1910. Approximately 42% of these immigrants came from Spanish-speaking countries; 33% from Asia; 17% from Europe; and 5% from Africa.

As indicated in Table 9.1, it is expected that minorities will comprise one third of the U.S. population by 2015 and nearly half of the population by 2050. The minority share of the U.S. population has more than doubled since 1950. By 2050, whites — who were an 87% majority in 1950 — will comprise only 53% of the U.S. population. Chiefly because of higher fertility rates, minorities represent a larger share of U.S. youth, whereas non-Hispanic whites constitute the bulk of the nation's elderly. About 35% of U.S. children under the age of 18 are minorities, while 84% of those over 65 are non-Hispanic whites. By 2025, nearly half of American children will be African American, Hispanic, or Asian.

- Asians (including Pacific Islanders) are the fastest-growing minority group, having increased by 179% since 1980. By 2050, Asians will comprise nearly 10% of the U.S. population.
- Since 1980, the number of Hispanics in the U.S. has grown five times faster than the rest of the population, making the U.S. the third largest Spanish-speaking country in the world. Hispanics passed African-Americans as the country's largest minority group. In 2005, the estimated number of undocumented immigrants was 10.3 million, an increase of 23% from the 8.4 million estimate of 2000. More than 50% of that growth was attributable to Mexican nationals living illegally in the U.S.[5]

TABLE 9.1
Current and Projected Population of the U.S. by Race and Hispanic Origin, 2000 to 2050

Population or Percent and Race or Hispanic Origin	2000	2010	2020	2030	2040	2050
Total Population	**282,125**	**308,936**	**335,805**	**363,584**	**391,946**	**419,854**
White only	228,548	244,995	260,629	275,731	289,690	302,626
Black only	35,818	40,454	45,365	50,442	55,876	61,361
Asian only	10,684	14,241	17,988	22,580	27,992	33,430
All other races[a]	7,075	9,246	11,822	14,831	18,388	22,437
Hispanic (of any race)	35,622	47,756	59,756	73,055	87,585	102,560
White only, not Hispanic	195,729	201,112	205,936	209,176	210,331	210,283
Percent of Total Population						
Total	**100.0**	**100.0**	**100.0**	**100.0**	**100.0**	**100.0**
White only	81.0	79.3	77.6	75.8	73.9	72.1
Black only	12.7	13.1	13.5	13.9	14.3	14.6
Asian only	3.8	4.6	5.4	6.2	7.1	8.0
All other races[a]	2.5	3.0	3.5	4.1	4.7	5.3
Hispanic (of any race)	12.6	15.5	17.8	20.1	22.3	24.4
White only, not Hispanic	69.4	65.1	61.3	57.5	53.7	50.1

Notes: In thousands except as indicated, resident population. Leading dots indicate sub-parts.

[a] Includes American Indian and Alaska Native only, Native Hawaiian and Other Pacific Islander alone, and Two or More Races.

Source: From *U.S. Census Bureau, Population Division, Population Projections Branch. Projected Population of the United States, by Race and Hispanic Origin: 2000 to 2050.* Last revised: March 18, 2004. Available at: http://www.census.gov/ipc/www/usinterimproj/natprojtab01a.pdf. Accessed August 4, 2004.

9.3.1 DISPARITIES IN THE HEALTH STATUS OF PEOPLE OF DIVERSE BACKGROUNDS

Despite recent progress in overall national health, there are continuing disparities in the incidence of illness and death among African Americans, Latino/Hispanic Americans, Native Americans, Asian Americans, Alaska Natives, and Pacific Islanders as compared with the U.S. population as a whole, as indicated in *Healthy People 2000*[6] and *Healthy People 2010*.[7]

Among the factors believed to be associated with health disparities are national origin and ethnicity; cultural, linguistic, and family backgrounds; individual experiences; age and gender; financial status; geographic location; educational level; and occupation. Lack of diversity in the workforce may also contribute to the challenge facing public health in meeting the needs of diverse populations, thereby affecting the quality of preventive care and contributing to health disparities.

9.3.1.1 Literacy, Language, and Healthcare

Culture and language have considerable impact on how patients access and respond to healthcare services. The Workforce Investment Act of 1998 (P.L. 105–220) defines literacy as "an individual's ability to read, write, speak in English, compute and solve problems at levels of proficiency necessary to function on the job, in the family of the individual, and in society." This is a broader view of literacy than just an individual's ability to read, the more traditional concept of literacy. As information and technology have increasingly shaped our society, the skills we need to function successfully have gone beyond reading, and literacy has come to include the skills cited in this definition. Nearly half of the adults in the U.S. have inadequate literacy skills. Not surprisingly, people who are older, disabled, have a poor education, or come from non-English speaking homes have an even higher percentage of difficulty.

More than 21 million people in the U.S. (8.1% of the population) reported during the 2000 Census that they spoke English "less than very well" or "not at all."[8] While regulations requiring adequate access to interpreters for patients covered by Medicare[9] will make the need for interpreters more acute, the use of untrained Spanish-speaking employees is not ideal. The National Alliance for Hispanic Health (http://www.hispanichealth.org), a Washington-based group that works to improve the health of Hispanics, maintains that relatives are less useful when they cannot accurately translate medical terms or when a patient has a condition he or she does not want disclosed to family.

To address the health needs of populations who speak limited English, in FY 1995 the Center for Cultural and Linguistic Competence in HealthCare (CCLCHC) — also known as the Center for Linguistic and Cultural Competence in HealthCare (CLCCHC) — was established within the Office of Minority Health (OMH). The center serves as a resource for healthcare professionals to help address the cultural and linguistic barriers to healthcare delivery and increase access to healthcare for people with limited English proficiency. Through CCLCHC, the OMH supports research, demonstrations, and evaluations to test new and innovative models aimed at increasing knowledge and providing a clearer understanding of health risk factors and successful prevention intervention strategies for minority populations.[10]

9.3.1.2 Age

The elderly population is expected to increase from 12.6% of the population in 2000 to 20% of the population by 2050.[11] Furthermore, the proportion of elderly within each of the 4 major race groups and the Hispanic origin population is expected to substantially increase during the first half of the 21st century, with the older population growing faster among minorities than among whites. From 1990 to 2050, the proportion of elderly is projected to increase from 13 to 23% for whites; from 8 to 14% for blacks; from 6 to 13% for American Indians, Eskimos, and Aleuts; from 6 to 15% for Asians and Pacific Islanders; and from 5 to 14% for Hispanics. In 1990, about 4.2 million persons or 13% of the population 65 years and over were nonwhite. By 2025, 25% of the elderly population is projected to be nonwhite, and 35% by 2050.[12]

9.3.1.3 Quality of Services and Health Outcomes

Differences among people arise from nationality, ethnicity, and culture, as well as from family background and individual experience, affecting health beliefs and behaviors of healthcare professionals and the people they serve. Critical factors in the provision of culturally competent healthcare include understanding of the:

- Beliefs, values, traditions, and practices of a culture
- Culturally-defined, health-related needs of individuals, families, and communities
- Culturally-based belief systems of the etiology of illness and disease and those related to health and healing
- Attitudes toward seeking help from healthcare providers

9.4 LEGISLATIVE, REGULATORY, AND ACCREDITATION MANDATES

Several factors have brought the need for cultural competence to the forefront. These factors include modifications in legislative and accreditation mandates, in addition to changes in U.S. demographics and the awareness of healthcare disparities already been discussed.

Title VI of the Civil Rights Act of 1964 mandates that no person in the U.S. shall, on ground of race, color, or national origin, be excluded from participation in, be denied the benefits of, or be subjected to discrimination under any program or activity receiving federal financial assistance. To ensure equal access to quality healthcare by diverse populations, Brach and Fraser (2000)[13] identified nine major techniques for achieving cultural competence. They encompass interpreter services, recruitment and retention policies, training, coordination with traditional healers, use of community health workers, culturally competent health promotion, including family/another culture, and administrative and organizational accommodations. A comprehensive report, *National Standards on Culturally and Linguistically Appropriate Services (CLAS) in HealthCare — Final Report,* describes 14 individual standards that healthcare organizations and providers should follow.[14] These are summarized in Box 9.2.

Box 9.2 Assuring Cultural Competence in HealthCare: Recommendations for National Standards and an Outcomes-Focused Research Agenda

- Promote and support the attitudes, behaviors, knowledge, and skills necessary for staff to work respectfully and effectively with patients and each other in a culturally diverse work environment.
- Have a comprehensive management strategy to address culturally and linguistically appropriate services, including strategic goals, plans, policies, procedures, and designated staff responsible for implementation.
- Utilize formal mechanisms for community and consumer involvement in the design and execution of service delivery, including planning, policy making, operations, evaluation, training and, as appropriate, treatment planning.
- Develop and implement a strategy to recruit, retain and promote qualified, diverse and culturally competent administrative, clinical, and support staff that are trained and qualified to address the needs of the racial and ethnic communities being served.
- Require and arrange for ongoing education and training for administrative, clinical, and support staff in culturally and linguistically competent service delivery.
- Provide all clients with limited English proficiency (LEP) access to bilingual staff or interpretation services.
- Provide oral and written notices, including translated signage at key points of contact, to clients in their primary language informing them of their right to receive interpreter services free of charge.
- Translate and make available signage and commonly-used written patient educational material and other materials for members of the predominant language groups in service areas.
- Ensure that interpreters and bilingual staff can demonstrate bilingual proficiency and receive training that includes the skills and ethics of interpreting, and knowledge in both languages of the terms and concepts relevant to clinical or nonclinical encounters. Family or friends are not considered adequate substitutes because they usually lack these abilities.
- Ensure that the clients' primary spoken language and self-identified race/ethnicity are included in the healthcare organization's management information system as well as any patient records used by provider staff.
- Use a variety of methods to collect and utilize accurate demographic, cultural, epidemiological, and clinical outcome data for racial and ethnic groups in the service area and become informed about the ethnic/cultural needs, resources, and assets of the surrounding community.
- Undertake ongoing organizational self-assessments of cultural and linguistic competence, and integrate measures of access, satisfaction, quality, and outcomes for CLAS into other organizational internal audits and performance improvement programs.

- Develop structures and procedures to address cross cultural ethical and legal conflicts in healthcare delivery and complaints or grievances by patients and staff about unfair, culturally insensitive or discriminatory treatment, or difficulty in accessing services or denial of services.
- Prepare an annual progress report documenting the organizations' progress with implementing CLAS standards, including information on programs, staffing, and resources.

Source: U.S. Department of Health and Human Services. Public Health Service. The Office of Minority Health. Assuring Cultural Competence in HealthCare: Recommendations for National Standards and an Outcomes-Focused Research Agenda. *Recommendations for National Standards and a National Public Comment Process.* Available at: http://www.omhrc.gov/clas/cultural1a.htm. Accessed August 2, 2004.

Watchdog and accrediting organizations have certain minimum requirements regarding cultural competence. For example, the Joint Commission on Accreditation of Healthcare Organizations (JCAHO, pronounced "jay-koe") views the delivery of services in a culturally and linguistically appropriate manner as an important healthcare safety and quality issue.[15] Accredited organizations are encouraged to provide equitable care, treatment, and services across diverse populations. At the federal level,[16] major policy initiatives have directly addressed cultural competence in a range of rules that cover nearly every healthcare provider in the country. For example, cultural competence is necessary in order for healthcare workers and patients to adhere to the 1998 Consumer Bill of Rights and Responsibilities[17] (available in its entirety at http://www.hcqualitycommission.gov/cborr/), which includes recommendations covering the patient's right to participate in all treatment decisions, the right to respect and nondiscrimination, and a set of responsibilities that all consumers should strive to meet.

Nevertheless, not everyone agrees that patients should be interviewed and assessed in their native language or even via use of an appropriate bilingual/bicultural interpreter (see Box 9.3).

9.4.1 Participation in Treatment Decisions

Consumers have the right and responsibility to fully participate in all decisions related to their healthcare. Consumers who are unable to fully participate in treatment decisions have the right to be represented by parents, guardians, family members, or other conservators. To ensure consumers' right and ability to participate in treatment decisions, healthcare professionals should provide patients with easily understood information and the opportunity to decide among treatment options consistent with the informed

---

Box 9.3 Executive Order 13,166

Executive Order 13,166: Improving Access to Services of Persons with Limited English Proficiency requires that federally funded hospitals, clinics, and doctors offer translation services for patients who speak limited English. According to the order, patients may use family members or volunteers but should be offered the option of a professional interpreter. But not everyone agrees with EO 13,166. In 2004, HHS was sued by several physicians and a physicians' group along with ProEnglish, a nonprofit advocacy organization dedicated to the preservation and promotion of state "official English" laws and policies, on the basis that EO 13,166 limits the free-speech rights of physicians, illegally intrudes into the practice of medicine, and improperly interprets civil rights law to include language as part of antidiscrimination based on national origin. As the policy is to be implemented at the physician's expense, the plaintiffs claimed that the order will result in doctors moving out of heavily immigrant communities or leaving the profession entirely.

Discussion question: What is your view on this issue?

consent process. Specifically, healthcare professionals should discuss all treatment options with a patient in a culturally competent manner, including the option of no treatment at all; discuss all current treatments a consumer may be undergoing, including those alternative treatments that are self-administered; and discuss all risks, benefits, and consequences to treatment or nontreatment.

Patients must be given the opportunity to refuse treatment and to express preferences about future treatment decisions. Healthcare providers must abide by the decisions made by their patients and/or their designated representatives consistent with the informed consent process.

9.4.2 Respect and Nondiscrimination

Consumers have the right to considerate, respectful care from all members of the healthcare system at all times and under all circumstances. An environment of mutual respect is essential to maintain a quality healthcare system. Consumers must not be discriminated against in the delivery of healthcare services consistent with the benefits covered in their policy or as required by law based on race, ethnicity, national origin, religion, sex, age, mental or physical disability, sexual orientation, genetic information, or source of payment.

Several ways in which clinicians work with multicultural patients and families can contribute to a positive experience. It is critical that healthcare providers recognize individual differences and do not participate in "cultural stereotyping." Because persons of the same ethnicity can have very different beliefs and practices, such as Hispanics from Puerto Rico or from Mexico, it is important to understand the particular circumstances of the patient or family by obtaining information on place of origin, social and economic background, degree of acculturation, and personal expectations concerning health and medical care.

Practitioners should reflect on their personal values when they are likely to interact with people whose appearance and lifestyle are different from their own. The first step is to be nonjudgmental about the patient's sexual orientation and appearance. This may require calling self-assessment and help from an expert familiar with the group's lifestyle.

9.4.2.1 Sexual Orientation

Gay affirmative practice models provide guidelines for behaviors and beliefs in work with gay and lesbian individuals. Scales have been developed to measure the professional's cultural competence for counseling patients and clients who are gay and lesbian.[18]

9.4.2.2 Body Size

Founded in 1969, the National Association to Advance Fat Acceptance (NAAFA) is a human rights organization. NAAFA works towards eliminating discrimination based on body size[19,20] and supports the concept of Health at Every Size[21] (see Box 9.4).

African American women consistently report greater acceptability for higher body weight than their white counterparts while still maintaining positive perceptions of body image.[22]

Box 9.4 Fat Women Daily Encounter Hostility and Discrimination

Fat women daily encounter hostility and discrimination. If we are fat, health practitioners often attribute our health problems to "obesity," postpone treatment until we lose weight, accuse us of cheating if we don't, make us so ashamed of our size that we don't go for help, and make all kinds of assumptions about our emotional and psychological state ("She must have emotional problems to be so fat").

Source: Boston Women's Health Book Collective. *Our Bodies, Our Selves for the New Century.* New York: Touchstone, 1998.

9.4.3 Consumer Responsibilities

In a healthcare system that protects consumers' rights, it is reasonable to expect and encourage consumers to assume reasonable responsibilities. Greater individual involvement by consumers in their care increases the likelihood of achieving the best outcomes and helps support a quality improvement, cost-conscious environment. Such responsibilities include:

- Taking responsibility for maximizing healthy habits, such as exercising, not smoking, and eating a healthy diet
- Becoming involved in specific healthcare decisions
- Working collaboratively with healthcare providers in developing and carrying out agreed-upon treatment plans
- Disclosing relevant information and clearly communicating wants and needs
- Recognizing the reality of risks and limits of the science of medical care and the human fallibility of the healthcare professional
- Being aware of a healthcare provider's obligation to be reasonably efficient and equitable in providing care to other patients and the community
- Showing respect for other patients and health workers

9.4.4 Marketplace Factors

To gain a competitive edge in the marketplace, programs need culturally competent policies, structures and practices to provide services for diverse populations. Additionally, cultural awareness decreases the likelihood of liability/malpractice claims. For example, providers may discover that they are liable for damages as a result of treatment in the absence of informed consent. Also, healthcare organizations and programs face potential claims that their failure to understand health beliefs, practices, and behavior on the part of providers or patients breaches professional standards of care. In some states, failure to follow instructions because they conflict with values and beliefs may raise a presumption of negligence on the part of the provider.

According to a report released by HRSA in 2004,[23] there are seven domains or performance areas for assessing cultural competence in community-oriented organizations.

- *Organizational values*: the worth of cultural competence to the organization and the organization's commitment to providing culturally competent care.
- *Governance:* the means an organization uses to deliver culturally competent care.
- *Planning and monitoring/evaluation:* the plans used for planning and assessing an organization's level of cultural competence.
- *Communication:* the exchange of information in ways that promote cultural competence between the organization/providers and the clients/population, and internally among staff.
- *Organizational infrastructure:* the organization's resources required to deliver culturally competent services.
- *Services/interventions:* an organization's delivery of clinical, public health, and health related services in a culturally competent manner.
- *Staff development*: organizations must ensure that their staff members have the requisite knowledge, attitudes, and skills for delivering culturally competent services.

9.5 NUTRITION STAFF DEVELOPMENT

Nutritionists play a role in developing the dietary component of the training for staff members. To do this, nutrition professionals should be aware of world views regarding food and nutrition practices of specific relevant cultural groups. According to Harris-Davis and

Haughton (2000),[24] the nutritionist with multicultural food and nutrition counseling knowledge should:

- Understand food selection, preparation, and storage within a cultural context
- Have knowledge of cultural eating patterns and family traditions such as core foods, traditional celebrations, and fasting
- Become familiar with relevant research and the latest findings regarding food practices and nutrition-related health problems of various ethnic and racial groups
- Possess specific knowledge of cultural values, health beliefs, and nutrition practices of particular groups served, including culturally different clients
- Have knowledge about within-group differences and understanding of variations in food practices
- Apply helping principle of "starting where the client is" by considering changes in eating patterns, such as the addition of American foods or substitution of foods

9.5.1 Strategies for Nutritionists in Clinical Practice

An important first step is to be sensitive to patients' cultural beliefs and practices and to convey respect for their cultural values. This may require calling for help in interpreting behavior, either from a provider who is from the same ethnic group as the patient or from an expert familiar with the group's language, lifestyle, and value preferences.

Box 9.5 offers a model for self-assessment of multicultural nutrition counseling competencies. This model focuses on multicultural nutrition counseling skills, multicultural awareness, and knowledge of foods from other cultures. The script in Box 9.6 may be used in assessing culturally diverse patients and families.

Box 9.5 Multicultural Skills

Multicultural Nutrition Counseling Skills

- Be able to differentiate between individual and universal similarities.
- Be experienced in application of medical nutrition therapy and nutrition-related health promotion/disease prevention strategies that are culturally appropriate.
- Have the ability to use cultural knowledge and sensitivity for appropriate nutrition intervention and materials.
- Take responsibility for collectively working with community leaders or members about unique knowledge or abilities for benefit of the culturally different client.
- Be able to evaluate new techniques, research, and knowledge as to validity and applicability in working with culturally different populations.

Multicultural Awareness

- Be aware of how own cultural background and experiences and attitudes, values, and biases influence nutrition counseling.
- Be able to recognize limits of own cultural competencies and abilities.
- Be aware and sensitive to own cultural heritage and to valuing and respecting differences.

Multicultural Food and Nutrition Counseling Knowledge

- Understand food selection, preparation, and storage with a cultural context.
- Have knowledge of cultural eating patterns and family traditions such as core foods, traditional celebrations, and fasting.

- Familiarize self with relevant research and latest findings regarding food practices and nutrition-related health problems of various ethnic and racial groups.

Source: Reprinted from Harris-Davis, E. and Haughton, B. Model for multicultural nutrition counseling competencies. *J Am Diet Assn.* 100, 1178–1185, 2000. With permission from The American Dietetic Association.

The culturally sensitive healthcare provider should also consider these additional suggestions regarding etiquette and communication:

- Speak slower than usual but not louder.
- Ask questions to increase your understanding of the patient's culture as it relates to healthcare practices. For example, ask what types of foods and medicines are administered or avoided under particular illness conditions or during physiological changes, such as those due to pregnancy. Then ask "If these are the rules, do you follow them? Why?" Make it clear to your respondents that "no" is a perfectly acceptable response.[25]
- Use drawings, models, and gestures to aid communication.
- Use empty packages of food to illustrate.
- Clearly communicate expectations.
- To ascertain understanding, ask the patient to repeat the information provided.
- Where appropriate, formulate treatment plans that take into account cultural beliefs and practices.
- Provide written instructions. Use handouts, if available. Be sure that all written materials are at the appropriate literacy level.

Box 9.6 Suggested Script for Interviewing a Culturally Diverse Family

So that I might be aware of and respect your cultural beliefs:

- Please tell me what languages are spoken in your home and the languages that you understand and speak.
- Please describe your usual diet. Are there times during the year when you change your diet in celebration of religious and other ethnic holidays?
- Please tell me about beliefs and practices including special events such as birth, marriage and death that you feel I should know.
- Please tell me about your experiences with healthcare providers in your native country. How often each year did you see a healthcare provider before you arrived in the U.S.? Have you noticed any differences between the type of care you received in your native country and the type you receive here? If yes, could you tell me about those differences?
- Please tell me if there is anything else I should know. Do you have any questions for me? (Encourage two-way communication.)
- Do you use any traditional remedies to improve your health?
- Is there someone, in addition to yourself, with whom you want us to discuss your medical condition?
- Are there certain foods or food combinations that your culture prohibits?
- Are there any other dietary considerations I should know about to serve your health needs?

Source: University of Michigan. Cultural Competence for Clinicians. *Enhancing Your Cultural Communication Skills.* Available at: http://www.med.umich.edu/pteducation/cultcomp.htm. Accessed August 1, 2006.

9.5.2 LOW LITERACY NUTRITION EDUCATION MATERIALS

Health People 2010 Objective 11–2 calls for improving the health literacy of the approximately 90 million adults with inadequate or marginal literacy skills. Until that has been accomplished, public and private organizations need to develop appropriate written materials. The knowledge exists to create effective, culturally, and linguistically appropriate, plain language health communications. Professional publications and federal documents provide the criteria to integrate and apply the principles of organization, writing style, layout, and design for effective communication. The National Cancer Institute (NCI) suggests a five-step process for developing publications for people with limited literacy skills: (1) define the target audience, (2) conduct target audience research, (3) develop a concept for the product, (4) develop content and visuals, and (5) pretest and revise draft materials (see Box 9.7).

Box 9.7 Five-Step Process for Developing Low-Literacy Publications

1. Define the target audience, which is the group of people the communicator wants to reach with a message. People with limited-literacy skills compose a broad target audience, crossing all ethnic and class boundaries. However, there are some common characteristics among low-literate audiences regarding how they interpret and process information.

   a. Tendency to think in concrete/immediate rather than abstract/futuristic terms
   b. Literal interpretation of information
   c. Insufficient language fluency to comprehend and apply information from written materials
   d. Difficulty with information processing, such as reading a menu, interpreting a bus schedule, following medical instructions, or reading a prescription label

2. Conduct target audience research.

   a. Age, sex, ethnicity, income and education levels, places of work, and residence
   b. Causative/preventive behaviors related to your topic
   c. Related knowledge, attitudes, and practices
   d. Patterns of use of related services
   e. Cultural habits, preferences, and sensitivities related to your topic
   f. Barriers to behavior change
   g. Effective motivators (e.g., benefits of change, fear of consequences, incentives, or social support)

3. Develop a concept for the product.

   a. Define the behavioral objective(s) of the material.
   b. Determine the key information points the reader needs to achieve the behavioral objective(s).
   c. Select the most appropriate presentation method(s) (e.g., audio, audiovisual, print, radio, TV, interactive computer programs).
   d. Decide on the reading level for the material if you select a print presentation.
   e. Organize topics in the order the person will use them.

4. Develop content and visuals.

   a. Content/style
      i. The material is interactive and allows for audience involvement.
      ii. The material presents "how-to" information.
      iii. Peer language is used whenever appropriate to increase personal identification and improve readability.
      iv. Words are familiar to the reader. Any new words are defined clearly.

   v. Sentences are simple, specific, direct, and written in the active voice.
   vi. Each idea is clear and logically sequenced (according to audience logic).
   vii. The number of concepts is limited per piece.
   viii. The material uses concrete examples rather than abstract concepts.
   ix. The text highlights and summarizes important points.

b. Layout

   i.   The material uses advance organizers or headers.
   ii. Headers are simple and close to text.
   iii. Layout balances white space with words and illustrations.
   iv. Text uses upper and lower case letters.
   v.   Underlining or bolding rather than all caps give emphasis.
   vi. Type style and size of print are easy-to-read; type is at least 12 point.

c. Visuals

   i.   Visuals are relevant to text, meaningful to the audience, and appropriately located.
   ii. Illustrations and photographs are simple and free from clutter and distraction.
   iii. Visuals use adult rather than childlike images.
   iv. Illustrations show familiar images that reflect cultural context.
   v.   Visuals have captions. Each visual illustrates and is directly related to one message.
   vi. Different styles, such as photographs without background detail, shaded line drawings, or simple line drawings, are pretested with the audience to determine which is understood best.
   vii. Cues, such as circles or arrows, point out key information. Colors used are appealing to the audience (as determined by pretesting)

d. Readability: Readability analysis is done to determine reading level.

5. Pretest and revise draft materials. Pretesting is a qualitative measure of audience response to a product. Pretesting helps ensure that materials are well understood, responsive to audience needs and concerns, and culturally sensitive. Pretest for comprehension, attraction, and acceptability.

   a. *Comprehension:* Does the respondent understand what the material is recommending and how and when to do it? Is anything unclear, confusing, or hard to believe? Suitability of the words used: "What does the educational piece mean when it says to eat balanced meals? How do you do that?" Distinguishing key details: "Which vegetables have lots of fiber?" Meaning or relationship of visuals to text: "Looking at this picture, how will you cut down on fat in your soups or stocks when cooking?"

   b. Attraction: What kind of feelings does the material generate? Enthusiasm, just OK, or a "turnoff"? For example, "Are the people in the material attractive to you? Is there anything you don't like about the people (or pictures) in this material? How about the color and the layout of the material?"

   c. Acceptability: Is the material compatible with local culture? Is it realistic? Would it offend people in any way? Are the hairstyles, clothing, etc., appropriate? Is it supportive of ethnic practices ("Do you think your friends and neighbors would be willing to cook their foods this way?") Does it invoke personal involvement? Can the respondent see himself or herself carrying out the actions called for in the materials?

Source: National Cancer Institute. *Clear & Simple: Developing Effective Print Materials for Low-literate Readers.* Pub. No. NIH 95-3594. 1995, updated 2002. Available at: http://www.nci.nih.gov/aboutnci/oc/clear-and-simple/allpages. Accessed August 1, 2006.

Box 9.8 Some Cuban Daily Fare

Breakfast: A typical Cuban breakfast consists of a *tostada* and *cafe con leche*. The tostada is a portion of Cuban bread that is buttered, then toasted on an electric grill. The *cafe con leche* is a combination of strong espresso coffee with warm milk. Cubans break the *tostada* into pieces, then dunk them into the *cafe con leche*, as Americans would dunk their doughnuts into their coffee. Additionally, some may eat ham *croquetas*, smoky creamed ham shaped in finger rolls, lightly breaded, and then fried. People in a hurry have *cafe cubano*, Cuban coffee.

Lunch: A Cuban lunch consists of *empanadas*, chicken or meat turnovers, or Cuban sandwiches. The sandwich could be a *media noche* (midnight sandwich), consisting of a slice of pork, ham, and swiss cheese and topped with pickles and mustard on sweetened egg bread. The *pan con bistec* is a thin slice of *palomilla* steak on Cuban bread garnished with lettuce, tomatoes, and fried potato sticks. *Mariquitas*, thinly sliced plantain chips, might accompany a hearty sandwich.

Snack: Cuban bakeries are famous for their finger foods, such as *pastelitos, croquetas, bocaditos*, and *empanadas*. *Pastelitos* are small flaky turnovers in various shapes filled with meat, cheese, guava, or a combination of guava and cream cheese. *Bocaditos* are small sandwiches layered with ham spread. *Tostones* are plantains deep fried in vegetable oil.

Dinner: Dinner might consist of a meat, chicken, or fish dish as the entree accompanied by white rice, black beans, and *maduros*, sweet fried plantains. *Ropa vieja* meaning "old shredded clothes" is a shredded beef stewed in a light tomato sauce with peppers and onions. A small salad of sliced tomatoes and onions or avocados might be added to the meal. Popular dessert options include the typical *flan*, a Cuban caramel-flavored custard, or bread or rice puddings.

Celebrations: For holidays or special occasions, the one dish that typifies Cuban cuisine would be a small pig, marinated with salt, garlic, and sour orange juice, then roasted over an open fire, and slowly cooked for several hours. The accompaniments for such a dish could consist of *congri,* a pork-flavored white rice and black bean mixture also known as *moros y cristianos* (Moors and Christians), *boniato* in a garlic dressing, and *maduros*. For refreshments, the most typical drinks are the *daiquiri* and the *mojito*. Both are made with lime juice and pure cane rum.

Sources:

Kittler, P.G., Sucher, K.P. *Food and Culture, Fourth Edition*. Belmont, CA: Thomson/Wadsworth. 2004.

Provenzo, E.E., Montes, R. *Exploring the Culture of Little Havana,* 1998. University of Miami. Available at: http://www.education.miami.edu/ep/LittleHavana/index.html. Accessed January 12, 2007.

9.6 FOODWAYS OF THE MAJOR ETHNIC/RACIAL GROUPS IN THE U.S.

This section contains generalizations about ethnic and cultural food practices of African Americans, Mexican Americans, Asians, and Hmong in the U.S., based, unless otherwise indicated, on information gathered by the Ohio State University Extension Department.[26] However, you cannot assume that the characteristics cited here apply to all individuals of a single cultural group. Not all people of a particular group have the same quality diets, have the same level of concern about their health, have the same understanding about the relationship of diet to health, or practice the same cooking techniques. Table 9.2 summarizes the food patterns, dietary strengths and weaknesses, and diet-related health concerns of African Americas, Asians, and Hispanics in the U.S. Continued reading and additional research into particular cultural groups is essential (see Table 9.3).

TABLE 9.2
Food Patterns, Dietary Strengths and Weaknesses, and Diet-Related Health Concerns of African Americans, Asians, and Hispanics in the U.S.

Country/Cultural Group	Food Pattern	Dietary Strengths	Dietary Weaknesses	Diet-Related Health Concerns
African American	The traditional African American diet emphasizes frying, boiling, and roasting dishes using pork, pork fat, corn, sweet potatoes, rice, and local green leafy vegetables. It also includes sausage, chicken, many kinds of fish, greens (mixtures of chard, collard greens, kale, mustard greens, spinach, and turnip greens), black-eyed peas, okra, grits, peas, tomatoes, and squash. Coffee and tea are more common beverages than milk or juice	Leafy green vegetables, legumes, and rice	Diet may be low in calcium and fiber and contain excesses of fat and sodium	Obesity, hypertension, diabetes, heart disease, lactose intolerance
Asian	Rice is the mainstay of the diet and is commonly eaten at every meal. Most Asian Americans use fresh food in their cooking, selecting live seafood, fresh meats, and seasonal fruits and vegetables from the local market to ensure freshness. Most Asians living in America adhere to a traditional Asian diet interspersed with American foods, particularly breads and cereals. Dairy products are not consumed in large quantities. Calcium is consumed through tofu and small fish (bones eaten). Fish, pork, and poultry are the main sources of protein. Significant amounts of nuts and dried beans are also eaten	Varied diet that is low in fat and sugar, and rich in fiber. Fruits and vegetables make up a large part of food intake	Diet may be low in calcium and contain an excess of sodium	Stroke, osteoporosis; risks of heart disease, obesity, and diabetes increase with acculturation
Hispanic	Diets vary by country and region of origin. Common elements include beans, rice, and (for some) corn. Foods are mainly fried or baked. Protein sources include eggs, legumes, fish, meats, and poultry. Soft drinks and sweetened beverages are favored	Rich in complex carbohydrates	Diet may be low in calcium and contain excessive fat and added sweeteners	Obesity, diabetes, heart disease, hypertension, dental caries, and undernutrition

TABLE 9.3
Food and Culture Resources

Food and Culture Resources for Nutritionists

Online Resources

Bibliographies

Food and culture. North America *(nonindigenous)*. Dirks R. *English-Language Resources for the Anthropology of Food and Nutrition*, Illinois State University. 2005. Available at: http://lilt.ilstu.edu/rtdirks/.

Ethnic and cultural food guide pyramids. USDA. Food and Nutrition Information Center. 2006. Available at: http://www.nal.usda.gov/fnic/etext/000023.html.

Cultural and ethnic food and nutrition education materials: *A Resource List for Educators*. USDA. Food and Nutrition Information Center. 2001. Available at: http://www.nal.usda.gov/fnic/pubs/bibs/gen/ethnic.html.

Food, nutrition, and culture. 2006. Part of *CulturedMed* at the State University of New York Institute of Technology, which is a Web site and a resource center of print materials promoting culturally-competent healthcare for refugees and immigrants. This project provides support to the healthcare community and newcomers to our country by providing practical information regarding culture and healthcare from both viewpoints. See: http://culturedmed.sunyit.edu/bib/food/index.html.

Other

National Center for Cultural Competence Georgetown University Center for Child and Human Development. http://www.mchgroup.org/nccc/index.html.

Americans at the Table: Reflections on Food and Culture. An electronic journal of the U.S. Department of State. 2004. Available at: http://usinfo.state.gov/journals/itsv/0704/ijse/ijse0704.htm.

Jones D.V. and Darling M.E. *Ethnic Foodways in Minnesota: Handbook of Food and Wellness Across Cultures*, 1998. Available online at http://www.agricola.umn.edu/foodways/. Accessed August 2, 2006.

Books and Pamphlets

General

Hauck-Lawson A., Deutsch J., eds. *Tastes of New York: Cultures through Food*. New York: Columbia University Press, in press.

Kittler P.G., Sucher K.P., *Food and Culture in America: A Nutrition Handbook*. 4th ed. Belmont, CA: West/Wadsworth, 2004.

Bryant C.A., DeWalt C.M., Courtney A., Schwartz J. *The Cultural Feast: An Introduction to Food and Society*, 2nd ed. Belmont, CA: Thomson/Wadsworth, 2003.

Kittler P.G., Sucher K.P. *Cultural Foods: Traditions and Trends*. Belmont, CA: Wadsworth/Thomson Learning, 2000.

Graves D.E., Suitor C.W. *Celebrating Diversity: Approaching Families through Their Food*. 2nd ed. Arlington, VA: National Maternal and Child Health Clearinghouse, 1998. Available through: National Maternal and Child Health Clearinghouse.

Hispanic

Sanjur D. *Hispanic Foodways, Nutrition, and Health*. Boston: Allyn and Bacon, 1995.

Rodriguez J.C. *Contemporary Nutrition for Latinos: A Latino Lifestyle Guide to Nutrition and Health*. New York: Writers Advantage, 2004.

The American Dietetic Association. Ethnic and Regional Food Practices Series:

  Filippino American Food Practices: Customs and Holidays (1994)
  Soul and Traditional Southern Food Practices, Customs, and Holidays (1995)
  Navajo Food Practices, Customs, and Holidays (1998)
  Northern Plains Indian Food Practices, Customs, and Holidays (1999)
  Chinese-American Food Practices, Customs, and Holidays (1998)
  Alaska Native Food Practices, Customs, and Holidays (1998)
  Cajun and Creole Food Practices, Customs, and Holidays (1996)
  Hmong American Food Practices, Customs, and Holidays (1999)
  Indian and Pakistani Food Practices, Customs, and Holidays (2000)
  Jewish Food Practices, Customs, and Holidays. 2nd ed. (1998)

9.6.1 AFRICAN AMERICANS

Unlike other immigrants, most Africans came to North America against their will. The centuries-long battle African Americans waged for freedom, for dignity, and for full participation in American society utterly transformed and shaped the nation. More than 35 million Americans claim African ancestry, and the number of African immigrants to the U.S. increases every year.

The present day African American population, like many other ethnic groups, is several generations removed from their original land. Thus, many practices and habits have been lost, dropped, simulated, or modified. The greatest influence on many African American families is the lifestyle of their parents or grandparents who lived in the southern U.S. Historically, African American rituals revolved around food. The society is based on religious ceremonies, feasting, cooking, and raising food.

The popular term for African American cooking with Southern roots is "soul food." Many soul food dishes are rich in nutrients, as found in collard greens and other leafy green and yellow vegetables, legumes, beans, rice, and potatoes. Other parts of the diet, however, are low in fiber, calcium, potassium, and high in fat. Common ways for African Americans to prepare food include frying, barbecuing, and serving foods with gravy and sauces. Home-baked cakes and pies prepared with lard are also common. A large selection and variety of food is prepared and much attention is given to an individual's favorite dishes.

Many African Americans are Protestant and have no specific food restrictions. However, a large number of families are members of religious groups that may have some restrictions or dietary preferences. These may include Seventh-Day Adventists (many of whom are vegetarian), Jehovah's Witnesses (some of whom are vegetarian), and Muslims (who are prohibited from taking food or drink from dawn to sunset during the holy month of *Ramadan*).

Taboos about child rearing and nursing are usually common or adhered to if older grandparents are heads of households. In 2003, the birth rate among African American adolescents was 63.7 births per 1,000 females aged 15–19 years (compared with 38.3 for whites).[27] Few teenage African American mothers breastfeed, but it is common with older mothers. Infant feeding methods vary with pressure from parents when babies are crying. Young mothers might give cereal along with formula because they think the infant is hungry.

Besides the formal and traditional American occasions and holidays, a large number of African Americans observe and celebrate Kwanza, an African American cultural holiday born out of the whirlwind of social and political changes of the 1960s, an era rich in expressions of freedom and self-identity. Kwanza was created in 1966 by Maulana Karenga, Ph.D. (chairperson from 1991–2002[28] of the Department of Black Studies at California State University in Long Beach), to provide an opportunity for the African American community to celebrate their heritage and reinforce positive community values through the principles of unity, self-determination, collective work and responsibility, cooperative economics, purpose, creativity, and faith.[29] Kwanza is observed for 7 days, starting December 26; December 31 is celebrated with ceremonies, a buffet, and festive attire.

9.6.1.1 Teaching Implications

Nutrition educators should focus on the way food is prepared, encouraging families to provide nutritious alternatives by modifying the sodium, fat, and sugar content of traditional foods. Cutting calories and eating smaller portions might need to be encouraged. Additional diet changes that might be suggested include substituting herbs for high sodium seasonings; substituting fresh fruits for fruit drink and fruit juice; increasing the amount of fresh vegetables consumed; substituting herbs for high-fat meat such as fatback and ham hocks when cooking dandelion, turnip, and collard greens; and decreasing the amount of meat consumed, removing the fat and skin from meat, and eating less of high-fat meat products, such as chicken wings, bologna, and sausage.[30] Some families may resist change because of family traditions.

9.6.2 HISPANICS

Mexico, Puerto Rico, and other Latin American countries have 500 years of separate history, as well as entirely different native populations present when the Spaniards arrived. Thus, the Mexican, Puerto Rican, and other Latin American cultures each has its own concept of what foods are appropriate and what these foods are called. Despite these differences, there are many similarities among these cultures, not the least of which is language. Another similarity is the "hot and cold" theory of disease, which has a profound influence on the health status of people from Latin America (as well as on people from Southeast Asia, the Philippines, and Malaysia). Hot and coldness are not determined by physical characteristics such as temperature,[31] and there is little agreement as to which foods are considered to be hot or cold.[32] Because of the great variability of this custom as practiced in the U.S.,[33] obtaining information about a client's individual hot–cold practices is an important component of the dietary interview.

It is estimated that the Hispanic population of the U.S. is 35 million. Of the total Hispanic population in the U.S., Mexicans make up 58.5%, Puerto Ricans 9.6%, Cubans 3.5%, and Dominicans 2.2%. Hispanics residing in the U.S. for a longer time tend to have macronutrient profiles more similar to those of the non-Hispanic whites. More acculturated Hispanics consume fewer ethnic foods and more foods related to the non-Hispanic-white eating patterns than those less acculturated. In general, efforts to promote better diets among Hispanics need to emphasize maintenance or adoption of healthful dietary patterns based on ethnic and modern foods that will satisfy their biological, emotional, and social needs.

9.6.2.1 Mexican American

Millions of people in the U.S. today identify themselves as Mexican immigrants or Mexican Americans. They are among both the oldest and newest inhabitants of the nation. Some Mexicans were already living in the Southern and Western regions of the North American continent centuries before the U.S. existed. Many more Mexicans came to the country during the 20th century, and Mexican immigrants continue to arrive today. See Section 3.3.4.1.2.1.

The multicultural inheritance of Mexican Americans is rich and complex. It reflects the influences of Spain, Mexico, and indigenous cultures, and has been shaped by hundreds of years of survival and adaptation in the crucible of North American history. Their history has also been shaped by wars and depressions, by the Treaty of Guadalupe Hidalgo and the Gadsden Purchase, and by shifting attitudes toward immigration.

Mexican immigration occupies a complex position in the U.S. legal system and in U.S. public opinion. Immigration law has swung back and forth throughout the 20th century, at times welcoming Mexican immigrants and at other times slamming the door shut on them. The public reception of this immigrant group has also been unpredictable; Mexican immigrants have been able to make a place for themselves in communities across the U.S. but frequently have had to battle hostile elements in those same communities to survive. In many ways, this push-and-pull dynamic continues today.

Mexican immigrants and their descendants now make up a significant portion of the U.S. population and have become one of the most influential social and cultural groups in the country, comprising 60% of the Hispanic/Latino population. Mexican Americans live predominantly in California, Texas, Arizona, New Mexico, and Colorado; their culture will likely continue to shape U.S. life in language, politics, food, and daily living and will help define the nation's identity for a new century.

The family unit is the single most important social unit in the life of Hispanics. Family responsibilities come before all others. Gender differentiation and male dominance are issues to consider while working with Hispanic families. The father is the leader of the family, and the mother runs the household, shops, and prepares the food. The traditional concepts of manhood and womanhood, however, appear to be changing toward a more egalitarian model with increased exposure to American society. The majority of Mexicans are Roman Catholic. Evangelical Protestantism is a fast-growing religion, especially among immigrants.

9.6.2.1.1 Mexican-American Foodways

The Mexican diet of today is rich in a variety of foods and dishes that represent a blend of pre-Columbian, Spanish, French, and more recently, American culture. The typical Mexican diet is rich in complex carbohydrates, provided mainly by corn and corn products, beans, rice, and breads. The typical Mexican diet contains an adequate amount of protein in the forms of beans, eggs, fish and shellfish, and a variety of meats, including beef, pork, poultry, and goat. Because of the extensive use of frying as a cooking method, the Mexican diet is also high in fat. The nutrients most likely to be inadequately provided are calcium, iron, vitamin A, folic acid, and vitamin C.

Traditionally, Mexicans ate four or five meals daily. The foods eaten varied with factors such as income, education, urbanization, geographic region, and family customs. The extent to which the traditional Mexican meal pattern continues among Mexicans in the U.S. has not been systematically studied. The three-meal pattern prevails, although whether or not the major meal of the day occurs in mid-afternoon is unclear. The daily meal pattern in the typical Mexican-American home varies according to the availability of traditional foods and the degree of assimilation into American society.

With emigration to the U.S., major changes occur in the Mexican-American diet. Healthy changes include a moderate increase in the consumption of milk, vegetables, and fruits, and a large decrease in the consumption of lard and Mexican cream. However, the introduction of salads and cooked vegetables has increased the use of fats, such as salad dressings, margarine, and butter. Other less healthy changes include a severe decline in the consumption of traditional fruit-based beverages in favor of high-sugar drinks. Consumption of inexpensive sources of complex carbohydrates, such as beans and rice, has also decreased as a result of acculturation. In addition to the negative impact on the health of this population, these dietary changes also may adversely affect the family's budget when low-priced foods are replaced with more expensive ones.

9.6.2.1.2 Teaching Implications

Healthcare providers need to understand Hispanic culture, beliefs, norms, food practices, and terminology to assist clients. Providers need to support and stimulate the preservation of healthy cultural food practices among Mexican-American clientele. When appropriate, suggest modifications of traditional dishes that are high in sodium, fat, and sugar. Increase clients' knowledge of healthy food selections from typical American fare. Gain support from clients' families to enhance their acceptance of the diet.

The diets of pregnant Mexican-American women of marginal social and economic standing are deficient in dietary iron, vitamin A, and calcium. Encourage the consumption of low-fat cheeses, lean red meat, fresh fruits, and vegetables. Monitor beverage intake, as carbonated soft drinks and presweetened drinks are widely consumed. Breastfeeding is widely practiced in Mexico, although most Mexican Americans use infant formula. Weaning children from the bottle at 1 year of age is not widely practiced. Baby bottle tooth decay is common in toddlers, suggesting that the child is put to bed with a bottle.

Efforts to promote better diets among the Hispanic elderly need to focus on maintenance or adoption of healthful dietary patterns based on ethnic and modern foods that will satisfy the biological, emotional, and social needs of the diverse Hispanic groups in the U.S. Continuing efforts to teach diverse groups of older adults about meeting current recommendations for macronutrient intake should consider the effects of acculturation and how migration factors may positively influence the use of certain foods and, perhaps negatively, affect others.[34]

The healthcare provider may intervene with Hispanic clients and communities in culturally sensitive ways, which includes viewing culture as an enabler rather than a resistant force, incorporating cultural beliefs into the plans of care, stressing familialism, and taking time for pleasant conversation.

9.6.2.2 Puerto Rican

Puerto Rico has been a possession of the U.S. for more than a century but has never been a state. Its people have been U.S. citizens since 1917, but they have no vote in Congress. As citizens, the people of Puerto Rico can move throughout the 50 states just as any other American can. This is considered internal migration, not immigration. However, in moving to the mainland, Puerto Ricans leave a homeland with its own distinct identity and culture, and the transition has involved many of the same cultural conflicts and emotional adjustments that most immigrants face. The Puerto Rican migration experience may be conceived as an internal immigration — as the experience of a people who move within their own country, but whose new home lies well outside of their emotional home territory.

At first, only very few Puerto Ricans came to the continental U.S. Although the U.S. tried to promote Puerto Rico as a glamorous tourist destination, in the early 20th century the island suffered a severe economic depression. Poverty was rife, and few of the island's residents could afford the long boat journey to the mainland. In 1910, there were fewer than 2,000 Puerto Ricans in the continental U.S., mostly in small enclaves in New York City. By the 1930s there were only 40,000 more.

After the end of World War II, however, Puerto Rican migration exploded. Although there were 13,000 Puerto Ricans in New York City in 1945, by 1946 there were more than 50,000. Over the next decade, more than 25,000 Puerto Ricans would come to the continental U.S. each year, peaking in 1953, when more than 69,000 arrived. By 1955, nearly 700,000 Puerto Ricans had migrated to the U.S., and by the mid-1960s, more than a million had. There were a number of reasons for this sudden influx. The continuing depression in Puerto Rico made many Puerto Ricans eager for a fresh start, and U.S. factory owners and employment agencies had begun recruiting heavily on the island. In addition, the postwar years saw the return home of thousands of Puerto Rican war veterans, whose service in the U.S. military had shown them the world. But perhaps the most significant cause was the sudden availability of affordable air travel. After centuries of immigration by boat, the Puerto Rican migration became the first great airborne migration in U.S. history.[35] Currently, the more than 3 million residents from Puerto Rico make up about 10% of the total Hispanic population of the U.S.

The meals of Puerto Ricans living on the mainland are similar to those of their relatives on the island. A light breakfast of strong coffee and bread may be followed by a light lunch of rice and beans (*arroz con gondules*) or a starchy vegetable such as potatoes or plantains with or without dried salt cod (*bacalo*). Americanized Puerto Ricans may substitute a sandwich and soft drink for the more traditional noonday meal. A late day dinner may consist of foods from the more traditional lunch. Salad consumption is erratic; snacking on low nutrient-dense foods is common.[36]

9.6.2.3 Cuban American

Cuban cuisine has been influenced by Spanish, French, African, Arabic, Chinese, and Portuguese cultures.[37] Traditional Cuban cooking is primarily peasant cuisine that has little concern with measurements, order, and timing. Mainstays of the Cuban diet are bananas and other tropical fruits, rice and black beans (*moros y cristianos*), pork, fried plantains, and strong, sweet coffee. Most of the food is sautéed or slow-cooked over a low flame. Very little is deep-fried and there are no heavy or creamy sauces.

Most Cuban cooking relies on a few basic spices, such as garlic, cumin, oregano, and bay laurel leaves. Many dishes use a *sofrito* as their basis. The sofrito consists of onion, green pepper, garlic, oregano, and ground pepper quick-fried in olive oil. The *sofrito*, which gives the food its flavor, is used when cooking black beans, stews, many meat dishes, and tomato-based sauces. Meats and poultry are usually marinated in citrus juices, such as lime or sour orange juices, and then roasted over low heat until the meat is tender and literally falling off the bone. Another common staple of the Cuban diet are root vegetables such as *yucca*, *malanga*, and *boniato*, which are found in most Latin markets. These vegetables are flavored with a marinade, called *mojo* that includes hot olive oil, lemon juice, sliced raw onions, garlic, cumin, and a little water. Box 9.8 provides a typical daily menu.

9.6.2.4 Dominican American

According to the 2000 census, more than 750,000 Dominicans live in the U.S. Immigration increased dramatically from the early 1960s (when just over 90,000 Dominicans were admitted to the U.S.) through the mid-1990s and began to decline thereafter. From 1988 to 1998 over 400,000 Dominicans migrated to the U.S. Two-thirds settled in New York and northern New Jersey; the remainder live primarily in Miami, Los Angeles, Boston, Houston, Chicago, Philadelphia, and Portland.[38] Dominicans in the U.S. suffer from low levels of education, income, and occupational status. Almost half are high school dropouts, and less than 10% are college graduates. On the other hand, only 8.8% of Dominicans born in the U.S. fail to complete high school and 21.7% are college graduates, indicating that second generation Dominicans will be less economically disadvantaged than their forebears.

Breakfast (*desayuno*) is usually light: strong, sweetened coffee and bread; people in urban areas may eat more. The evening meal (*cena*) is also light, often not more than a snack or leftovers from the midday meal (*comida*). Lunch (*almuerzo*), the main meal of the day, consists of large portions of rice and beans (*habichuelas*), along with such favorites as cassava (*yucca*) that is boiled, prepared as fritters, or baked into rounds of crisp cracker bread called *casabe*. Tropical fruits such as banana, mango, papaya, pineapple, guava, and avocado are relished. People may eat small quantities of chicken, beef, pork, goat, or *bacalau* with a meal. Popular beverages include beer, rum, sweetened fruit juices, and soft drinks.[39]

9.6.3 ASIAN AMERICANS

Food preparation in the Asian culture is meticulous, and consumption is ceremonious and deliberate. Two key elements draw the diverse cultures of the Asian region together: the composition of meals (emphasis on vegetables and rice, with relatively little meat) and cooking techniques. Asian Americans have emigrated from the Philippines, China, Hong Kong, Cambodia, Vietnam, Laos, Thailand, Korea, and Japan. The religions they practice include Confucianism, Buddhism, Taoism, and Shintoism (Japanese only). A large number of native Filipinos are Roman Catholic. Bowing is important, but most Asian Americans will shake hands. The elderly, children, and pregnant women are held in high esteem. The Vietnamese and Hmong cultures are discussed separately.

Most Asians living in the U.S. adhere to a traditional Asian diet interspersed with American foods, particularly breads and cereals. Dairy products are not consumed in large amounts, except for ice cream. Calcium is consumed through tofu and small fish (bones eaten). Fish, pork, and poultry comprise the main proteins. Significant amounts of nuts and dried beans are also eaten. Vegetables and fruits make up a large part of their food intake. Rice is the mainstay of the diet and is commonly eaten at every meal. Asian food preparation techniques include stir-frying, barbecuing, deep-frying, boiling, and steaming. All ingredients are carefully prepared (chopped, sliced, and so on) prior to starting the cooking process. A typical day's menu might include hot cereal, bread, fruit juice, soy milk, fruit, nuts, and rice for breakfast; rice or bread with vegetables or fruits for lunch; and rice, vegetable soup mixed with tofu, vegetables, fish, or meat for dinner.

- Thai food is generally spicy, hot, and high in sodium. Hot peppers are used daily. Thai women usually breastfeed their children up to age two.
- The Japanese are very concerned about the visual appeal of the food and the "separateness" of the foods and tastes. Garlic and hot pepper are not common ingredients. Most Japanese women in the U.S. breastfeed their babies.

- Koreans make kimchee in October or November for use throughout the winter. Kimchee is cabbage marinated in salt water, layered with peppers and spices in crockery, and left to ferment through November and December. Kimchee is eaten with every meal. Many Korean parents bottle feed their babies. New Korean mothers eat seaweed soup for the first month after delivery; the soup is believed to cleanse the blood.

9.6.3.1 Vietnamese

The Vietnamese come from both remote agricultural and fast-paced urban areas of Southeast Asia. Most Vietnamese practice Buddhism, but some practice Confucianism or Taoism. Vietnamese Americans are one of the fastest growing American Asian Pacific Islander (AAPI) groups in the U.S. From 1990 to 2000, the Vietnamese population in the U.S. grew by 83% (614,547 to 1,122,528),[40] and is expected to reach 3 million by 2030. California, with 450,000 Vietnamese, is the state with the largest population, most of whom live in Los Angeles, Riverside, Orange County; San Francisco, Oakland, San Jose, and San Diego. Texas, with 135,000, has the second largest Vietnamese population, notably in Houston, Galveston, and Brazoria and the Dallas–Fort Worth area. Additional cities with 30,000–46,000 Vietnamese residents include Seattle, Tacoma, and Bremerton (Washington), Washington, D.C., and Boston.

The Vietnamese population has encountered significant social challenges since their immigration to the U.S. Compared with other AAPI groups, the Vietnamese have lower socioeconomic status and many have difficulty with the English language. Culturally, many Vietnamese rely on traditional beliefs about health and medicine. Social isolation is also a major problem in Vietnamese-American communities. Low reading levels and limited access to culturally and literacy-appropriate education materials may contribute to inadequate dietary intake.

The basic food in Vietnam is dry, flaky rice supplemented with vegetables, eggs, and small amounts of meat and fish. Although similar to Chinese cooking, Vietnamese cooking uses little fat or oil for frying. *NuocMam* fish sauce is a principle ingredient in almost every Vietnamese dish. Vietnamese are fond of fruits — bananas, mangos, papayas, oranges, coconuts, and pineapple. They are accustomed to little milk and cheese, and many exhibit varying degrees of lactose intolerance. They drink a large amount of hot green tea and coffee without adding sugar, milk, or lemon.

The Vietnamese eat three meals a day with some snacking on fruits and soups. A light breakfast may consist of soup (*pho*), rice, or rice noodles; thin slices of beef, chicken, or pork, bean sprouts, greens, green tea or green coffee, boiled eggs, and crusty bread. Lunch and dinner are similar in food content — rice, fish, or meat, a vegetable dish with *nuoc mam* or fish sauce, plus tea or coffee. Smaller portions are served at dinner. Chopsticks and small bowls are used for eating, with bowls brought to the mouth to eat.

In their home country, Vietnamese either grow food or purchase it daily. There are few refrigerators. Teaching Vietnamese living in the U.S. proper food storage of perishable foods is important. Encourage home and community gardening as a source of native vegetables.

Vietnamese eat a wide variety of vegetables. Soybeans, mung beans, and peanuts are used extensively. New, inexpensive legumes should be introduced. Encourage variety in their diet through introducing unfamiliar vegetables and fruits. Discourage low-nutrient foods such as soft drinks, candy, and chips.

Pregnant women do not increase their caloric intake. Milk consumption is low or nonexistent during pregnancy and lactation. Infants are breastfed to about one year. Rice gruel (rice flour and water) is the only food introduced in the first year, sometimes as early as one month.

9.6.3.1.1 Teaching Implications

Education is extremely important to the Vietnamese. Their learning system emphasizes memorization and repetition, not critical study. Vietnamese show great respect to elders, superiors, and strangers. They clasp both hands against their chests in welcome. Shaking hands is seldom done;

a smile and nod would suffice. Beckoning with a finger is a sign of contempt used toward an animal or inferior.

Vietnamese people tend to be polite and delicate. Because frankness and outspokenness are usually considered rude, true feelings are often veiled. Vietnamese people may just smile and nod when they do not understand you. Keep in mind that this means, "Yes, I hear you," or, "Yes, I see what you mean even though I don't truly understand it!" Vietnamese are typically friendly and giving people, and hospitality and food are related. A Vietnamese person might not ask, "How are you?" but rather, "Have you eaten yet?" Although they love to give gifts, it is considered rude to open them in front of people.

Respect for parents and ancestors is a key virtue in Vietnamese families. The oldest male in the family is the head of the household and the most important family member. His oldest son is the second leader of the family. Sometimes, related families live together in a big house and help each other.

Even though Vietnamese immigrants range from farmers to urban dwellers, their move to the U.S. is one of enormous cultural change. They are a people of tradition yet are open to try new "American" ways. Unfamiliar with most of our grocery items, they not only need to be retaught words and techniques for their own cooking but need a total introduction to American food culture.

9.6.3.2 Hmong

The Hmong were a highly developed people with a rich culture who lived in northeast China under the leadership of the Hmong king Chiyou. They were invaded over 5000 years ago and forced to migrate to southern China, some eventually arriving in Southeast Asia, principally the rural mountain areas of Laos. In 1975 when Laos was taken over by communists, the Hmong began to disperse to many parts of the world, including the U.S. In 2000, there were 186,310 Hmong in the U.S.,[41] principally in Minneapolis/St. Paul (MN),[42] Fresno (CA), and Milwaukee (WI). Hmong families are typically large, with four to eight children per household.

The Hmong follow an animist religion, believing in spirits in all places and every aspect of life. They also have close family and clan relationships and are divided into clans or tribes that share the same paternal ancestry. Each clan has a leader who oversees all relations. Clans will move to the same area in the U.S. to maintain their closeness. Each clan has a shaman (wise man/medicine man) who deals with spiritual and physical problems, similar to the functions of a minister, psychologist, and doctor. As the clan leader and the shaman are important to the Hmong family members, it is important for the healthcare worker to gain their respect.

9.6.3.2.1 Hmong Foodways

The Hmong staple food is white rice. Their diet is enhanced by a variety of vegetables, fish, meat, and traditional spices. They eat three meals a day. Snacking is not part of their native culture. A typical day's menu might include light soup with rice, pumpkin, vegetables, chicken, or pork (eaten very early, for breakfast) and nonglutinous rice, fried or steamed meat, pork, chicken, or beef (eaten at noon or before for lunch and eaten late in the evening for dinner).

Most of a Hmong's daily calories are from the carbohydrates/grain group. Native vegetables are also consumed in large amounts. The Hmong diet could be enhanced with the addition of a variety of inexpensive, available vegetables. Meats and fish are used in small amounts as enhancements. The amounts are sufficient, however, to provide ample protein. Popular fruits are bananas, mangos, pineapples, coconuts, lichees, and jackfruit. As with vegetables, additional varieties of fruit could enhance the Hmong diet. In particular, citrus fruits should be emphasized for their vitamin C content.

Fresh milk and cheese are typically unavailable to Hmongs in their native country. This, along with lactose intolerance, discourages the consumption of dairy products. Overall fat content in the diet is low. Relatively few households in Laos eat sweets. A steamed rice cake may be eaten occasionally.

Hmong food is usually home grown. Meats are usually fresh, home butchered, and shared among clan members to keep storage time short. Meals are served in a communal style. Food is placed (and replenished) in the middle of the table, and each person eats from the center with a spoon or fork. Using fingers to eat is impolite. Cooking methods include stir-frying, boiling, steaming, and roasting over an open fire. Vegetable oils and pork fat are the principal fats used in cooking. Food is usually chopped in uniform pieces before cooking. Seasonings are an essential aspect of Hmong cooking. Fish sauce and soy sauce, both of which are high in sodium, replace table salt. Hot peppers, ginger, garlic, coriander, coconut, and lemon grass contribute to the robust flavor.

Mothers nurse infants for one to two years. An infant's first solid food is rice flour and water made into a gruel. This may be started as early as one month but other foods are not introduced until one year. During pregnancy and lactation many women do not increase their caloric intake. Many do not include milk in their diet.

9.6.3.2.2 Teaching Implications

The Hmong do not feel comfortable with direct eye contact and do not like to be touched on their heads. Hmong education is oral, which explains why many of the elders do not read. They are a willing group of learners. The Hmong are a happy and hospitable people. Many times in teaching situations they will nod and say, "Yes," which means, "Yes, I am listening to you," not, "Yes, I understand." The Hmong people have experienced an enormous cultural change in their move to the U.S. No longer can they have the fresh variety of food available in their homeland. The Hmong mother is caught between her husband who wants homeland cooking and her children who are becoming "Americanized" and expect her to cook American meals.

9.7 CONCLUSION

Working within a rapidly diversifying society requires the health professional to become culturally competent, not just culturally sensitive. Understanding the cultural context in which a client lives can positively affect communication and improve health status. Achieving cultural competence and practicing in a culturally competent manner are difficult and time-consuming, but important, goals. This chapter has explored the traditions and foodways of several large immigrant groups in the U.S. Fortunately, through the Internet, academic, and cultural organizations, information about these and other groups within our society is readily available.

9.8 ACRONYMS

CCLCHC	Center for Cultural and Linguistic Competence in HealthCare
CDC	Centers for Disease Control and Prevention
CLAS	Culturally and Linguistically Appropriate Services
CLCCHC	Center for Linguistic and Cultural Competence in HealthCare
HHS	U.S. Department of Health and Human Services
HRSA	Health Resources and Services Administration
MHI	Minority Health Initiative
NAAFA	National Association for the Advance of Fat Acceptance
NCCC	National Center for Cultural Competence
NCMHD	National Center on Minority Health and Health Disparities
NIH	National Institutes of Health
OMH	Office of Minority Health
P.L.	Public Law

REFERENCES

1. Cross, T., Bazron, B., Dennis, K., and Isaacs, M. *Towards a Culturally Competent System of Care: A Monograph on Effective Services for Minority Children Who Are Severely Emotionally Disturbed: Volume I.* Washington, D.C.: Georgetown University Child Development Center, 1989.

2. *National Center for Cultural Competence Policy Brief. Rationale for Cultural Competence in Primary Care. 1999.* Available at: http://www.mchgroup.org/nccc/documents/Policy_Brief_1_2003.pdf. Accessed August 1, 2006.

3. U.S. Department of Health and Human Services. Indicators of Cultural Competence in HealthCare Delivery Organizations: An Organizational Cultural Competence Assessment Profile. Health Resources and Services Administration. Available at: http://www.hrsa.gov/culturalcompetence/indicators. Accessed August 1, 2006.

4. Betancourt, J.R. Cultural competence — marginal or mainstream movement? *N Eng J Med.* 351, 953–955, 2004.

5. PEW Hispanic Center. Available at: http://pewhispanic.org/. Accessed July 31, 2006.

6. U.S. Department of Health and Human Services. *Healthy People 2000.* GPO No. 017-001-00474-0. 1991.

7. U.S. Department of Health and Human Services. *Healthy People 2010.* 2nd ed. With Understanding and Improving Health and Objectives for Improving Health. 2 Vols. Washington, D.C., November 2000. Available at: http://www.healthypeople.gov/document. Accessed August 1, 2006.

8. Census Bureau. Language use and English-speaking ability: 2000. Census 2000 Brief. Available at: http://www.census.gov/prod/2003pubs/c2kbr-29.pdf. Accessed May 31, 2005.

9. Guidance to Federal Financial Assistance Recipients Regarding Title VI Prohibition against National Origin Discrimination Affecting Limited English Proficient Persons. Washington, D.C.: Department of Health and Human Services, 2003. Available at: http://www.hhs.gov/ocr/lep/revisedlep.html. Accessed May 31, 2005.

10. U.S. Department of Health and Human Services. About the Center of Cultural and Linguistic Competence in HealthCare. Office of Minority Health. Available at: http://www.omhrc.gov/templates/browse.aspx?lvl=1&lvlID=3. Accessed August 6, 2006.

11. Day, J.C. *Population Projections of the United States by Age, Sex, Race, and Hispanic Origin: 1995 to 2050,* U.S. Bureau of the Census, Current Population Reports, P25-1130, Washington, D.C., 1996. Available at: http://www.census.gov/prod/1/pop/p25-1130/p251130.pdf. Accessed July 31, 2006.

12. Executive Summary: A Population Perspective of the United States. Population Resource Center. Available at: http://www.prcdc.org/summaries/uspopperspec/uspopperspec.html. Accessed July 31, 2006.

13. Brach, C. and Fraser, I. Can cultural competency reduce racial and ethnic health disparities? A review and conceptual model. *Med Care Res Rev.* 57(S1), 181–217, 2000.

14. U.S. Department of Health and Human Services. Office for Minority Health. Final CLAS Report: *National Standards for Culturally and Linguistically Appropriate Services in HealthCare.* Available at: http://www.omhrc.gov/omh/programs/2pgprograms/finalreport.pdf. Accessed January 17, 2005.

15. Joint Commission on Accreditation of Healthcare Organizations homepage. Available at: http://www.jcaho.org/index.htm. Accessed August 22, 2004.

16. U.S. Department of Health and Human Services. Public Health Service. The Office of Minority Health. Assuring Cultural Competence in HealthCare: *Recommendations for National Standards and an Outcomes-Focused Research Agenda.* Recommendations for National Standards and a National Public Comment Process. Available at: http://www.omhrc.gov/clas/cultural1a.htm. Accessed August 2, 2004.

17. President's Advisory Commission on Consumer Protection and Quality in the HealthCare Industry. *Quality First: Better HealthCare for All Americans.* 1998. Available at: http://www.hcqualitycommission.gov/ final/. Accessed August 22, 2004.

18. Crisp, C. The Gay Affirmative Practice Scale (GAP): a new measure for assessing cultural competence with gay and lesbian clients. *Soc Work.* 51, 115–126, 2006.

19. National Association to Advance Fat Acceptance (NAAFA) homepage: http://www.naafa.org/. Accessed August 1, 2006.

20. Powell, A.D. and Kahn, A.S. Racial differences in women's desire to be thin. *Int J Eating Dis.* 17, 191–195, 1995.

21. Bacon, L., Keim, N.L., Van Loan, M.D., et al. Evaluating a "non-diet" wellness intervention for improvement of metabolic fitness, psychological well-being and eating and activity behaviors. *Int J Obes Relat Metab Disord.* 26, 854–865, 2002.

22. Gore, S.V. African-American women's perceptions of weight: paradigm shift for advanced practice. *Holistic Nurs Pract.* 13, 71–79, 1999.

23. Linkins, K.W., McIntosh, S., Bell, J., and Chong, U. *Indicators of Cultural Competence in HealthCare Delivery Organizations: An Organizational Cultural Competence Assessment Profile.* A report prepared for the U.S. Department of Health and Human Services, The Health Resources and Services Administration. April 2002. Available at http://www.hrsa.gov/OMH/cultural1.htm/. Accessed August 22, 2004.

24. Harris-Davis, E. and Haughton, B. Model for multicultural nutrition counseling competencies. *J Am Diet Assoc.* 100(10), 1178–1185, 2000.

25. Pelto, G.H., Pelto, P.J., and Messer, E. Symbolic, folkloric and medicinal factors, Appendix C in *Research Methods in Nutritional Anthropology.* Toyko: The United Nations University. 1989.

26. Ohio State University Extension Fact Sheets. Family and Consumer Sciences. Cultural Diversity — Eating in America. Available at: http://ohioline.osu.edu/lines/food.html#FOODF. Accessed August 2, 2006. (a) Ewing, J. African-American. HYG-5250-95. http://ohioline.osu.edu/hyg-fact/5000/5250. html. (b) Warrix, M. Mexican-American. HYG-5255-95.. http://ohioline.osu.edu/hyg-fact/5000/5255. html. (c) Syracuse, C.J. Puerto Rican. HYG-5257-95. http://ohioline.osu.edu/hyg-fact/5000/5257. html. (d) Hill, P. Asian. HYG-5253-95. http://ohioline.osu.edu/hyg-fact/5000/5253.html. (e) Betancourt, D. Hmong. HYG-5254-95. http://ohioline.osu.edu/hyg-fact/5000/5254.html. (f) Betancourt, D. Vietnamese. HYG-5258-95. http://ohioline.osu.edu/hyg-fact/5000/5258.html.

27. Federal Interagency Forum on Child and Family Statistics. *America's Children: Key National Indicators of Well-Being, 2005.* Washington, D.C.: The Federal Interagency Forum on Child and Family Statistics. Washington, D.C., 2005.

28. Clark, M.L. Vision marks black studies chairman's legacy. On-Line 49er. 10(20) October 3, 2002. Available at http://www.csulb.edu/~d49er/archives/2002/fall/news/v10n20-vis.shtml. Accessed September 4, 2004.

29. The Official Kwanzaa Web site. Available at: http://www.officialkwanzaaweb site.org/index.html. Accessed September 4, 2004.

30. Burke, C.B. and Raia, S.P. *Ethnic and Regional Food Practices. A Series. Soul and Traditional Southern Food Practices and Customs.* Chicago, IL: The American Dietetic Association, 1995.

31. Bryant, C.A., DeWalt, K.M., Courtney, A., and Schwartz, J. Worldview, religion, and health beliefs: the ideological basis of food practices. *The Cultural Feast: An Introduction to Food and Society,* 2nd ed. Belmont, CA: Thomson/Wadsworth, 2003, chap. 8.

32. Algert, S.J. and Ellison, T.H. *Ethnic and Regional Food Practices. A Series. Mexican American Food Practices, Customs, and Holidays.* Chicago, IL: The American Dietetic Association, 1989.

33. Grivetti, L.E. Nutrition past — nutrition today. Prescientific origins of nutrition and dietetics. Part 4. Aztec patterns and Spanish Legacy. *Nutr Today.* 27, 13–25, 1992.

34. Bermudez, O.L., Falcon, L.M., and Tucker, K.L. Intake and food sources of macronutrients among older Hispanic adults: association with ethnicity acculturation, and length of residence in the United States. *J Am Diet Assoc.* 100, 665–673, 2000.

35. Library of Congress. Immigration…Puerto Rico/Cuba. American Memory, 2004. Available at http://memory.loc.gov/learn/features/immig/cuban3.html. Accessed August 2, 2006.

36. Kittler, P.M. and Sucher, K.P. Caribbean Islanders and South Americans, *Food and Culture,* 4th ed. Belmont, CA: Thomson/Wadsworth, 2004, chap. 10.

37. Rosario, D. Cuban Cuisine. Available at: http://www.education.miami.edu/ep/littlehavana/cuban_food/cuban_cuisine/cuban_cuisine.html. Accessed August 2, 2006.

38. Castro, M.J. and Boswell, T.D. The Dominican diaspora revisited: Dominicans and Dominican-Americans in a new century. North-South Agenda Paper No. 53. January 2002. Available at: http://www.miami.edu/nsc/pages/pub-ap-pdf/53AP.pdf. Accessed September 7, 2004.

39. Available at http://www.ason.org/dominicanrepublic.pdf. Accessed September 9, 2004.

40. Barnes, J.S. and Bennett, C.E. Census Brief 2000. The Asian Population 2000. February 2002. Available at http://www.census.gov/prod/2002pubs/c2kbr01-16.pdf. Accessed September 6, 2004.

41. Barnes, J.S. and Bennett, C.E. Census Brief 2000. The Asian Population 2000. February 2002. Available at http://www.census.gov/prod/2002pubs/c2kbr01-16.pdf. Accessed September 6, 2004.

42. Jones, D.V. and Darling, M.E. *Ethnic Foodways in Minnesota: Handbook of Food and Wellness Across Cultures.* St. Paul, MN: University of Minnesota Extension Service, 1996. Available at: http://www.agricola.umn.edu/foodways/. Accessed September 22, 2004.

10 Food and Nutrition Politics, Policy, and Legislation

I think it is important to realize that nutrition as such is not a science. Rather, nutrition is an agenda for action based on a number of sciences: physiology, organic chemistry, biochemistry, epidemiology, psychology, sociology, and economics, as well as a number of other fields like agriculture, food technology, political science, and human relations. While the scientific basis is indispensable if nutritionists are going to be authoritative in what they do, the science by itself does not constitute nutrition unless and until a program of action is incorporated as part of the discipline.

Jean Mayer, president of Tufts University, 1989.[1]

U.S. food policy affects the safety, integrity, nutritional quality, and accessibility of the nation's food supply as well as the nutritional guidance given to the American population. Food and nutrition policymakers advocate for policies, regulations, and programs designed to protect and advance the health and nutritional status of the American public.

Food and nutrition advocates focus on the particular needs of vulnerable segments of the population: low-income children and families; populations with special needs due to age or physiologic status; ethnic, linguistic, and racial minorities; immigrants; and groups at risk due to undernutrition, obesity, disability, and other conditions. Food and nutrition advocates also aim to protect the environment by encouraging the consumption of locally produced, minimally processed food. Goals of food and nutrition advocacy include:

- Education and training
- Monitoring and modifying food and nutrition policy
- Developing intervention models
- Field application of methods
- Identifying the most successful approaches to alleviating problems of food insecurity and hunger, and to improving the nutritional health of the American population
- Monitoring and evaluating programs
- Communicating food and nutrition advice to nutrition and health professionals, policy makers in government and in the private sector, and the American public
- Advocacy for policy, regulation, and programs designed to advance the health and nutritional status of the American public
- Advocacy for policy and regulations to protect the environment

National nutrition policy includes such disparate programs as the nation's food and nutrition guidelines issued jointly by the U.S. Department of Agriculture (USDA) and the Department of Health and Human Services (DHHS), as well as the micronutrient fortification of table salt, milk, grain products, and water. It is not surprising, then, that federal nutrition policies exert considerable influence on state and local decision makers, stakeholders, and consumers.

This chapter examines policy at the federal and state levels. We examine the history of U.S. nutrition policy and current national health policies aimed at increasing physical activity, in addition

Box 10.1 Definitions

Polis is the Greek word for city-state. In classical Greece, a *polis* was a unit of governmental and social organization through which Greek citizens identified themselves by means of their common language, customs, history, religion, and a nearby city-center or metro*polis*. Derived from the Greek word *polis* are the English words *politics* and *policy* (and also *polite*).

Politics may be thought of as the activity through which people make, preserve, and amend the rules under which they live. Although politics usually refers to government, it is observed in all human group interactions, including corporate, academic, and religious. Institutions arrive at decisions through their politics. As the method of making decisions for groups, politics is the process by which rules for group behavior are established, competition for positions of leadership is regulated, the disruptive effects of disputes are minimized, a community's decisions are made, and policies are established.

Policy, on the other hand, may be regarded as a principle (basic generalization that is accepted as true) or rule (formal regulation that has the force of law) to guide decision-making; statements, plans, practices, principles, or rules adopted by a government or other organization for the purpose of guiding or controlling institutional and community behavior; or an established plan or course of action adopted to address specific issues or achieving particular goals.

In the context of government and public service, a *regulation* (as a process) is the control of something by rules. A *rule* is a principle or condition that customarily governs behavior ("it was his rule to take a walk before breakfast;" "short haircuts were the regulation"). And a *ruling* is an interpretation of a regulation (an authoritative rule).

to other prevention efforts. We also look at state guidelines, such as local wellness policies mandated in schools participating in the National School Lunch Program. Chapter 12 explores federal food and nutrition policy embodied in the Dietary Guidelines for Americans and the USDA's food guidance system known as MyPyramid.

10.1 MAKING POLICY

Suggesting a new policy or suggesting revisions to an existing policy is initiated by a politician or political party, by a professional or professional organization, or by other stakeholders or special interest groups that have enlisted political support. The case study in the following section illustrates the genesis of a nutrition policy.

Very briefly, the process of introducing a policy includes these activities.[2,3]

1. Documenting needs through assessments, surveillance, monitoring, literature review, and so on.
2. Drafting a preliminary statement that refers to past and existing policies.
3. Seeking support from stakeholders, as well as key legislators and policymakers.
4. Mobilizing a grassroots constituency. Policy is made, in part, through the visibility and organization of public interest constituencies. (President Franklin Delano Roosevelt once told a group of businessmen who had come to lobby him: "I agree with everything you say. Now go out there and *make* me do it!")
5. Securing public and professional comments and input.
6. Implementing the policy.
7. Monitoring the policy, once it has been implemented.
8. Evaluating the policy. To what extent does it produce the desired results? When it is no longer serving its purpose, return to step number one.

10.1.1 CASE STUDY: DEVELOPING A NATIONAL NUTRITION POLICY

This case study examines the process of developing a national nutrition policy for the labeling of foods eaten away from home.[4,5,6,7,8] At the time of this writing, the legislation is still pending.

In 2002, Americans spent about 46% of their total food budget on food eaten away from home, an increase from 27% in 1962. Foods eaten in chain restaurants tend to be less nutritious and higher in calories than foods prepared at home.[9,10] Current nutrition labeling law exempts much of the food-away-from-home sector from mandatory labeling regulations. Because consumers are less likely to be aware of the ingredients and nutrient content of away-from-home food than of foods prepared at home, public health advocates have called for mandatory nutrition labeling for major sources of food eaten away from home, such as fast-food and chain restaurants.[11]

A USDA Economic Research Service (ERS) assessment of a food-away-from-home nutrition labeling policy indicates that even if a labeling policy has no direct effect on consumer intake, it could still benefit consumers through producer-initiated reformulation of products. If a labeling policy required disclosure of nutritionally negative attributes such as calories, fat, and sodium content, companies selling products with high amounts of energy and these nutrients may choose to reformulate their products rather than risk losing sales. Thus, product reformulation may benefit all consumers who use the products, not just those who read the label. In fact, healthier restaurant fare resulting from reformulation may prove to be the largest benefit of menu labeling.[12]

In 2002, the Surgeon General recommended that nutrition information be available to customers at restaurants. In 2004, the FDA's Obesity Working Group released a comprehensive report entitled Calories Count, outlining a series of key recommendations for ways FDA can help stem the rising tide of obesity in areas within its authority. A major set of recommendations in the report calls on the FDA to encourage the restaurant industry to provide nutrition information. As a result, the FDA urged the restaurant industry to launch a nationwide, voluntary, point-of-sale nutrition information campaign for customers that includes information on calories.

The report also calls on the FDA to work with a third-party facilitator to begin a national policy dialogue to seek consensus-based solutions to specific aspects of the obesity problem involving foods consumed away from home. To implement this recommendation, the FDA hired a nonprofit organization that assists diverse participants achieve consensus on pressing public policy issues to convene a forum on away-from-home foods. This forum, consisting of a broad range of key stakeholders, met to consider what could be done to support consumers' ability to manage their energy intake, within the scope of away-from-home foods, to prevent undue weight gain and obesity. The final report was delivered to the FDA on June 2, 2006. Recommendation 4.1 states that "away-from-home food establishments should provide consumers with calorie information in a standard format that is easily accessible and easy to use."

Not coincidentally, on June 6, 2006, Tom Harkin (D-Iowa) reintroduced in the Senate the Menu Education and Labeling Act or the MEAL Act (S. 3484) "to amend the Federal Food, Drug, and Cosmetic Act to extend the food labeling requirements of the Nutrition Labeling and Education Act [NLEA] of 1990 to enable customers to make informed choices about the nutritional content of standard menu items in large chain restaurants." The purpose of the MEAL Act is to close a loophole created by the NLEA, which requires most retail food packages to provide nutrition information, but exempts restaurant food from these requirements. The MEAL Act would require chain restaurants with 20 or more business locations to provide consumers with information about calories, sodium, fat, and *trans* fat on standard menu items. Just two weeks after the MEAL Act was introduced, the American Heart Association (AHA) gave menu labeling a tacit endorsement in their diet and lifestyle recommendations for cardiovascular disease risk reduction: "when you eat food that is prepared outside of the home, follow the AHA Diet and Lifestyle Recommendations." One would need to know what is in the food in order to follow the AHA recommendation; the only way to know that would be through nutrient disclosure. On June 8, 2006 the bill was referred to the Senate Committee on Health, Education, Labor, and Pensions.

The final report of the *Keystone Forum on Away-From-Home Foods: Opportunities for Preventing Weight Gain and Obesity* (May 2006) is available at http://www.keystone.org/spp/documents/ forum_

Box 10.2 Politics

Politics is who gets what, when and how.

Source: Lasswell, H. *Politics: Who Gets What, When and How.* New York: McGraw-Hill, 1936.

---

report_fINAL_5-30-06.pdf. The text of S. 3484 is available at: http://thomas.loc.gov/cgi-bin/query/z?c109:S.3484.IS.

10.2 TYPES OF FOOD AND NUTRITION POLICY

Food and nutrition policy may take the form of a law, a rule or regulation (interpreting law), a practice, a plan (for a course of action), or even a statement. Examples of the various types of policy are illustrated here.

- *Policy statement*: The *Dietary Guidelines for Americans*
- *Comprehensive action plans*: *Healthy People 2010:* Understanding and Improving Health and the HealthierUS Initiative.
- *Law:* The Food Allergen Labeling and Consumer Protection Act of 2004 (FALCPA)[13]
- *Local policies:*[14] School food is controlled by local wellness policies, required in all schools that participate in the federal food program.
- *Federal regulation*: FDA regulates nutrient fortification of foods.

10.2.1 THE *DIETARY GUIDELINES FOR AMERICANS*

The *Dietary Guidelines* are literally a set of guidelines that form the basis for carrying out food, nutrition, and health programs. The sixth edition of the guidelines was released in 2005.[15] Whereas the *Dietary Guidelines* are not themselves a law, but rather a statement of the nation's nutrition policy, Public Law 101–445, Title III, 7 U.S.C. 5301 *et seq.* requires that a panel of experts be chosen every 5 years to review them (see Box 10.3). This panel examines the scientific literature that has been published since the last review and, if necessary, recommends updates to the guidelines. The law also requires the Secretaries of the USDA and HHS to review all federal dietary guidance-related publications for the general public. Table 10.1 provides a chronology for the development of the 2005 *Dietary Guidelines.*[16]

Box 10.3 Public Law 101–445

Public Law 101–445, Section 301 (7 U.S.C. 5341) directs the Secretaries of the U.S. Departments of Agriculture (USDA) and Health and Human Services (HHS) to issue at least every 5 years a joint report entitled *Dietary Guidelines for Americans*. The law instructs that this publication contain nutritional and dietary information and guidelines for the general public, be based on the preponderance of scientific and medical knowledge current at the time of publication, and be promoted by each federal agency in carrying out any federal food, nutrition, or health program. Issued voluntarily by USDA and HHS in 1980, 1985, and 1990, the 1995 edition was the first statutorily mandated report.

Source: USDA. Departmental Regulation No. 1042-128. September 23, 1999. Subject: Dietary Guidelines Advisory Committee. OPI: Agricultural Research Service. Available at: http://www.ocio.usda.gov/directives/files/dr/DR1042-128.htm. Accessed June 23, 2006.

TABLE 10.1
Development of the 2005 Dietary Guidelines — A Chronology

September 2003	The U.S. Department of Health and Human Services (HHS) and the U.S. Department of Agriculture (USDA) publish in the Federal Register the official notice of the first meeting of the Dietary Guidelines Advisory Committee (DGAC) and solicit written comments on the review of the Dietary Guidelines for Americans.
September 2003	The advisory committee holds its first meeting.
December 2003	HHS and USDA provide notice of the second meeting of the committee, and request oral testimony and written comments.
January 2004	The DGAC meets to consider issues including energy balance, fatty acids, nutrient adequacy, food safety, and alcohol.
March 2004	The DGAC meets to consider issues including energy balance, physical activity, and fluids and electrolytes.
May 2004	The DGAC meets and formulates major conclusions regarding food choices, energy balance, fats, fruits and vegetables, whole grains, and dairy.
August 2004	The DGAC meets and formulates major conclusions regarding energy balance, carbohydrates, fats, selected fluids and electrolytes, alcohol, selected food groups, discretionary calories, and food safety.
August 2004	The DGAC report is published in the Federal Register. Public comment period begins.
September 2004	Oral comments from the public are presented at HHS headquarters in Washington, D.C., and public comments are reviewed.
Fall/Winter 2004	HHS and USDA conduct internal scientific review of the advisory committee's report.
January 2005	Release of The *2005 Dietary Guidelines for Americans*.

Source: U.S. Department of Health and Human Services and U.S. Department of Agriculture. *Dietary Guidelines for Americans 2005*. Development of the 2005 Dietary Guidelines — A Chronology. Available at: www.health.gov/dietary guidelines/dga2005/chronology.htm. Accessed June 13, 2006.

The Dietary Guidelines are intended primarily for use by policymakers, healthcare providers, nutritionists, and nutrition educators. In particular, the information in the guidelines is useful for developing educational materials, aiding policymakers in designing and implementing nutrition-related programs, and improving the regulation of food by providing guidance for the inclusion of health claims and nutrient content claims on food labels.

10.2.2 THE HEALTHY PEOPLE INITIATIVE

Healthy People 2010[17], released in 2000, is a roadmap for improving the health of all people in the U.S. during the first decade of the 21st century. It presents a comprehensive, nationwide health promotion and disease-prevention agenda, focusing on desired outcomes, such as increasing the proportion of worksites that offer nutrition or weight management classes or counseling, or increasing food security among U.S. households. Box 10.4 lists the *Healthy People 2010* objectives for Focus Area 19: Nutrition and Overweight. Box 10.5 contains food- and nutrition-related objectives from four additional focus areas: diabetes (area 5); food safety (area10); heart disease and stroke (area 12); and maternal, infant, and child care (area 16).

Box 10.4 *Healthy People 2010*, Nutrition and Overweight Objectives, Focus Area 19

Weight Status and Growth

19-1. Increase the proportion of adults who are at a healthy weight. Target: 60%.
Baseline: 42% of adults aged 20 years and older were at a healthy weight (defined as a

body mass index [BMI] equal to or greater than 18.5 and less than 25) in 1988–1994 (age adjusted to the year 2000 standard population). Data source: NHANES

19-2. Reduce the proportion of adults who are obese. Target: 15%. Baseline: 23% of adults aged 20 years and older were identified as obese (defined as a BMI of 30 or more) in 1988–1994 (age adjusted to the year 2000 standard population). Data source: NHANES

19-3. Reduce the proportion of children and adolescents who are overweight or obese.

Target and baseline:

Objective	Reduction in Overweight or Obese Children and Adolescents*	1988–1994 Baseline %	2010 Target %
19-3a.	Children aged 6 to 11 years	11	5
19-3b.	Adolescents aged 12 to 19 years	11	5
19-3c.	Children and adolescents aged 6 to 19 years	11	5

*Defined as at or above the gender- and age-specific 95th percentile of BMI based on the revised CDC growth charts for the U.S. *Data source:* NHANES.

19-4. Reduce growth retardation among low-income children under age 5 years. Target: 4%. Baseline: 6% of low-income children under age 5 years were growth retarded in 1997 (defined as height for age below the 5th percentile in the age-gender appropriate population using the 2000 CDC growth charts; preliminary data; not age adjusted). Data source: PedNSS

Food and Nutrient Consumption

19-5. Increase the proportion of persons aged 2 years and older who consume at least 2 daily servings of fruit. Target: 75%. Baseline: 28% of persons aged 2 years and older consumed at least 2 daily servings of fruit in 1994–1996 (age adjusted to the year 2000 standard population). Data source: CSFII (2-day average)

19-6. Increase the proportion of persons aged 2 years and older who consume at least 3 daily servings of vegetables, with at least being dark green or orange vegetables. Target: 50%. Baseline: 3% of persons aged 2 years and older consumed at least three daily servings of vegetables, with at least of these servings being dark green or orange vegetables in 1994–1996 (age adjusted to the year 2000 standard population). Data source: CSFII (2-d average)

19-7. Increase the proportion of persons aged 2 years and older who consume at least 6 daily servings of grain products, with at least 3 being whole grains. Target: 50%. Baseline: 7% of persons aged 2 years and older consumed at least 6 daily servings of grain products, with at least 3 being whole grains in 1994–1996 (age adjusted to the year 2000 standard population). Data source: CSFII (2-day average)

19-8. Increase the proportion of persons aged 2 years and older who consume less than 10% of calories from saturated fat. Target: 75%. Baseline: 36% of persons aged 2 years and older consumed less than 10% of daily calories from saturated fat in 1994–1996 (age adjusted to the year 2000 standard population). Data source: CSFII (2-d average)

19-9. Increase the proportion of persons aged 2 years and older who consume no more than 30% of calories from total fat. Target: 75%. Baseline: 33% of persons aged 2 years and older consumed no more than 30% of daily calories from total fat in 1994–1996 (age adjusted to the year 2000 standard population). Data source: CSFII (2-d average)

19-10. Increase the proportion of persons aged 2 years and older who consume 2400 mg or less of sodium daily. Target: 65%. Baseline: 21% of persons aged 2 years and older consumed 2,400 mg or less of sodium daily (from foods, dietary supplements, tap water, and salt use at the table) in 1988–1994 (age adjusted to the year 2000 standard population). Data source: NHANES

19-11. Increase the proportion of persons aged 2 years and older who meet dietary recommendations for calcium. Target: 74%. Baseline: 45% of persons aged 2 years and older were at or above approximated mean calcium requirements (based on consideration of calcium from foods, dietary supplements, and antacids) in 1988–1994 (age adjusted to the year 2000 standard population). Data source: NHANES

Iron Deficiency and Anemia

19-12. Reduce iron deficiency among young children and females of childbearing age. Target and baseline:

Objective	Reduction in Iron Deficiency (iron deficiency is defined as having abnormal results for two or more of the following tests: serum ferritin concentration, erythrocyte protoporphyrin, or transferrin saturation.)	1988–1994 Baseline	2010 Target
		%	
19-12a.	Children aged 1–2 years	9	5
19-12b.	Children aged 3–4 years	4	1
19-12c.	Nonpregnant females aged 12–49 years	11	7

Data source: NHANES

19-13. Reduce anemia among low-income pregnant females in their third trimester. Target: 20%. Baseline: 29% of low-income pregnant females in their third trimester were anemic (defined as hemoglobin < 11.0 g/dL) in 1996. Data source: PedNSS

19-14. (Developmental) Reduce iron deficiency among pregnant females. Potential data source: NHANES

Schools, Worksites, and Nutrition Counseling

19-15. (Developmental) Increase the proportion of children and adolescents aged 6 to 19 years whose intake of meals and snacks at school contributes to good overall dietary quality. This objective was proposed for deletion due to lack of a suitable data source that would provide at least two sets of nationally representative estimates this decade. Ten comments were received in response to the proposal to delete this objective. All the submissions, including one from the American Dietetic Association, agreed that the objective should be retained in one form or another.

19-16. Increase the proportion of worksites that offer nutrition or weight management classes or counseling. Target: 84%. Baseline: 54% of worksites with 50 or more employees offered nutrition or weight management classes or counseling at the worksite or through their health plans in 1998–1999. Data source: NWHPS

19-17. Increase the proportion of physician office visits made by patients with a diagnosis of cardiovascular disease, diabetes, or hyperlipidemia that include counseling or education related to diet and nutrition. Target: 75%. Baseline: 42% of physician office visits made by patients with a diagnosis of cardiovascular disease, diabetes, or hyperlipidemia included ordering or providing counseling or education on diet and nutrition in 1997 (age adjusted to the year 2000 standard population). Data source: NAMCS

Food Security

19-18. Increase food security among U.S. households and in so doing reduce hunger. Target: 94%. Baseline: 88% of all U.S. households were food secure in 1995. Target setting method: 6% age point improvement (50% decrease in food insecurity; consistent with the U.S. pledge to the 1996 World Food Summit). Data source: Food Security Supplement to the Current Population Survey (from the Bureau of the Census in the U.S. Department of Commerce)

Source: All 10 written submissions are available on the Healthy People 2010 Midcourse Review page at: http://www. healthypeople.gov/data/midcourse/comments/reports/viewobjective.asp?oldTopicID=19&TopicID=19&SubopicID= 113&submit1=Submit. Accessed June 20, 2006.

Box 10.5 *Healthy People 2010*, Food and Nutrition Related Objectives in the Areas of Diabetes, Food Safety, Heart Disease and Stroke, and Maternal, Infant, and Child Care

Diabetes. Goal: Through prevention programs, reduce the disease and economic burden of diabetes, and improve the quality of life for all persons who have or are at risk for diabetes.

- 5-1. Increase to 60% the proportion of persons with diabetes who receive formal diabetes education. In 1998, 45% of persons with diabetes received formal diabetes education (age adjusted to the year 2000 standard population).
- 5-2. Prevent diabetes by decreasing to 3.8 new cases per 1000 population per year. In 1997–1999, there were 5.5 new cases of diabetes per 1000 population aged 18 to 84 years (3-year average; age adjusted to the year 2000 standard population).
- 5-3. Reduce to 25 cases per 1000 population the overall rate of diabetes that is clinically diagnosed. In 1997, 40 overall cases (including new and existing cases) of diabetes per 1000 population occurred (age adjusted to the year 2000 standard population).

Food Safety. Goal: Reduce foodborne illnesses.

- 10-1. Reduce by 50% infections caused by key foodborne pathogens.
- 10-4. Reduce deaths caused by food allergies.
- 10-5. Increase from 72% to 79% the proportion of consumers who follow key food safety practices.
- 10-6. Improve by 25% food employee behaviors and food preparation practices that directly relate to foodborne illnesses in retail food establishments.

Heart Disease and Stroke. Goal: Improve cardiovascular health and quality of life through the prevention, detection, and treatment of risk factors, and prevention of recurrent cardiovascular events.

- 12-9. Reduce to 16% the proportion of adults with high blood pressure. 28% of adults aged 20 years and older had high blood pressure in 1988–1994 (age adjusted to the year 2000 standard population).
- 12-11. Increase to 95% the proportion of adults with high blood pressure who are taking action (for example, losing weight, increasing physical activity, or reducing sodium intake) to help control their blood pressure. In 1998, 82% of adults aged 18 years and older with high blood pressure were taking action to control it (age adjusted to the year 2000 standard population).
- 12-15. Increase to 80% the proportion of adults who have had their blood cholesterol checked within the preceding 5 years. In 1998, 67% of adults aged 18 years and older had their blood cholesterol checked within the preceding 5 years (age adjusted to the year 2000 standard population).
- Increase to 75% the proportion of worksites with 50 or more employees that offer a comprehensive employee health promotion program to their employees.

Maternal, Infant, and Child Health. Goal: Improve the health and well-being of women, infants, children, and families.

- 16-6. Increase to 90% the proportion of pregnant women who receive early and adequate prenatal care. Baseline: 74%
- 16-10. Reduce low birth weight (LBW) and very low birth weight (VLBW) to 5% and 0.9%, respectively. Baseline: 7.6 and 1.4%, respectively.
- 16-15. Reduce by 50% to 3 new cases per 10,000 live births the occurrence of spina bifida and other neural tube defects (NTDs). 1996 Baseline: 6/100,000
- 16-16a. Increase to 80% the proportion of pregnancies begun with an optimum folic acid level (consumption of at least 400 µg folic acid). Baseline 1991–1994: 21%.
- 16-17. Increase abstinence to 94%, 100%, 99%, and 100% from alcohol, cigarettes, and illicit drugs, respectively, among pregnant women. Baseline 1996–1997: 86%, 99%, 87% (1998) and 98%, respectively.
- 16-18. Reduce the occurrence of fetal alcohol syndrome (FAS). Estimates of the cases of FAS vary from 0.2 to 1.0 per 1000 live births. CDC studies have documented FAS prevalence rates ranging from 0.2 to 1.5/1000 live births. (developmental)
- 16-19. Increase the proportion of mothers who breastfeed their babies in the early post partum period, at 6 months, and at 1 year to 75%, 50%, and 25%, respectively. 1999 baseline: 64%, 29%, and 16%, respectively.

Source: Weber, M.K., Floyd, R.L., Riley, E.D., and Snider, D.E. National Task Force on Fetal Alcohol Syndrome and Fetal Alcohol Effect. Defining the National Agenda for Fetal Alcohol Syndrome and Other Prenatal Alcohol-Related Effects. *MMWR.* 51(RR14), 9–12, 2002. Available at: http://www.cdc.gov/mmwr/preview/mmwrhtml/rr5114a2.htm. Accessed June 20, 2006.

Since 1979, DHHS has supported a nationwide effort to formulate and monitor national disease prevention and health promotion objectives The Healthy People initiative is at the forefront of this agenda.[18]

10.2.2.1 Origins: 1979–1990

The Healthy People initiative began in 1979 with *Healthy People: The Surgeon General's Report on Health Promotion and Disease Prevention*.[19] The report contained general goals for reducing preventable death and injury in different age groups by the year 1990. Healthy People was a landmark in the history of public health, as it presented for the first time a national public health agenda developed as a consensus among the health community. In 1980, a companion piece — *Promoting Health/Preventing Disease: Objectives for the Nation*[20] — set forth 226 measurable health objectives organized into 15 strategic areas. These objectives, referred to as "the 1990 health objectives," called for improvements in health status, risk reduction, public and professional awareness, health services and protective measures, and surveillance and evaluation. These companion reports served as the blueprint for future decennial health priorities.

10.2.2.2 *Healthy People 2000*

In 1990, DHHS published *Healthy People 2000*,[21] which established three overarching goals and grew to 319 objectives in 22 priority areas. The Healthy People 2000 goals were to (1) increase the span of healthy life, (2) reduce health disparities, and (3) provide access to preventive health services. (See Box 10.6.)

Box 10.6 Government Policies and Funding Priorities

One way a government indicates its policies is through its funding priorities and to this end, one way the U.S. manifests its health agenda is by requiring that the National Institutes of Health within the Public Health Service support only projects that address one or more *Healthy People 2010* objectives. Therefore, every program announcement (PA), request for proposals (RFP), and request for applications (RFA) the NIH publishes contains a statement such as this:

The Public Health Service (PHS) is committed to achieving the health promotion and disease prevention objectives of *Healthy People 2010,* a PHS-led national activity for setting priority areas. This PA is related to one or more of the priority areas. Potential applicants may obtain a copy of *Healthy People 2010* at http://www.health.gov/healthypeople.

10.2.2.3 *Healthy People 2010*

Building on the experiences of the first two decades of objectives, on public hearings, and on a public comment process that generated more than 11,000 public comments, in January 2000, DHHS issued *Healthy People 2010,* the third generation of 10-year disease prevention and health promotion objectives for the nation. *Healthy People 2010* is a comprehensive set of national health objectives, based on scientific evidence, for the first decade of the 21st century. It identifies two overarching goals — to increase the quality and years of healthy life, and to eliminate health disparities — amplified by 467 objectives in 28 focus areas.[22-23]

DATA 2010 is the data system used to track all the 467 Healthy People objectives. Data on each objective in all the 28 focus areas are available, as well as data on specific population groups. Updates are made quarterly. DATA 2010 also includes data on specific objectives related to the Steps to a HealthierUS initiative (see Section 10.2.3).[24] (See Box 10.7.)

10.2.2.4 Midcourse Review

Each decennial edition of Healthy People is subject to a midcourse review to assess the status of the objectives. Through this review, DHHS, other federal agencies, and subject matter experts assess the data trends during the first half of the decade, consider new science and available data, and make changes to ensure that Healthy People remains current, accurate, and relevant, while simultaneously assessing emerging public health priorities.[25]

Through the *Healthy People 2010* Midcourse Review, the lead agencies for the 28 *Healthy People 2010* focus areas proposed revisions to the agenda, made available for public review and comment. The Office of Disease Prevention and Health Promotion (ODPHP) within the Office of the Public Health Service served as the overall coordinator for the dissemination and processing of public comments. The public was invited to comment on the proposed deletion of the objectives and subobjectives listed below which, except where indicated, lacked data sources. (See Box 10.8.)

Box 10.7 The Nation's Progress

Many of the nutrition and overweight (focus area 19) objectives in *Healthy People 2010* measure the nation's progress in implementing the recommendations of the *Dietary Guidelines for Americans.*

Box 10.8 Midcourse Review Comments

It is instructive to read the comments submitted by the public as part of the midcourse review of *Healthy People 2010*. The comments are posted on the Midcourse Review Web site: www.healthypeople.gov/data/midcourse/default.asp.

- 5-8: Gestational diabetes. Decrease the proportion of pregnant women with gestational diabetes (developmental objective).
- 7-11j: Increase the proportion of local health departments that have established culturally appropriate and linguistically competent community health promotion and disease prevention programs in food safety.
- 10-1e and 10-1g: Reduce infections caused by (10-1e) *Cyclospora cayetanensis* and by (10-1g) congenital *Toxoplasma gondii* (proposed for deletion due to change in science).
- 19-15: Meals and snacks at school. Increase the proportion of children and adolescents aged 6 to 19 years whose intake of meals and snacks at school contributes to good overall dietary quality (developmental objective).

Objective 19-15 is proposed for deletion because no data source can provide at least two sets of nationally representative estimates for evaluation. ODPHP received 10 letters in response to the proposal to delete the objective. Some respondents suggested that the objective be reworded; all agreed that *Healthy People 2010* should contain an objective that addresses meals and snacks at school. The American Dietetic Association (ADA) was one of the responders, offering two alternatives to deleting the objective.

As a first choice, ADA suggested rewording Objective 19-15 to shift the focus from individual intake to school or district level measures. One possible objective would be, "Increase the proportion of school districts that promote healthy options for all foods sold on the school campus throughout the day." A data source for this objective is the School Health Policies and Programs Study (SHPPS),[26] a national survey that collects data on school health policies and programs at the state, district, school, and classroom levels. Two sets of nationally representative estimates will be available: 2000 data to serve as a baseline and 2006 data for comparison. Alternatively, if DHHS proceeds with deleting Objective 19-15, then ADA suggests that the department address the school nutrition environment in a companion document or white paper.

Similarly, another respondent suggested rewording the objective to: "Reduce sweetened beverage consumption at school among children and adolescents aged 5 to 9 years," using Continuing Survey of Food Intake of Individuals/National Health and Nutrition Examination Survey (CSFII/NHANES) data for monitoring.

The 2010 midcourse review, released in 2006, features revisions and a status report on progress from 2000 to 2005 toward achieving the targets for the year 2010.

10.2.3 THE PRESIDENT'S HEALTHIERUS INITIATIVE

Another comprehensive, nationwide health promotion and disease prevention agenda is the Healthier US initiative, launched by President Bush in 2002 "to help Americans live longer, better, and healthier lives."[27] As such, its goal is indistinguishable from the first of the two overarching goals of *Healthy People 2010*, which is "to increase quality and years of healthy life." Despite their similar goals, these two broad initiatives differ in scope. Healthy People presents a comprehensive nationwide health promotion and disease prevention agenda for the first decade of the 21st century. It includes family planning (objective 9), HIV (objective 13), immunizations and infectious diseases (objective 14), injury and violence prevention (objective 15), and vision and hearing (objective 28).

Box 10.9 *Healthy People 2010* and the HealthierUS Initiative

Healthy People 2010 and the HealthierUS Initiative represent comprehensive action plans developed by the U.S. Department of Health and Human Services. Both plans focus on health promotion, and primary and secondary prevention.

Source: Healthier US. Available at: http://www.whitehouse.gov/infocus/fitness/. Accessed June 24, 2005.

In contrast, HealthierUS focuses on health promotion through four key prevention objectives: increased physical activity, responsible dietary habits, increased use of preventive health screenings, and healthy choices concerning alcohol, tobacco, drugs, and safety.

10.2.3.1 Steps to a HealthierUS Initiative

Steps to a HealthierUS[29] is the DHHS component of the HealthierUS initiative. As its name implies, Steps is concerned with decreasing the burden of chronic disease by identifying and promoting programs that encourage small behavior changes. (See Box 10.9.)

At the heart of the Steps initiative lie both *personal responsibility* for the choices Americans make and *social responsibility* to ensure that policymakers support programs that foster healthy behaviors and prevention.[30] Steps works through public–private partnerships at the community level to support community-based programs. These programs seek the full engagement of schools, businesses, faith-communities, healthcare purchasers and providers, health plans, academic institutions, senior centers, and many other community sectors.

In FY 2003 and FY 2004, NCCDPHP (under the aegis of CDC within DHHS) allocated almost $50 million to 40 demonstration programs in states, cities, and tribal entities throughout the U.S. These programs implemented chronic disease prevention efforts focused on reducing the burden of diabetes, overweight, obesity, and asthma by addressing three related risk factors — physical inactivity, poor nutrition, and tobacco use. Diabetes, asthma, overweight, and obesity were chosen as targets because of their rapidly increasing prevalence in the U.S. and the ability for individuals to control and even prevent these diseases through exercise, diet, and other strategies. One of the major focuses of this funding program is to design, test, and disseminate effective prevention research strategies. Measurable outcomes of the program include supporting prevention research to develop sustainable and transferable community-based behavioral interventions.

10.2.3.2 SmallStep.gov

In keeping with its goal to strengthen individual knowledge and skills and capitalizing on the power of the Internet, DHHS has developed an information program called SmallStep.gov,[31] which offers separate online sites targeting adults, children, and educators. The adult site offers strategies, such as "100 small steps," for making individual lifestyle and behavior changes. An interactive component allows the participant to e-mail small step reminders to friends and relatives and provides information about linking up with community programs funded by the Steps to a HealthierUS program. SmallStep KIDS provides interactive activities for young children. The educator's site offers a language arts and math curriculum for second through fourth grade students with materials that focus on health and fitness.

10.2.4 FEDERAL ACTION STEPS

The USDA's Food and Nutrition Service (FNS) works with other federal agencies to coordinate the federal government's efforts in promoting healthy eating and active lifestyles. One of the first actions in HealthierUS was the signing of the three memoranda of understanding (MOUs) among federal agencies detailed below.

- *Partnership to improve nutrition, physical activity and health of the nation's children.* The Department of Education (ED), USDA, and DHHS are working together to expand school-based efforts to help children and young people develop healthy eating and physical activity skills.
- *Promoting public health and recreation.* The Department of the Interior, the Army, USDA, and DHHS work in concert to promote healthy lifestyles through sound nutrition, physical activity, and recreation in America's great outdoors.
- *Promoting the consumption of fruits and vegetables: The 5 A Day Program.* USDA and DHHS are developing a general framework for enhancing and more effectively coordinating the national 5 A Day for Better Health Program, whose goal is to increase fruit and vegetable consumption to 5 to 9 servings per day.

10.2.5 STATE AND LOCAL ACTION STEPS

On the local level, a goal of Steps is to expand community efforts and effective strategies for building private–public collaborations to support disease prevention, preparedness, and health promotion. From the standpoint of pubic health nutrition, three of the most important goals of the initiative are: (1) to encourage state and local governments and the private sector to promote health and wellness programs at schools and work sites and other community-based settings, including faith-based organizations; (2) to educate the public effectively about their health; and (3) to enact policies that promote healthy environments.[32]

Promoting wellness at work,[33] in schools,[34] and in community-based settings is an important step in helping people to help themselves. Education and social support can induce people to take charge of their health. Examples of such initiatives include physical activity strategies such as motivational signs and reminders placed near elevators and escalators encouraging the use of stairs for health benefits or weight loss;[35] school health programs that provide environments and instruction that promote healthy eating and daily physical activity, such as the HealthierUS School Challenge;[36] and community-based programs that bring together health advisors, nurses, nutritionists, and representatives of faith-based organizations to support, encourage, and help people obtain the information they need for health promotion, and primary and secondary disease prevention.

Policy and environmental changes can affect large segments of the population simultaneously. People are more likely to adopt healthy behaviors when supportive community norms and health policies are in place, such as safe walking and cycling trails, including a safe walk to school program such as the Walking School Bus[37] and the CDC's KidsWalk-to-School initiative[38] (see Box 7.3); incentives to schools to increase physical education; low-fat/high-fruit-and-vegetable menu selections in restaurants, schools, and employee cafeterias; and menu labeling in chain restaurants. See Box 10.10 for a discussion of the ecological approach to public health.

10.2.6 HEALTHIERUS SCHOOL CHALLENGE

In 2004, the Secretary of Agriculture launched the HealthierUS School Challenge. This federal-level strategy provides incentives to increase participation in the National School Lunch Program and to address the problems of childhood overweight and obesity. As its name implies, the HealthierUS School Challenge is an extension of HealthierUS (Section 10.2.3), which encourages all Americans to eat a nutritious diet and become physically active each day.

The HealthierUS School Challenge recognizes K-12 schools that meet voluntary nutrition and physical activity standards established by the USDA's FNS at two levels of accomplishment (gold and sliver). The program was designed to build upon the USDA's Team Nutrition program. To be

Box 10.10 An Ecological Approach

Behavior change is more likely to endure when a person's environment also changes in a manner that supports the behavior change, requiring public health practitioners to move beyond a strictly educational approach to broader efforts that produce environmental change. Interventions should address not only the intentions and skills of individuals, but also their social and physical environments, including the social networks and organizations that affect them.[1] The "spectrum of prevention" is a paradigm that promotes a multifaceted range of activities for effective prevention. It consists of six levels of increasing scope, beginning with a focus on the individual and family, on community norms, institutional practices, and finally laws. The specific activity levels included in the spectrum are:

- Strengthening individual knowledge and skills
- Promoting community education
- Educating providers
- Fostering coalitions and networks
- Changing organizational practices
- Influencing policy and legislation

The levels are complementary and, when used together, result in greater effectiveness than would be possible by implementing just any single activity. The spectrum assists practitioners and community-based organizations develop comprehensive, multifaceted prevention initiatives that result in environmental and norms change.[2] The spectrum paradigm provides the basis for the HealthierUS Initiative.

Sources:

[1] U.S. Department of Health and Human Services. The Power of Prevention. 2003. Available at: http://www.healthierus.gov/steps/summit/prevportfolio/power/index.html#meeting. Accessed June 27, 2005.

[2] Cohen, L. and Swift, S. The spectrum of prevention: developing a comprehensive approach to injury prevention. *Injury Prev.* 5, 203–207, 1999. Available at: http://www.preventioninstitute.org/spectrum_injury.html. Accessed June 27, 2005.

recognized by the HealthierUS School Challenge, schools must enroll in Team Nutrition and then meet higher standards than those required by the National School Lunch Program. Schools that meet the challenge are awarded a plaque and the school name is posted on the Team Nutrition Web site to showcase their success and encourage others to follow their lead (see Box 10.11).

Box 10.11 Team Nutrition

To be designated a Team Nutrition school, the administration of a school that participates in the National School Lunch Program must support the USDA's Team Nutrition goal and values; demonstrate a commitment to help students meet the Dietary Guidelines for Americans; designate a Team Nutrition School Leader who will establish a school team; distribute Team Nutrition materials to teachers, students, and parents; involve teachers, students, parents, food service personnel, and the community in interactive and entertaining nutrition education activities; demonstrate a well-run Child Nutrition Program; and share their successful strategies and programs with other schools. Team Nutrition provides schools with nutrition education materials for children and families; technical assistance materials for school food service directors, managers and staff; and materials to build school and community support for healthy eating and physical activity.

To attain silver certification, schools must serve National School Lunch Program meals that meet nutritional standards, offer nutrition education, maintain National School Lunch participation above the national average, offer physical activity for students, and ensure that all foods offered throughout the school meet healthy standards as outlined in the Dietary Guidelines for Americans. Gold certification is awarded to schools that meet the silver criteria and serve or sell only food that meets healthy standards during the day if the food is not already included in school meals. School lunches must include a fresh fruit or raw vegetable, a whole grain product, and low- or nonfat milk every day.

10.2.7 LOCAL WELLNESS POLICY

The Child Nutrition and WIC Reauthorization Act of 2004 (P.L. 108–265, Sec. 204) requires that each local educational agency participating in a federal school food program develop and implement a local wellness policy.[39] This legislation, which supports the HealthierUS initiative, formalizes it and encourages schools to promote student health, including preventing obesity and combating problems associated with poor nutrition and physical inactivity. The legislation places the locus of responsibility for developing a wellness policy at the local level. This policy is endorsed by the Department of Education (ED) as well as DHHS and USDA.

10.2.7.1 Components of a Local Wellness Policy

At a minimum, the local wellness policy must include these components:

1. Goals for nutrition education, physical activity, and other school-based activities designed to promote student wellness
2. Nutrition guidelines for all foods available on each school campus during the school day, with the objectives of promoting student health and reducing childhood obesity
3. An assurance that guidelines for reimbursable school meals shall not be less restrictive than regulations and guidance for the USDA's school food programs
4. A plan for evaluating the implementation of the wellness policy, including designating at least one person with operational responsibility for ensuring that the school meets the local wellness policy
5. The involvement of parents, students, the public, and representatives of the school food authority, school board, and school administrators in developing the school wellness policy

10.2.7.2 Assistance

The USDA has been allotted $4 million (July 1, 2006–September 30, 2009) to assist schools in establishing healthy school nutrition environments, reducing childhood obesity, and preventing diet-related chronic diseases. The assistance includes relevant and applicable examples of schools and local educational agencies that have taken steps to offer healthy options for foods sold or served in schools. See Box 10.12 for a summary of strategies for establishing healthy school nutrition environments.

Box 10.12 Strategies to Establish Healthy School Nutrition Environments

The primary approaches being used in schools to promote healthy eating are summarized below. These activities are intended to establish healthy nutrition environments as a normal expectation of schools.

Establish nutrition standards for competitive foods. Nutrition standards list criteria that determine which foods and beverages can and cannot be offered on a school campus. Strategies for establishing nutrition standards include:

- Ensuring that available foods adhere to healthful nutrient and portion size specifications.
- Prohibiting the use of "foods of minimal nutritional value" (for example, soft drinks, gum, and some candies) in schools or as fund-raisers.
- Adopting a "fruits and vegetables only" snack policy for snacks brought from home.
- Instituting nutrition standards as part of a comprehensive nutrition policy. Such policies may address nutrition education, healthy school nutrition environments, staff development on nutrition, parent and community involvement, and school-based screening, counseling, and referrals for nutrition.

Influence food and beverage contracts. Food and beverage contracts give vendors selling rights in return for cash and noncash benefits to the school or district. Schools and school districts can influence vending contracts by canceling them, not signing them, not renewing them, or negotiating contracts that promote healthful eating. Strategies for influencing food and beverage contracts include:

- Transferring the management of vending machines to the school food service program, giving it the opportunity to improve the nutritional quality and increase revenue without external contracts.
- Improving the nutritional quality of beverages available under an existing contract.
- Writing an RFP for vending that pays a higher commission to the district for healthful beverages, increases the percentage of healthful items available, and charges a lower price for the healthier beverages.

Make more healthful foods and beverages available. Making available more healthful foods and beverages enables students to choose healthful food. Healthful foods and beverages can be added wherever food is available, including à la carte lines, vending machines, snack bars, student stores, concession stands at extracurricular events, and school parties. A wide variety of healthful food and beverage choices exists, including: water, 100% fruit juices, fresh fruit and vegetables, yogurt (reduced fat and lowfat), cheese (reduced fat), milk (lowfat and skim), vegetable salads, fruit salads, whole grain breads and crackers, unsalted dry-roasted nuts, air-popped popcorn, dried fruit, and fruit smoothies. At the same time, it is important to remove items such as candy, soft drinks, sweetened drinks, fried chips, deep fried foods, and snack cakes.

Adopt marketing techniques to promote healthful choices. Schools can promote the consumption of healthful foods and beverages by using the principles of social marketing discussed in Chapter 14: (1) identify and offer healthful *products* that are appealing and meet student needs, (2) use product *placement* to make healthful products easy to choose, (3) use promotion strategies so that students know about these products and are motivated to try them, and (4) set their *price* at a level that encourages students to purchase them. Schools and school districts may adopt a variety of marketing techniques, such as:

- Conduct surveys to determine student opinions about healthful products.
- Offer samples of potential items to assess student response.
- Install state-of-the-art vending machines and place them in high traffic locations.
- Place healthier items in vending machines at eye level and less healthful items on the bottom row.
- Involve students and staff in promotional activities using signs, contests, games, health fairs, advertisements, flyers, banners, and other means.
- Price healthful foods lower than the less healthful items.

Limit student access to competitive foods. Limiting access means making it more difficult for students to obtain competitive foods or beverages sold outside of federal meal programs. Schools can limit access by reducing the number of places where students can obtain the foods, changing the location where food is sold so it is less accessible, or prohibiting the sale of foods and beverages at certain times during the school day. Currently, federal regulations only require that schools prohibit access to "foods of minimal nutritional value" in food service areas during meal times, but states are adopting stricter regulations. Access to less desirable food choices can be limited in a number of ways, such as:

- Limit the number of snacks that elementary students can purchase.
- Reduce the portion size of dessert items.
- Reduce the number of soft drink vending machines.
- End student access to "foods of minimal nutritional value" in all school locations throughout the school day.
- Have vending-machine free elementary schools.

Use fundraising activities and rewards that support student health. Fundraising supports student health when it involves selling nutritious foods and beverages or selling nonfood items. Reward programs support student health when they involve using nonfood items or activities to recognize students for their achievements or good behavior. Schools and districts can implement these healthy alternatives:

- Reward students by organizing walks with the principal rather than holding pizza parties.
- Sell fruit and gift wrap rather than candy or nonnutritious items as a fundraiser.
- Add juice, water, cheese trays, and fresh fruit and vegetable trays to classroom parties, and remove soft drinks and chips.
- Switch from selling items from a candy cart to selling items from a breakfast cart to raise money for a school student council.

Source: Food and Nutrition Service, U.S. Department of Agriculture; Centers for Disease Control and Prevention, U.S. Department of Health and Human Services; and U.S. Department of Education. FNS-374, Making It Happen! School Nutrition Success Stories. Alexandria, VA, January 2005. Available at: http://teamnutrition.usda.gov/ Resources/ makingithappen.html. Accessed June 29, 2006.

10.2.8 Team Nutrition

Team Nutrition is an initiative of FNS within USDA to support the Child Nutrition programs through training and technical assistance for food service, nutrition education for children and their caregivers, and school and community support for healthy eating and physical activity. (See Box 10.13.) Team Nutrition supplies assistance in developing, implementing, and evaluating local wellness policies.

In 2006, Team Nutrition training grants were authorized at $4 million in funding by P.L. 109–97; approximately $2 million was used in support of four Team Nutrition Local Wellness Demonstration Projects for a period of 3 years (2006–2009). State agencies were given 2 months

---

Box 10.13 Team Nutrition's Goals

One of Team Nutrition's goals for 2006 was to provide support for healthy eating and physical activity by involving school administrators and other school and community partners.

(from March 16th through May 11th) to complete the applications. Rewards were announced at the beginning of September, with funds available for implementation of the projects starting September 30th.

The Team Nutrition Local Wellness Demonstration Projects provided states with the opportunity to:

- Assess local wellness policy activities in individual districts or local educational agencies (LEA).
- Document the processes used by LEAs to develop, implement, and measure the implementation of a local wellness policy.
- Assess the level and types of technical assistance necessary at the state level.
- Document any school environmental changes.
- Assist FNS in developing a Team Nutrition technical assistance guide to assist other states and LEAs in implementing and measuring the impact of local wellness policies. This allows FNS, at the conclusion of the project, to assess how well local wellness policies were implemented at the local level and what types of technical assistance and resources are needed at the federal level.

10.2.9 POLICY REGARDING FOOD ALLERGIES

Food allergy is an immunologic disease responsible for substantial morbidity and some mortality in the U.S. population. It occurs in 6 to 8% of children and 2% of adults. Approximately 30,000 anaphylactic episodes and 150 deaths per year are due to food allergy. Published reports document the increasing prevalence of food allergy and food-induced anaphylaxis, but the reasons for these increases are poorly understood. (See also Section 15.1.1.2.3 for additional information on food allergies.)

Six foods (milk, egg, peanuts, tree nuts, fish, and shellfish) cause 90% of all allergic reactions to foods. The most effective strategy to prevent an allergic episode is strict food avoidance. Since its founding, the Food Allergy and Anaphylaxis Network (FAAN) has advocated for simple, clear, and accurate food labels that would allow allergic people to make informed choices about the foods they eat.[40] (See Box 10.14.) Due in part to FAAN's advocacy, the Food Allergen Labeling and

---

Box 10.14 The Food Allergy and Anaphylaxis Network (FAAN)

Founded in 1991 by Anne Muñoz-Furlong, FAAN is the world's largest nonprofit organization providing information about food allergy to the media, schools, health professionals, pharmaceutical companies, the food industry, government officials, and the food-allergic community. Ms. Muñoz-Furlong established the organization because of the lack of information available when her own daughter was diagnosed with milk and egg allergy as an infant. Based in Fairfax, VA, FAAN's mission is to raise public awareness, to provide advocacy and education, and to advance research on behalf of all those affected by food allergies and anaphylaxis. Paid membership is close to 30,000 in the U.S., Canada, and 63 other countries. Members include people who have food allergy, parents of children who have food allergies, school officials, and medical and food industry professionals. FAAN's medical advisory board reviews the materials published by the organization. Of particular interest to nutrition professionals are their materials regarding the following public health topics.

- School guidelines for managing children with food allergies
- College and university guidelines for managing students with food allergies
- Guidelines for managing food allergies at summer camps
- Managing students with food allergy during a shelter-in-place emergency
- Travel tips for flying with a peanut allergy, including a list of airlines that do not serve peanut snacks

---

Box 10.15 The FALCPA

FDA's Food Allergen Labeling and Consumer Protection Act (FALCPA) requires allergens to be listed on food labels in easily understood language.

Consumer Protection Act (FALCPA) was passed in 2004.[41] The law, implemented in 2006, requires the labeling of any food containing a protein derived from one or more of the following: peanuts, soybeans, cow's milk, eggs, fish, crustacean shellfish, tree nuts, and wheat. (See Box 10.15.)

10.2.10 POLICY REGARDING MICRONUTRIENTS

FDA, as a public health agency, is charged with protecting American consumers by enforcing the Federal Food, Drug, and Cosmetic Act and several related public health laws. To carry out this mandate of consumer protection, the FDA has some 1,100 investigators and inspectors who cover the country's almost 95,000 FDA-regulated businesses. These employees are located in district and local offices in 157 cities across the country.

Fortification of the food supply has long been a nutrition policy tool to help meet people's nutrient needs.[42] Fortification is governed by FDA rules. An example of this nutrition policy is the practice of micronutrient fortification of salt, milk, grain products, and water. Although the terms *enrichment* and *fortification* are often used interchangeably to indicate the addition of nutrients to foods, enrichment more accurately refers to nutrient additions based on FDA standards of identity, whereas fortification refers to other voluntary additions of nutrients to foods.[43]

10.2.10.1 Iodization of Salt

Fortification in the U.S. began in 1924 when iodized salt was introduced in Michigan, resulting in a decrease from 38.6 to 9% in the prevalence of goiter in that state. The success of these efforts made the Michigan experience with iodized salt one of the most noteworthy food fortification programs in applied public health in the twentieth century. Between 1924 and 1928, the use of iodized salt spread rapidly throughout the country. Salt manufacturers were eager to produce the iodized product because, from a marketing perspective, it made sense to offer the, literally, new and improved salt. Doing so was an assurance the salt producers would not lag behind the competition.[44] Table salt continues to be available without iodide as well as in the iodized form.

10.2.10.2 Fortification of Milk with Vitamins D and A

In 1921, it was estimated that 75% of infants in New York City were afflicted with rickets. By the 1930s, rickets was recognized a major public health problem in the U.S., particularly in the northeastern states. When a milk fortification program was implemented to combat rickets, it nearly eliminated this disorder in the U.S.

The concentration of vitamin D_3 in cow's milk is roughly 35–80 International Units (IU), rather low from the perspective of the 200–400 IU per day recommended by the Food and Nutrition Board of the Institute of Medicine (IOM). The Adequate Intake (AI) is 5 micrograms or the equivalent of 200 μg from birth through 50 years of age, 10 μg for ages 51 through 70 years, and 15 μg for ages 71 years and above.[45] Accordingly, the practice of supplementing cow's milk with chemically synthesized vitamin D_3 was initiated. At the present time, approximately 98% of all milk sold commercially in the U.S. has 400 IU of chemically synthesized vitamin D_3 added per quart. FDA requires any vendor of milk containing added vitamin D_3 to include a notice on the carton to the effect that the product contains 400 IU of added vitamin D3.[46] Most fat-free milk and dried nonfat milk solids sold in the U.S. are also fortified with vitamin A (a fat-soluble vitamin) to replace the amount lost when the fat is removed from the whole milk.

10.2.11 ENRICHMENT AND FORTIFICATION OF GRAIN PRODUCTS

In 1941, President Franklin D. Roosevelt convened the National Nutrition Conference for Defense, which led to the first recommended dietary allowances of nutrients, and resulted in issuance of War Order Number 1, a program to enrich wheat flour with vitamins and iron.[47] With the end of World War II, the FDA established formal standards of identity for enriched pasta (1946), white bread (1952), corn meal and grits (1955), and white rice (1958).

Folic acid was added to the "enrichment formula" for cereal and other grain products in order to prevent neural tube defects. The FDA introduced mandatory fortification of all grain products with folic acid at a dose of 140 µg per 100 g of grain (about double what was originally attended).[48] The prevalence of low serum folate in the population has decreased from a range of 16 to 22% prior to the fortification program to 0.5 to 1.7% subsequent to fortification.[49]

How long will the fortification of grains with folic acid continue? Vitamin B_{12} deficiency is common in older people, with prevalence increasing from about 5% at 65 years of age to 20% at the age of 80. Clinicians have voiced concern about the safety of elevated intakes of folate in older people who have low vitamin B_{12} status. Such people appear to have a more rapid deterioration of cognitive function in the presence of a high folate intake. This concern has delayed the introduction of mandatory folic acid fortification in the U.K.[50]

10.2.12 WATER

Fluoridation of community drinking water, begun in 1945, is a major contributor to the decline in dental caries (tooth decay) during the second half of the 20th century. The history of water fluoridation is a classic example of clinical observation leading to epidemiologic investigation and community-based public health intervention. Although other fluoride-containing products are available (such as toothpastes, gels, mouth rinses, tablets, and drops), water fluoridation remains the most equitable and cost-effective method of delivering fluoride to most members of most communities regardless of age, educational attainment, or income level. Water fluoridation is especially beneficial for communities of low socioeconomic status, which have a disproportionate burden of dental caries and have less access than higher-income communities to dental-care services and other sources of fluoride. Water fluoridation may help reduce such dental health disparities.

Slightly more than half of the people in the U.S. (56% or 144 million) were receiving fluoridated water in 1992, including 10 million people served by almost 4000 public water systems that have natural fluoride levels greater than or equal to 0.7 ppm. However, approximately 42,000 public water systems and 153 U.S. cities with populations greater than or equal to 50,000 have not instituted fluoridation. There is no universal consensus on the desirability of fluoridating the water supply; concomitant with the decline in dental caries prevalence and incidence in developed countries has been an increase in the prevalence of dental fluorosis.[51]

Since the early days of community water fluoridation, the prevalence of dental caries has declined in communities both with and without fluoridated water in the U.S. This trend has been attributed largely to the diffusion of fluoridated water to areas without fluoridated water through bottling and processing of foods and beverages in areas with fluoridated water as well as the widespread use of fluoride toothpaste.[52] On the other hand, the increased consumption of bottled water, with its variable fluoride content, can lead to a decreased exposure to fluoride among some segments of the population. Solely drinking bottled water may not provide sufficient fluoride to maintain optimal dental health.[53,54,55] FDA requires that fluoride be listed on the label of bottled waters only if the bottler adds fluoride during processing; the concentration of fluoride is regulated but does not have to be stated on the label. Few bottled water brands have labels listing the fluoride concentration.[56]

10.2.13 POLICY REGARDING DOMESTIC HUNGER

The federal government initially responded to hunger among the low-income U.S. population during the Depression. Interest waned during the Second World War and the Korean War. In the 1960s, the federal government was again forced to acknowledge hunger's presence in the U.S. by a study entitled Hunger USA and a documentary called *Hunger in America*. This resulted in a "nutrition safety net," comprised of programs such as WIC.

The face of hunger has changed during the past century, from that of the rail-thin Appalachian farmer to that of the overweight, minority urbanite. During this time, the concept of food insecurity and the contradiction of food deprivation and obesity, rather than frank malnutrition have become the dominant issues facing victims of domestic hunger.

10.2.13.1 First Half of the 20th Century

At the beginning of the 20th century, matters pertaining to the well-being of poor citizens in the U.S. were left to local charities rather than the federal government. With the advent of the Depression in the 1930s, the conditions of the poor, particularly widespread hunger, became a national concern. In response, President Franklin D. Roosevelt launched the New Deal, a suite of federal programs designed to alleviate the widespread unemployment and suffering caused by the prevailing economy conditions. Major initiatives to deal with hunger introduced by the way of the New Deal involved the purchase and distribution of surplus agricultural products, which were given to needy families, and Aid to Dependent Children (ADC) that provided cash assistance (welfare) for the care of widows and orphaned children.

Scant attention was paid to the lives and living conditions of Americans in local communities while the government was preoccupied with the external threats occasioned by the Second World War and throughout the 1940s while the U.S. helped to rebuild war-torn Europe and Japan. As the nation made the transition from World War II into the Korean War, communism became the dominant interest of political leaders in the mid- to late-1950s. However, with the resumption of economic prosperity and the demise of perceived external threats in the late 1950s to early 1960s, the federal government refocused its attention on internal conditions.[57]

10.2.13.2 Second Half of the 20th Century

The road to U.S. national nutrition policy in the 1970s was paved by media coverage of hunger in America during the raised consciousness era of the Civil Rights Movement and the War on Poverty. In the late 1960s, the nation was stunned to learn of chronic hunger and malnutrition in the South.[58] In 1968, the Citizens' Board of Inquiry into Hunger and Malnutrition issued a study, *Hunger USA*,[59] reporting that millions of citizens suffered from hunger, even extreme malnutrition like that experienced by people in the Third World. Also in 1968, CBS televised the award-winning documentary *Hunger in America*, which showed the faults of the Food Stamp Program in combating hunger in the Mississippi Delta, on Indian reservations, in migrant camps, and inner cities. Existing food programs were either insufficient or not reaching people who needed them most and, as a result, hunger was widespread.[60] (See Box 10.16.) By the end of the decade, the government's failure to adequately address hunger in America was being heavily criticized.[61]

Within this climate President Nixon convened the 1969 White House Conference on Food, Nutrition, and Health.[62] The conference, a seminal event that focused public attention on the importance of nutrition in the life and well-being of the U.S. population, led to an action-oriented

---

Box 10.16 Hunger Is a Concept

Hunger is a concept that is measured at the individual level. Food insecurity is a household-level concept. Wunderlich G.S., Norwood J.L.

Source: Food Insecurity and Hunger in the United States: An Assessment of the Measure. Washington, D.C.: National Academies Press, 2006.

---

agenda that helped shape the "nutrition safety net." For example, the conference proposed a specific recommendation of food supplementation for high-risk pregnant women and their infants, one of the major factors leading to the creation of what is now known as the Special Supplemental Nutrition Program for Women, Infants, and Children (WIC). Initiatives for food labeling and the feeding program for the elderly were also developed at the conference.

In 1999, the 30th anniversary of this landmark conference, planning began for a year 2000 National Nutrition Summit. While considerable progress had been made since 1969 in solving the problem of hunger in the U.S., there remained serious concerns about household food security in some segments of the population, and there has been a troubling rise in the prevalence of overweight and obesity. Thus, the 2000 National Nutrition Summit was convened to develop human nutrition policy for the 21st century. The summit identified continuing challenges and emerging opportunities for the U.S., focusing on nutrition and lifestyle issues across the lifespan, particularly those relevant to overweight and obesity. A number of overarching themes emerged from the National Nutrition Summit (see Table 10.2), which paved the way for current national nutrition policy regarding

---

TABLE 10.2
National Nutrition Summit 2000: General Overarching Themes and Themes Regarding Obesity

	Nutrition Summit 2000	
Area	**General Recommendations[a]**	**Obesity Recommendations[b]**
Federal agency coordination	Improve Federal agency coordination and increase partnerships among and between public and private interests to create more visibility for healthy lifestyle behaviors. Draw on the strengths of communities and build partnerships at all levels (e.g., federal, state, local, public, private) to eliminate hunger, improve nutrition, encourage physical activity, and enhance community food environment	Better federal agency coordination is needed along with more partnerships of public and private interests at the federal, state, and local levels
Targeted national campaigns	Based on the research outcomes to identify cost-effective and exemplary health promotion practices and programs, promote national campaigns that	National campaigns are needed that target specific behavioral change
Behavior change	target specific behavioral changes (e.g., obesity prevention and treatment, dietary and physical	Interventions should use multichannel and culturally relevant approaches to
High-risk groups	activity habits, behavioral change barriers) among high-risk groups (e.g., elderly citizens, reproductive-aged women, physically inactive adolescents, and children) and employ multichannel and culturally relevant methodologies. Piggyback campaigns on existing national media and education campaigns involving the healthcare system, schools, worksites, and communities	target high-risk groups such as inactive children and youth who consume diets rich in fat and added sugar

TABLE 10.2 (Continued)
National Nutrition Summit 2000: General Overarching Themes
and Themes Regarding Obesity

	Nutrition Summit 2000	
Area	**General Recommendations[a]**	**Obesity Recommendations[b]**
Education	Educate the public about the various nutrition and physical activity requirements for different populations (e.g., infants, children, reproductive-aged women, and elderly) to facilitate the appropriate implementation of prevention and intervention strategies	Interventions should use multichannel and culturally relevant approaches to target high-risk groups such as inactive children and youth who consume diets rich in fat and added sugar
Supportive environments	Supportive environments to promote and practice healthy behaviors are needed	Prevent overweight and obesity among U.S. citizens through creation of a supportive environment for promoting healthy lifestyles and encouraging people to practice appropriate nutrition and activity behaviors, including changes in the physical environment, health policy, and social norms
Diet and exercise as primary prevention	Encourage and support healthy dietary and physical activity behaviors across all levels of society to improve health status	Interventions should use multichannel and culturally relevant approaches to target high-risk groups such as inactive children and youth who consume diets rich in fat and added sugar
Awareness	Deliver more expertly effective communication of nutrition and health messages intended to raise awareness that hunger continues to exist Deliver more expertly effective communication of nutrition and health messages intended to raise recognition that poor dietary practices, overweight, and lack of physical activity contribute to poor health	Prevention and treatment of obesity must become a healthcare priority if the obesity epidemic is to be reversed
Economics	Conduct economic analyses of the ramifications of poor nutrition and physical inactivity. Food insecurity and the epidemic of obesity may increase the burden on our healthcare system because of comorbidity and related losses in production. Conduct this analytic research through Federal agencies and the use of grant programs as a broader base of issues come forward. Examples of economic analyses include the increment in healthcare cost related to obesity, the impact on productivity of workers due to co-morbidities, the impact that recruiting physically unfit soldiers places on the military, the impact on Medicare, and the role of food assistance in making the transition from poverty	Prevention and treatment of obesity must become a healthcare priority if the obesity epidemic is to be reversed

(continued)

TABLE 10.2 (Continued)
National Nutrition Summit 2000: General Overarching Themes
and Themes Regarding Obesity

	Nutrition Summit 2000	
Area	**General Recommendations[a]**	**Obesity Recommendations[b]**
Research	Conduct applied and behavioral research to identify cost-effective and exemplary health promotion practices and programs	
	Conduct basic and clinical research to determine how dietary constituents and physical activity influence pathways to health and to identify those who will benefit from dietary change and increased physical activity	
	Conduct research in the areas of behavioral change, cost-effectiveness of interventions, and identification of exemplary practices and programs to change population behaviors	
	Conduct research to understand which factors act as barriers to behavioral change and identify the changes that can be made to facilitate positive behavioral change	
	Conduct research and evaluation to determine how to best communicate these messages to individuals and specific populations	
Food security	Publicize the message that food security is the foundation of a healthy lifestyle by raising awareness of the links among poverty, hunger, and health to better engage the public in the fight against hunger and poor nutrition. Maintain and strengthen Federal nutrition assistance programs as an integral part of every community's nutrition safety net	

Sources:

[a] Picciano, M.F., Coates, P.M., and Cohen, B.E. The National Nutrition Summit: history and continued commitment to the nutritional health of the U.S. population. *J Nutr.* 133, 1949–1452, 2003. Available at: http://www.nutrition.org/cgi/content/full/133/6/1949. Accessed July 2, 2005.

[b] Stockmyer, C., Kuester, S., Ramsey, D., and Dietz, W.H. National Nutrition Summit, May 30, 2000: Results of the obesity discussion groups. *Obes Res.* 9, S41–S52, 2001. Available at: http://www.obesityresearch.org/cgi/content/full/9/4/S41. Accessed July 2, 2005.

nutrition assistance programs and the obesity crisis. Chapter 13 contains an in-depth discussion of the various programs that comprise the nation's nutrition safety net, and Chapter 7 examines programs developed in response to escalating rates of obesity.

10.3 U.S. FARM POLICY AND HEALTH

In an effort to help the American farmer gain economic stability and drive down the price of food, the USDA created and continues to support farm policies that encourage the overproduction of a select few multiple-use agricultural products (bulk agricultural commodities). Grains, meats, soybeans, and dairy are examples of these products. Farmers receive economic subsidies from the USDA's Farm Services Agency to offset the cost of producing these agricultural commodities. (See Box 10.17.)

Box 10.17 Corn and Its Derivatives

Corn is one example of an inexpensive bulk agricultural commodity crop that can be developed into many other products.[1,2,3] Corn on the cob is sold in its unprocessed state or is minimally processed to produce corn products such as flours and meals used as an ingredient in home cooking and in mass production of cereals, breads, and other starchy foods. But corn in itself is not a high value commodity until it is transformed into other items, such as high fructose corn syrup (HFCS) or animal feed, and then becomes more valuable at a cheaper price.

HFCS has become a food industry staple used as a sweetener to replace sugar in many products. In the 1970s, the price of sugar increased, which led the food industry to explore other options for food sweeteners. Food scientists learned that corn can be converted into a sweetener that is six times sweeter than regular sucrose at a fraction of the cost. HFCS also gives food a longer shelf life, helps avoid freezer burn in frozen foods, gives items a more "natural and fresh" look and, most importantly, is inexpensive to produce. This discovery led the food industry to begin replacing sugar with HFCS in many processed foods, including bread and canned vegetables, over the past 30 years because of its economic benefits. Today, HFCS has replaced sugar as the sweetener in most sweetened carbonated beverages sold in the U.S.

Corn can also be manufactured into inexpensive animal feed that allows varying livestock industries to lower their production costs. By using an inexpensive feed to raise livestock the varying industries are able to sell their product, such as chicken and beef, at a lower price to the food industry. This in turn allows fast food restaurants to sell hamburgers and chicken nuggets on their dollar menu.

Sources:

[1] Haddad, L. Redirecting the diet transition: what can food policy do? *Devt Policy Rev.* 21, 599–614, 2003.

[2] Critser, G. *Fat Land: How Americans Became the Fattest People in the World.* Houghton Miffin Company, New York, New York. 2003.

[3] Tillotson, J. America's obesity: conflicting public policies, industrial economic development, and unintended consequences. *Annu Rev Nutr.* 24, 617–643, 2004.

10.3.1 BACKGROUND

The first American agricultural assistance programs addressed the increased yield patterns these farmers had developed in support of the World War I effort. At the end of the war, farmers continued to grow crops at a record pace, resulting in an oversupply, followed by plummeting prices. The severe economic problems faced by this large segment of society, where about 25% of the U.S. population then resided, needed mitigation. Relief came in the form of the first Agricultural Adjustment Act (AAA) in 1933, which helped stabilize the agricultural sector through guaranteed minimum farm prices and other supply management techniques. This system helped to ensure an abundant supply of food at artificially reduced prices. In effect, government was encouraging continued increased production by buying the surplus. Since then, farm price and income support programs have formed the core of agricultural policy in the U.S.

Box 10.18 U.S. Farm and Nutrition Policies

U.S. farm policies and nutrition policies often lack coherence and are not designed specifically to improve the health of U.S. consumers.

TABLE 10.3
A Century of Structural Changes in U.S. Agriculture

	1900	1930	2000/2002
U.S. rural population as a share of the nation's overall population	60%	48%	28%
U.S. farm population as a share of the overall U.S. population	39%	28%	1%
Percent of workforce employed in agriculture	41	21.5	1.9
Average size of farms (in acres)	146	151	441
Number of farms (in millions)	5.7	6.3	2.17
Average number of commodities produced per farm	5	4.5	1

Source: Dimitri, C., Effland, A., Conklin, N. The 20th Century Transformation of U.S. Agriculture and Farm Policy, EIB-3 USDA, Economic Research Service, June 2005. Available at: http://www.ers.usda.gov/ publications/ eib3/. Accessed June 25, 2006.

A common topic in the debate over U.S. farm programs is that current policies were tailored for a time in American agriculture that no longer exists. The U.S. is no longer a nation of farmers. Furthermore, the change in the structure of farms over the last century raises questions about the efficacy of policies with roots in an agriculturally based economy.[63] As indicated in Table 10.3, at the beginning of the 20th century most of the nation's approximately six million farms were small and diversified. Today they are confined to fewer, larger, and more specialized operations. In 1900, 41% of the workforce was employed in agriculture; a century later, that percentage had dropped to 1.9. Over the same period, both the U.S. farm population and rural population dwindled as a share of the nation's overall population.

Farming continues to move toward fewer, larger operations producing the bulk of farm commodities, complemented by a growing number of smaller farms. Today, farm residents account for less than two percent of the total U.S. population, and most of the nation's two million farmers are mainly part-timers who rely on off-farm sources for most of their income. In 1997, about 157,000 large farms, with annual agricultural sales averaging about $900,000, accounted for only 8% of all U.S. farms, but 72% of all farm sales.[64]

The current larger farms are more productive than were the agricultural operations at the middle of the 20th century. Advances in plant and animal breeding have facilitated mechanization and increased yields, enhanced by the rapid development of inexpensive chemical fertilizers and pesticides since 1945. As a result, growth in agricultural productivity averaged 1.9% annually between 1948 and 1999, compared with a 1.3% average annual growth in manufacturing over the same period. (Manufacturing growth ranged from 0 to 2.3%, depending on the industry.)[63]

10.3.2 FARM SUBSIDIES

Despite these changes, government continues to encourage American farming to overproduce by assuring farmers of a predetermined price for their harvest. The U.S. government subsidizes agricultural commodities — corn, wheat, and soybeans — through a direct payment to the farmer. This drives down the price of the commodities, making vast quantities available to the food industry at artificially low prices. In particular, the low cost of corn, wheat, and soybeans results in the low prices of their by-products, which include high-fructose corn syrup (HFCS), hydrogenated fats, and corn-fed meats[65] (see Box 10.17).

10.3.3 HEALTH IMPLICATIONS OF CURRENT U.S. FARM POLICY

Because corn sweeteners and soy- and corn-based fats are inexpensive to produce, the food industry has an incentive to use these inexpensive ingredients in the processed foods they create. The result is a food supply that contains a large and ever-increasing number of relatively inexpensive, highly caloric food products. These foods fall into the very dietary categories that have been linked to

---

Box 10.19 Michael Pollan Quote

Corn products are not fresh food. To make them, you're using corn as an industrial raw material...I avoid foods with more than five ingredients on the label, and I eat as few processed foods as I can — in particular, anything made with high-fructose corn syrup. It's not evil, but it's a marker of a highly processed food.

Source: Q & A Michael Pollan. Think global, eat local. *Washington Post.* June 28, 2006, p. F01

---

obesity. In 1998, of the 11,000 new food products introduced into the market, about three-quarters were candies, condiments, breakfast cereals, baked goods, and beverages — all foods high in added sugars and fats. Such products taste good, have a long shelf life, and on a per-calorie basis, cost much less than fruits and vegetables. Low-income people find these foods particularly attractive because they are often more available and more affordable than healthier choices.[66]

A dichotomy, therefore, exists between

U.S. nutrition policies that attempt to guide food consumption in the interests of human health, such as the *Dietary Guidelines for Americans*	and	U.S. farm policies that encourage increased food production and food industry objectives that promote increased food consumption.

Obesity is one marker of how the conflict is proceeding.[67] As a result of this tension, contemporary critics of the system, such as Nestle and Pollan, argue that U.S. farm policy is one (though not the only) cause of the obesity epidemic. (See Box 10.19.)

10.3.3.1 Corn and Soy

The ability of fast-food restaurants to sell hamburgers inexpensively (for example, the dollar meal) can be linked to cheap commodities. Corn and soybeans are also used to produce low cost animal feed for the animals that become fried chicken and hamburger patties. Animal feed in the form of soy meal also produces soy oil as a by-product. It therefore contributes not only to the burger but also to the side orders of fried potatoes and fried onion rings. Thus, in the short run, U.S. farm policy (see Boxes 10.20 and 10.21) makes poor eating habits an economically sensible choice.[65]

10.3.3.2 Produce

As discussed, a number of USDA farm policies function as disincentives for American farmers to grow healthier foods. For example, more subsidies focus on bulk commodities, whereas few have been instituted to encourage the production of fruits and vegetables. High value produce crops receive a smaller level of government economic support and risk management insurance, resulting in more farmers focusing on high bulk agricultural commodities rather than produce. Although a farmer might

---

Box 10.20 U.S. Per Capita Calories

From 1970 to 1997, *per capita* calories from the U.S. food supply increased from 2220 to 2680 (adjusted for spoilage and waste).

Source: USDA's Economic Research Service.

Box 10.21 U.S. Farm Policy and Obesity

U.S. farm policy geared towards driving down prices for corn and soybeans is a significant contributor to the nation's obesity epidemic. Low prices for corn and soybeans over the last several decades has spurred investment in high fructose corn syrup (HFCS) and hydrogenated vegetable oils (trans fats). The introduction of HFCS and trans fats directly mirrors alarming increases in obesity rates in the U.S. While prices for crop ingredients for HFCS and trans fats have decreased, contributing to low-priced, calorie-dense processed foods, prices for fruits and vegetables, grown with relatively little government support, have steadily increased.

Source: Schoonover H, Muller M. Food Without Thought: how U.S. Farm Policy Contributes to Obesity. Institute for Agriculture and Trade Policy, 2006. Available at: http://www.iatp. org/iatp/ publications.cfm?accountID=421&refID=80627. Accessed June 29, 2006.

---

generate a higher return in market for high value produce, the lack of support makes growing fruits and vegetables a riskier proposition for the farmer. Thus, the production of agricultural commodities leads to an artificially depressed production of fruits and vegetables. In the U.S., the cost of fresh fruits and vegetables has increased by 40% over the past 20 years while that of food with dubious nutritional value ("junk food") has decreased by 25% when taking inflation into consideration.[68] (See Box 10.22.)

10.3.4 ENVIRONMENTAL IMPLICATIONS OF CURRENT U.S. FARM POLICY

Bulk commodity subsidies also discourage farmers from focusing on diverse crops for local consumption. Many rural farm communities are unable to sustain themselves because they concentrate on one bulk commodity. Rural areas now depend on food imports in order to have a diverse food supply in their community. For example, in an agricultural region of southeastern Minnesota, only $2 million of the total $500 million local residents spent on food went directly to local farmers. This situation has become the norm in many American agricultural communities as a consequence of farm policies that reward bulk agricultural commodity products rather than diverse crops to feed local communities.[69] See Box 10.22 for a discussion of sustainable agriculture. (See Box 10.23.)

10.3.5 POLICY CHANGES

As we have seen, current policies that encourage overproduction and provide subsidies for bulk agricultural commodities leave farmers of fresh produce at an economic disadvantage.[65] The challenge to economists, public health experts, and the USDA is to institute changes that will help reverse the effects of current U.S. agricultural policy and provide the general public with a healthier food supply that remains affordable. To succeed, any new farm policies must consider both the health and well-being of the population as well as the economic exigencies of the agricultural and food industry sectors.

Economic subsidies to encourage farmers to produce healthy foods that are in turn economically affordable for the American public could lead to higher consumption of fruits and vegetables and place U.S. farm policy in line with the current dietary guidelines. Creating economic subsidies for

---

Box 10.22 Marion Nestle

The government does not subsidize fruit and vegetable production the way it supports corn, soybeans, sugar cane, and sugar beets.

Source: Nestle M. *What to Eat.* New York: North Point Press, 2006.

Box 10.23 Sustainable Agriculture

Sustainable agriculture enhances environmental quality; is economically viable; enhances the quality of life for farmers, farm workers, and society as a whole; and provides for basic human food and fiber needs.[1] Robinson and Smith's report on a survey of members of the Minnesota Dietetic Association states "a relocalized and sustainable agricultural system could enhance community food security." Presently, most food in the U.S. travels an average of 1300 miles to reach the dinner table, using large amounts of nonrenewable fossil fuels in the process.[2]

That our diets can contribute to both personal health and to sustainability was first suggested by Gussow and Clancy in 1986 and more recently by Wilkins.[2,3,4] In a commentary for the ADA, Peters suggests that promoting a more sustainable food system may be part of the roles and responsibilities of dietetics professionals. She encourages pilot projects to identify and overcome barriers to purchasing locally grown food.[2]

Without exploring the environmental or political ramifications of sustainablity, purchasing and eating locally produced food presents an important approach for low-income neighborhoods to increase access to fresh fruits and vegetables. Gussow states, "we will not have sustainable food systems merely by working to improve the environment or even by keeping local farmers in business with a two-tiered system: healthy, fresh, local food for the well-off and cheap industrialized food for the poor. Truly sustainable food systems will be those that provide good jobs for all of those working with food and good food for everyone who eats."[3]

Can a sustainable diet be nutritionally adequate, particularly considering seasonal eating? Creative growing techniques and, more significantly, creative thinking and consumer education can answer issues such as those raised by the more limited food production of the winter and early spring months.[3,4]

Increasingly, state and local efforts to foster food security emphasize sustainable, system-wide approaches.[5] Policies that support education about how to purchase, plan, and prepare meals based on locally available foods are needed.[4]

Sources:

[1]Robinson, R. and Smith, C. Integrating issues of sustainably produced foods into nutrition practice: a survey of Minnesota Dietetic Association members. *J Am Diet Assoc.* 103(5), 608–611, 2003.

[2]Peters, J. Community food systems: working toward a sustainable future. *J Am Diet Assoc.* 97(9), 955–956, 1997.

[3]Gussow, J.D. and Clancy, K.L. Dietary guidelines for sustainability. *J Nutr Educ.* 18, 1–5, 1986.

[4]Feenstra, G. Seasonal and local diets: consumers' role in achieving a sustainable food system. University of California, Sustainable Agriculture Research and Education Program. www.sarep.ucdavis.edu/NEWSLTR/v8n3/sa-12.htm. Accessed February 27, 2004.

[5]McCullum, C., Pelletier, D., Barr, D., and Wilkins, J. Use of a particular planning process as a way to build community food security. *J Am Diet Assoc.* 102, 962–967, 2002.

---

high-value produce would also drive down the price of high-value crops, making purchase and production of healthier foods an economically sensible choice for the food industry. For example, the USDA could help improve public health by creating a retail-based mechanism to provide participants in its Food Stamp Program (FSP) with significant monetary incentives to purchase health-promoting foods, such as minimally processed fruits, vegetables, and whole-grain products. This incentive program could be underwritten by redirecting some of the funds currently allocated to annual commodity support payments. The redirected funds could be used to reimburse retailers and wholesaler-distributors for lost revenues, and to provide growers and processors with direct payments.

10.3.5.1 Proposals for the Next U.S. Farm Bill

Each new federal farm bill provides an opportunity to influence the overall direction of U.S. farm policy. The bill, which expires every four to five years (the most recent ones were enacted in 2002 and 2007), serves as the major U.S. agricultural legislation that outlines provisions on commodity programs, trade, conservation, credit, agricultural research, food stamps, and marketing. Because the farm bill contains hundreds of programs and provisions that impact the U.S. food system, it provides a unique opportunity to institute policies that foster systemic changes that could lead to a healthier food supply. The following policy goals have been recommended by the Institute for Agriculture and Trade Policy:

- Emphasize the connections between public health, food, and farm policy to broaden the discussion, and form a diverse base of people to develop and implement local, state, and national policies that benefit both public health and family farmers.
- Develop market incentives for increasing healthy food consumption. From 1985–2000, the real price of fresh fruits and vegetables increased almost 40% in the U.S., while the real price of added fats and sugars declined. Government policies need to be developed that make buying healthy foods an economically sensible choice.
- Encourage school and government procurement policies that favor healthy foods. Improving the quality of school lunch — such as through higher nutrition standards for the National School Lunch Program and healthier selections in the USDA commodity donations to schools — would increase demand for fruits and vegetables, providing an even greater incentive for American farmers to grow these crops.
- Reward farmers for "producing" health benefits. Programs should be developed that provide farmers with financial incentives for raising produce crops and grass-fed dairy and livestock.

In sum, overproduction and the consequent reduction in the cost of some foods is an environmental force favoring the occurrence of obesity. U.S. farm policy, specifically crop subsidies and incentives for bulk agricultural commodities, promote obesity by creating a relatively inexpensive, high-calorie food source for the food industry to use in the production of low-cost foods replete with added fats and sugars. This creates an environment that conflicts with the Dietary Guidelines' suggestion to limit the amount of sugars and fats in one's diet and makes eating unhealthy foods less expensive in the short term. To improve the food environment in which we live, economists, health experts, and policymakers must promote new farm policies that result in a healthier food supply while not undermining economic prosperity for both the food industry and the American farmer.

10.4 TAKING ACTION

Different approaches are available to effect nutrition policy. Activists can propose new policies, as well as support policies they believe in that have been introduced by others. As an example, the following case study describes the steps taken by the Center for Science in the Public Interest (CSPI) to promote passage of a bill designed to improve school food. CSPI followed the steps necessary for making policy that are outlined at the beginning of this chapter.

10.4.1 Case Study: Promoting the Child Nutrition Promotion and School Lunch Protection Act

1995

- S 1074, the Healthy Lifestyles and Prevention America or the HeLP America Act is introduced in the Senate by Tom Harkin (D-Iowa) on May 18th. The legislation was designed as a comprehensive bill to improve the health of Americans and reduce healthcare costs by reorienting the nation's healthcare system toward prevention, wellness, and self-care. Section 102, entitled "Child Nutrition Promotion and School Lunch Protection," would require the USDA to apply the same standards for competitive foods as for school lunches, and to apply those standards to all foods sold on campus throughout the school day. The bill was sent to the Committee on Finance where it remained because it received no Congressional support in the form of cosponsors.

- In anticipation of Sec.102 being resubmitted as a separate bill entitled the Child Nutrition Promotion and School Lunch Protection Act, CSPI called on nutrition activists to support the legislation. Through the National Alliance for Nutrition and Activity (NANA) and the Internet, CSPI signed on more than 80 national, state, and local organizations to support the bill (see http://www.cspinet.org/new/pdf/nana_coalition.pdf for the list of supporters).

2006
- In April, bipartisan S 2592/HR 5167 was introduced in the Senate and the House.
- In June, CSPI released a compendium of state policies regarding competitive foods. The report demonstrates that most state nutrition policies fail to keep nutrition-poor foods and sugary drinks out of schools. The report, School Foods Report Card is posted on the CSPI Web site: http://cspinet.org/new/pdf/school_foods_ report_card.pdf. (See Box 10.24.)
- Also in June, CSPI mounted a letter-writing campaign to Congress. Activists on CSPI's e-mail lists were asked to encourage their legislators to co-sponsor (support) the bill. CSPI even provided a model letter that could be used (see Box 10.25).

Box 10.24 Model Letter

Dear:

As your constituent, I urge you to cosponsor the bipartisan Child Nutrition Promotion and School Lunch Protection Act, (S 2592 / HR 5167).

The bill would require the USDA to bring its nutrition standards for foods sold out of vending machines, school stores, and a la carte in line with current nutrition science, and to apply those standards to all foods sold on campus throughout the school day.

In a state-by-state review of school food and beverage policies published in June 2006 (http://cspinet.org/ new/pdf/school_foods_report_card.pdf), the Center for Science in the Public Interest found that most states allow far too much "junk food" to be sold in schools through vending machines and school stores, and on a la carte lines. With junk foods tempting children at nearly every other public place in America, school should be one locale where parents do not need to worry about what their children are eating. Just as Congress has enacted strong nutrition standards for school lunch and breakfast programs, it should take similar steps to assure that all school foods are healthy.

Children's poor diets and rising rates of pediatric obesity are national problems that need a national response. Please let me know if I can count on you to cosponsor S. 2592 and H.R. 5167.

Sincerely,
Name, professional credentials
Contact information
Note: The Center for Science in the Pubic Interest generously made their materials available for inclusion in this chapter.

Box 10.25 Activities

- Read "School Foods Report Card," posted at: http://cspinet.org/new/pdf/school_foods_report_card.pdf.
- Access the full text of S 2592 or HR 5167 through THOMAS at: http://thomas.loc.gov/ to determine the current status of the proposed legislation.
- Use Google or another search engine to investigate the portrayal of the proposed legislation in the mass media. Explain why certain interest groups are in favor of the legislation and others are opposed to it.
- Discuss how the proposed legislation might overlap school local wellness policies established in response to P.L. 108–265.
- Predict how local wellness policies could be affected if this legislation is enacted.

In your opinion, should the federal government determine what kinds of foods can be sold in vending machines in schools? Explain.

10.5 CONCLUSION

What people choose to eat is affected by far more than personal selection. The foods available through our food system are determined by agricultural and economic policies. Because our agricultural policies encourage overproduction of energy-dense, low-nutrient foods, they are in direct conflict with federal nutritional guidelines, which advocate nutrient-dense, low-energy foods.

Although the focus of the nation's nutritional guidelines and support has shifted from malnutrition in the 1930s to over-nutrition presently, the low-income segment of our population remains most negatively affected. Clearly, the federal government is capable of affecting positive change as evidenced by mandates for the fortification of grains and iodization of salt. Legislation such as the Farm Bill as well as local wellness policies can be an effective tool for encouraging production and consumption of fresh fruits and vegetables rather than processed foods dense with added fats and sugars.

10.6 ACRONYMS

AAA	Agricultural Adjustment Act
ADA	American Dietetic Association
ADC	Aid to Dependent Children
AHA	American Heart Association
AI	Adequate intake
CDC	Centers for Disease Control and Prevention (DHHS)
CSFII	Continuing Survey of Food Intake of Individuals
CSPI	Center for Science in the Public Interest
DHHS	U.S. Department of Health and Human Services
ED	U.S. Department of Education
ERS	Economic Research Service
FAAN	Food Allergy and Anaphylaxis Network
FALCPA	Food Allergen Labeling and Consumer Protection Act of 2004
FDA	Food and Drug Administration
FNS	Food and Nutrition Service (USDA)
FRAC	Food Research and Action Center
FSP	Food Stamp Program
FY	Fiscal year
H.R.	U.S. House of Representatives
HFCA	Hunger-Free Communities Act

HFCS	High fructose corn syrup
IU	International units
LEA	Local educational agencies
MEAL Act	Menu Education and Labeling Act
MOUs	Memorandum of understanding
NAMCS	National Ambulatory Medical Care Survey
NANA	National Alliance for Nutrition and Activity (at CSPI)
NCCDPHP	National Center for Chronic Disease Prevention and Health Promotion (CDC)
NHANES	National Health and Nutrition Examination Survey
NLEA	Nutrition Labeling and Education Act
NSLP	National School Lunch Program
NWHPS	National Worksite Health Promotion Survey (from the Partnership for Prevention and the Office of Disease Prevention and Health Promotion in the Office of Public Health and Science)
ODPHP	Office of Disease Prevention and Health Promotion
OPHS	Office of the Public Health Service
PedNSS	Pediatric Nutrition Surveillance System
P.L.	Public law
RFA	Request for applications
S.	U.S. Senate
SHPPS	School Health Policies and Program Study
TN	Team nutrition
U.S.	United States
USDA	U.S. Department of Agriculture
WIC	Special Supplemental Nutrition Program for Women, Infants, and Children (USDA)

REFERENCES

1. Mayer, J. National and International Issues in Food Policy. Lowell Lecture, May 15, 1989. Available at: http://www.dce.harvard.edu/pubs/lowell/jmayer.html. Accessed August 30, 2006.
2. Chapman, N. Developing agency, community, and state policies. In Kaufman, M. *Nutrition in Public Health: A Handbook for Developing Programs and Services*. Rockville, MD: Aspen Publishers, 1990, chap. 5.
3. Chapman, N. and Edmonds, M.T. Develop agency, community, and state nutrition policies. In Kaufman, M. *Nutrition in Promoting the Public's Health. Strategies, Principles, and Practice*. Sudbury, MA: Jones and Bartlett Publishers, 2007, chap. 5.
4. U.S. Department of Health and Human Services. The Surgeon General's call to action to prevent and decrease overweight and obesity. U.S. Department of Health and Human Services, Public Health Service, Office of the Surgeon General, Rockville, MD, 2001. Available at: http://www.surgeon-general.gov/topics/obesity/calltoaction/CalltoAction.pdf. Accessed June 22, 2006.
5. Food and Drug Administration. Center for Food Safety and Applied Nutrition. Calories Count: Report on the Working Group on Obesity, February 11, 2004. Available at: http://www.cfsan.fda.gov/~dms/owg-toc.html. Accessed July 3, 2005.
6. Crawford, L.M. Speech before the 2nd National Forum on Obesity Policy, Regulation, and Litigation, May 11, 2005. Available at: http://www.fda.gov/oc/speeches/2005/obesity0511.html. Accessed July 2, 2005.
7. The Keystone Forum on Away-From-Home Foods: Opportunities for Preventing Weight Gain and Obesity. Final Report. May 2006. Available at: http://www.keystone.org/spp/documents/forum_report_ FINAL_5-30-06.pdf. Accessed June 22, 2006.
8. Lichtenstein, A.H., Appel, L.J., Brands, M., et al. Diet and lifestyle recommendations revision 2006. A scientific statement from the American Heart Association Nutrition Committee. *Circulation*. 114, 82–96, 2006. Published online before print June 19, 2006. Available at: http://circ.ahajournals.org/cgi/reprint/CIRCULATIONAHA.106.176158. Accessed June 23, 2006.
9. Lin, B.-H., Frazao. Food Allergen Labeling and Consumer Protection Act of 2004. 21 USC 301. Available at: http://www.cfsan.fda.gov/~dms/alrgact.html. Accessed June 24, 2006.

10. Guthrie, J. *Away-From-Home Foods Increasingly Important to Quality of American Diet.* Agriculture Information Bulletin No. 749. U.S. Department of Agriculture, Economic Research Service, January 1999. Available at: http://www.ers.usda.gov/publications/aib749/. Accessed June 30, 2005.

11. Center for Science in the Public Interest. Anyone's Guess: The Need for Nutrition Labeling at Fast-Food and Other Chain Restaurants. Washington, D.C.: Center for Science in the Public Interest, November 2003. Available at: http://cspinet.org/new/pdf/anyone_s_guess_final_web.pdf. Accessed June 27, 2005.

12. Variyam, J.N. Nutrition Labeling in the Food-Away-From-Home Sector: An Economic Assessment. U.S. Department of Agriculture, Economic Research Service. Economic Research Report No. (ERR4), April 2005. Available at: http://www.ers.usda.gov/publications/ERR4/. Accessed June 30, 2005.

13. Food Allergen Labeling and Consumer Protection Act of 2004. 21 USC 301. Available at: www.cfsan. fda.gov/~dms/alrgact.html. Accessed June 24, 2006.

14. Excerpt from P.L. 108-265 Child Nutrition and WIC Reauthorization Act of 2004. Sec. 204. Local Wellness Policy. Available at: http://schoolmeals.nal.usda.gov/Training/CO_Middle_School_Marketing/ 1-2004_Middle_School_Marketing_Memos_and_Notices/WellnessPolicyRequirement.pdf. Accessed June 24, 2005.

15. U.S. Department of Agriculture; U.S. Department of Health and Human Services. *Dietary Guidelines for Americans.* 6th ed. Washington, D.C. January 2005. HHS Publication number: HHS-ODPHP-2005-01-DGA-A USDA Publication number: Home and Garden Bulletin No. 232. 2005. Available at: http://www.health.gov/dietaryguidelines/dga2005/document/pdf/DGA2005.pdf/. Accessed June 17, 2005.

16. P.L. 105–115. Food and Drug Administration Modernization Act of 1997. Title III: Improving regulation of food. Available at: http://www.fda.gov/cder/guidance/105-115.htm. Accessed June 23, 2006.

17. Healthy People 2010. Available at: http://www.healthypeople.gov/default.htm. Accessed June 20, 2006.

18. For more information about *Healthy People 2010* and its history, visit the *Healthy People 2010* Internet Web site at http://www.healthypeople.gov.

19. Public Health Service. Healthy people: the Surgeon General's report on health promotion and disease prevention. Washington, D.C.: U.S. Department of Health, Education, and Welfare, Public Health Service, 1979; DHEW publication no. (PHS) 79-55071. Available at: http://profiles.nlm.nih.gov/ NN/B/B/G/K/_/nnbbgk.pdf. Accessed June 21, 2006.

20. Public Health Service. Promoting health/preventing disease: objectives for the nation. Washington, D.C.: U.S. Department of Health and Human Services, Public Health Service, 1980.

21. *Healthy People 2000.* Available at: http://www.cdc.gov/nchs/about/otheract/hp2000/hp2000.htm. Accessed June 21, 2006

22. *Healthy People 2010.* Available at: http://www.healthypeople.gov/. Accessed June 21, 2006.

23. U.S. Department of Health and Human Services. *Healthy People 2010: Understanding and Improving Health,* 2nd ed. Washington, D.C., November 2000. Available at: http://www.healthypeople.gov/document/. Accessed June 24, 2005.

24. Centers for Disease Control and Prevention. DATA 2010. Available at: http://wonder.cdc.gov/data2010. Accessed June 24, 2006.

25. U.S. Department of Health and Human Services. Solicitation for written comments on the proposed changes to *Healthy People 2010* through the Midcourse Review. *Federal Register.* 70(August 12), 47206–47207, 2005.

26. Centers for Disease Control and Prevention. The School Health Policies and Programs Study (SHPPS). Available at: http://www.cdc.gov/HealthyYouth/shpps/index.htm. Accessed June 24, 2006.

27. HealthierUS.gov. Available at: http://www.healthierus.gov/ Accessed June 24, 2005.

28. U.S. Department of Health and Human Services. *Healthy People 2010.* 2nd ed. 2 Vols. Washington, D.C., 2000. Available at: http://www.healthypeople.gov/document/. Accessed June 28, 2005.

29. U.S. Department of Health and Human Services. Steps to a HealthierUS. Available at: http://www.healthierus.gov/STEPS/. Accessed June 14, 2006.

30. U.S. Department of Health and Human Services. *The Power of Prevention.* 2003. Available at: http:// www.healthierus.gov/steps/summit/prevportfolio/power/index.html#meeting. Accessed June 27, 2005.

31. U.S. Department of Health and Human Services. *SmallStep.gov.* Available at: http://smallstep.gov/ index.html. Accessed June 24, 2006.

32. U.S. Department of Health and Human Services. *The Power of Prevention*. 2003. Available at: http://www.healthierus.gov/steps/summit/prevportfolio/power/index.html#meeting. Accessed June 27, 2005.
33. U.S. Department of Health and Human Services. *Prevention Makes Common "Cents."* September 2003. Available at: http://aspe.hhs.gov/health/prevention/index.shtml#BUSINESSES. Accessed June 27, 2005.
34. Centers for Disease Control and Prevention. School Health Index. Available at: http://apps.nccd.cdc.gov/shi/HealthyYouth/intro.htm. Accessed June 27, 2005.
35. Andersen, R.E., Franckowiak, S.C., Snyder, J., Bartlett, S.J., and Fontaine, K.R. Can inexpensive signs encourage the use of stairs? Results from a community intervention. *Ann Intern Med.* 129, 363–369, 1998. Available at: http://www.annals.org/cgi/content/full/129/5/363. Accessed June 28, 2005.
36. USDA Food and Nutrition Service. HealthierUS School Challenge. Available at: http://www.fns.usda.gov/tn/HealthierUS/index.htm. Accessed June 28, 2005.
37. The Walking School Bus Information Web site. Available at: http://www.walkingschoolbus.org/. Accessed June 27, 2005.
38. Division of Nutrition and Physical Activity, National Center for Chronic Disease Prevention and Health Promotion KidsWalk-to-School. Centers for Disease Control and Prevention. Available at: http://www.cdc.gov/nccdphp/dnpa/kidswalk/. Accessed July 2, 2005.
39. Programs authorized by the Richard B. Russell National School Lunch Act (42 U.S.C. 1751 et seq) or the Child Nutrition Act of 1966 (42 U.S.C. 1771 et seq).
40. Food Allergy and Anaphylaxis Network (FAAN) homepage. Available at: http://www.foodallergy.org/about.html. Accessed June 24, 2006.
41. Food Allergen Labeling and Consumer Protection Act of 2004. 21 USC 301. Available at: www.cfsan.fda.gov/~dms/alrgact.html. Accessed June 24, 2006.
42. Gerrior, S., Bente, L., and Hiza, H. Nutrient Content of the U.S. Food Supply, 1909–2000. (Home Economics Research Report No. 56). U.S. Department of Agriculture, Center for Nutrition Policy and Promotion, 2004. Available at: http://www.cnpp.usda.gov/Pubs/Food%20Supply/FoodSupply2003Rpt/FoodSupply1909-2000.pdf. Accessed July 1, 2005.
43. Berner, L.A., Clydesdale, F.M., and Douglass, J.S. Fortification contributed greatly to vitamin and mineral intakes in the United States, 1989–1991. *J Nutr.* 131, 2177–2183, 2001. Available at: http://www.nutrition.org/cgi/content/full/131/8/2177. Accessed July 1, 2005.
44. Bishai, D. and Nalubola, R. The History of food fortification in the United States: its relevance for current fortification efforts in developing countries. *Econ Dev Cult Change.* 51, 37–53, 2002.
45. Institute of Medicine, Food and Nutrition Board. Dietary Reference Intakes: Calcium, Phosphorus, Magnesium, Vitamin D and Fluoride. National Academy Press, Washington, D.C., 1999. Available at: http://www.nap.edu/books/0309063507/html/. Accessed July 1, 2005.
46. Dietary Supplement Fact Sheet: Vitamin D. Office of Dietary Supplements, Warren G. Magnuson Clinical Center, National Institutes of Health. http://ods.od.nih.gov/factsheets/vitamind.asp.
47. Ten great public health achievements — United States, 1900–1999. *MMWR.* 48, 241–243, 1999. Available at: http://www.cdc.gov/mmwr/preview/mmwrhtml/00056796.htm. Accessed August 14, 2005.
48. U.S. Department of Health and Human Services. Food and Drug Administration. Food Standards: Amendment of Standards of Identity for Enriched Grain Products to Require Addition of Folic Acid. *Federal Register.* 61, 8781–8797, 1996. 21 CFR Parts 136, 137, and 139. Available at: http://www.cfsan.fda.gov/~lrd/fr96305b.html. Accessed July 1, 2005.
49. Pfeiffer, C.M., Caudill, S.P., Gunter, E.W., Osterloh, J., and Sampson, E.J. Biochemical indicators of B vitamin status in the U.S. population after folic acid fortification: results from the National Health and Nutrition Examination Survey 1999–2000. *Am J Clin Nutr.* 82, 442–450, 2005.
50. Clarke, R. Vitamin B_{12}, folic acid, and the prevention of dementia. *N Eng J Med.* 354, 2817–2819, 2006.
51. Warren, J.J. and Levy, S.M. Current and future role of fluoride in nutrition. *Dent Clin North Am.* 47, 225–243, 2003.
52. Achievements in public health, 1900–1999: Fluoridation of drinking water to prevent dental caries. *MMWR.* 48, 933–940, 1999. Available at: http://www.cdc.gov/mmwr/preview/mmwrhtml/mm4841a1.htm. Accessed August 14, 2005.
53. Johnson, S.A. and DeBiase, C. Concentration levels of fluoride in bottled drinking water. *J Dent Hyg.* 77, 161–167, 2003.

54. Bartels, D., Haney, K., and Khajotia, S.S. Fluoride concentrations in bottled water. *J Okla Dent Assoc.* 91, 18–22, 2000.

55. Lalumandier, J.A. and Ayers, L.W. Fluoride and bacterial content of bottled water vs tap water. *Arch Fam Med.* 9, 246–250, 2000. Available at: http://archfami.ama-assn.org/cgi/content/full/9/3/246. Accessed July 1, 2005.

56. Centers for Disease Control and Prevention. Recommendations for Using Fluoride to Prevent and Control Dental Caries in the United States. *MMWR.* 50(RR-14), 1–42, 2001. Available at: http://www.cdc.gov/mmwr/PDF/RR/RR5014.pdf. Accessed July 1, 2005.

57. Brown, L.J. Hunger in the U.S.: A Brief History, from Chapter I of *Know Hunger: Challenging Youth to be Leaders in the Fight Against Hunger*, 2003. Available at: http://www.knowhunger.org/ knowhunger/frames/toPrint/kNOwHungerNew.pdf. Accessed July 2, 2005.

58. Galer-Unti, R. *Hunger and Food Assistance Policy in the United States.* New York: Garland Publishing, 1995.

59. Citizens' Board of Inquiry into Hunger and Malnutrition in the United States. HUNGER, U.S.A. Boston, MA: Beacon Press, 1998.

60. Eisinger, P.K. *Toward an End to Hunger in America.* Washington, D.C.: The Brookings Institution Press, 1998. Available at: http://brookings.nap.edu/books/0815722818/html/. Accessed August 14, 2005.

61. Kotz, N. *Let Them Eat Promises: The Politics of Hunger in America.* Englewood Cliffs, NJ: Prentice-Hall, 1969.

62. White House Conference on Nutrition and Health. Available at: http://www.nns.nih.gov/1969/full_report/PDFcontents.htm. Accessed June 5, 2005.

63. Dimitri, C., Effland, A., and Conklin, N. The 20th Century Transformation of U.S. Agriculture and Farm Policy. ERS Electronic Information Bulletin Number 3, June 2005. Available at: www.ers.usda.gov/publications/EIB3/EIB3.htm. Accessed June 27, 2006.

64. Miner, J. Marketplace Incentives Could Bring U.S. Agriculture and Nutrition Policy into Accord While Improving Diets of Low-Income Americans. *California Agriculture.* 60, 2006, pp. 8–13.

65. Schoonover, H. and Muller, M. Food without Thought: How U.S. Farm Policy Contributes to Obesity. Minneapolis, MN: The Institute for Agricultural and Trade Policy; 2006. Available at: http://www.iatp.org/iatp/publications.cfm?accountID=421&refID=80627. Accessed June 20, 2006.

66. Drewnowski, A. and Darmon, N. The economics of obesity: dietary energy density and energy cost. *Am J Clin Nutr.* 82(Suppl.), 265s–273s, 2005.

67. Tillotson, J.E. Pandemic obesity: unintended policy consequences. *Nutr Today.* 38, 116–119, 2003.

68. Tillotson, J. America's obesity: conflicting public policies, industrial economic development, and unintended consequences. *Ann Rev Nutr.* 24, 617–643, 2004.

69. Waltner-Toews, D. and Lang, T. A new conceptual base for food and agricultural policy: the emerging model of links between agriculture, food, health, environment, and society. *Glob Change Hum Policy,* 1, 116–129, 2000. Available at: http://www.ovc.uoguelph.ca/popmed/ecosys/DWT-Lang.PDF. Accessed June 20, 2006.

11 Food and Nutrition Guidance

Eat food. Not too much. Mostly plants.

Michael Pollan, 2007

Everyone, it seems, offers advice about what we should eat. Diet books are perennial best sellers, with the eating plans they espouse providing the basis for endless articles in women's consumer magazines and fitness and health magazines, and are the subject for television talk shows and newspaper columns. Perhaps less well known is the more credible advice issued by the U.S. Department of Agriculture (USDA) and the Department of Health and Human Services (DHHS) and from voluntary health organizations such as the American Heart Association (AHA) and the American Cancer Society (ACS). Population-based recommendations from the government include the *Dietary Guidelines for Americans* and the MyPyramid food guidance system. Research funded by the government has produced the Dietary Approaches to Stop Hypertension (DASH) eating plan. Organizations dedicated to preventing the major chronic diseases have developed their own diet and lifestyle advice. This chapter examines federal food and nutrition policy aimed at health promotion and guidelines from voluntary as well as federal health associations for the primary and secondary prevention of cardiovascular diseases, cancer, and diabetes.

11.1 HISTORY OF FEDERAL FOOD AND NUTRITION GUIDANCE

It is instructive to review the history of dietary guidance in the U.S. in order to appreciate the genesis and maturing of our current system. Federal dietary guidance began in the early 20th century with early messages focused on avoiding dietary deficiency diseases.

11.1.1 FOOD-BASED DIETARY GUIDANCE — 1900s THROUGH THE 1980s

The USDA has been issuing food and nutrition recommendations for more than 100 years.[1] USDA food scientist W.O. Atwater's research on food composition and nutritional needs ushered in the USDA's long history of food guides. By emphasizing variety, proportionality, and moderation in food intake in 1902, he set the stage for all future work in the field of dietary recommendations (see Box 11.1).

A food guide translates nutrient intake recommendations into food intake recommendations and provides a conceptual framework for selecting the kinds and amounts of foods that will provide a nutritionally sound diet. The USDA's first food guide, published in 1916 (see Table 11.1), categorized foods into five groups: milk and meat, cereals, vegetables and fruits, fats and fatty foods, and sugars and sugary foods. That guide was followed in 1917 by dietary recommendations that were based on these five food groups.*

In the 1920s, guides were released using these same five food groups to suggest amounts of foods to purchase each week for families of varying sizes. During the Depression, economic constraints influenced dietary guidance. In 1933, the USDA developed its first food plans at four cost levels to help people with food shopping. The plans were organized into 12 major food groups to buy and use within a week to meet nutritional needs. Research to provide guidance on selecting a healthful diet at different cost levels continues at the USDA. (See Box 11.2.)

---

* A century later, this pattern was reversed when the 1990 and 2005 Dietary Guidelines preceded the Food Guide Pyramid and MyPyramid, respectively.

Box 11.1 Atwater Quote

Unless care is exercised in selecting food, a diet may result which is one-sided or badly balanced, that is, one in which either protein or fuel ingredients (carbohydrate and fat) are provided in excess.... The evils of overeating may not be felt at once, but sooner or later they are sure to appear, perhaps in an excessive amount of fatty tissue, perhaps in general debility, perhaps in actual disease.

W.O. Atwater, as quoted in Davis and Saltos, 1999

Source: Davis, C. and Saltos, E. Dietary recommendations and how they have changed over time. In Frazao, E., ed. *America's Eating Habits: Changes and Consequences*. Washington, D.C.: Economic Research Service, U.S. Department of Agriculture, Agriculture Information Bulletin No. 750, 1999, pp. 33–50, chap. 2.

At the beginning of the U.S. entry into World War II, President Franklin D. Roosevelt convened the National Nutrition Conference for Defense, a meeting notable to the nutrition community for at least two reasons. The conference resulted in the development in 1941 of the first Recommended Dietary Allowances (RDAs), published in 1943 by the Food and Nutrition Board of the National Academy of Sciences (NAS). The first edition of the RDAs listed specific recommended intakes for calories and nine essential nutrients: protein, iron, calcium, vitamin A, vitamin C, vitamin D, thiamine, riboflavin, and niacin. The conference also addressed the need for public nutrition education and provided suggestions for an effective nutrition education program. The suggestions provided in 1941 reflect essential program characteristics that remain applicable today. Effective nutrition education must:

- Reach the whole population — all groups, all races, both sexes, all creeds, all ages
- Recognize motives for action and include suggestions on what to do and how to do it
- Develop qualified leadership
- Drive home the same ideas many times and in many ways
- Employ every suitable education tool available
- Adapt those tools to the many and varied groups to be reached and use them with intelligence and skill
- Consider all phases of individual, family, and group situations that have a bearing upon the ability to produce, buy, prepare, conserve, and consume food
- Afford opportunity for participation in making, putting into effect, and evaluating local nutrition programs
- Enlist the fullest participation of all citizens and work through every possible channel to reach the people
- Be adequately financed

As part of national defense efforts, the USDA released the Basic Seven food guide in 1943 in the form of a leaflet entitled *National Wartime Nutrition Guide*. This was revised in 1946 as the *National Food Guide*. This guide specified a foundation diet that would provide a major share of the RDAs for nutrients but only a portion of caloric needs. It was assumed that people would include more foods than the guide recommended to meet their energy and nutrient requirements. In those days, little guidance was provided on the use of fats and sugars. The wartime version of the Basic Seven was intended to help people cope with limited supplies of certain foods.

The 1946 version suggested numbers of servings within each food group and was widely used for over a decade. However, its complexity and lack of specifics regarding serving sizes necessitated modification. In 1956 the USDA released what became known as its Basic Four Food Groups (dairy, grains, meat and alternates, and fruits and vegetables). (See Box 11.3.) Used for the next two decades, the focus of this foundation diet was on getting adequate nutrients.

TABLE 11.1
Principal USDA Food Groups, 1916 through 2005

Year	Type of Food Guide	Title	Food Groups
1916	Buying guides	*Food for Young Children,* developed by Caroline Hunt	1. Meat and other protein-rich foods, including milk 2. Cereals and other starchy foods 3. Vegetables and fruit 4. Fatty food 5. Sugars
1930s	Buying guides	Food plans at four cost levels, developed by Hazel K. Stiebeling	1. Milk 2. Lean meat/poultry/fish 3. Dry mature beans, peas, nuts 4. Eggs 5. Flours and cereals 6. Leafy green and yellow vegetables 7. Potatoes and sweet potatoes 8. Other vegetables and fruits 9. Tomatoes and citrus 10. Butter 11. Other facts 12. Sugars
1940s	Foundation diet	Basic 7	1. Milk and milk products 2. Meat, poultry, fish, eggs, dried beans, peas, nuts 3. Bread, flour, and cereals 4. Leafy green and yellow vegetables 5. Potatoes and other fruits and vegetables 6. Citrus, tomato, cabbage, salad greens 7. Butter, fortified margarine
1956–1970s	Foundation diet	Basic 4	1. Milk group 2. Meat group 3. Bread and cereal group 4. Vegetable and fruit group
1979	Foundation diet	*Hassle-Free Food Guide*	1. Milk–cheese group 2. Meat, poultry, fish, and beans group 3. Breads, cereal, rice, pasta 4. Vegetable-fruit group 5. Fats, sweets, alcohol
1984–2005	Total diet	*Food Guide Pyramid*	1. Milk, yogurt, cheese 2. Meat, poultry, fish, eggs, dry beans, nuts 3. Breads, cereals, rice, pasta 4. Vegetables: dark green/deep yellow, starchy legumes, other 5. Fruit: citrus and others 6. Fats, oils, sweets
2005–present	Total diet	*MyPyramid*	1. Milk group 2. Meat and beans group, including eggs, fish, poultry, dry beans, nuts and seeds, and peanut butter 3. Grain group 4. Vegetables group, including dark green and orange vegetables, starchy vegetables, other vegetables, and legumes 5. Fruits group 6. Oils 7. Discretionary calorie allowance

Source: Davis, C. and Saltos, E. Dietary Recommendations and How They Have Changed Over Time. In Frazao, E., ed. *America's Eating Habits: Changes and Consequences.* Agriculture Information Bulletin No. AIB-750. May 1999, chap. 2. Available at: http://www.ers.usda.gov/Publications/aib750. Accessed July 6, 2006; U.S. Department of Agriculture. MyPyramid Food Intake Patterns. April 2005. Available at: http://www.mypyramid.gov/downloads/MyPyramid_Food_Intake_Patterns.pdf. Accessed July 6, 2006.

Box 11.2 Illustrations

Illustrations of historical guides are available in the online slide collection that traces the USDA's food guides from the 1890s to the present. www.nal.usda.gov/fnic/history/index.html.

By the 1970s, research had implicated over-consumption of fat, saturated fat, cholesterol, and sodium in the development of some chronic diseases. The USDA's Dietary Goals for the United States heralded a new direction for dietary advice that shifted the focus of recommendations from obtaining enough nutrients to decreasing intakes of food components associated with heart disease, stroke, and some forms of cancer. The dietary goals specified quantitative goals for intakes of protein, carbohydrate, fatty acids, cholesterol, sugars, and sodium and drew attention to the need for new guidance on diet and health. In addition, the USDA began addressing the role of fats, sugars, and sodium in risks for chronic diseases in its 1979 *Hassle-Free Guide to a Better Diet*, a modified Basic Four plan that added and highlighted a fifth food group — fats, sweets, and alcoholic beverages — targeted for moderation.

With the release of the first edition of its dietary guidelines, the USDA began work on developing a new food guide, *A Pattern for Daily Food Choices,* designed to help consumers implement the guidelines in their daily food choices. Focusing on the total diet rather than the foundation diet described by earlier guides, the new food guide emphasized making food selections both to meet nutrient objectives and to moderate intake of those components related to risk of chronic diseases. It suggested numbers of servings from each of five major food groups (bread, cereal, rice, and pasta; vegetables; fruit; milk, yogurt, and cheese; and meat, poultry, fish, dry beans, eggs, and nuts) and recommended sparing use of a sixth food group — fats, oils, and sweets. The food guide was initially presented as a food wheel graphic but also appeared as a table in several USDA publications published in the 1980s.

11.1.2 THE FOOD GUIDE PYRAMID, 1992–2005

In 1992, the USDA's Food Guide Pyramid was released with the objective of translating the Dietary Guidelines into food choices. The pyramid recommended that choices come primarily from the grains, vegetables, and fruit groups (plant foods), with less from the meat and dairy groups (animal foods), and even less from fats, oils, and sweets. Within the pyramid, food groups were arranged to indicate proportionality of servings, with accompanying text that provided the recommended numbers of servings from each group. For more than a decade (1992–2005), the Food Guide Pyramid was widely used by nutrition and health professionals, educators, media, and the food industry, and helped to disseminate the nutritional messages of the Dietary Guidelines.[2]

Box 11.3 Basic Four Foundation Diet

The Basic Four Foundation Diet (released in 1956 by the USDA)

- Milk group — 2 cups or more
- Meat group — 2 or more 2- to 3-oz servings
- Bread, cereal — 4 or more (1 oz dry cereal, 1 slice of bread, $1/_2$ – $3/_4$ cup cooked cereal
- Vegetable–fruit — 4 or more (includes dark green/yellow vegetables frequently and citrus daily; $1/_2$ cup or average-size piece)

The philosophical goals[3] that guided the process of developing the Food Guide Pyramid continue to be relevant today. The principles of designing a food guide ensure that it:

- Promotes overall health and well-being (rather than prevents a particular disease)
- Is based on up-to-date research
- Focuses on the total diet, not a core or foundation diet
- Is useful to the target audience, builds on previous food guides, and contains recognizable food groups based on a conceptual framework
- Meets its nutritional goals in a realistic manner, based on the incorporation in the diet of commonly used foods
- Permits maximum flexibility, allowing consumers to eat in a manner that suits their tastes
- Presents practical ways to meet nutritional needs, which might mean using different plans for different activity and age levels; however, because families generally eat the same foods, members should be able to meet their needs by choosing different serving sizes from each of the food groups

The 1990 Dietary Guidelines and the Food Guide Pyramid reflect the key concepts of variety, proportionality, and moderation introduced by Atwater a century ago. Table 11.2 illustrates how the Food Guide Pyramid serves as a mechanism for translating the key concepts of the Dietary Guidelines.

11.1.3 Nutrient-Based Guidance

By the 1970s, it was generally recognized that dietary guidance should not only target adequacy but should also provide guidance related to moderation of those dietary components being consumed in excess. This paved the way for nutrient-based dietary guidance, which focuses primarily on nutrients and other food factors, such as cholesterol, saturated fats, and *trans* fats. A food-based

---

TABLE 11.2
The Food Guide Pyramid as a Mechanism for Translating the Key Concepts of the Dietary Guidelines

Dietary Guidelines for Americans, 1990	Key Concepts of the USDA Food Guide Pyramid, 1992			
	Variety	Proportionality	Moderation	Usability
Eat a variety of foods	√	√		
Choose a diet with plenty of vegetables, fruits, and grain products	√	√		
Maintain a healthy weight		√	√	
Choose a diet low in fat, saturated fat, and cholesterol			√	
Use sugars only in moderation			√	
Use salt and sodium only in moderation			√	
If you drink alcoholic beverages, do so in moderation			√	

Source: Welsh, S.O., Davis, C., and Shaw, A. *USDA's Food Guide: Background and Development.* USDA Human Nutrition Information Service. Nutrition Education Division. Miscellaneous Publication No. 1514. September 1993. Available at: www.usda.gov/cnpp/Pubs/Pyramid/FoodGuideDevt.pdf. Accessed June 19, 2005.

approach presents recommendations in terms of number of servings (the Food Guide Pyramid) or amounts (MyPyramid) of food to be consumed from each of the food groups. In contrast, nutrient-based guidance presents recommendations for single food factors. Recommendations are stated in terms of either the weight (in grams) or percentage of calories that should be provided by one or more of the energy nutrients (carbohydrate, protein, fat). Nutrient-based recommendations also specify the amounts to be consumed of fiber (grams) and vitamins and minerals (milligrams and micrograms).

11.1.3.1 *Dietary Goals for the United States*, 1977

In February of 1977, the Senate Select Committee on Nutrition and Human Needs released the *Dietary Goals for the United States*,[4] which recommended that Americans:

- Increase carbohydrate intake to 55 to 60% of calories
- Decrease dietary fat intake to no more than 30% of calories, with a reduction in intake of saturated fat, and recommended approximately equivalent distributions among saturated, polyunsaturated, and monounsaturated fats to meet the 30% target
- Decrease cholesterol intake to 300 mg/d
- Decrease sugar intake to 15% of calories
- Decrease salt intake to 3 g/d

These goals were the focus of so much controversy among some nutritionists, industry groups, the scientific community, and others concerned with food, nutrition, and health that the Committee released Supplemental Views to the report in November 1977[5] and a second edition in December 1977.[6] Table 11.3 summarizes the goals of the first and second editions. It is instructive to note the differences in the recommendations of the two reports although released in the same calendar year. Developing dietary guidelines and the political processes involved can never be completely separated because the outcomes are not simply scientific statements. Dietary recommendations have economic consequences for many different groups.[7]

When the quantitative recommendations of the dietary goals and of the 1977 U.S. diet are represented in side-by-side bar graphs, it is evident that the goals advocate a more plant-based diet (see Figure 11.1). Key to this interpretation is the recommended protein distribution. To decrease consumption of total fats, one needs to consume less vegetable oil and fat derived from animal sources. For example, the dietary modification to decrease fats would require using less oil in cooking and salad dressings, switching from high-fat to lower-fat meat and poultry products, and replacing the reduction in calories with an increased intake of foods rich in complex carbohydrates and naturally occurring sugars such as grain products, fruits, and vegetables. To maintain the proportion of calories derived from protein, as illustrated in the bar graph, the source of protein calories should switch from animal to plant products.

In essence, the 1997 dietary goals recommended replacing some higher biological value protein (from animal products) with lower biological value protein (from plants). Similarly, the recommendation to decrease cholesterol, derived exclusively from animal products and principally from egg yolks, would be achieved by decreasing intake of whole eggs and/or meat. In other words, the dietary goals advocated a diet that approached vegetarianism. The message to reduce consumption of meat and eggs would result in negative economic consequences for producers and marketers of these products, arousing their opposition to the recommendations.

11.1.3.2 *Dietary Guidelines for Americans*, 1980–2004

In response to the public's burgeoning interest in nutrition and health, in 1980 the federal government published the *Dietary Guidelines for Americans*.[8] This document was based on the most up-to-date information available at the time and was directed to healthy Americans. These guidelines

TABLE 11.3
Dietary Goals for the U.S., 1997

Dietary Goals for the U.S., February 1977	Dietary Goals for the U.S., 2nd Edition, December 1977
	To avoid overweight, consume only as much energy (calories) as is expended; if overweight, decrease energy intake and increase energy expenditure
Increase carbohydrate intake to 55–60% of calories	Increase the consumption of complex carbohydrates and "naturally occurring" sugars from about 28% to about 48% of energy intake
Decrease sugar intake to 15% of calories	Reduce the consumption of refined and processed sugars by about 45% to account for about 10% of total energy intake
Decrease dietary fat intake to no more than 30% of calories, with a reduction in intake of saturated fat, and recommended approximately equivalent distributions among saturated, polyunsaturated, and monounsaturated fats to meet the 30% target	Reduce overall fat consumption from approximately 40% to about 30% of energy intake
	Reduce saturated fat consumption to account for about 10% of total energy intake, and balance that with polyunsaturated and monounsaturated fats, which should account for about 10% of energy intake each
Decrease cholesterol intake to 300 mg/d	Reduce cholesterol consumption to about 300 mg/d
Decrease salt intake to 3 g/d	Limit the intake of sodium by reducing the intake of salt to about 5 g/d

Source: U.S. Congress. Senate. Select Committee on Nutrition and Human Needs. *Dietary Goals for the United States* [1st edition]. Washington, DC: U.S. Government Printing Office, 1977. [Description: Congressional report with references and statements by scientists.] Also, United States Senate. Select Committee on Nutrition and Human Needs. *Dietary Goals for the United States*, 2nd ed. Washington, D.C., December 1977.

generated considerable discussion by nutrition scientists, consumer groups, the food industry, and others. A report by a U.S. Senate appropriations committee directed that a committee be established to review scientific evidence and recommend revisions to the guidelines.[9]

In 1983, a federal advisory committee of nine nutrition scientists selected from outside the federal government was convened to review and make recommendations about the first edition of the Dietary Guidelines. Based on the committee's recommendations, DHHS and USDA jointly issued a second edition of the guidelines in 1985.[10] Although nearly identical to the first edition, some changes were made for clarity; others reflected advances in scientific knowledge of the associations between diet and a range of chronic diseases. The second edition received wide acceptance and was used as a framework for consumer education messages.

In 1989, USDA and DHHS established a second advisory committee that considered whether the 1985 Dietary Guidelines needed revision and then proceeded to make recommendations for revision in a report to the Secretaries. *The Surgeon General's Report on Nutrition and Health* (1988)[11] and the National Research Council's report *Diet and Health: Implications for Reducing Chronic Disease Risk* (1989)[12] were key resources used by this committee.

The 1990 Dietary Guidelines[13] contained additional refinements to reflect increased understanding of the science of nutrition and how best to communicate this to consumers. The language of the new *Dietary Guidelines for Americans* was more positive, was oriented toward the total diet,

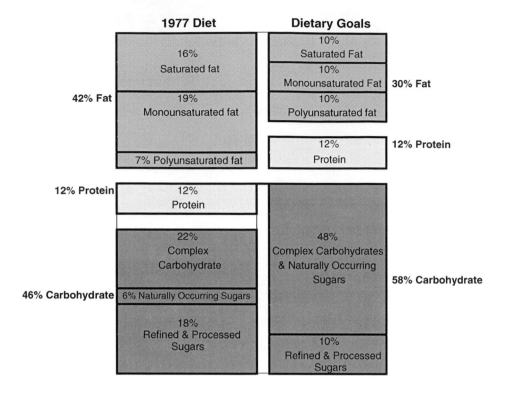

FIGURE 11.1 Comparison of the1977 Diet and the Dietary Goals.

and provided more specific information regarding food selection. For the first time, numerical recommendations were made for intakes of total dietary fat and of saturated fat.

In 1990, with the passage of P.L.101–445,[14] Congress formally instructed the two departments to issue the guidelines every 5 years. The legislation directed that the guidelines must (1) contain nutritional and dietary information and guidelines for the general public; (2) be based on the preponderance of current scientific and medical knowledge; and (3) be promoted by each federal agency in carrying out any federal food, nutrition, or health program. In other words, the act made the report official federal policy on nutrition guidance. Thus, while the government voluntarily issued the Dietary Guidelines in 1980, 1985, and 1990, editions published in 1995, 2000, and 2005 were statutorily mandated.

Since 1980, the *Dietary Guidelines for Americans* have been updated every 5 years. A Dietary Guidelines Advisory Committee was established to assist in the preparations of the 1995, 2000, and 2005 editions of the guidelines. Although the guidelines have remained consistent, there have been changes through the years that reflect emerging science. The guidelines have evolved into a document that attempts to reflect scientific consensus and provides the statutory basis of federal nutrition education efforts.

The 1995 edition of the guidelines[15] continued to support the concepts elucidated in earlier editions. New information included the Food Guide Pyramid, Nutrition Facts Labels, and boxes highlighting good food sources of key nutrients. Starting with the second edition of the Dietary Goals and continuing through the first four editions of the guidelines, recommendations have been presented as seven individual guidelines. The 2000 edition[16] offers 10 guidelines, created by separating physical activity from the weight guideline, splitting the grains from fruits and vegetables for greater emphasis, and introducing a new guideline about safe food handling. The progression from 7 to 10 guidelines is illustrated in the guidelines summary (1980 through 2000) in Table 11.4.

TABLE 11.4
Dietary Guidelines for Americans, 1980–2000

1980	1985	1990	1995	2000	
7 Guidelines	7 Guidelines	7 Guidelines	7 Guidelines	10 Guidelines, clustered into 3 groups	
Eat a variety of foods	Eat a variety of foods	Eat a variety of foods	Eat a variety of foods		
Maintain ideal weight	Maintain desirable weight	Maintain healthy weight	Balance the food you eat with physical activity—maintain or improve your weight	Aim for a healthy weight	Aim for Fitness
				Be physically active each day	
Avoid too much fat, saturated fat, and cholesterol	Avoid too much fat, saturated fat, and cholesterol	Choose a diet low in fat, saturated fat, and cholesterol		Let the Pyramid guide your food choices	Build a Healthy Base
Eat foods with adequate starch and fiber	Eat foods with adequate starch and fiber	Choose a diet with plenty of vegetables, fruits, and grain projects	Choose a diet with plenty of grain products, vegetables, and fruits	Choose a variety of grains daily, especially whole grains	
				Choose a variety of fruits and vegetables daily	
				Keep food safe to eat	
		Choose a diet low in fat, saturated fat, and cholesterol		Choose a diet that is low in saturated fat and cholesterol and moderate in total fat	Choose Sensibly
Avoid too much sugar	Avoid too much sugar	Use sugars only in moderation	Choose a diet moderate in sugars	Choose beverages and foods to moderate your intake of sugars	
Avoid too much sodium	Avoid too much sodium	Use salt and sodium only in moderation	Choose a diet moderate in salt and sodium	Choose and prepare foods with less salt	
If you drink alcohol, do so in moderation	If you drink alcoholic beverages, do so in moderation	If you drink alcoholic beverages, do so in moderation	If you drink alcoholic beverages, do so in moderation	If you drink alcoholic beverages, do so in moderation	

Shading indicates how the order in which the guidelines are presented has changed over time

Source: Center for Nutrition Policy and Promotion, USDA. May 30, 2000. Available at: www.usda.gov/cnpp/Pubs/DG2000/Dgover.PDF. Accessed July 6, 2006.

11.1.3.2.1   Healthy Eating Index

To assess and monitor the dietary status of Americans, in 1995 the USDA's Center for Nutrition Policy and Promotion (CNPP) developed the Healthy Eating Index (HEI). Designed to measure compliance with the 1990 edition of the Dietary Guidelines, the HEI gauges relative intake of the key dietary components identified in the guidelines. The 1995 index comprises 10 components, each representing different aspects of a healthful diet. Components 1–5 measure the degree to which a person's diet conforms to serving recommendations for the five major food groups of the 1992 Food Guide Pyramid (grains, vegetables, fruits, milk, and meat). Components 6–9 conform to recommendations in the 1995 Dietary Guidelines for total fat and saturated fat consumption as a percentage of total food energy intake and total cholesterol and sodium intake. Lastly, component 10 measures variety in a person's diet. Scores for each component are given equal weight; the maximum combined score for the 10 components is 100. An HEI score above 80 implies a good diet; a score between 51 and 80 suggests the diet needs to be improved; and a score below 51 indicates a poor diet.[17,18]

The HEI has been used for developing nutrition education and evaluating interventions. The USDA uses the HEI to monitor diet quality. For example, as indicated in Table 11.5, the USDA has been using the HEI to evaluate children's diets since 1989. According to the statistics in the table, most children have a diet that is poor or needs improvement. As children get older, their diet quality declines. The lower quality diets of older children are linked to declines in their fruit and sodium scores.

TABLE 11.5
Healthy Eating Index — Overall and Component Mean Scores and Percentages for Children, 1989–2000

| | 1989–1990 | | | 1994–1996 | | | 1998–2000 | | |
| | Ages | | | Ages | | | Ages | | |
Component	2–6	7–12	13–18	2–6	7–12	13–18	2–6	7–12	13–18
HEI Score									
Overall	70.2	66.6	59.2	69.4	64.6	59.9	70.3	64.1	61.0
1. Grains	7.6	7.0	6.3	7.7	7.5	6.9	8.0	7.5	6.8
2. Vegetables	5.2	5.0	5.6	5.3	5.2	5.9	5.6	4.8	5.3
3. Fruits	6.2	4.6	3.1	6.0	4.1	3.2	5.8	3.7	3.1
4. Milk	8.6	8.3	6.7	7.3	7.1	5.3	7.3	6.9	7.5
5. Meat	6.6	7.0	7.1	5.7	5.7	6.3	5.4	5.5	6.0
6. Total fat	6.7	6.9	6.1	7.3	7.1	7.0	7.3	7.2	7.1
7. Saturated fat	3.7	4.2	4.0	5.5	5.7	6.2	5.8	6.2	6.2
8. Cholesterol	9.4	8.7	8.1	9.0	8.6	7.6	9.0	8.6	8.1
9. Sodium	9.1	7.3	5.8	8.4	6.6	5.6	8.0	6.4	5.7
10. Variety	7.2	7.7	6.5	7.3	7.1	6.0	8.1	7.5	7.2

Source: Forum on Child and Family Statistics: *Healthy Eating Index: Overall and Component Mean Scores and Percentages for Children Ages 2–18, 1989–90, 1994–96, and 1999–2000.* Available at: http://www.childstats.gov/ amchildren05/ xls/ econ4d.xls. Accessed August 17, 2006.

11.1.3.3   Recommended Dietary Allowances (RDAs) and Dietary Reference Intakes (DRIs)

Until 1997, the RDAs served as a benchmark for nutritional adequacy. They were designed to suggest the levels of nutrients adequate to meet the nutrient needs of the majority of healthy people. Subsequently, the DRIs reflect a shift in emphasis from preventing deficiency to decreasing the risk of chronic disease.

11.1.3.3.1   RDA History

During World War II, the National Research Council (NRC) determined that a set of dietary standards was needed in the event that food would have to be rationed. These standards would be used to make nutrition recommendations for the armed forces, civilians, and the overseas population who might need food relief. All available data concerning nutrient needs was surveyed to create a tentative set of allowances, which was then reviewed by experts before being accepted in 1941. The allowances were meant to provide superior nutrition for civilians and military personnel; therefore, they included a "margin of safety." The first edition, published in 1943, was intended to provide "standards to serve as a goal for good nutrition." The RDAs were revised nine times; the 10th and last edition was published in 1989.

Box 11.4 Activity

Based on the data presented in Table 11.5, what other observations and interpretations can you make?

Box 11.5 The Dietary Reference Intake Reports Issued by the Institute of Medicine, 1997–2004

1. Dietary Reference Intakes: Water, Potassium, Sodium, Chloride, and Sulfate (February 11, 2004)
2. Dietary Reference Intakes: Guiding Principles for Nutrition Labeling and Fortification (December 11, 2003)
3. Dietary Reference Intakes: Applications in Dietary Planning (February 6, 2003)
4. Dietary Reference Intakes for Energy, Carbohydrate, Fiber, Fat, Fatty Acids, Cholesterol, Protein, and Amino Acids (September 5, 2002)
5. Dietary Reference Intakes for Energy, Carbohydrate, Fiber, Fat, Fatty Acids, Cholesterol, Protein, and Amino Acids (September 5, 2002)
6. Dietary Reference Intakes: Proposed Definition of Dietary Fiber (May 2, 2001)
7. Dietary Reference Intakes for Vitamin A, Vitamin K, Arsenic, Boron, Chromium, Copper, Iodine, Iron, Manganese, Molybdenum, Nickel, Silicon, Vanadium, and Zinc (January 9, 2001)
8. Dietary Reference Intakes for Vitamin C, Vitamin E, Selenium, and Carotenoids (August 3, 2000)
9. Dietary Reference Intakes for Thiamin, Riboflavin, Niacin, Vitamin B6, Folate, Vitamin B12, Pantothenic Acid, Biotin, and Choline (June 12, 2000)
10. Dietary Reference Intakes: Applications in Dietary Assessment (May 1, 2000)
11. Dietary Reference Intakes: Proposed Definition and Plan for Review of Dietary Antioxidants and Related Compounds (August 5, 1998)
12. Dietary Reference Intakes for Calcium, Phosphorus, Magnesium, Vitamin D, and Fluoride (January 1, 1997)

In 1997, at the suggestion of the Institute of Medicine (IOM) of the National Academy of Sciences (NAS), the RDAs were incorporated into a broader set of dietary guidelines called the DRIs and are used by both the U.S. and Canada. The DRIs have been published in seven separate volumes covering the macro- and micro-nutrients, two reports addressing the definitions of fiber and dietary antioxidants and related compounds, and three reports that examine the use of DRIs in dietary assessment, diet planning, and labeling and fortification (see Box 11.5). The DRIs appear in Figure 11.2.

11.1.3.3.2 DRIs

The DRIs are a set of nutrient-based reference values that have replaced the 1989 RDAs in the U.S. and the Recommended Nutrient Intakes (RNIs) in Canada. The reference values, collectively referred to as the DRIs, include the Estimated Average Requirement (EAR), the Recommended Dietary Allowance (RDA), the Adequate Intake (AI), and the Tolerable Upper Intake Level (UL). The RDA represents the average daily dietary nutrient intake level sufficient to meet the nutrient requirements of almost all healthy individuals (97.5%) in a particular life stage and gender group. AI is used when a definitive RDA cannot be determined from the scientific data. The UL is the maximum amount of a nutrient at which no adverse effects have been observed (see Boxes 11.6 and 11.7).

Because the DRIs also focus on chronic disease risk, the Acceptable Micronutrient Distribution Ranges (AMDRs) recommend percentage ranges of calories for daily macronutrients (protein, fat, carbohydrate). For adults, the recommended range for carbohydrates is 45–65% of calories, for fat 20–35% of calories, and for protein 5–10% of calories.

The DRIs differ from the 1989 RDAs in at least two respects: DRIs are based on a reduction in the risk of chronic disease, rather than merely the absence of signs of deficiency; when data are available, ULs are established to avoid the risk of adverse effects from excess consumption.

Dietary Reference Intakes (DRIs): Recommended Intakes for Individuals, Macronutrients

Food and Nutrition Board, Institute of Medicine, National Academies

Life Stage Group	Total Water[a] (L/d)	Carbohydrate (g/d)	Total Fiber (g/d)	Fat (g/d)	Linoleic Acid (g/d)	α-Linolenic Acid (g/d)	Protein[b] (g/d)
Infants							
0–6 mo	0.7*	60*	ND	31*	4.4*	0.5*	9.1*
7–12 mo	0.8*	95*	ND	30*	4.6*	0.5*	**11.0[c]**
Children							
1–3 y	1.3*	**130**	19*	ND	7*	0.7*	**13**
4–8 y	1.7*	**130**	25*	ND	10*	0.9*	**19**
Males							
9–13 y	2.4*	**130**	31*	ND	12*	1.2*	**34**
14–18 y	3.3*	**130**	38*	ND	16*	1.6*	**52**
19–30 y	3.7*	**130**	38*	ND	17*	1.6*	**56**
31–50 y	3.7*	**130**	38*	ND	17*	1.6*	**56**
51–70 y	3.7*	**130**	30*	ND	14*	1.6*	**56**
> 70	3.7*	**130**	30*	ND	14*	1.6*	**56**
Females							
9–13 y	2.1*	**130**	26*	ND	10*	1.0*	**34**
14–18 y	2.3*	**130**	26*	ND	11*	1.1*	**46**
19–30 y	2.7*	**130**	25*	ND	12*	1.1*	**46**
31–50 y	2.7*	**130**	25*	ND	12*	1.1*	**46**
51–70 y	2.7*	**130**	21*	ND	11*	1.1*	**46**
> 70 y	2.7*	**130**	21*	ND	11*	1.1*	**46**
Pregnancy							
14–18 y	3.0*	**175**	28*	ND	13*	1.4*	**71**
19–30 y	3.0*	**175**	28*	ND	13*	1.4*	**71**
31–50 y	3.0*	**175**	28*	ND	13*	1.4*	**71**
Lactation							
14–18 y	3.8*	**210**	29*	ND	13*	1.3*	**71**
19–30 y	3.8*	**210**	29*	ND	13*	1.3*	**71**
31–50 y	3.8*	**210**	29*	ND	13*	1.3*	**71**

Note: This table presents Recommended Dietary Allowances (RDAs) in **bold type** and Adequate Intakes (AIs) in ordinary type followed by an asterisk (*). RDAs and AIs may both be used as goals for individual intake. RDAs are set to meet the needs of almost all (97 to 98 percent) individuals in a group. For healthy infants fed human milk, the AI is the mean intake. The AI for other life stage and gender groups is believed to cover the needs of all individuals in the group, but lack of data or uncertainty in the data prevent being able to specify with confidence the percentage of individuals covered by this intake.

[a] *Total* water includes all water contained in food, beverages, and drinking water.
[b] Based on 0.8 g/kg body weight for the reference body weight.
[c] Change from 13.5 in prepublication copy due to calculation error.

Dietary Reference Intakes (DRIs): Additional Macronutrient Recommendations

Food and Board, Institute of Medicine, National Academies

Macronutrient	Recommendation
Dietary cholesterol	As low as possible while consuming a nutritionally adequate diet
Trans fatty acids	As low as possible while consuming a nutritionally adequate diet
Saturated fatty acids	As low as possible while consuming a nutritionally adequate diet
Added sugars	Limit to no more than 25% of total energy

Source: Dietary Reference Intakes for Energy, Carbohydrate, Fiber, Fat, Fatty Acids, Cholesterol, Protein, and Amino Acids (2002).

FIGURE 11.2 DRI Charts.

Dietary Reference Intakes (DRIs): Recommended Intakes for Individuals, Vitamins

Food and Nutrition Board, Institute of Medicine, National Academies

Life Stage Group	Vit A (µg/d)[a]	Vit C (mg/d)	Vit D (µg/d)[b,c]	Vit E (mg/d)[d]	Vit K (µg/d)	Thiamin (mg/d)	Riboflavin (mg/d)	Niacin (mg/d)[e]	Vit B6 (mg/d)	Folate (µg/d)[f]	Vit B12 (µg/d)	Pantothenic Acid (mg/d)	Biotin (µg/d)	Choline[g] (mg/d)
Infants														
0–6 mo	400*	40*	5*	4*	2.0*	0.2*	0.3*	2*	0.1*	65*	0.4*	1.7*	5*	125*
7–12 mo	500*	50*	5*	5*	2.5*	0.3*	0.4*	4*	0.3*	80*	0.5*	1.8*	6*	150*
Children														
1–3 y	300	15	5*	6	30*	0.5	0.5	6	0.5	150	0.9	2*	8*	200*
4–8 y	400	25	5*	7	55*	0.6	0.6	8	0.6	200	1.2	3*	12*	250*
Males														
9–13 y	600	45	5*	11	60*	0.9	0.9	12	1.0	300	1.8	4*	20*	375*
14–18 y	900	75	5*	15	75*	1.2	1.3	16	1.3	400	2.4	5*	25*	550*
19–30 y	900	90	5*	15	120*	1.2	1.3	16	1.3	400	2.4	5*	30*	550*
31–50 y	900	90	5*	15	120*	1.2	1.3	16	1.3	400	2.4	5*	30*	550*
51–70 y	900	90	10*	15	120*	1.2	1.3	16	1.7	400	2.4[h]	5*	30*	550*
>70 y	900	90	15*	15	120*	1.2	1.3	16	1.7	400	2.4[h]	5*	30*	550*
Females														
9–13 y	600	45	5*	11	60*	0.9	0.9	12	1.0	300	1.8	4*	20*	375*
14–18 y	700	65	5*	15	75*	1.0	1.0	14	1.2	400[i]	2.4	5*	25*	400*
19–30 y	700	75	5*	15	90*	1.1	1.1	14	1.3	400[i]	2.4	5*	30*	425*
31–50 y	700	75	5*	15	90*	1.1	1.1	14	1.3	400[i]	2.4	5*	30*	425*
51–70 y	700	75	10*	15	90*	1.1	1.1	14	1.5	400	2.4[h]	5*	30*	425*
>70 y	700	75	15*	15	90*	1.1	1.1	14	1.5	400	2.4[h]	5*	30*	425*
Pregnancy														
14–18 y	750	80	5*	15	75*	1.4	1.4	18	1.9	600[j]	2.6	6*	30*	450*
19–30 y	770	85	5*	15	90*	1.4	1.4	18	1.9	600[j]	2.6	6*	30*	450*
31–50 y	770	85	5*	15	90*	1.4	1.4	18	1.9	600[j]	2.6	6*	30*	450*
Lactation														
14–18 y	1,200	115	5*	19	75*	1.4	1.6	17	2.0	500	2.8	7*	35*	550*
19–30 y	1,300	120	5*	19	90*	1.4	1.6	17	2.0	500	2.8	7*	35*	550*
31–50 y	1,300	120	5*	19	90*	1.4	1.6	17	2.0	500	2.8	7*	35*	550*

FIGURE 11.2 (Continued).

Note: This table (taken from the DRI reports, see www.nap.edu) presents Recommended Dietary Allowances (RDAs) in **bold type** and Adequate Intakes (AIs) in ordinary type followed by an asterisk (*). RDAs and AIs may both be used as goals for individual intake. RDAs are set on meet the needs of almost all (97 to 98 percent) individuals in a group. For healthy breastfed infants, the AI is the mean intake. The AI for other life stage and gender groups is believed to cover needs of all individuals in the group, but lack of data or uncertainty in the data prevent being able to specify with confidence the percentage of individuals covered by this intake.

[a] As retinol activity equivalents (RAEs). 1 RAE = 1 μg retinol, 12 μg β-carotene, 24 μg α-carotene, or 24 μg β-cryptoxanthin. The RAE for dietary provitamin A carotenoids is twofold greater than retinol equivalents (RE), whereas the RAE for preformed vitamin A is the same as RE.

[b] As cholecalciferol. 1 μg cholecalciferol = 40 IU vitamin D.

[c] In the absence of adequate exposure to sunlight.

[d] As α-Tocopherol. α-Tocopherol includes RRR-α-tocopherol, the only form of a-tocopherol that occurs naturally in foods, and the 2R-stereoisomeric forms of α-tocopherol (RRR-, RSR-, RRS-, and RSS-α-tocopherol) that occur in fortified foods and supplements. It does not include the 2S-stereoisomeric forms of α-tocopherol (SRR-, SSR-, SRS-, and SSS-α-tocopherol), also found in fortified foods and supplements.

[e] As niacin equivalents (NE). 1 mg of niacin = 60 mg of tryptophan; 0–6 months = preformed niacin (not NE).

[f] As dietary folate equivalents (DFE). 1 DFE = 1 μg food folate = 0.6 μg of folic acid from fortified food or as a supplement consumed with food = 0.5 μg of a supplement taken on an empty stomach.

[g] Although AIs have been set for choline, there are few data to assess whether a dietary supply of choline is needed at all stages of the life cycle, and it may be that the choline requirement can be met by endogenous synthesis at some of these stages.

[h] Because 10 to 30 percent of older people may malabsorb food-bound B_{12}, it is advisable for those older than 50 years to meet their RDA mainly by consuming foods fortified with B_{12} or a supplement containing B_{12}.

[i] In view of evidence linking folate intake with neural tube defects in the fetus, it is recommended that all women capable of becoming pregnant consume 400 μg from supplements of fortified foods in addition to intake of food folate from a varied diet.

[j] It is assumed that women will continue consuming 400 μg from supplements or fortified food until their pregnancy is confirmed and they enter prenatal care, which ordinarily occurs after the end of the periconceptional period—the critical time for formation of the neural tube.

Copyright 2004 by the National Academy of Sciences. All rights reserved.

FIGURE 11.2 (Continued).

Dietary Reference Intakes (DRIs): Recommended Intakes for Individuals, Elements
Food and Nutrition Board, Institute of Medicine, National Academies

Life Stage Group	Calcium (mg/d)	Chromium (µg/d)	Copper (µg/d)	Fluoride (mg/d)	Iodine (µg/d)	Iron (mg/d)	Magnesium (mg/d)	Manganese (mg/d)	Molybdenum (µg/d)	Phosphorus (mg/d)	Selenium (µg/d)	Zinc (mg/d)	Potassium	Sodium (g/d)	Chloride (g/d)
Infants															
0–6 mo	210*	0.2*	200*	0.01*	110*	0.27*	30*	0.003*	2*	100*	15*	2*	0.4*	0.12*	0.18*
7–12 mo	270*	5.5*	220*	0.5*	130*	11	75*	0.6*	3*	275*	20*	3	0.7*	0.37*	0.57*
Children															
1–3 y	500*	11*	340	0.7*	90	7	80	1.2*	17	460	20	3	3.0*	1.0*	1.5*
4–8 y	800*	15*	440	1*	90	10	130	1.5*	22	500	30	5	3.8*	1.2*	1.9*
Males															
9–13 y	1,300*	25*	700	2*	120	8	240	1.9*	34	1,250	40	8	4.5*	1.5*	2.3*
14–18 y	1,300*	35*	890	3*	150	11	410	2.2*	43	1,250	55	11	4.7*	1.5*	2.3*
19–30 y	1,000*	35*	900	4*	150	8	400	2.3	45	700	55	11	4.7*	1.5*	2.3*
31–50 y	1,000*	35*	900	4*	150	8	420	2.3*	45	700	55	11	4.7*	1.5*	2.3*
51–70 y	1,200*	30*	900	4*	150	8	420	2.3*	45	700	55	11	4.7*	1.3*	2.0*
>70 y	1,200*	30*	900	4*	150	8	420	2.3*	45	700	55	11	4.7*	1.2*	1.8*
Females															
9–13 y	1,300*	21*	700	2*	120	8	240	1.6*	34	1,250	40	8	4.5*	1.5*	2.3*
14–18 y	1,300	24*	890	3*	150	15	360	1.6*	43	1,250	55	9	4.7*	1.5*	2.3*
19–30 y	1,000*	25*	900	3*	150	18	310	1.8*	45	700	55	8	4.7*	1.5*	2.3*
31–50 y	1,000*	25*	900	3*	150	18	320	1.8*	45	700	55	8	4.7*	1.5*	2.3*
51–70 y	1,200*	20*	900	3*	150	8	320	1.8*	45	700	55	8	4.7*	1.3*	2.0*
>70 y	1,200*	20*	900	3*	150	8	320	1.8*	45	700	55	8	4.7*	1.2*	1.8*
Pregnancy															
14–18 y	1,300*	29*	1,000	3*	220	27	400	2.0*	50	1,250	60	12	4.7*	1.5*	2.3*
19–30 y	1,000*	30*	1,000	3*	220	27	350	2.0*	50	700	60	11	4.7*	1.5*	2.3*
31–50 y	1,000*	30*	1,000	3*	220	27	360	2.0*	50	700	60	11	4.7*	1.5*	2.3*
Lactation															
14–18 y	1,300*	44*	1,300	3*	290	10	360	2.6*	50	1,250	70	13	5.1*	1.5*	2.3*
19–30 y	1,000*	45*	1,300	3*	290	9	310	2.6*	50	700	70	12	5.1*	1.5	2.3*
31–50 y	1,000*	45*	1,300	3*	290	9	320	2.6*	50	700	70	12	5.1*	1.5*	2.3*

Note: This table presents Recommended Dietary Allowances (RDAs) in **bold type** and Adequate Intakes (AIs) in ordinary type followed by an asterisk (*). RDAs and AIs may both be used as goals for individual intake. RDAs are set to meet the needs of almost all (97 to 98 percent) individuals in a group. For healthy breastfed infants, the AI is the mean intake. The AI for other life stage and gender groups is believed to cover needs of all individuals in the groups, but lack of data or uncertainty in the data prevent being able to specify with confidence the percentage of individuals covered by this intake.

Sources: Dietary References Intakes for Calcium, Phosphorous, Magnesium, Vitamin D, and Fluoride (1997); Dietary Reference Intakes for Thiamin, Riboflavin, Niacin, Vitamin B6, Folate, Vitamin B12, Pantothenic Acid, Biotin, and Choline (1998); Dietary Reference Intake for Vitamin C, Vitamin E, Selenium, and Carotenoids (2000); Dietary Reference Intakes for Vitamin A, Vitamin K, Arsenic Baron, Chromium, Copper, Iodine, Iron, Manganese, Molybdenum, Nickel, Silicon, Vanadium, and Zinc (2001); and Dietary Reference Intakes for Water, Potassium, Sodium, Chloride, and Sulfate (2004). These reports may be accessed via. http://www.nap.edu.

Copyright 2004 by the National Academy of Sciences. All rights reserved.

FIGURE 11.2 (Continued).

Dietary Reference Intake (DRIs): Estimated Average Requirement for Groups

Food and Nutrition Board, Institute of Medicine, National Academies

Life Stage Group	CHO (g/d)	Protein (g/d)ᵃ	Vit A (μg/d)ᵇ	Vit C (mg/d)	Vit E (mg/d)ᶜ	Thiamin (mg/d)	Riboflavin (mg/d)	Niacin (mg/d)ᵈ	Vit B₆ (mg/d)	Folate (μg/d)ᵇ	Vit B₁₂ (μg/d)	Copper (μg/d)	Iodine (μg/d)	Iron (mg/d)	Magnesium (mg/d)	Molybdenum (μg/d)	Phosphrous (mg/d)	Selenium (μg/d)	Zinc (mg/d)
Infants																			
7–12 mo		9*												6.9					2.5
Children																			
1–3 y	100	11	210	13	5	0.4	0.4	5	0.4	120	0.7	260	65	3.0	65	13	380	17	2.5
4–8 y	100	15	275	22	6	0.5	0.5	6	0.5	160	1.0	340	110	4.1	65	17	405	23	4.0
Males																			
9–13 y	100	27	445	39	9	0.7	0.8	9	0.8	250	1.5	540	73	5.9	200	26	1,055	35	7.0
14–18 y	100	44	630	63	12	1.0	1.1	12	1.1	330	2.0	685	95	7.7	340	33	1,055	45	8.5
19–30 y	100	46	625	75	12	1.0	1.1	12	1.1	320	2.0	700	95	6	330	34	580	45	9.4
31–50 y	100	46	625	75	12	1.0	1.1	12	1.1	320	2.0	700	95	6	350	34	580	45	9.4
51–70 y	100	46	625	75	12	1.0	1.1	12	1.4	320	2.0	700	95	6	350	34	580	45	9.4
>70 Y	100	46	625	75	12	1.0	1.1	12	1.4	320	2.0	700	95	6	350	34	580	45	9.4
Females																			
9–13 y	100	28	420	39	9	0.7	0.8	9	0.8	250	1.5	540	73	5.7	200	26	1,055	35	7.0
14–18 y	100	38	485	56	12	0.9	0.9	11	1.0	330	2.0	685	95	7.9	300	33	1,055	45	7.3
19–30 y	100	38	500	60	12	0.9	0.9	11	1.1	320	2.0	700	95	8.1	255	34	580	45	6.8
31–50 y	100	38	500	60	12	0.9	0.9	11	1.1	320	2.0	700	95	8.1	265	34	580	45	6.8
51–70 y	100	38	500	60	12	0.9	0.9	11	1.3	320	2.0	700	95	5	265	34	580	45	6.8
>70 y	100	38	500	60	12	0.9	0.9	11	1.3	320	2.0	700	95	5	265	34	580	45	6.8
Pregnancy																			
14–18 y	135	50	530	66	12	1.2	1.2	14	1.6	520	2.2	785	160	23	335	40	1,055	49	10.5
19–30 y	135	50	550	70	12	1.2	1.2	14	1.6	520	2.2	800	160	22	290	40	580	49	9.5
31–50 y	135	50	550	70	12	1.2	1.2	14	1.6	520	2.2	800	160	22	300	40	580	49	9.5
Lactation																			
14–18 y	160	60	885	96	16	1.2	1.3	13	1.7	450	2.4	985	209	7	300	35	1,055	59	10.9
19–30 y	160	60	900	100	16	1.2	1.3	13	1.7	450	2.4	1,000	209	6.5	255	36	580	59	10.4
31–50 y	160	60	900	100	16	1.2	1.3	13	1.7	450	2.4	1,000	209	6.5	265	36	580	59	10.4

FIGURE 11.2 (Continued).

Note: This table presents Estimated Average Requirements (EARs), which serve two purposes: for assessing adequacy of population intakes, and as the basis for calculating Recommended Dietary Allowances (RDAs) for individuals for those nutrients. EARs have not been established for vitamin D, vitamin K, pantothenic acid, biotin, choline, calcium, chromium, fluoride, manganese, or other nutrients not yet evaluated via the DRI process.

a For individual at reference weight (Table 1–1). * indicates change from prepublication copy due to calculation error.

b As retinol activity equivalents (RAEs). 1 RAE = 1 μg retinol, 12 μg β-carotene, 24 μg α-carotene, or 24 μg β-cryptoxanthin. The RAE for dietary provitamin A carotenoids is twofold greater than retinol equivalents (RE), whereas the RAE for preformed vitamin A is the same as RE.

c As α-tocopherol. α-Tocopherol includes RRR-α-tocopherol, the only form of α-tocopherol that occurs naturally in foods, and the $2R$-stereoisomeric forms of α-tocopherol (RRR-, RSR-, RRS-, and RSS-α-tocopherol) that occur in fortified foods and supplements. It does not include the $2S$-stereoisomeric forms of α-tocopherol (SRR-, SSR-, SRS-, and SSS-α-tocopherol), also found in fortified foods and supplements.

d As niacin equivalents (NE). 1 mg of niacin = 60 mg of tryptophan.

e As dietary folate equivalents (DFE). 1 DFE = 1 μg food folate = 0.6 μg of folic acid from fortified food or as a supplement consumed with food = 0.5 μg of a supplement taken on an empty stomach.

Sources: Dietary Reference Intakes for Calcium, Phosphorous, Magnesium, Vitamin D, and Fluoride (1997); Dietary Reference Intakes for Thiamin, Riboflavin, Niacin, Vitamin B$_6$, Folate, Vitamin B$_{12}$, Pantothenic Acid, Biotin, and Choline (1998); Dietary Reference Intakes for Vitamin C, Vitamin E, Selenium, and Carotenoids (2000); Dietary Reference Intakes for Vitamin A, Vitamin K, Arsenic, Boron, Chromium, Copper, Iodine, Iron, Manganese, Molybdenum, Nickel, Silicon, Vanadium, and Zinc (2001), and Dietary Reference Intakes for Energy, Carbohydrate, Fiber, Fat, Fatty Acids, Cholesterol, Protein, and Amino Acids (2002). These reports may be accessed via www.nap.edu.

FIGURE 11.2 (Continued).

Dietary Reference Intake (DRIs): Estimated Energy Requirements (EER) for Men and Women 30 Years of Age[a]

Food and Nutrition Board, Institute of Medicine, National Academies

Height (m[in])	PAL[b]	Weight for BMI[c] of 18.5 kg/m² (kg[ib])	Weight for BMI of 24.99 kg/m² (kg[ib])	EER, Men[d] (kcal/day) BMI of 18.5 kg/m²	EER, Men[d] (kcal/day) BMI of 24.99 kg/m²	EER, Women[d] (kcal/day) BMI of 18.5 kg/m²	EER, Women[d] (kcal/day) BMI of 24.99 kg/m²
1.50 (59)	Sedentary	41.6 (92)	56.2 (124)	1,848	2,080	1,625	1,762
	Low active			2,009	2,267	1,803	1,956
	Active			2,215	2,506	2,025	2,198
	Very active			2,554	2,898	2,291	2,489
1.65 (65)	Sedentary	50.4 (111)	68.0 (150)	2,068	2,349	1,816	1,982
	Low active			2,254	2,566	2,016	2,202
	Active			2,490	2,842	2,267	2,477
	Very Active			2,880	3,296	2,567	2,807
1.80 (71)	Sedentary	59.9 (132)	81.0 (178)	2,301	2,635	2,015	2,211
	Low active			2,513	2,884	2,239	2,459
	Active			2,782	3,200	2,519	2,769
	Very active			3,225	3,720	2,855	3,141

[a] For each year below 30, add 7 kcal/day for women and 10 kcal/day for men. For each year above 30, subtract 7 kcal/day for women and 10 kcal/day for men.

[b] PAL = physical activity level.

[c] BMI = body mass index.

[d] Derived from the following regression equations based on doubly labeled water data:

Adult man: FER = 662 − 9.53 × age (y) + PA × (15.91 × wt [kg] + 539.6 × ht [m])

Adult woman: FER = 354 − 6.91 × age (y) + PA × (9.36 × wt [kg] + 726 × ht [m])

Where PA refers to coefficient for PAL.

PAL = total energy expenditure ÷ basal energy expenditure

PA = 1.0 if PAL ≥ 1.0 < 1.4 (sedentary)

PA = 1.12 if PAL ≥ 1.4 < 1.6 (low active)

PA = 1.45 if PAL ≥ 1.9 < 2.5 (very active)

Dietary Reference Intakes (DRIs): Acceptable Macronutrient Distribution Ranges

Food and Nutrition Board, Institute of Medicine, National Academies

Macronutrient	Range (Percent of Energy) Children, 1–3 y	Range (Percent of Energy) Children, 4–18 y	Range (Percent of Energy) Adults
Fat	30–40	25–35	20–35
n-6 polyunsaturated fatty acids[a] (linoleic acid)	5–10	5–10	5–10
n-3 polyunsaturated fatty acids[a] (α-linolenic acid)	0.6–1.2	.0.6–1.2	0.6–1.2
Carbohydrate	45–65	45–65	45–65
Protein	5–20	10–30	10–35

[a] Approximately 10% of the total come from longer-chain n-3 or n-6 fatty acids.

Source: Dietary Reference Intakes for Energy, Carbohydrate, Fiber, Fat, Fatty Acids, Cholesterol, Protein, and Amino Acids (2002).

FIGURE 11.2 (Continued).

Dietary Reference Intakes (DRIs): Tolerable Upper Intake Levels (UL[a]), Vitamins

Food and Nutrition Board, Institute of Medicine, National Academies

Life Stage Group	Vitamin A (μg/d)[b]	Vitamin C (mg/d)	Vitamin D (μg/d)	Vitamin E (mg/d)[c,d]	Vitamin K	Thiamin	Riboflavin	Niacin (mg/d)[d]	Vitamin B₆ (mg/d)	Folate (μg/d)[d]	Vitamin B₁₂	Pantothenic Acid	Biotin	Choline (g/d)	Carotenoids[e]
Infants															
0–6 mo	600	ND[f]	25	ND	ND	ND	ND	ND	ND	ND	ND	ND	ND	ND	ND
7–12 mo	600	ND	25	ND	ND	ND	ND	ND	ND	ND	ND	ND	ND	ND	ND
Children															
1–3 y	600	400	50	200	ND	ND	ND	10	30	300	ND	ND	ND	1.0	ND
4–8 y	900	650	50	300	ND	ND	ND	15	40	400	ND	ND	ND	1.0	ND
Males, Females															
9–13 y	1,700	1,200	50	600	ND	ND	ND	20	60	600	ND	ND	ND	2.0	ND
14–18 y	2,800	1,800	50	800	ND	ND	ND	30	80	800	ND	ND	ND	3.0	ND
19–70 y	3,000	2,000	50	1,000	ND	ND	ND	35	100	1,000	ND	ND	ND	3.5	ND
>70 y	3,000	2,000	50	1,000	ND	ND	ND	35	100	1,000	ND	ND	ND	3.5	ND
Pregnancy															
14–18 y	2,800	1,800	50	800	ND	ND	ND	30	80	800	ND	ND	ND	3.0	ND
19–50 y	3,000	2,000	50	1,000	ND	ND	ND	35	100	1,000	ND	ND	ND	3.5	ND
Lactation															
14–18 y	2,800	1,800	50	800	ND	ND	ND	30	80	800	ND	ND	ND	3.0	ND
19–50 y	3,000	2,000	50	1,000	ND	ND	ND	35	100	1,000	ND	ND	ND	3.5	ND

[a] UL = The maximum level of daily nutrient intake that is likely to pose no risk of adverse effects. Unless otherwise specified, the UL represents total intake from food, water, and supplements. Due to lack of suitable data, ULs could not be established for vitamin K, thiamin riboflavin, vitamin B₁₂, pantothenic acid, biotin, carotenoids. In the absence of ULs, extra caution may be warranted in consuming levels above recommended intakes.

[b] As preformed vitamin A only.

[c] As α-tocopherol; applies to any form of supplemental α-tocopherol.

[d] The ULs for vitamin E, niacin, and folate apply to synthetic forms obtained from supplements, fortified foods, or a combination of the two.

[e] β-Carotene supplements are advised only to serve as a provitamin A source for individuals at risk of vitamin A deficiency.

[f] ND = Not determinable due to lack of data of adverse effects in this age group and concern with regard to lack of ability to handle excess amounts. Source of intake should be from food only to prevent high levels of intake.

Source: Dietary Reference Intakes for Calcium, Phosphorous, Magnesium, Vitamin D, and Fluroide (1997); Dietary Reference Intake for Thiamin, Riboflavin, Niacin, Vitamin B₆, Folate, Vitamin B₁₂, Pantothenic Acid, Biotin, and Choline (1998); Dietary Reference Intakes for Vitamin C, Vitamin E, Selenium, and Corotenoids (2000); and Dietary Reference Intakes for Vitamin A, Vitamin K, Arsenic, Boron Chromium, Copper, Iodine, Iron, Manganese, Molybdenum, Nickel, Silicon, Vanadium, and Zinc (2001). These reports may be accessed via http://www.nap.edu.

FIGURE 11.2 (Continued).

Dietary Reference Intakes (DRIs): Tolerable Upper Intake Levels (UL^a), Elements

Food and Nutrition Board, Institute of Medicine, National Academies

Life Stage Group	Arsenic^b	Boron (mg/d)	Calcium (g/d)	Chromium	Copper (µg/d)	Fluoride (mg/d)	Iodine (mg/d)	Iron (mg/d)	Magnesium (mg/d)^c	Manganese (mg/d)	Molybdenum (µg/d)	Nickel (g/d)	Phosphorus (g/d)	Potassium	Selenium (µg/d)	Silicon^d	Sulfate	Vanadium (mg/d)^e	Zinc (mg/d)	Sodium (g/d)	Chloride (g/d)
Infants																					
0–6 mo	ND^f	ND	ND	ND	ND	0.7	ND	40	ND	ND	ND	ND	ND	ND	45	ND	ND	ND	4	ND	ND
7–12 mo	ND	ND	ND	ND	ND	0.9	ND	40	ND	ND	ND	ND	ND	ND	60	ND	ND	ND	5	ND	ND
Children																					
1–3 y	ND	3	2.5	ND	1,000	1.3	200	40	65	2	300	0.2	3	ND	90	ND	ND	ND	7	1.5	2.3
4–8 y	ND	6	2.5	ND	3,000	2.2	300	40	110	3	600	0.3	3	ND	150	ND	ND	ND	12	1.9	2.9
Males, Females																					
9–13 y	ND	11	2.5	ND	5,000	10	600	40	350	6	1,100	0.6	4	ND	280	ND	ND	ND	23	2.2	3.4
14–18 y	ND	17	2.5	ND	8,000	10	900	45	350	9	1,700	1.0	4	ND	400	ND	ND	ND	34	2.3	3.6
19–70 y	ND	20	2.5	ND	10,000	10	1,100	45	350	11	2,000	1.0	4	ND	400	ND	ND	1.8	40	2.3	3.6
>70 y	ND	20	2.5	ND	10,000	10	1,100	45	350	11	2,000	1.0	3	ND	400	ND	ND	1.8	40	2.3	3.6
Pregnancy																					
14–18 y	ND	17	2.5	ND	8,000	10	900	45	350	9	1,700	1.0	3.5	ND	400	ND	ND	ND	34	2.3	3.6
19–50 y	ND	20	2.5	ND	10,000	10	1,100	45	350	11	2,000	1.0	3.5	ND	400	ND	ND	ND	40	2.3	3.6
Lactation																					
14–18 y	ND	17	2.5	ND	8,000	10	900	45	350	9	1,700	1.0	4	ND	400	ND	ND	ND	34	2.3	3.6
19–50 y	ND	20	2.5	ND	10,000	10	1,100	45	350	11	2,000	1.0	4	ND	400	ND	ND	ND	40	2.3	3.6

[a] UL = The maximum level of daily nutrient intake that is likely to pose no risk of adverse effects. Unless otherwise specified, UL represents total intake from food, water, and supplements. Due to lack of suitable data, ULs could not be established for arsenic, chromium, silicon, potassium, and sulfate. In the absence of ULs, extra caution may be warranted in consuming levels above recommended intakes.

[b] Although the UL was not determined for arsenic, there is no justification for adding arsenic to food or supplements.

[c] The ULs for magnesium represent intake from a pharmacological agent only and do not include intake from food and water.

[d] Although silicon has not been shown to cause adverse effects in humans, there is no justification for adding silicon to supplements.

[e] Although vanadium in food has not been shown to cause adverse effects in humans, there is no justification for adding vanadium to food and vanadium supplements should be used with caution. The UL is based on adverse effects in laboratory animals and this data could be used to set a UL for adults but not children and adolescents.

[f] ND = Not determinable due to lack of data of adverse effects in this age group and concern with regard to lack of ability to handle excess amounts. Source of intake should be from food only to prevent high levels of intake.

Sources: Dietary Reference Intakes for Calcium, Phosphorous, Magnesium, Vitamin D, and Fluoride (1997); Dietary Reference Intakes for Thiamin, Riboflavin, Niacin, Vitamin B₆, Folate, Vitamin B₁₂, Pantothenic Acid, Biotin, and Choline (1998); Dietary Reference Intakes for Vitamin C, Vitamin E, Selenium, and Carotenoids (2000); Dietary Reference Intakes for Vitamin A, Vitamin K, Arsenic, Boron, Chromium, Copper, Iodine, Iron, Manganese, Molybdenum, Nickel, Silicon, Vanadium, and Zinc (2001); and Dietary Reference Intakes for Water, Potassium, Sodium, Chloride, and Sulfate (2004). These reports may be accessed via http://www.nap.edu.

FIGURE 11.2 (Continued).

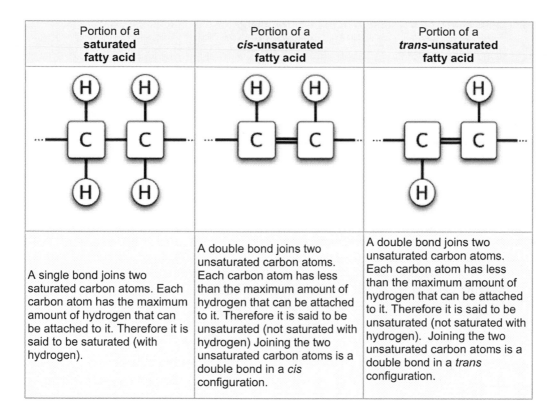

Portion of a **saturated fatty acid**	Portion of a ***cis*-unsaturated fatty acid**	Portion of a ***trans*-unsaturated fatty acid**
A single bond joins two saturated carbon atoms. Each carbon atom has the maximum amount of hydrogen that can be attached to it. Therefore it is said to be saturated (with hydrogen).	A double bond joins two unsaturated carbon atoms. Each carbon atom has less than the maximum amount of hydrogen that can be attached to it. Therefore it is said to be unsaturated (not saturated with hydrogen) Joining the two unsaturated carbon atoms is a double bond in a *cis* configuration.	A double bond joins two unsaturated carbon atoms. Each carbon atom has less than the maximum amount of hydrogen that can be attached to it. Therefore it is said to be unsaturated (not saturated with hydrogen). Joining the two unsaturated carbon atoms is a double bond in a *trans* configuration.

FIGURE 11.3 Diagram of the molecular structures of fatty acids. The same molecule, containing the same number of atoms, with a double bond in the same location, can be either a *trans* or a *cis* fatty acid depending on the conformation of the double bond. In most naturally occurring unsaturated fatty acids, the hydrogen atoms are on the same side of the double bonds of the carbon chain (*cis* configuration — meaning "on the same side" in Latin). However, partial hydrogenation reconfigures most of the double bonds that do not become chemically saturated, twisting them so that the hydrogen atoms end up on different sides of the chain. This type of configuration is called *trans,* which means "across" in Latin. (From Henein C. Trans fat. Wikipedia®. November 9, 2006. Available at: http://en.wikipedia.org/wiki/Trans_fat. Page last modified February 16, 2007. Accessed February 16, 2007.)

Box 11.6 The Four Components of the Dietary Reference Intakes

- **Estimated Average Requirement (EAR):** The usual nutrient intake level estimated to meet the requirements of half the healthy individuals in a life stage and gender group. It is used to plan and assess dietary adequacies for population groups.
- **Recommended Dietary Allowance (RDA):** The usual daily dietary nutrient intake level sufficient to meet the nutrient requirements of nearly all (97.5%) healthy individuals in a particular life stage and gender group. It is derived from the EAR: if the distribution of requirements in the group is assumed to be normal, the RDA can be derived as the EAR plus two standard deviations of requirements.
- **Adequate Intake (AI):** The recommended average daily intake level based on experimentally determined approximations or estimates of nutrient intake assumed to be adequate for a group (or groups) of apparently healthy people. It is used when an RDA and EAR cannot be determined.

- **Tolerable Upper Intake Level (UL):** The highest usual daily nutrient intake level that is likely to pose no risk of adverse health effects for almost all individuals in the general population. As intake increases above the UL, the potential risk of adverse health effects for almost all individuals in the general population. As intake increases above the UL, the risk increases of developing adverse effects.

Source: Dietary Reference Intakes for Energy, Carbohydrate, Fiber, Fat, Fatty Acids, Cholesterol, Protein and Amino Acids, 2002.

11.1.3.3.2.1   Micronutrients

The DRIs for micronutrients (vitamins and minerals) include the EAR, RDA, AI, and UL. When sufficient information is available on the distribution of nutrient requirements, a nutrient will have both an EAR and an RDA. When information is not sufficient to determine an EAR (and, thus, an RDA), an AI is set for the nutrient. In addition, many nutrients have a UL. For some nutrients, however, data are insufficient to estimate the UL reliably. The absence of a UL indicates that the current evidence does not permit its estimation.

The RDA component of the DRIs differs from the 1989 RDAs for vitamins A, B_{12}, and C, and for the minerals calcium, magnesium, and sodium. The RDA for sodium was reduced whereas the RDAs for the remaining nutrients were increased. The RDAs now also recommend that foods fortified with vitamins D and B_{12} be included in meals for older adults. The old RDAs for infants have been replaced with AIs.

11.1.3.3.2.2   Energy, Fiber, and the Macronutrients

A different set of DRIs has been developed for energy, fiber, and the macronutrients (carbohydrate, protein, and fat). [19]

Energy. The food energy (calorie) requirement is expressed in terms of estimated energy requirements (EER). An adult EER is the dietary energy intake needed to maintain energy balance in a healthy adult of a given age, gender, weight, height, and level of physical activity. In children, the EER is the sum of the dietary energy intake predicted to maintain energy balance for a child's age, weight, height, and activity level, with allowance for normal growth and development.

Fiber. For fiber, the DRI is expressed as an AI. The fiber AI increases from 19 g/d for children through the age of 3 years to 25 g/d for females and 38 g/d for males aged 19 to 50 years. For adults, this is the equivalent of 14 g per 1,000 calorie intake. Many legumes such as baked beans, black beans, kidney beans, navy beans, and pinto beans deliver about 6 to 8 grams of fiber per $^1/_2$ cup serving. Other legumes such as garbanzo beans, great northern beans, lentils, lima beans, and split peas provide slightly less fiber, at 5 g for a $^1/_2$-cup serving. The online Nutrient Data Laboratory (NDL) database is a convenient tool for looking up the micro- and macro-nutrient value of food, including fiber content. (See Table 11.6 and Box 11.8).

Box 11.7 DRIs for Nutrients and Food Energy

Vitamins and minerals	EAR, RDA, AI, UL, AMDR
Protein	EAR, RDA, AMDR
Carbohydrate	EAR, RDA, AMDR
Fiber	AI
Fat	AMDR
Food energy	EER

TABLE 11.6
DRI: Adequate Intake for Total Fiber (grams/day)

Age, in Years	Female	Male
1–3	19	19
4–8	25	25
9–13	26	31
14–18	26	38
19–50	25	38
Pregnancy, 14–50	28	—
Lactation, 14–50	29	—
> 51	21	30

Source: Dietary Reference Intakes for Energy, Carbohydrate, Fiber, Fat, Fatty Acids, Cholesterol, Protein, and Amino Acids, 2002.

Macronutrients. For intake of fat, protein, and carbohydrate, the DRIs include AMDRs, expressed as a percentage of energy intakes.

Additional recommendations. Saturated fatty acids, *trans* fatty acids, and dietary cholesterol have no known role in preventing chronic disease and are not required at any level in the diet, although many of the foods containing these fats do provide valuable nutrients. Meats, bakery items, and full-fat dairy products are the primary sources of these fats. As there is no intake level of saturated fatty acids, *trans* fatty acids, or dietary cholesterol at which there is no adverse effect, no UL is set for them. Instead, the DRI calls for intakes of dietary cholesterol, *trans* fatty acids, and saturated fatty acids "as low as possible while consuming a nutritionally adequate diet." (See Box 11.9.)

11.1.3.3.2.3 Added Sugar

Whereas the acceptable range for carbohydrates is 45 to 65% of total calories, almost inexplicably, the DRI also recommends that added sugars be limited to 25% or less of total energy intake, as shown in Figure 11.2 (or one-half of the carbohydrates consumed). It is difficult to consume a nutritionally adequate diet when added sugar provides more than one-fourth of energy intake. In contrast, the World Health Organization recommends 10% or less of total calories come from added sugars.[20] As early as 1977, reducing the consumption of refined and processed sugars to about 10% of energy intake was one of the Dietary Goals. (See Table 11.3 and Box 11.10.)

11.1.3.3.2.4 Uses of the Dietary Reference Intakes

The introduction of the DRIs, especially the EAR and the UL, provided better tools for use in dietary assessment and planning for individuals and for groups than did the RDAs published through

---

Box 11.8 Nutrient Data Laboratory

The Nutrient Data Laboratory (NDL), housed in the Beltsville Human Nutrition Research Center of the Agricultural Research Service (ARS), is responsible for developing and maintaining the USDA's National Nutrient Database for Standard Reference. NDL's nutrient database is used in food policy, research, and nutrition monitoring, and is the foundation of most food and nutrition databases in the U.S. The public and scientific community can access their online database at www.ars.usda.gov/ba/bhnrc/ndl to search for the nutrient content of food.

TABLE 11.7
DRI: Acceptable Macronutrient Distribution Ranges and
Additional Macronutrient Recommendations in Percentages

Macronutrient	Children, 1–3 Years	Children, 4–18 years	Adults
Fat [a]	30–40	25–35	20–35
Carbohydrate [a]	45–65	45–65	45–65
Protein [a]	5–20	10–30	10–35
Added sugars [b]	Age not specified 25		

[a] DRI: Acceptable Macronutrient Distribution Ranges.
[b] DRI: Additional Macronutrient Recommendations.

Source: Dietary Reference Intakes for Energy, Carbohydrate, Fiber, Fat, Fatty Acids, Cholesterol, Protein and Amino Acids, 2002.

Box 11.9 *Trans* Fatty Acids and the Law of Unintended Consequences

Trans fatty acids (also known as *trans* fats) are chemically classified as unsaturated fatty acids; however, once in the body, they behave more like saturated fatty acids. Both *trans* and saturated fatty acids increase the risk of heart disease in vulnerable people by raising low-density lipoprotein cholesterol levels. The magnitude of this effect may be greater for *trans* fatty acids than for saturated fats.

Trans fats are found in partially hydrogenated vegetable oils, such as margarine and shortening, with lower levels found in meats and dairy products. For the food industry, partially hydrogenated vegetable oils are attractive because of their long shelf life, their stability during deep-frying, and their semisolidity, which can be customized to enhance the palatability of baked goods and sweets.[1]

Fatty acids are the chemical compounds that comprise fats. They are chains of carbon atoms with attached hydrogen atoms. A saturated fatty acid has the maximum possible number of hydrogen atoms attached to every carbon atom. It is therefore said to be "saturated" with hydrogen atoms. Sometimes a pair of hydrogen atoms in the middle of a chain is missing, creating a gap that leaves two carbon atoms connected by a double bond, rather than a single bond. The missing hydrogen atoms cause the chain to be unsaturated. A fatty acid that has one double bond is said to be monounsaturated. Those having more than one double bond are called *polyunsaturated*. When the hydrogen atoms at a double bond are positioned on the same side of the carbon chain, it is described as a *cis* (meaning "same" in Latin) configuration. In nutrition labeling, all monounsaturated and polyunsaturated fatty acids are in the *cis* configuration.

Trans fatty acids are produced from vegetable oils through a manufacturing process known as *partial hydrogenation*. Hydrogen atoms are added to unsaturated sites on fatty acids, eliminating double bonds and resulting in a more solid fat with a longer shelf life. Some double bonds and hydrogen atoms end up on opposite sides of the carbon chain. This type of configuration is called *trans* (meaning "across" in Latin). The structures of saturated and unsaturated fatty acids are depicted in Figure 11.2.

At the time the FDA ruled that effective 2006, *trans* fatty acids be declared in the nutrition label of conventional foods and dietary supplements, the average consumption of industrially produced *trans* fatty acids in the U.S. was 2–3 % of total calories consumed.[2,3] In response, many food companies have removed *trans* fat from their products and replaced it with palm oil, a saturated fat that was taken out of many products in the late 1980s after an effective campaign waged in part by the American Soybean Association and CSPI helped turn Americans away from all forms of tropical oils.[4] This is an example of the "law of unintended consequences."

Sources:

[1] Mozaffarian, D., Katan, M.B., Ascherio, A., Stampfer, M.J., and Willett, W.C. Trans fatty acids and cardiovascular disease. *N Engl J Med.* 354, 1601–1613, 2006.

[2] Allison, D.B., Egan, S.K., Barraj, L.M., Caughman, C., Infante, M., and Heimbach, J.T. Estimated intakes of trans fatty and other fatty acids in the U.S. population. *J Am Diet Assoc.* 99, 166–174, 1999.

[3] FDA. Food Labeling: trans Fatty Acids in Nutrition Labeling, Nutrient Content Claims, and Health Claims. Center for Food Safety and Applied Nutrition. August 2003. Available at: http://www.cfsan.fda.gov/~dms/transgui.html. Accessed July 22, 2006.

[4] Severson, K. and Warner, M. Fat substitute is pushed out of the kitchen. *New York Times.* February 13, 2005.

Box 11.10 DRI and Added Sugar

Almost inexplicably, the DRI also recommends that added sugars be limited to 25% or less of total energy intake.

1989 (the "old" RDAs). The DRIs were developed anticipating a variety of uses, such as assessment of diets of individuals and groups, design and evaluation of diets in a variety of institutions, creation of nutrition guidelines and education programs, and development of regulations around the nutritional quality of the food supply. Indeed, separate IOM reports have been published addressing the role of the DRIs in dietary assessment[21] and planning[22] as well as labeling and fortification.[23]

It is likely that FDA will adopt many of IOM's recommendations regarding changes in nutrition labeling. An example of one of the recommendations is that the DVs for saturated fatty acids, *trans* fatty acids, and cholesterol should be set at a level that is as low as possible in keeping with an achievable health-promoting diet. (See Box 11.11.)

If FDA does adopt the recommendations regarding discretionary fortification, food manufacturers will be required to document the public health need for the addition of a particular nutrient. (See Box 11.12.)

Box 11.11 Guiding Principles for Nutrition Labeling

Read all 10 principles for nutrition labeling online at: http://darwin.nap.edu/books/ 0309091438/ html/5.html.

Box 11.12 Guiding Principles for Discretionary Fortifications

Read all 10 principles online at: http://darwin.nap.edu/books/0309091438/html/5.html.

11.2 CURRENT FEDERAL FOOD, NUTRITION, AND LIFESTYLE GUIDANCE

In accordance with federal mandate, an updated *Dietary Guidelines for Americans* is published every 5 years, the latest in 2005. In the same year, the Food Guide Pyramid was replaced by MyPyramid, a more individualized and interactive food guidance tool.

11.2.1 DIETARY GUIDELINES FOR AMERICANS, 2005

The sixth and most recent edition of the *Dietary Guidelines* was released in January 2005[24] (see Table 11.8). The document is also available in its entirety online. An abbreviated Executive Summary appears in Table 11.9. (See also Box 11.14.)

The *Dietary Guidelines* provide dietary advice for Americans ages 2 years and over. The recommendations are based on current scientific knowledge about the relationship between dietary intake and health promotion and reduction of risk for major chronic diseases. The document forms the basis for federal nutrition policy, sets standards for nutrition assistance programs, and guides nutrition education programs. In particular, the guidelines are the source of the information contained in the USDA's food guidance system, MyPyramid.

The guidelines provide the rationale for food and nutrition legislation and play a role in developing policies aimed at preventing disease and promoting optimal health as well as in assessing the impact of prevention policies on population behavior and health outcomes.[25] Federal nutrition assistance programs such as the USDA's School Meal and Food Stamp Programs, and the Supplemental Food Program for Women, Infants, and Children (WIC) use the principles in the *Dietary Guidelines* as the scientific underpinning for designing benefit structures.

All federal dietary guidance for the public must be consistent with the *Dietary Guidelines*. The CNPP chairs the USDA Dietary Guidance Working Group, which reviews the USDA and dietary guidance materials to ensure consistency with the Guidelines. In sum, the guidelines enable the federal government to speak with "one voice" on nutrition issues for the health of the American public.

11.2.1.1 The Guidelines and Steps to a HealthierUS

The integrated messages that comprise the guidelines are meant to be implemented as a whole. When taken together, they encourage most Americans to eat fewer calories, be more active, and make wiser food choices. Being more active and making wiser food choices are also themes of Steps to a HealthierUS, discussed in Section 10.2.3.1. Steps is a federal health and fitness initiative to help Americans

---

TABLE 11.8
2005 *Dietary Guidelines for Americans*: Topic Areas and Recommendations

Topic Area	Recommendation
Adequate nutrients within calorie needs	Consume a variety of foods within and among the basic food groups while staying within energy needs
Weight management	Control calorie intake to manage body weight
Physical activity	Be physically active every day
Food groups to encourage	Increase daily intake of fruits and vegetables, whole grains, and nonfat or low-fat milk and milk products
Fats	Choose fats wisely for good health
Carbohydrates	Choose carbohydrates wisely for good health
Sodium and potassium	Choose and prepare foods with little salt
Alcoholic beverages	If you drink alcoholic beverages, do so in moderation
Food safety	Keep food safe to eat

TABLE 11.9
Dietary Guidelines, 2005: Topic Areas, Goals, and Key Recommendations for the General Population

Topic Area	Goal	Key Recommendations for the General Population (Objectives)
Adequate nutrients within calorie needs	Consume a variety of foods within and among the basic food groups while staying within energy needs	Consume a variety of nutrient-dense foods and beverages within and among the basic food groups while choosing foods that limit the intake of saturated and *trans* fats, cholesterol, added sugars, salt, and alcohol Meet recommended intakes within energy needs by adopting a balanced eating pattern, such as the U.S. Department of Agriculture (USDA) Food Guide or the Dietary Approaches to Stop Hypertension (DASH) Eating Plan
Weight management	Control calorie intake to manage body weight	To maintain body weight in a healthy range, balance calories from foods and beverages with calories expended To prevent gradual weight gain over time, make small decreases in food and beverage calories and increase physical activity
Physical activity	Be physically active every day	Engage in regular physical activity and reduce sedentary activities to promote health, psychological well-being, and a healthy body weight To reduce the risk of chronic disease in adulthood, engage in at least 30 min of moderate-intensity physical activity, beyond usual activity at work or home on most days of the week For most people, greater health benefits can be obtained by engaging in physical activity of more vigorous intensity or longer duration To help manage body weight and prevent gradual, unhealthy body weight gain in adulthood: Engage in approximately 60 min of moderate- to vigorous-intensity activity on most days of the week while not exceeding caloric intake requirements To sustain weight loss in adulthood, participate in at least 60 to 90 min of moderate-intensity physical activity daily while not exceeding caloric intake requirements. Some people may need to consult with a healthcare provider before participating in this level of activity Achieve physical fitness by including cardiovascular conditioning, stretching exercises for flexibility, and resistance exercises or calisthenics for muscle strength and endurance
Food groups to encourage	Increase daily intake of fruits and vegetables, whole grains, and nonfat or low-fat milk and milk products	Consume a sufficient amount of fruits and vegetables while staying within energy needs. Two cups of fruit and 2 $1/_2$ cups of vegetables per day are recommended for a reference 2000-calorie intake, with higher or lower amounts depending on the calorie level Choose a variety of fruits and vegetables each day. In particular, select from all five vegetable subgroups (dark green, orange, legumes, starchy vegetables, and other vegetables) several times a week Consume 3 or more 1-oz equivalents of whole-grain products per day, with the rest of the recommended grains coming from enriched or whole-grain products. In general, at least half the grains should come from whole grains Consume 3 cups per day of fat-free or low-fat milk or equivalent milk products

TABLE 11.9 (Continued)
Dietary Guidelines, 2005: Topic Areas, Goals, and Key Recommendations
for the General Population

Topic Area	Goal	Key Recommendations for the General Population (Objectives)
Fats	Choose fats wisely for good health	Consume less than 10% of calories from saturated fatty acids and less than 300 mg/d of cholesterol, and keep *trans* fatty acid consumption as low as possible
		Keep total fat intake between 20–35% of calories, with most fats coming from sources of polyunsaturated and monounsaturated fatty acids, such as fish, nuts, and vegetable oils
		When selecting and preparing meat, poultry, dry beans, and milk or milk products, make choices that are lean, low-fat, or fat-free
		Limit intake of fats and oils high in saturated and/or *trans* fatty acids, and choose products low in such fats and oils
Carbohydrates	Choose carbohydrates wisely for good health	Choose fiber-rich fruits, vegetables, and whole grains often
		Choose and prepare foods and beverages with little added sugars or caloric sweeteners. Aim for amounts suggested by the USDA Food Guide and the DASH Eating Plan
		Reduce the incidence of dental caries by practicing good oral hygiene and consuming sugar- and starch-containing foods and beverages less frequently
Sodium and potassium	Choose and prepare foods with little salt	Consume less than 2300 mg of sodium (approximately 1 tsp of salt) per day
		Choose and prepare foods with little salt. At the same time, consume potassium-rich foods, such as fruits and vegetables
Alcoholic beverages	If you drink alcoholic beverages, do so in moderation	Those who choose to drink alcoholic beverages should do so sensibly and in moderation — defined as the consumption of up to one drink per day for women and up to two drinks per day for men
		Alcoholic beverages should not be consumed by some individuals, including those who cannot restrict their alcohol intake, women of childbearing age who may become pregnant, pregnant and lactating women, children and adolescents, individuals taking medications that can interact with alcohol, and those with specific medical conditions
		Alcoholic beverages should be avoided by individuals engaging in activities that require attention, skill, or coordination, such as driving or operating machinery
Food safety	Keep food safe to eat	To avoid microbial foodborne illness:
		Clean hands, food contact surfaces, and fruits and vegetables. Meat and poultry should not be washed or rinsed
		Separate raw, cooked, and ready-to-eat foods while shopping, preparing, or storing foods
		Cook foods to a safe temperature to kill microorganisms
		Chill (refrigerate) perishable food promptly and defrost foods properly
		Avoid raw (unpasteurized) milk or any products made from unpasteurized milk, raw or partially cooked eggs or foods containing raw eggs, raw or undercooked meat and poultry, unpasteurized juices, and raw sprouts

live longer, better, healthier lives. The initiative promotes increased physical activity, the consumption of nutritious foods, regular preventive health screenings, and the avoidance of risk behaviors — especially those involving alcohol, tobacco, and illegal drugs. The Dietary Guidelines support two of the four pillars of the HealthierUS initiative — eating a nutritious diet and being physically active every day.

Box 11.13 Dietary Guidelines URL

Read the 2005 edition of the *Dietary Guidelines for Americans* at: http://www.health.gov/dietaryguidelines/dga2005.

11.2.1.2 Dietary Advice

Presented in the guidelines are key recommendations, based on a preponderance of the scientific evidence, regarding nutritional factors important for lowering risk of chronic disease and promoting health. To optimize the beneficial impact of these recommendations on health, the guidelines should be implemented in their entirety. The key recommendations are grouped into nine general topic areas (see Table 11.9).

11.2.1.2.1 Nutrient Density

The 2005 Dietary Guidelines recommend consuming a variety of nutrient-dense foods and beverages within and among the basic food groups. Nutrient-dense foods provide more nutrients and generally fewer calories per unit volume than energy-dense, nutrient-poor foods. (See Box 11.13.) Foods low in nutrient density supply calories but relatively small amounts of micronutrients, sometimes none at all.

The greater the consumption of foods or beverages low in nutrient density, the more difficult it is to consume enough nutrients without gaining weight, especially for sedentary individuals. Selecting low-fat forms of foods in each group and foods free of added sugars — in other words, nutrient-dense versions of foods — allows an individual to meet his or her nutrient needs without over-consuming calories. However, the U.S. food supply is replete with foods such as potato chips, buttered popcorn, deep-fat fried chicken, and whole milk that are not in their most nutrient-dense forms. Most people will exceed calorie recommendations if they consistently choose higher fat foods within the food groups.

Based on NHANES III data (see Section 5.1.9), adults who consumed energy-dense, nutrient-poor foods were likely to have a high energy intake, marginal micronutrient intake, poor compliance

---

Box 11.14 Slightly More Than Half …

Slightly more than half of the 2005 Dietary Guidelines recommendations address the general public; the rest target special populations:

- Children and adolescents
- Women of childbearing age who may become pregnant
- Pregnant women, including women in the first trimester of pregnancy
- Breastfeeding women
- Middle-aged adults, people over age 50, and older adults
- Blacks and people with dark skin
- People exposed to insufficient ultraviolet band radiation (i.e., sunlight)
- Those who need to lose weight, including overweight children, overweight adults, and overweight children with chronic diseases and/or on medication
- Individuals with hypertension
- Those who are immunocompromised

Box 11.15 Nutrient Density

Foods low in calories and high in nutrients are *nutrient dense,* while foods high in calories and low in nutrients are *nutrient poor* (or *energy dense*). A healthful diet for adults and children includes mostly nutrient-dense foods.

Source: U.S. Department of Agriculture and Health and Human Services. *Dietary Guidelines for Americans,* 6th ed. 2005.

---

with nutrient- and food group-related dietary guidance, and low serum concentrations of vitamins and carotenoids (the precursors to vitamin A).[26] Similarly, in children, a high intake of low-nutrient-dense foods is related to an overall higher energy intake and a lower intake of the major food groups and micronutrients. Nearly one-third of the daily energy intake of American children and adolescents comes from relatively energy-dense, low-nutritional-value foods.[27]

11.2.1.3   The Revised Healthy Eating Index (HEI)

The HEI (see Section 11.1.3.2.1) was revised to reflect the 2005 *Dietary Guidelines for Americans* and is based on nutrient density of the diet (density standards per 1000 calories)[28] (see Box 11.15). In the new version, the recommendation to limit discretionary calories is addressed by crediting the absence of solid fats, alcohol, and added sugars (SoFAAS) in the diet. This category accounts for 20 out of the total 100 possible points. The recommendation to consume a variety of vegetables is addressed by crediting consumption of dark green and orange vegetables and legumes, as well as total vegetables.

11.2.1.4   *Codex Alimentarius*

The *Dietary Guidelines* are intended primarily for use by policymakers, healthcare providers, nutritionists, and nutrition educators. It provides the foundation for food and nutrition policy and the government's position on standards in the *Codex Alimentarius,* an international mechanism intended to promote the health and economic interests of consumers while encouraging fair international food trade. (See Box 11.16.)

Box 11.16 *Codex Alimentarius*

The *Codex Alimentarius* Commission (CAC), or Codex, was created in 1962 by two United Nations organizations [the Food and Agriculture Organization (FAO) and the World Health Organization (WHO)]. The CAC provides a forum for its more than 150 member countries as well as international organizations to discuss issues relative to food safety and commerce. The main purpose of the CAC is to promote consumer protection and facilitate global food trade through the development of food standards, codes of practice, and other guidelines, which taken together constitute the *Codex Alimentarius.*

Source: Food and Agriculture Organization of the United Nations. World Health Organization. Understanding the *Codex Alimentarius.* 1999. Available at: http://www.fao.org/documents/show_cdr.asp?url_ file=/docrep/ W9114E/ W9114E00.htm. Accessed June 22, 2005.

11.2.1.5 Authoritative Statements

The Dietary Guidelines may be used to provide "authoritative statements" as described in the Food and Drug Administration Modernization Act (FDAMA) of 1997.[29] Only statements included in the Executive Summary (see Table 11.9), which reflect the preponderance of scientific evidence, will be used for identification of authoritative statements.

11.2.1.5.1 Health and Nutrient Content Claims

Prior to the passage of FDAMA, companies could not use a health claim or nutrient content claim in food labeling unless the Food and Drug Administration (FDA) had published a regulation authorizing such a claim.[30] Two new provisions of FDAMA, specifically Section 303 and Section 304, permit nutrient claims in food labeling and in dietary supplements based on current published, authoritative statements from "a scientific body of the United States with official responsibility for public health protection or research directly related to human nutrition … or the National Academy of Sciences (NAS) or any of its subdivisions." These provisions are intended to expedite the process by which the scientific basis for such claims is established.

The National Institutes of Health (NIH) and the Centers for Disease Control and Prevention (CDC) are federal government agencies specifically identified as scientific bodies by FDAMA. Other federal agencies may also qualify as appropriate sources for such authoritative statements. Along with NAS (or any of its subdivisions), these federal scientific bodies may be sources of authoritative statements: CDC; NIH; the Surgeon General within DHHS; and the Food and Nutrition Service, the Food Safety and Inspection Service (FSIS), and the Agricultural Research Service (ARS) within USDA.

11.2.2 MyPyramid Food Guidance System, 2005

In 2005 MyPyramid replaced the Food Guide Pyramid. The 2-page graphic (see Figure 11.4a and Figure 11.4b), available at: http://www.mypyramid.gov/downloads/MiniPoster.pdf, was developed by the Center for Nutrition Policy and Promotion. MyPyramid is both a symbol and an interactive food guidance system designed to assist Americans in identifying healthier lifestyle choices to improve their overall health. MyPyramid is an educational tool intended to translate recommendations from the 2005 Dietary Guidelines into concrete recommendations concerning the kinds and amounts of food to eat. In addition, MyPyramid is designed to make consumers aware of the health benefits of simple, modest improvements in nutrition, physical activity, and lifestyle behavior. The central message of MyPyramid is "Steps to a Healthier You," which is consistent with the HealthierUS initiative that emphasizes nutrition combined with physical activity, prevention, and a healthier lifestyle.[31] (See Box 11.17.)

The MyPyramid symbol is meant to encourage consumers to make healthier food choices and to be active every day. Stairs on the pyramid represent the importance of exercise and the steps consumers can take each day to improve their health and that of their families. The MyPyramid graphic was designed to illustrate:

- *Variety*, symbolized by the six different colored stripes representing the five food groups and the oils and fats group that should be consumed each day. Orange represents grains; green, vegetables; red, fruits; blue, dairy and calcium-rich foods; purple, nondairy, protein-rich foods (such as meat, poultry, fish, eggs, and dried beans and legumes); and yellow, fats and oils. *Recommendation*: Eat foods from all food groups and subgroups.
- *Moderation*, represented by the narrowing of each food group from bottom to top. The wider base stands for foods with little or no solid fats, added sugars, or caloric sweeteners, which should be selected more often to obtain the most nutritionally-dense diet. *Recommendation*: Choose forms of foods that limit intake of saturated and *trans* fats, added sugars, cholesterol, salt, and alcohol.

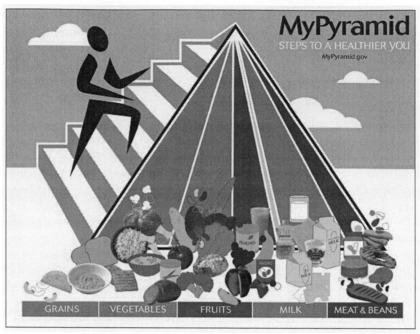

(A)

FIGURE 11.4A MyPyramid page 1.

GRAINS Make half your grains whole	VEGETABLES Vary your veggies	FRUITS Focus on fruits	MILK Get your calcium-rich foods	MEAT & BEANS Go lean with protein
Eat at least 3 oz. of whole-grain cereals, breads, crackers, rice, or pasta every day 1 oz. is about 1 slide of bread, about 1 cup of breakfast cereal, or ½ cup of cooked rice, cereal, or pasta	Eat more dark-green veggies like broccoli, spinach, and other dark leafy greens Eat more orange vegetables like carrots and sweetpotatoes Eat more dry beans and peas like pinto beans, kidney beans, and lentils	Eat a variety of fruit Choose fresh, frozen, canned, or dried fruit Go easy on fruit juices	Go low-fat or fat-free when you choose milk, yogurt, and other milk products If you don't or can't consume milk, choose lactose-free products or other calcium sources such as fortified foods and beverages	Choose low-fat or lean meats and poultry Bake it, broil it, or grill it Vary your protein routine – choose more fish, beans, peas, nuts, and seeds

For a 2,000-calories diet, you need the amounts below from each food group. To find the amounts that are right for you, go to MyPyramid.gov.

Eat 6 oz. every day	Eat 2½ cups every day	Eat 2 cups every day	Get 3 cups every day; for kids aged 2 to 8, it's 2	Eat 5½ oz. every day

Find your balance between food and physical activity
- Be sure to stay within your daily calorie needs.
- Be physically active for at least 30 minutes most days of the week.
- About 60 minutes a day of physical activity may be needed to prevent weigh gain.
- For sustaining wight loss, at least 60 to 90 minutes a day of physical activity may be required.
- Children and teenagers should be physically active for 60 minutes every day, or most days.

Know the limits on fats, sugars, and salt (sodium)
- Make most of your fat sources from fish, nuts, and vegetable oils.
- Limit solid fats like butter, margarine, shortening, and lard, as well as foods that contain these.
- Check the Nutrition Facts label to keep saturated fats, trans fats, and sodium low.
- Choose food and beverages low in added sugars. Added sugars contribute calories with few, if any, nutrients.

MyPyarmid enphasized the basics.

Keep good nutrition simple – be physically active, stay within calorie limits and enjoy foods rich in essential nutrients from all five food groups.

Shop the perimeter of the store to power your plate with nutrient-rich foods.

MyPyramid.gov
STEPS TO A HEALTHIER YOU

(B)

FIGURE 11.4B MyPyramid page 2.

Box 11.17 Food Guidance System

The Food Guidance System is the working name for all the elements of the USDA's dietary guidance system. These elements include the graphic MyPyramid image, core messages, and educational materials.

- *Proportionality*, suggested by the varied widths of the stripes. *Recommendation*: Eat more of some foods (fruits, vegetables, whole grains, fat-free or low-fat milk products), and less of others (foods high in saturated or *trans* fats, added sugars, cholesterol, salt, and alcohol).
- *Physical activity*, represented by the steps and the person climbing them, as a reminder of the importance of daily physical activity. *Recommendation*: Be physically active every day.
- *Personalization*, operationalized by the MyPyramid Web site at MyPyramid.gov, which can be accessed by consumers who want to obtain more in-depth information about food choices that would match their own needs. Consumers can also use MyPyramid Tracker to maintain a log of daily food intake and check improvement over time.
- *Gradual improvement*, encouraged by the slogan "Steps to a Healthier You," which suggests that small steps can lead to improved diet and lifestyle. The Steps theme, introduced by DHHS in 2003, is discussed in Section 10.2.3.1.

Numerous components of the food guidance system have already been developed or are forthcoming. These include:

- An educator's toolkit, designed to orient health professionals and educators to the system
- A child-friendly version of MyPyramid for teachers and children 6 to 11 years of age
- Other enhancements such as features that make it possible for consumers to make specific food choices by group, look at everyday portions of favorite foods, and adjust their choices to meet their daily needs

Key concepts comprise part of the educator's portion of the food guidance system (see Box 11.18). These 12 messages, designed for the general public, illustrate the scope of the food guidance and clearly establish what topics and recommendations are included. If adhered to, the recommendations would result in these desirable changes in a typical diet:

- Increased intake of vitamins, minerals, dietary fiber, and other essential nutrients, especially those that are often low in typical diets
- Lowered intake of saturated fats, *trans* fats, and cholesterol, and increased intake of fruits, vegetables, and whole grains to decrease risk for some chronic diseases
- Calorie intake balanced with energy needs to prevent weight gain and/or promote a healthy weight

11.2.3 DISSENSION AND CONTROVERSY

The process of guideline development should be transparent and iterative (see Box 11.19). The pursuit of consensus is driven by an evidence-based review based on the science, coupled with discussion, formulation, and evaluation of guidelines. During the process and, indeed, in the final report, failure to achieve unanimous agreement is inevitable. All parties will not agree when issues of emerging science are being considered and when one segment or another of the food industry is threatened. These points are illustrated when one reviews the comments received by the Dietary Guidelines Advisory Committee.[32]

Box 11.18 Key Recommendations in the 2005 USDA Food Guidance System

1. Balance calorie intake from foods and beverages with calories expended.
2. Engage in regular physical activity and reduce sedentary activities.
3. Make at least half of the total grains eaten whole grains.
4. Eat recommended amounts of vegetables, and choose a variety of vegetables each day.
5. Eat recommended amounts of fruit, and choose a variety of fruits each day.
6. Consume 3 cups of fat-free or low-fat (1%) milk, or an equivalent amount of yogurt or cheese, per day. Children 2 to 8 years old should consume 2 cups of fat-free or low-fat milk, or an equivalent amount of yogurt or cheese, per day. Consume other calcium-rich foods if milk and milk products are not consumed.
7. Make choices that are low-fat or lean when selecting meats and poultry.
8. Choose most fats from sources of monounsaturated and polyunsaturated fatty acids, such as fish, nuts, seeds, and vegetable oils. Keep the amount of oils consumed within the total allowed for caloric needs.
9. Choose and prepare foods and beverages with little added sugars or caloric sweeteners. Keep the amount of sugars and sweets consumed within the discretionary calorie allowance, after taking into account other discretionary calories that have been consumed.
10. Choose and prepare foods with little salt. Keep sodium intake less than 2300 mg/d. At the same time, consume potassium-rich foods, such as fruits and vegetables.
11. If one chooses to drink alcohol, consume it in moderation. Some people, or people in certain situations, should not drink. Keep consumption of alcoholic beverages within daily discretionary calorie allowance.
12. Clean hands, contact surfaces, and fruits and vegetables. To prevent cross contamination, meat and poultry should not be washed or rinsed. Separate raw, cooked, and ready-to-eat foods while shopping, preparing, or storing foods. Cook foods to a safe temperature to kill microorganisms. Chill (refrigerate) perishable foods promptly and defrost foods properly. Avoid raw (unpasteurized) milk or any products made from unpasteurized milk, raw or partially cooked eggs, or foods containing raw eggs, raw or undercooked meat and poultry, unpasteurized juices, and raw sprouts.

Public comments were solicited five times during the development of the 2005 Guidelines. For the final solicitation, the public was asked to provide oral or written comments on the *Report of the Dietary Guidelines Advisory Committee on the Dietary Guidelines for Americans, 2005 to the Secretaries of Health and Human Services and Agriculture*. In all, more than 400 responses were received. As a means of keeping the development process "transparent," these comments were posted on the Internet and can be viewed online: http://www.health.gov/dietaryguidelines/dga2005/comments/ViewAll.asp#10.

Box 11.19 Iteration

Iteration is the repetition of a process. It describes a procedure that repeats until some condition is satisfied. Successive approximations, each based on the preceding approximations, are processed in such a way as to arrive at the desired solution. Iteration describes the systematic process used for development of the Dietary Guidelines. The previous guidelines are reviewed and critiqued by nutrition specialists along with healthcare professionals, industry, consumers, and other stakeholders. The resulting revised guidelines are reviewed again by stakeholders, and revised again before being reviewed by USDA and DHHS and released to the public.

Box 11.20 Position of The Sugar Association, Inc.

In August 2004, the Department of Health and Human Services (HHS) and Department of Agriculture (USDA) announced that public comments were being accepted on the *Report of the Dietary Guidelines Advisory Committee on the Dietary Guidelines for Americans, 2005 to the Secretaries of Health and Human Services and Agriculture*. Individuals and organizations were encouraged to provide written comments within the month. The Committee received 42 comments regarding carbohydrates and sugars.

These statements were extracted from the comments submitted by The Sugar Association.

... There is no validated body of irrefutable evidence that corroborates the popular theory that added sugars reduce the nutrient adequacy of the American diet ...

Terminology — sugar-sweetened drinks. The Food and Drug Administration has defined sugar to mean sucrose for the purpose of ingredient labeling, 21 C.F.R. 101.4(b)(20). For the purposes of ingredient labeling, the term sugar *shall refer to sucrose, which is obtained from sugar cane and sugar beets, in accordance with the provisions of 184.1854. The term* sugars *(plural) is used to designate all mono- and disaccharides. Therefore, The Association (i.e., The Sugar Association, Inc.) takes strong issue with the use of the term* "sugar-sweetened drinks" *to denote caloric beverages throughout the Committee's final recommendations and asks that the Agencies not allow this terminology in the messages developed to communicate dietary guidance to the American public.*

Very few beverages, and all major soft drinks, have not contained sugar since the mid-1980s. High fructose corn syrup (HFCS) is the major sweetener in nearly all caloric beverages and to use the term "sugar-sweetened drinks" *is not only inaccurate but misleads the consuming public ... the sucrose share of the U.S. caloric sweetener market has fallen from nearly 86% in 1970 to 43% in 2003.*

Source: Comments of The Sugar Association, Inc. September 2007, 2004. Available at: http://www.health.gov/ dietaryguidelines/dga2005/comments/ViewTopics.asp?TopicID=5&SubTopicID=21&submit1=Submit. Accessed September 2, 2006.

In the past, the Dietary Guidelines settled for minor tweaks. The "avoid too much sugar" guideline in 1980 and 1985 evolved into "use sugars only in moderation" in 1990, "choose a diet moderate in sugars" in 1995, and "choose beverages and foods to moderate your intake of sugars" in 2000. In the 2005 revision, however, Americans are urged to "choose food and beverages low in added sugars. Added sugars contribute calories with few, if any, nutrients." Despite the impassioned and lengthy, 1700-word statement submitted by the Sugar Association, Inc., to the 2005 Dietary Guidelines Advisory Committee (see Box 11.20), the 2005 Dietary Guidelines take a harder line on sugars than ever before.

On the other hand, the recommendation that individuals in the U.S. should increase their dairy intake from 2 to 3 cups per day has been met with skepticism by some who believe the recommendation is the result of intense lobbying by the National Dairy Council.[33] The chairman of the Nutrition Department at the Harvard University School of Public Health argues that "dairy products shouldn't occupy the prominent place they do in the USDA Food Pyramid, nor should they be the centerpiece of the national strategy to prevent osteoporosis."[34] Other sources of calcium are available such as collards, tofu, spinach, calcium-fortified orange juice, and calcium supplements. The evidence, some of the milk critics say, is scant to support nutrition guidelines focused specifically on increasing milk or other dairy product intake for bone health.[35] (See Boxes 11.21 and 11.22.)

Other stakeholders that weighed in heavily during the Dietary Guidelines revision process were the United Fresh Fruit and Vegetable Association, Soft Drink Association, American Meat Institute, National Cattlemen's Beef Association, and Wheat Foods Council.[36] Understandably, various other interest groups such as vegetarians representing varying levels of strictness and supporters of organic or pesticide-free agriculture also want their principles represented in the Guidelines. Not all points are included.

Box 11.21 Calcium Content URL

An extensive list of the calcium content of foods is available online from the USDA (http://www.nal.usda.gov/fnic/foodcomp/Data/SR17/wtrank/sr17w301.pdf).

Box 11.22 Nestle Reference

In-depth discussions about the pressure exerted by various special interest groups and the economic ramifications of national nutrition policy are available in Nestle M. *Food Politics*. New York: Oxford University Press, 2002 and Light L. *What to Eat*. New York: McGraw-Hill Trade Books, 2006.

As the government should deliver state-of-the-art nutrition advice unfettered by special interests, one former Washington insider suggested the responsibility for developing nutrition guidance be moved solely to the DHHS as their policymakers do not represent agricultural interests and are therefore less likely than USDA employees to be influenced by pressures from food lobbies.[37]

Box 11.23 Strategies for Facilitating Adoption of the AHA Diet and Lifestyle Recommendations

1. Practitioners should promote the AHA Diet and Lifestyle Recommendations to their patients, along with encouraging regular physical activity, discussing BMI, and encouraging alcohol and tobacco control.
2. Restaurants should facilitate their customers' adherence to AHA recommendations by offering menu labeling; reducing portion sizes; reformulated recipes to reduce fat and sodium, providing more fruit and vegetable options prepared with minimally-added salt, fat, and sugar; allowing patrons to substitute reduced fat options for high-fat side dishes (such as french fries and potato salad); and providing whole-grain products.
3. Food industry should reduce the salt and sugar content of processed foods, replace saturated and *trans* fats in prepared foods and baked goods with low-saturated fat liquid vegetable oils, increase the proportion of whole-grain foods available, package foods in smaller individual portion sizes, and develop packaging that allows for greater stability, preservation, and palatability of fresh fruits and vegetables without added sodium and reduces refrigeration needs in grocery stores.
4. Schools should adopt HealthierUS School Challenge policies, such as limiting foods high in added sugar, saturated and *trans* fat, sodium, and calories while encouraging consumption of fruits, vegetables, whole-grain foods, and low-fat or fat-free dairy in all food sold outside of the reimbursable school lunch.
5. Local government should develop and implement a Safe Routes to School plan, implement land-use practices that promote nonmotorized transportation (walking and biking), and promote policies that increase availability of healthy foods, for example, use of public land for farmers' markets and full-service grocery stores in low-income areas.

Source: Lichtenstein, A.H., Appel, L.J., Brands, M., et al. Diet and lifestyle recommendations revision 2006: a scientific statement from the American Heart Association Nutrition Committee. *Circulation*. 2006;114:82–96. Available at: http://circ.ahajournals.org/cgi/reprint/114/1/82. Accessed February 16, 2007.

11.3 DISEASE PREVENTION GUIDANCE FROM FEDERAL AND VOLUNTARY HEALTH ORGANIZATIONS

The six leading causes of death in the U.S. are, in order, heart disease, cancer, stroke, chronic lower respiratory diseases, accidents, and diabetes. Of these, heart disease, some forms of cancer, and type 2 diabetes correlate to poor nutrition. Escalating rates of obesity and the corresponding increases in morbidity, mortality, and healthcare costs necessitate a focus by public health practitioners on prevention of cardiovascular disease, cancer, and diabetes through education and outreach.

11.3.1 CARDIOVASCULAR DISEASE (CVD)

The American Heart Association's (AHA's) 2006 Diet and Lifestyle Recommendations provide a foundation for a public health approach to CVD risk reduction. The plan includes recommendations for healthy eating and other health-promoting behaviors for healthy Americans 2 years of age and older. The recommendations are intentionally flexible to meet the unique needs for growth, development, and aging. In particular, the document presents guidelines for a healthy diet; healthy weight; cholesterol, blood pressure, and fasting blood sugar control; physical activity; and avoidance of tobacco.[38] Compared to the AHA's previous guidelines released in 2000, the 2006 edition includes a significantly more restrictive fat intake recommendation. The recommendation for saturated fat was reduced from less than 10% of energy in 2000 to less than 7% of energy in 2006.[39]

In addition to recommendations for individuals, the 2006 AHA statement contains strategies for practitioners, restaurants, the food industry, schools, and local governments to facilitate adoption of the AHA Diet and Lifestyle Recommendations. (See Box 11.24 and Table 11.10.). Thus, AHA has been informed by the ecological model of health behavior change (see Box 10.10), which identifies multiple levels of influence on a person's behavior. These multiple levels include intrapersonal factors, interpersonal processes and primary groups, institutional factors, community factors, and public policy. The ecological model has been found to bring about population improvements in health, as we have learned so well from the campaigns for tobacco control.[40]

Box 11.24 The Diabetes Prevention Program

The Diabetes Prevention Program (DPP), conducted at 27 centers nationwide, is the first major trial to show that lifestyle changes can effectively delay diabetes in a diverse population of overweight American adults with impaired glucose tolerance.

Sponsored by the National Institute of Diabetes and Digestive and Kidney Diseases (NIDDK), an Institute within the National Institutes of Health, the DPP compared three approaches to normalizing blood sugar — lifestyle modification, treatment with an oral hypoglycemic agent (metformin), and standard medical advice — in 3234 overweight people with impaired glucose tolerance (IGT). The Lifestyles manuals used in the study are available on the DPP Web site at http://www.bsc.gwu.edu/dpp/index.htmlvdoc. DPP volunteers were randomly assigned to one of the following groups:

- Lifestyle modification with the aim of reducing weight by 7% through a low-fat diet and exercising for 150 min a week
- Treatment with the drug metformin (850 mg twice a day), approved in 1995 to treat type 2 diabetes, plus information about diet and exercise
- A standard group taking placebo pills in place of metformin, plus information about diet and exercise

A fourth arm of the study, treatment with the drug troglitazone (Rezulin) combined with standard diet and exercise recommendations, was discontinued in June 1998 due to the potential for liver toxicity.

Forty-five percent of DPP participants were from minority groups that suffer disproportionately from type 2 diabetes: African Americans, Hispanic Americans, Asian Americans and Pacific Islanders, and American Indians. The trial also recruited other groups at higher risk for type 2 diabetes, including individuals age 60 and older, women with a history of gestational diabetes, and people with a first-degree relative with type 2 diabetes.

Diet and exercise that achieved a 5–7% weight loss reduced diabetes incidence by 58% in participants randomized to the study's lifestyle intervention group. Participants in this group exercised at moderate intensity, usually by walking an average of 30 min a day 5 days a week, and lowered their intake of fat and calories. Volunteers randomly assigned to treatment with metformin had a 31% lower incidence of type 2 diabetes. Metformin lowers blood glucose mainly by decreasing the liver's production of glucose.

Lifestyle intervention worked equally well in men and women and in all the ethnic groups. It was most effective in people age 60 and older, who lowered the risk of developing diabetes by 71%. Metformin was also effective in both sexes and in all the ethnic groups, but it was relatively ineffective in older volunteers and in those who were less overweight.

Both interventions lowered fasting blood glucose levels, but lifestyle changes more effectively lowered blood glucose levels 2 h after a glucose drink. Also, about twice as many people in the lifestyle group compared to placebo regained normal glucose tolerance, showing that diet and exercise can reverse IGT.

DPP participants ranged from age 25 to 85, with an average age of 51. Upon entering the study, all had impaired glucose tolerance as measured by an oral glucose tolerance test, and all were overweight, with an average body mass index (BMI) of 34. About 29% of the DPP standard group developed diabetes during the average follow-up period of 3 years. In contrast, 14% of the diet and exercise arm and 22% of the metformin group developed diabetes. Volunteers in the diet and exercise arm met the study goal, on average a 7% — or 15 lb — weight loss, in the first year and generally sustained a 5% total loss for the study's duration. Participants in the lifestyle intervention arm received training in diet, exercise (most chose walking), and behavior modification skills.

Source: Knowler, W.C., Barrett-Connor, E., Fowler, S.E., Hamman, R.F., Lachin, J.M., Walker, E.A., and Nathan, D.M. Diabetes Prevention Program Research Group. Reduction in the incidence of type 2 diabetes with lifestyle intervention or metformin. *N Engl J Med.* 346, 393–403, 2002.

11.3.1.1 Hypertension

Hypertension (blood pressure of 140/90 mm Hg or higher) affects approximately 50 million individuals in the U.S. and approximately 1 billion worldwide. As the population ages, the prevalence of hypertension will increase even more unless broad and effective preventive measures are implemented. The relationship between high blood pressure and risk of CVD events is independent of other risk factors. The higher the blood pressure, the greater the chance of heart attack, heart failure, stroke, and kidney disease.

11.3.1.1.1 Prehypertension

Prehypertension (blood pressure between 120/80 mm Hg and 139/89 mm Hg) signals the need for increased education of both healthcare professionals and the public to reduce blood pressure levels and prevent the development of hypertension in the general population. Hypertension prevention strategies are available to achieve this goal.[41]

Public health approaches, such as reducing calories, saturated fat, and salt in processed foods; increasing community and school opportunities for physical activity; and other recommendations

TABLE 11.10
AHA 2006 Recommendations and Strategies for CVD Risk Reduction

Strategy (Process Objective)	Recommendation (Outcome Objective)
Choose lean meats and vegetable alternatives, select fat-free (skim), 1% fat, and low-fat dairy products, and minimize intake of partially hydrogenated fats	Reduce saturated to < 7% of energy, *trans* fatty acids to < 1% of energy, and cholesterol to < 300 mg/d
Choose and prepare foods with little or no salt	Reduce sodium intake to no more than 2300 milligrams daily. Middle-aged and older adults, African Americans, and those with hypertension are advised to reduce sodium intake to 1500 mg of sodium daily
Minimize the intake of food and beverages with added sugars	Read labels to minimize consumption of foods with one or more of these ingredients: HFCS, corn syrup, raisin syrup, dextrose, honey, sucrose, fructose, maltose, concentrated fruit juice
Strive to be physically activity and control weight	Adults should aim for > 30 min of physical activity most days of the week. At least 60 min of physical activity most days of the week is recommended for adults who are attempting to lose weight or maintain weight loss and for children
Aim for a diet rich in vegetables, fruits (not fruit juices), and whole-grain foods	Follow the eating plan. Blood pressure may be further lowered by replacing some carbohydrates with either protein from plant sources or with monounsaturated fat.
Achieve and maintain healthy cholesterol, blood pressure and blood glucose levels	Achieve and maintain an LDL cholesterol level of < 100 mg/dL; blood pressure of 120 mm Hg and a diastolic BP 80 mm Hg or less; and a fasting blood glucose level of < 100 mg/dL
	Avoid use of and exposure to tobacco products
If alcohol is consumed, it should be at a moderate level	Limit alcohol intake to not more than 1 drink per day for women and 2 drinks per day for men (1 drink = 12 oz of beer, 4 oz of wine, 1.5 oz of 80-proof distilled spirits, or 1 oz of 100-proof spirits)
Follow AHA Diet and Lifestyle Recommendations even when eating food that is prepared outside of the home	See all of the above

Source: Lichtenstein, A.H., Appel, L.J., Brands, M., et al. Diet and lifestyle recommendations revision 2006, a scientific statement from the American Heart Association Nutrition Committee. *Circulation.* 114, 82–96, 2006. Available at: http://circ.ahajournals.org/cgi/reprint/CIRCULATIONAHA.106.176158. Accessed July 2, 2006.

proposed by the AHA (see Section 11.3.1) can achieve a downward shift in the distribution of the blood pressure in the U.S. population, potentially reducing morbidity, mortality, and the lifetime risk of an individual's becoming hypertensive. A population-based approach is an important component for any comprehensive plan to prevent hypertension. Even a small decrement in the distribution of systolic blood pressure is likely to result in a substantial reduction in the burden of blood pressure-related illness.[42]

11.3.1.2 Primary Prevention

Adoption of healthy lifestyles by all persons is critical for the prevention of high blood pressure and is an indispensable part of the management of those with hypertension. Major lifestyle modifications shown to lower blood pressure include weight reduction in those individuals who are overweight or obese, dietary sodium reduction, physical activity, moderation of alcohol consumption,

TABLE 11.11
DASH Eating Plan

Food Groups	Servings per Day				Serving Sizes
	1600 cal/d	2000 cal/d	2600 cal/d	3100 cal/d	
Grains[a]	6	6–8	10–11	12–13	1 slice bread; 1 oz dry cereal;[b] $1/_2$ cup cooked rice, pasta, or cereal
Vegetables	3–4	4–5	5–6	6	1 cup raw leafy vegetable; $1/_2$ cup cut-up raw or cooked vegetable; $1/_2$ cup vegetable juice
Fruits	4	4–5	5–6	6	1 medium fruit; $1/_4$ cup dried fruit; $1/_2$ cup fresh, frozen, or canned fruit; $1/_2$ cup fruit juice
Fat-free or low-fat milk and milk products	2–3	2–3	3	3–4	1 cup milk or yogurt; $1^1/_2$ oz cheese
Lean meats, poultry, and fish	3–6	6 or less	6	6–9	1 oz cooked meats, poultry, or fish; 1 egg[c]
Nuts, seeds, and legumes	3 per week	4–5 per week	1	1	cup or $1^1/_2$ oz nuts; 2 tbsp peanut butter; 2 tbsp or $1/_2$ oz seeds; $1/_2$ cup cooked legumes (dry beans and peas)
Fats and oils	2	2–3	3	4	1 tsp soft margarine; 1 tsp vegetable oil; 1 tbsp mayonnaise; 2 tbsp salad dressing[d]
Sweets and added sugars	0	5 or less per week	less than 2	less than 2	1 tbsp sugar; 1 tbsp jelly or jam; $1/_2$ cup sorbet or gelatin; 1 cup lemonade

[a] Whole grains are recommended for most grain servings.

[b] Serving sizes vary between $1/_2$ cup and $1/_4$ cups, depending on cereal type. Check the product's nutrition facts label.

[c] Limit egg yolk intake to no more than 4 per week; 2 egg whites have the same protein content as 1 oz of meat.

[d] Fat content determines the serving size for fats and oils, e.g., 1 tbsp of regular salad dressing = 1 serving; 1 tbsp of low-fat dressing = $1/_2$ serving; and 1 tbsp of a fat-free dressing = 0 servings.

Source: U.S. Department of Health and Human Services. National Institutes of Health. National Heart, Lung, and Blood Institute. *Your Guide to Lowering Your Blood Pressure With DASH.* NIH Publication No. 06–4082. Originally printed 1998; revised April 2006. Available at: http://www.nhlbi.nih.gov/health/public/heart/hbp/dash/new_dash.pdf. Accessed July 3, 2006.

and adoption of the Dietary Approaches to Stop Hypertension (DASH) eating plan, which is rich in potassium and calcium. (See Table 11.11.)

Lifestyle modifications reduce blood pressure, enhance antihypertensive drug efficacy, and decrease cardiovascular risk. A 1,600-mg-sodium DASH eating plan has effects similar to single-drug therapy and can decrease systolic blood pressure 8–14 mm Hg; combinations of two or more lifestyle modifications can achieve even better results, as indicated in Table 11.12.[43]

11.3.2 DIABETES

All recommendations to prevent the development of diabetes are based on the Diabetes Prevention Program (DPP) (see Box 11.24), a major clinical trial that found that decreasing diabetes risk factors can prevent diabetes. The DPP demonstrated that for every 7 people with prediabetes who are treated for 3 years, 1 case of diabetes can be prevented. Thus, it should also be possible to delay or prevent the development of complications, substantially reducing the individual and public health burden of diabetes.[44]

TABLE 11.12
Lifestyle Modifications Recommended by the Joint National Committee 7 (JNC 7) to Manage Hypertension

Modification	Recommendation	Approximate Range of Systolic BP Reduction
Weight reduction	Maintain normal body weight (BMI = 18.5–24.9 kg/m^2)	5–20 mm Hg per 10 kg weight loss
DASH eating plan	Consume a diet rich in fruits, vegetables, and low-fat dairy products with a reduced content of saturated and total fat	8–14 mm Hg
Dietary sodium reduction	Reduce dietary sodium intake no more than 2.4 g sodium or 6 g sodium chloride	2–8 mm Hg
Physical activity	Engage in regular aerobic physical activity such as brisk walking at least 30 min per day, most days of the week	4–9 mm Hg
Moderation of alcohol	Limit consumption to no more than 2 drinks per day in most men and to no more than 1 drink per day in women and lighter weight persons. 1 drink is the equivalent of 1 oz or 30 mL ethanol; e.g., 24 oz beer, 10 oz wine, or 3 oz 80-proof whiskey	2–4 mm Hg

Source: National High Blood Pressure Education Program. *Prevention, Detection, Evaluation, and Treatment of High Blood Pressure.* The Seventh Report of the Joint National Committee (JNC 7). U.S. Department of Health and Human Services. National Institutes of Health. National Heart, Lung, and Blood Institute. NIH Publication Number 03-5233. December 2003. Available at: http://www.nhlbi.nih.gov/guidelines/hypertension/express.pdf. Accessed July 3, 2006.

Community screening programs, as well as primary care physicians, have an opportunity to identify individuals at high risk for developing diabetes and provide primary prevention strategies. The American Diabetes Association (ADA) recommends that individuals with normoglycemia have repeat screenings at 3-year intervals. However, for people with prediabetes, modest weight loss and regular physical is advised in order to prevent or delay diabetes.

11.3.2.1 Prediabetes

Information learned thus far about the natural history and pathogenesis of diabetes indicates that this disease has a prolonged prediabetic phase. The ADA has identified an intermediate group of patients who have blood glucose values higher than the defined normal level but not high enough to meet the diagnostic criteria for diabetes. This group includes patients with impaired glucose tolerance (IGT) or impaired fasting glucose (IFG).

- IGT is defined as 2-h, 75-g oral glucose tolerance test values of 140 to 199 mg per dL (7.8 to 11.0 mmol per L); normal values on this test are below 140 mg per dL.
- IFG is defined as fasting plasma glucose values (FPG) of 100 to 125 mg per dL (5.6 to 6.9 mmol per L); normal fasting glucose values are below 100 mg per dL.
- Diabetes is diagnosed when FPG levels are 126 mg/dl (7.0 mmol/L) or higher on two different days.

People with IGT or IFG are at significant risk for diabetes. Other risk factors include history of diabetes in a first-degree relative, overweight, sedentary lifestyle, hypertension, dyslipidemia, history of gestational diabetes or large-for-gestational-age infant, and polycystic ovary syndrome (PCOS). Blacks, Latin Americans, Native Americans, and Asian-Pacific Islanders also are at increased risk for diabetes (see Box 11.25).

Box 11.25 Modifiable and Nonmodifiable Conditions Associated with Diabetes

Nonmodifiable factors
- Age (at least 45 years)
- Diabetes in a first-degree relative (any relative who is one meiosis away from a particular individual in a family, i.e., parent, sibling, offspring) with diabetes
- Family background (Alaska Native, American Indian, African American, Hispanic/Latino American, Asian American, or Pacific Islander)
- History of CVD

Modifiable lifestyle factors
- Overweight (BMI greater than 25 kg per m^2)
- Inactive (exercise < 3 times per week)

Clinical conditions
- IGT or IFG
- Prehypertension (BP at least 140/90 mm Hg)
- Dyslipemia (HDL-cholesterol > 35 mg/dL or triglycerides > 250 mg/dL)
- History of gestational diabetes or LGA baby
- PCOS
- *Acanthosis nigricans* (A dermatalogic presentation characterized by hyperpigmented, velvety plaques of body folds. Caused by hyperinsulinemia, a consequence of insulin resistance that occurs associated with obesity.)

Source: Rao, S.S., Disraeli, P., and McGregor, T. Impaired glucose tolerance and impaired fasting glucose. *Am Fam Physician.* 69, 1961–1968, 2004.

Adults with a Body Mass Index (BMI) of 25 kg/m^2 or greater who are at least 45 years of age are candidates for screening to detect IFG or IGT. Children with a BMI 25 kg/m^2 or greater who have one or more other risk factors should be considered for screening:

Screening should be carried out only as part of a healthcare office visit. Either a fasting plasma glucose (FPG) test or 2-h oral glucose tolerance test (OGTT) with 75-g glucose load is appropriate, and positive test results should be confirmed on another day.

11.3.2.2 Primary Prevention

People with IFG or IGT should be given counseling on weight loss as well as instruction for increasing physical activity. Follow-up counseling appears important for success. Monitoring for the development of diabetes should be performed every 1–2 years. Close attention should be given to, and appropriate treatment given for, other CVD risk factors such as hypertension and dyslipidemia, as well as for tobacco use.

11.3.2.2.1 The National Diabetes Education Program (NDEP)

The NDEP is jointly sponsored by DHHS's National Institute of Diabetes and Digestive and Kidney Diseases (NIDDKD) of the National Institutes of Health (NIH) and CDC's Division of Diabetes Translation, with the participation of over 200 partner organizations. NDEP's "Small Steps. Big Rewards. Prevent Type 2 Diabetes" initiative is the first national diabetes prevention campaign (Figure 11.5). Its goal is to promote sub-federal primary prevention programs and to develop and disseminate tailored materials that can be adopted for use in those diabetes prevention programs. NDEP has produced copyright-free campaign tools to help promote diabetes prevention and control (see Box 11.26). Organizations are encouraged to download and reproduce these tools from the NDEP Web site at: http://ndep.nih.gov/campaigns/SmallSteps/SmallSteps_index.htm.

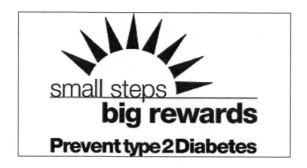

FIGURE 11.5 Small Steps logo. (From U.S. Department of Health and Human Services. National Institutes of Health. National Diabetes Education Program. *Small Steps. Big Rewards. Prevent Type 2 Diabetes.* Campaign logo. Available at: http://www.ndep.nih.gov/campaigns/SmallSteps/SmallSteps_index.htm. Accessed February 16, 2007.)

11.3.3 Cancer

Because there is a proven association between increased consumption of fruits and vegetables and a decreased incidence of some cancers, organizations such as the National Cancer Institute (NCI) and the American Institute for Cancer Research (AICR) work to promote dietary change, based on the Dietary Guidelines. These organizations also support research into detection, prevention, and cures.

11.3.3.1 National Cancer Institute (NCI)

Founded in 1991 as a partnership between NCI and the Produce for Better Health Foundation (PBHF), the 5 a Day for Better Health Program was a national initiative to increase consumption of fruits and vegetables by all Americans to 5 to 9 servings a day as a means of reducing the risk of many cancers, high blood pressure, heart disease, diabetes, stroke, and other chronic diseases. The program sought to do this by increasing public awareness of the importance of eating 5 to 9 servings of fruits and vegetables every day, by providing consumers with specific information about how to include more servings of fruits and vegetables in their daily routines, and by increasing the availability of fruits and vegetables at home, school, work, and other places where food is served. NCI is the lead federal agency for the program.[45]

As the Dietary Guidelines' recommended intake of fruits and vegetables increased, the campaign followed suit by increasing its recommendations from a daily intake of at least five to the suggested intake of five to nine. In 2007 the PBHF relaunched its campaign to reflect the escalating recommendation. Effective 2007, the rebranded slogan exhorts "More Matters."

Box 11.26 Small Steps Recommendation

The "Small Steps Big Rewards Prevent Type 2 Diabetes" diet and lifestyle recommendation is summarized in one sentence: By losing a modest amount of weight by getting 30 min of physical activity 5 days a week and eating healthier, people with prediabetes can delay or prevent the onset of the disease.

Box 11.27 AICR's Diet and Health Guidelines for Cancer Prevention

1. Choose a diet rich in a variety of plant-based foods.
2. Eat plenty of vegetables and fruits.
3. Maintain a healthy weight and be physically active.
4. Drink alcohol only in moderation, if at all.
5. Select foods low in fat and salt.
6. Prepare and store foods safely.
7. *And, always remember* ... do not use tobacco in any form.

11.3.3.2 American Institute for Cancer Research (AICR)

Founded in 1982, AICR offers cancer prevention education programs and supports research into the role of diet and nutrition in the prevention and treatment of cancer. Their *Diet and Health Guidelines for Cancer Prevention* to reduce the risk of developing cancer is strikingly similar to the 1995 *Dietary Guidelines for Americans.* (See Box 11.27.)

Three strategies are suggested for achieving the cancer prevention and weight management components of AICR's Guidelines: eat a greater proportion of plant foods, keep physically active, and maintain a healthy weight. AICR developed the "New American Plate" as way to help people achieve these goals. The New American Plate promotes a healthy proportion of plant foods to protein, attained by gradually making the transition to a plate that contains at least two-thirds vegetables, fruits, whole grains and beans, and no more than one-third meat or dairy products. The second step of the New American Plate suggests gradually reducing portion size as an additional way to reduce calories.[46] For portion control, a medium-sized plate about the size of a Frisbee® is suggested. As a weight-loss strategy, the "healthy plate" (half vegetables and fruit, a quarter healthy starches, and a quarter lean meats and alternates) has been adopted by *MOVE!* — a national weight management program designed by the Veterans Administration's National Center for Health Promotion and Disease Prevention, Capital Health (Canada), and the New York State Department of Health.

See also Section 6.1.1.1 for a discussion of collaborative prevention efforts by the American Cancer Society, the American Diabetes Association, and the American Heart Association.

11.4 CONCLUSION

The federal government has been providing food and nutrition guidance to the public and for use by public health professionals since the early 20th century. Although guidance originally focused on food and prevention of deficiency, it gradually refocused on nutrients and prevention, with the nature of the guidance changing in response to the nutritional status of the population.

Primary tools for nutrition guidance include the *Dietary Guidelines for Americans* and MyPyramid. The process of maintaining and updating this information is complex and ongoing, requiring input from both subject-matter experts and the general public.

Because the guidelines set the standard for federal nutrition policy, nutrition assistance programs (such as WIC), and assessment (such as HEI), the federal government is able to speak with one consistent voice on nutrition issues. At present, a major focus of both private and public health organizations is on chronic diseases such as cardiovascular disease, cancer, and diabetes, the risks for which are strongly correlated with poor diet and lifestyle choices.

Michael Pollan, the coauthor of the quotation on the beginning of this chapter, offers his own irreverent dietary guidance in Box 11.28.

Box 11.28 Flagrantly Unscientific Rules of Thumb Regarding How to Eat

- Eat food. Don't eat anything your great-great-grandmother wouldn't recognize as food.
- Avoid even those food products with health claims. Not only are they likely to be heavily processed, but the claims on them are often questionable.
- Avoid food products containing more than five ingredients that are unfamiliar and poly-syllabic. Also avoid foods that contain HFCS. All of these ingredients indicate the food is highly-processed.
- Get out of the supermarket whenever possible so you can find fresh whole foods picked at the peak of nutritional quality.
- Pay more (better food costs more) and eat less (stop when you're 80% full).
- Eat mostly plants, especially leaves.
- Eat by following the dietary rules of a traditional culture; copy how the cultural group eats as well as what they eat.
- Cook and (if you can) plant a garden.
- Eat like an omnivore. Try to add new species, not just new foods, to your diet.

Source: Pollan, M. Unhappy meals. *The New York Times Magazine*, January 28, 2007, p. 38.

11.5 ACRONYMS

ACS	American Cancer Society
ADA	American Diabetes Association
AHA	American Heart Association
AI	Adequate intake
AICR	American Institute for Cancer Research
AMDR	Acceptable Micronutrient Distribution Range
ARS	Agricultural Research Service
BMI	Body Mass Index
CAC	*Codex Alimentarius* Commission
CBE	Clinical breast exam
CDC	Centers for Disease Control and Prevention
CNPP	Center for Nutrition Policy and Promotion (within USDA)
CVD	Cardiovascular disease
DASH	Dietary Approaches to Stop Hypertension
DHHS	Department of Health and Human Services
DPP	Diabetes Prevention Program
DRI	Dietary Reference Intake
EAR	Estimated average requirement (for groups)
EER	Estimated energy requirements
FAO	Food and Agriculture Organization (of the United Nations)
FDA	U.S. Food and Drug Administration (within DHHS)
FDAMA	Food and Drug Administration Modernization Act of 1997
FPG	Fasting plasma glucose
FSIS	Food Safety and Inspection Service (within USDA)
HEI	Healthy Eating Index
Hg	Mercury
IFG	Impaired fasting glucose
IGT	Impaired glucose tolerance
IOM	Institutes of Medicine
mm	Millimeter
NAS	National Academy of Sciences
NCI	National Cancer Institute
NDEP	National Diabetes Education Project

NDL	Nutrient Data Laboratory
NIDDKD	National Institute of Diabetes and Digestive and Kidney Diseases
NIH	National Institutes of Health
NHANES	National Health and Nutrition Examination Survey
NRC	National Research Council
OGTT	Oral glucose tolerance test
PBHF	Produce for Better Health Foundation
PCOS	Polycystic ovary syndrome
RDA	Recommended Dietary Intake
SoFAAS	Solid fats, alcohol, and added sugars
UL	Tolerable upper intake levels
USDA	U.S. Department of Agriculture
WHO	World Health Organization (of the United Nations)

REFERENCES

1. This discussion about the history of food guidance is adapted from these two USDA sources: Davis, C., Saltos, E. Dietary recommendations and how they have changed over time. In Frazao, E., Ed. *America's Eating Habits: Changes and Consequences.* Washington, D.C.: Economic Research Service, U.S. Department of Agriculture, Agriculture Information Bulletin No. 750, 999, pp. 33–50, chap. 2; Welsh, S.O. and Shaw. A. *USDA's Food Guide: Background and Development.* USDA Human Nutrition Information Service. Nutrition Education Division. Miscellaneous Publication No. 1514. September 1993. Available at: www.usda.gov/cnpp/Pubs/Pyramid/FoodGuideDevt.pdtf. Accessed June 19, 2005.

2. Davis, C. and Saltos, E. Dietary recommendations and how they have changed over time. In Frazao, E., Ed. *America's Eating Habits: Changes and Consequences.* Washington, D.C.: Economic Research Service, U.S. Department of Agriculture, Agriculture Information Bulletin No. 750, 1999, pp. 33–50, chap. 2.

3. Welsh, S.O., Davis, C., and Shaw, A. *USDA's Food Guide: Background and Development.* USDA Human Nutrition Information Service. Nutrition Education Division. Miscellaneous Publication No. 1514. September 1993. Available at: http://www.usda.gov/cnpp/Pubs/Pyramid/FoodGuideDevt.pdf. Accessed June 19, 2005.

4. U.S. Congress. Senate. Select Committee on Nutrition and Human Needs. *Dietary Goals for the United States* [1st edition]. Washington, D.C., 1977. [Description: Congressional report with references and statements by scientists.]

5. U.S. Congress. Senate. Select Committee on Nutrition and Human Needs. *Dietary Goals for the United States* [1st edition], supplemental views. Washington, D.C., 1977.

6. U.S. Congress. Senate. Select Committee on Nutrition and Human Needs. *Dietary Goals for the United States* [2nd edition]. Washington, D.C., December 1977.

7. Dwyer, J.T. Nutrition guidelines and education of the public. *J Nutr.* 131(11 S): 3074S–3077S, 2001. Available at: http://www.nutrition.org/cgi/content/full/131/11/3074S. Accessed June 20, 2005.

8. U.S. Department of Agriculture; U.S. Department of Health and Human Services. *Nutrition and Your Health: Dietary Guidelines for Americans.* February 1980. Home and Garden Bulletin No. 232. Available at: http://www.health.gov/dietaryguidelines/1980thin.pdf. Accessed June 17, 2005.

9. The discussion about the history of the Dietary Guidelines is adapted from: 2005 Dietary Guidelines Advisory Committee. Report of the Dietary Guidelines Advisory Committee on the *Dietary Guidelines for Americans,* 2005. August 19, 2004. Available at: http://www.health.gov/dietaryguidelines/dga2005/report/. Accessed June 19, 2005.

10. U.S. Department of Agriculture; U.S. Department of Health and Human Services. *Nutrition and Your Health: Dietary Guidelines for Americans,* 2nd ed. Home and Garden Bulletin No. 232. 1985. Available at: http://www.health.gov/dietaryguidelines/1985thin.pdf. Accessed June 17, 2005.

11. U.S. Department of Health and Human Services, Public Health Service. *The Surgeon General's Report on Nutrition and Health.* DHHS (PHS) Publication No. 88-50215, 1988.

12. National Academy of Sciences, National Research Council, *Food and Nutrition Board. Diet and Health: Implications for Reducing Chronic Disease Risk.* Washington, D.C.: National Academy Press, 1989.

13. U.S. Department of Agriculture; U.S. Department of Health and Human Services. *Nutrition and Your Health: Dietary Guidelines for Americans,* 3rd ed. Home and Garden Bulletin No. 232. Revised November 1990. Available at: http://www.health.gov/dietaryguidelines/1990thin.pdf. Accessed June 17, 2005.

14. *National Nutrition Monitoring and Related Research Act of 1990* (7 U.S.C. 5341), Public Law 101–445. Available at: http://uscode.house.gov/download/pls/7C84.txt. Accessed June 16, 2005.

15. U.S. Department of Agriculture; U.S. Department of Health and Human Services. *Nutrition and Your Health: Dietary Guidelines for Americans,* 4th ed. Home and Garden Bulletin No. 232. December 1995. Available at: http://www.health.gov/dietaryguidelines/dga95/default.htm. Accessed June 17, 2005.

16. U.S. Department of Agriculture; U.S. Department of Health and Human Services. *Nutrition and Your Health: Dietary Guidelines for Americans,* 5th ed. Home and Garden Bulletin No. 232. 2000. Available at: http://www.health.gov/dietaryguidelines/dga2000/document/frontcover.htm. Accessed June 17, 2005.

17. Basiotis, P.P., Carlson, A., Gerrior, S.A., Juan, W.Y., Lino, M. *The Healthy Eating Index: 1999–2000.* U.S. Department of Agriculture, Center for Nutrition Policy and Promotion. CNPP-12. 2002. Available at: http://www.cnpp.usda.gov/publications/HEI/HEI99-00report.pdf. Accessed July 12, 2006.

18. Kennedy, E.T., Ohls, J., Carlson, S., and Flemming, K. The healthy eating index: design and applications. *J Am Diet Assoc.* 95, 1103–1108, 1995.

19. Institute of Medicine. *Dietary Reference Intakes for Energy, Carbohydrate, Fiber, Fat, Fatty Acids, Cholesterol, Protein, and Amino Acids.* Washington, D.C.: National Academy Press, 2002.

20. Report of a Joint FAO/WHO Consultation. Diet, Nutrition and the Prevention of Chronic Diseases. Geneva: World Health Organization; 2003 (WHO Technical Report Series 916). Available at: http://www.fao.org/docrep/005/AC911E/AC911E00.HTM. Accessed August 17, 2006.

21. *Dietary Reference Intakes: Applications in Dietary Assessment,* May 1, 2000.

22. *Dietary Reference Intakes: Applications in Dietary Planning.* February 6, 2003.

23. *Dietary Reference Intakes: Guiding Principles for Nutrition Labeling and Fortification.* December 11, 2003.

24. U.S. Department of Agriculture; U.S. Department of Health and Human Services. *Dietary Guidelines for Americans.* 2005. 6th ed. Washington, D.C. January 2005. HHS Publication number: HHS-ODPHP-2005-01-DGA-A USDA Publication number: Home and Garden Bulletin No. 232. 2005. Available at: http://www.health.gov/dietaryguidelines/dga2005/document/pdf/DGA2005.pdf/. Accessed June 17, 2005.

25. Schneeman, B.O. and Mendelson, R. Dietary guidelines: past experience and new approaches. *J Am Diet Assoc.* 102, 1498–1500, 2002.

26. Kant, A.K. Consumption of energy-dense, nutrient-poor foods by adult Americans: nutritional and health implications. The third National Health and Nutrition Examination Survey, 1988–1994. *Am J Clin Nutr.* 72, 929–936, 2000.

27. Kant, A.K. Reported consumption of low-nutrient-density foods by American children and adolescents. Nutritional and health correlates, NHANES III, 1988 to 1994. *Arch Pediatr Adolesc Med.* 157, 789–796, 2003.

28. Zelman, K. and Kennedy, E. Naturally nutrient rich...putting more power on Americans' plates. *Nutrition Today.* 40, 60–68, 2005.

29. Food and Drug Administration Modernization Act of 1997. Public Law 105–115. Available at: http://www.fda.gov/cder/guidance/105-115.htm#SEC.%20301. Accessed June 21, 2005.

30. Center for Food Safety and Applied Nutrition. Office of Food Labeling (HFS-150). Guidance for Industry: Notification of a Health Claim or Nutrient Content Claim Based on an Authoritative Statement of a Scientific Body. Washington, D.C.: U.S. Food and Drug Administration. June 11, 1998. Available at: http://www.cfsan.fda.gov/~dms/hclmguid.html. Accessed June 21, 2005.

31. HealthierUS.Gov. Available at: http://www.healthierus.gov/. Accessed June 18, 2005.

32. Overview of the Sugar Association, Inc. position on sugars. September 27, 2004. Available at: http://www.health.gov/dietaryguidelines/dga2005/comments/ViewTopics.asp?TopicID=5&SubTopicID=21&submit1=Submit. Accessed June 25, 2005.

33. Kuehn, B.M. Experts charge new U.S. dietary guidelines pose daunting challenge for the public. *JAMA*. 293, 918–920, 2005.

34. Willett, W.C. *Eat, Drink, and Be Healthy*. New York: Simon and Schuster Source, 2001, p. 139.

35. Lanou, A.J., Berkow, S.E., and Barnard, N.D. Calcium, dairy products, and bone health in children and young adults: a reevaluation of the evidence. *Pediatrics*. 115, 736–743, 2005.

36. Nestle, M. *Food Politics: How the Food Industry Influences Nutrition and Health*. Berkeley, CA: University of California Press, 2002.

37. Light, L. A fatally flawed food guide. *Whole Life Times*. November 2004. Available at: http://www. wholelifetimes.com/2004/wlt2611/wh_lead2611.html. Accessed June 26, 2005.

38. Lichtenstein, A.H., Appel, L.J., Brands, M., et al. Diet and lifestyle recommendations revision 2006 a scientific statement from the American Heart Association Nutrition Committee. *Circulation*. 114, 82–96, 2006. Available at: http://circ.ahajournals.org/cgi/reprint/CIRCULATIONAHA.106.176158. Accessed July 2, 2006.

39. Krauss, R.M., Eckel, R.H., Howard, B., et al. AHA Dietary Guidelines: revision 2000: a statement for healthcare professionals from the Nutrition Committee of the American Heart Association. *Circulation*. 102, 2284–2299, 2000.

40. Sallis, J.F. and Owen, N. Ecological models of health behavior. In Glanz, K., Lewis, M.L., and Rimer, B.K., Eds. *Health Behavior and Health Education*, 3rd ed. San Francisco, CA: Jossey-Bass, 2002, chap. 20.

41. National High Blood Pressure Education Program. *Prevention, Detection, Evaluation, and Treatment of High Blood Pressure. The Seventh Report of the Joint National Committee (JNC 7)*. U.S. Department of Health and Human Services. National Institutes of Health. National Heart, Lung, and Blood Institute. NIH Publication Number 03-5233. December 2003. Available at: http://www.nhlbi.nih.gov/ guidelines/hypertension/express.pdf. Accessed July 3, 2006.

42. Whelton, P.K., He, J., Appel, L.J., et al. Primary prevention of hypertension: clinical and public health advisory from The National High Blood Pressure Education Program. *JAMA*. 288, 1882–1888, 2002.

43. National High Blood Pressure Education Program. *Prevention, Detection, Evaluation, and Treatment of High Blood Pressure. The Seventh Report of the Joint National Committee (JNC 7)*. U.S. Department of Health and Human Services. National Institutes of Health. National Heart, Lung, and Blood Institute. NIH Publication Number 03-5233. December 2003. Available at: http://www.nhlbi.nih. gov/ guidelines/ hypertension/express.pdf. Accessed July 3, 2006.

44. Knowler, W.C., Barrett-Connor, E., Fowler, S.E., et al. Reduction in the incidence of type 2 diabetes with lifestyle intervention or metformin. *N Engl J Med*. 346, 393–403, 2002.

45. National Cancer Institute. Eat 5 to 9 a Day. U.S. Department of Health and Human Services. National Institutes of Health. http://www.5aday.gov/. Accessed July 5, 2006.

46. American Institute for Cancer Research. The New American Plate. Available at: http://www.aicr.org/ site/PageServer?pagename=pub_nap_index_21. Accessed July 5, 2006.

12 Food and Nutrition Assessment of the Community

Assessment, policy development, and assurance are the three core functions of public health, whether at the federal, state, or local level. Assessment, the focus of this chapter, refers to the systematic collection, assembly, analysis, and dissemination of information about the health of a community. Policy development involves the creation of comprehensive public health policies based on scientific knowledge. Assurance is the pledge to constituents that services necessary to achieve agreed-upon goals are provided by encouraging the action of others (private or public), by stipulating action through regulation, or by providing the service directly.[1]

Every public health agency must ensure that assessment occurs either directly or through intergovernmental or interagency cooperation. Accurate information on the health status of a community and a clear understanding of the available resources is requisite to making informed decisions about which areas should have priority, which policies might be effective, or which interventions might be possible to implement. In addition, monitoring must be either ongoing or undertaken at regular intervals to provide a baseline understanding of the community's health in order to evaluate how well any new policies or interventions improve health, how cost-effective one option is over another, or how long a program might continue.[2]

Community health assessment, of which assessments of food and nutrition status are an extension, includes the following:

- Determining the health needs of the community by establishing a systematic process that periodically provides pertinent health information.
- Investigating adverse health events and health hazards by conducting timely investigations that identify the magnitude of health problems, including their duration, trends, location, and at-risk populations.
- Analyzing the determinants of identified health problems to discover the reasons why certain populations are at risk for adverse health outcomes.

More specific to this chapter, public health agencies — in performing their role of assessment — monitor food and nutrition-related health status to identify and solve nutrition-related health problems. Activities of state and local public health agencies include:

- Diagnosis of a community's health status
- Identification of food and nutrition-related threats to health
- Periodic collection, analysis, and publication of information on access, utilization, costs, and outcomes of nutrition services
- Attention to the vital statistics and nutrition-related health status of specific groups at higher risk than the total population.

Because Chapter 5 offers a comprehensive discussion of data-gathering performed at the national level, the primary goal of this chapter is to introduce the information needed to conduct food and nutrition assessments within a community. A secondary goal is to help readers appreciate the value of ongoing collaboration between local health assessment coordinators and nutritionists, and state and local food and nutrition assessment efforts. (See Box 12.1.)

Box 12.1 The Community Toolbox

The Community Toolbox is a project that promotes community health and development by connecting people, ideas, and resources. The toolbox provides practical skill-building information on over 250 different topics, including step-by-step instruction, examples, check-lists, and related resources. Maintained by the Work Group on Health Promotion and Community Development at the University of Kansas in Lawrence, the Web site has been online since 1995 and continues to grow on a weekly basis: http://ctb.ku.edu/.

12.1 COMMUNITY ASSESSMENT

Three types of assessment discussed in this chapter focus on food and nutrition-related matters in the community: the *nutrition assessment,* the *food assessment* (sometimes referred to as a *food system assessment*), and the *food security assessment.* In clinical practice, the counterparts to the community nutrition assessment and food assessment would be the nutritional assessment and the diet history, respectively. The food security assessment collects information to determine the extent to which existing community resources provide adequate, culturally acceptable foods to households in the area.

The purpose of any kind of assessment is to collect and analyze information in order to identify problems and suggest solutions to ameliorate them. In the clinic, assessment forms the basis for developing and implementing an individual's care plan or course of medical nutrition therapy. In the community, assessment forms the basis for subsequent program planning and evaluation.

Regardless of the specific focus of the assessment — or who initiates the process or assumes major responsibility for carrying it out — the goals of food and nutrition assessments in the community are to:

- Improve the health of the people in a defined area by building the capacity of local health jurisdictions to reduce nutritional risk and promote optimal nutritional health of community members
- Raise official awareness of food and nutrition issues to promote the inclusion of nutrition questions in local health assessments and otherwise get food and nutrition issues on the local agenda
- Determine how to allocate limited resources
- Evaluate the efficacy of food and nutrition programs and services in the community
- Identify current and potential food and nutrition problems in the community

Three basic kinds of information are gathered during any community assessment. These include a statistical community profile (Section 12.2.2), qualitative data on the experiences of the population

---

Box 12.2 Community Health Assessment Clearinghouse

The New York State Department of Health (NYSDOH) has compiled resources to use when performing a community health assessment (CHA). The NYSDOH Community Health Assessment Clearinghouse is a "one-stop" resource for community health planners, practitioners, and policy developers. From 2003 through 2006 the New York State Assessment Initiative (NYAI) was funded through a cooperative agreement with the Centers of Disease Control and Prevention (CDC) Assessment Initiative. The NYAI works with four partner states (Maine, New Hampshire, New Jersey, Vermont) and CDC-funded assessment initiative states to develop and disseminate assessment methods, systems, and approaches. The Community Health Assessment Clearinghouse is available at: http://www.health.state.ny.us/statistics/chac/

Box 12.3 Washington State Community Nutrition Education Assessment Project

When planning a community nutrition assessment, be sure to investigate the Washington State Community Nutrition Assessment Project Web site, which was developed in 1999 by the Washington State Department of Health. The site is available at: http://depts.washington.edu/commnutr/home/.

(Section 12.2.3.1.1), and an assessment of local resources and assets (Section 12.2.3.2).[3] Termed an *assets-based approach*,[4] this type of assessment recognizes and employs individual and community talents, skills, and assets, rather than focusing on problems and needs. Such an approach imparts a sense of ownership to community members participating in the process. In every community there are groups who care about nutrition: churches, healthcare institutions, government agencies, breastfeeding support groups, Head Start, schools, parents, and healthcare providers. A thoughtful compilation of assets prevents an assessment from becoming a compendium of morbidity and mortality statistics.

The successful community assessment includes understanding current issues confronting families and individuals, evaluating local capacities for supporting health and nutrition needs, and building community support for implementing changes. To conduct a community assessment, it is necessary to:[3]

1. Organize a planning group
2. Define community boundaries
3. Gather quantitative data that includes a statistical profile of the community and a compendium of community resources
4. Collect qualitative data that reflects the food and nutrition concerns of representatives of key community groups
5. Analyze and prioritize common issues, high-risk individuals and populations, and unmet needs

12.1.1 THE COMMUNITY NUTRITION ASSESSMENT

A nutrition assessment of a community is initiated and implemented by professionals to examine a broad range of nutrition-related issues and assets in order to improve the community's nutrition services system. The nutrition assessment is part of the larger community health assessment. During the assessment process, relationships are forged between individuals and organizations that may result in enhanced opportunities for collaboration and funding. An overarching goal of the community nutrition assessment is a movement away from a categorical and programmatic view of nutrition services and programs to a focus on the role of nutrition in the community as a whole.

A nutrition assessment examines, in particular, the health and nutrition status of community members, including:

- Pregnancy-related status, including prepregnancy weight, weight gain during pregnancy, and anemia
- Prevalence of diseases affected by nutrition such as diabetes, cardiovascular disease, and HIV/AIDS
- Physical activity and food-related behaviors
- Food intake, such as amount of fruits and vegetables consumed
- Dental health
- Food security (see Section 12.5)

The Washington State Community Nutrition Assessment Project[3] has compiled knowledge, skills, tools, and resources for nutrition professionals and local health assessment coordinators to use when conducting a community nutrition assessment.

Box 12.4 New York State Nutrition Surveillance Link

Additional information about the New York State Nutrition Surveillance Program can be found at: http://www.cardi.cornell.edu/health_and_safety/nutrition/000266.php.

12.1.1.1 Local Nutrition Surveillance

For effective nutrition programming, planning, and policymaking, state and community leaders require timely, objective information on the current and changing nutrition condition of the populations they serve. Providing such information is the goal of nutrition surveillance, which collects nutrition indicators from a representative sample of a particular locality (see also Chapter 5: Food and Nutrition Surveys). Examples of measurements used in nutrition surveillance include self-reported height and weight and brief food frequency questionnaires. The inclusion in surveillance studies of questions regarding knowledge, attitudes, and behavior can help in developing target strategies for dietary messages. Indicators of dietary practices in the community, such as comparing the amount of supermarket shelf space for whole vs. low-fat and fat-free milk, may also be used. The problems identified through surveillance can help generate timely interventions.[5]

Nutrition surveillance comprises four types of activities: timely warning and intervention, problem identification, policy and program planning, and management and evaluation. As an example, in 1984, New York State began a Nutrition Surveillance Program (NSP), the first phase of which was connected to the Supplemental Nutrition Assistance Program (SNAP), a new program that supported over 1000 emergency food and WIC programs in the state, and expanded home-delivered meals to the elderly. NSP gathered information about the characteristics and unmet nutrition needs of these populations, which was then used for funding requests and program development. The second phase of NSP began in 1988, identifying and characterizing populations at nutritional risk and evaluating the status of current nutrition programs. Results of this assessment included the addition of a nutrition component to the Dental Survey of School Children and the development of an inventory of information sources in all state agencies. The third phase, a policy and planning phase, also monitors HealthyPeople objectives and the 5-year plan of the state's Food and Nutrition Policy Council.[6] (See Box 12.4.)

12.1.2 THE COMMUNITY FOOD ASSESSMENT

A community food assessment is a participatory and collaborative process spearheaded by members of the community rather than health professionals. Community members along with officials representing public and private agencies examine a broad range of food-related issues and community assets in order to improve the community's food system. Through such an assessment, diverse stakeholders work together to research their local food system, publicize their findings, and take action.[7] A number of communities (see Section 12.1.2.1) have successfully planned and implemented community food assessments, gathered a wide range of data, and used the results to

---

Box 12.5 Food is Central to Our Lives

"Despite how central food is to our lives, most of us know very little about where the food we eat comes from, how it is grown, and how it reaches our plates. This lack of knowledge is true not only for individuals, but also for communities as a whole."

Source: Our Foodshed in Focus: Missoula County Food and Agriculture by the Numbers. Available at: www.umt. edu/cfa/indicator.htm. Accessed August 23, 2006.

---

generate tangible outcomes. Their endeavors demonstrate that assessments in diverse settings can generate a variety of results, including new policies and programs, as well as process benefits such as new partnerships and capacity development.[8]

A community food assessment relies on the participation of diverse stakeholders, including community residents, to plan and implement the assessment and emphasizes shared leadership and collaborative decision-making. In addition, it fosters education and empowerment strategies, such as training young people in survey methods. Significantly, this type of assessment focuses on meeting the needs of low-income and other marginalized populations, examines a variety of issues and the connections between them, and generates specific recommendations and actions aimed at improving the local food system.[9]

A community food assessment includes four components:[10]

- *Organization* to identify key stakeholders, arrange initial meetings, determine the group's interest in conducting an assessment, identify and recruit other participants representing diverse interests and skills, and continue to coordinate and engage constituents throughout the project.
- *Planning* to review other assessments that have been conducted, determine assessment purpose and goals, develop an overall plan and decision-making process and clarify roles, define geographic population boundaries, and identify and secure grants, in-kind resources, and/or project sponsors.
- *Research* to develop questions and indicators, identify existing data and information needed, develop research tools, collect and analyze data, and compile and summarize findings.
- *Advocacy* to discuss findings with community and develop recommendations, create action plans to implement priority recommendations, determine whether additional partners should be recruited, develop media strategy, disseminate findings to the public, policymakers and journalists, urge policymakers and others to take action based on recommendations, and evaluate the assessment project.

12.1.2.1 Community Food Assessment Projects

Whereas community food assessments are undertaken for a variety of reasons and in diverse communities, a review of nine community food assessment projects — from Austin, TX to Somerville, MA (see Table 12.1) — conducted between 1993–2003[11] revealed these common characteristics:

- *Focused on the needs of low-income residents* and shared a concern for the problems they face with respect to food security. Recommendations from the studies included such strategies as instituting a new bus route connecting low-income neighborhoods to large supermarkets, the development of year-round farmers' markets, and improved coordination of food assistance efforts throughout the county.
- *Shared concerns about the sustainability of the food system* relevant to their own communities. In these studies, sustainability included creating closer links between two or more food system activities (for example, production, processing, distribution, consumption, and waste disposal); making specific food system practices more environmentally friendly; including previously excluded categories, such as low-income consumers and small farmers; and educating community residents about their participation in food systems and ways to enhance sustainability.
- *Viewed the community as a source of strength* that held solutions to problems of food access.
- *Focused on assets in the community,* such as existing resources, infrastructure, and motivated and talented individuals and their networks.
- *Relied on extant data from myriad sources,* including: social, economic, demographic, and health data from censuses; community directories; and primary information derived from surveys, focus groups, and interviews.

TABLE 12.1
Nine Community Food Assessments

Site	Goals	Issues Examined	Outcomes
Austin, TX	Raise awareness of community needs, problems; Inform systematic action on community food problems	Food access problems in central Austin, coping strategies; Quality of food available in a poor neighborhood	New "grocery" bus route; Legislation allowing public lands for community gardens, farmers' markets; Grocery store renovation; Awareness of food access; Food policy council established
Berkeley, CA	Enhance community knowledge, awareness of local food systems; Study feasibility of new ways to link farmers' markets and communities	Local food production: farms and urban gardens; Food retail; Role of educational institutions; Public policies related to above issues	Formalized collaboration between Berkeley Food Policy Council and area producers, retailers, and community-based nonprofit (including youth) organizations; Links between local producers and Berkeley school cafeterias; Dissemination of study tools nationally
Detroit, MI	Support community food security planning actions; Create university–community partnerships on community food issues	Food in local economy (including contribution to local economy; grocery store locations; food access, availability in poor neighborhoods; Regional agriculture	Collaboration by nonprofit organizations in nutrition, social services, greening, community development, etc., to develop community food projects; Greater public, private, nonprofit, university collaboration on community food issues; National dissemination of study tools, findings; Production, dissemination of *Detroit Food Handbook* for local planning
Los Angeles, CA	Assess food insecurity in inner city, following 1993 unrest, adequacy of federal food programs, and role of food industry in inner city community based strategies for change; Propose framework for community food security planning	Community food access, availability, prices; Hunger and food insecurity; Food retail structure; Sustainable production, distribution models; Current food policies; alternative approaches	Formation of Los Angeles Community Food Security Network, Los Angeles food policy council; Growth of community gardens, farmers markets, food stamp outreach; Food assessments in other communities; Catalyst for community food security movement in the U.S.
Madison, WI	Increase knowledge, understanding of local food system; Inform strategies for improving food security; Establish university, community partnerships	Conventional food system (production, processing, wholesale, retail) and its impacts on environment, food access, availability; Antihunger resources; Coping strategies of low-income residents; Alternatives to conventional system; Policies helping, hurting community food security	Development of Dane County REAP (Research, Education, Action, and Policy) Food Group; Greater visibility of food issues in Madison; Increased networking, collaboration among individuals and organizations around food issues; Madison Food System Working Paper series; National dissemination of assessment tools

Location	Goals	Assessment data gathered	Outcomes/recommendations
Milwaukee, WI	Examine the root causes of hunger Develop partnerships to promote food security and systemic change in Milwaukee County	Population characteristics Food access and transportation Food retail: locations, availability, prices Antihunger and alternative food sources Perceptions and experiences of poor individuals and families	Formation of Milwaukee Farmers' Market Association Development of Fondy Food Center Project (market, kitchen incubator, information center) Overhaul of emergency pantry network, community meal program coalition, and inclusion of new types of technical assistance and guidelines Expansion of WIC Farmers' Market Nutrition Program (FMNP) to all farmers markets Increased university–community partnerships National dissemination of study tools, finding
North Country Region, NY	Mobilize and engage a broad network of country residents Improve access to healthful, locally produced foods while strengthening economic viability of regional agricultures	Demographics, health, economy, agriculture, food availability Sources of food, eating patterns Ways to build a stronger community through alternative management of local food resources Visions for how local food system should look and work in 5 years Visions for 20 years	Development of an Extension staff position to continue work Increased networks among community, agency members Creation of a fellowship kitchen to serve all community members, including needy and vulnerable households in Essex County Program to provide donations of venison and beef to local food pantries in Lews and St. Lawrence counties Establishment of weekly farmers market in Jefferson County Improved food distribution networks between the community action programs of Jefferson and Franklin Counties Increased storage and trucking facilities through joint efforts of a food security committee
San Francisco, CA	Identify and promote strategies to improve food access to nutritious foods in Bayview Hunters Point neighborhood Provide job training for neighborhood youth	Food sources for residents, barriers to access, consumption Preferred alternatives for food procurement	Creation of a new Bayview Community Farmers Market Commitments on the part of corner store owners to stock fresh produce Transit authority agreement to provide transit shuttles to food sources Skills development, empowerment of neighborhood youth
Somerville, MA	Strengthen planning and policy for community-based food and nutrition resources for low-income residents	Food and nutrition needs, resources	Publication of an extensive community food and nutrition guide Cooking classes for low-income residents Implementation of a Community Kitchen Task Force to examine the feasibility of commercial kitchen facilities Formation of a Public Health Nutrition Task Force to conduct community food and nutrition strategic planning

Source: Table adapted from Pothukuchi, K. Community food assessment: a first step in planning for community food security. *Jour Plant Edn Rsch.* 23, 356–377, 2004.

Beneficial and tangible outcomes from these community food assessments are reviewed in *What's Cooking in Your Food System?*[12] In addition, this guide, available from the Community Food Security Coalition (www.foodsecurity.org), discusses problems with our present food system and their relevance to food security, details the process of planning and conducting a community assessment (see Section 12.2), and reviews how to implement changes based on assessment results. Process-oriented benefits resulting from the featured programs include development of networks and coalitions, community participation and collaboration, and capacity development.

12.1.2.2 Food and Farming in Montana

In 2003, two University of Montana professors formed a steering committee of stakeholders from the community that included farmers, county planning officials, and food bank representatives to identify the most vital research questions related to food and farming in Missoula County. Next, the faculty members designed a multidisciplinary university course, engaging 21 students in gathering information regarding food production, distribution, and consumption in the county.[13] The results of this research are compiled in two reports: Foodshed[14] uses existing statistical data, primarily from U.S. census reports and other government sources, to describe patterns in the local food system, and how these have changed over time. Seven chapters, all authored by students, detail relevant trends in the following areas: demographics, agricultural production, environment, food distribution, employment in farming and food-related businesses, consumption, and food security and access. Each chapter also discusses why these trends might be occurring and explains why these measures are important. Appendices include both the raw data and the data sources used for each chapter. Additional reference material is provided at the end of each chapter. *Grow, Eat, Know*[15] is a resource guide of food and farming in the county.

The next phase of the project sought input from county agricultural producers and county residents. Representatives of the agricultural community were asked to comment on the future of farming in the county, whereas residents of various income levels were asked to identify their concerns regarding food quality, cost, and access. The research was designed to answer questions that the steering committee asked about Missoula County's food system. It includes the following:

- What is needed for viable and sustainable commercial food production in the county?
- What are the existing assets and barriers to creating a more viable and sustainable production system?
- What concerns do county residents at various income levels have about food, including quality, access, transportation to food outlets, cost, eating behaviors and choices?
- What do residents perceive as their county's food-related assets?

Original data was collected during the spring of 2004. The results of these interviews and recommendations for action are compiled in a report entitled *Food Matters.*[16] The report also offers recommendations designed to generate a community dialogue about the future of the food and farming system in the county.

12.1.3 THE COMMUNITY FOOD SECURITY ASSESSMENT

Although many elements overlap, a community food security assessment more specifically focuses on communities at risk for food insecurity than does a community food assessment. (See Box 12.6.)

The USDA has developed a toolkit of instructions and materials for conducting a community food security assessment.[17] The kit contains standardized measurement tools for assessing various aspects of community food security. These tools focus on examining basic assessment components: profiling general community characteristics and community food resources, assessment of household food security, food resource accessibility, food availability and affordability, and food production resources. Appendices to the toolkit provide tips for developing data tables, materials and guides for conducting focus groups, and materials for conducting food store surveys.

Box 12.6 What Is a Community Food Security Assessment?

"A community food security (CFS) assessment is a unique type of community assessment. It includes the collection of various types of data to provide answers to questions about the ability of existing community resources to provide sufficient and nutritionally sound amounts of culturally acceptable foods to households in the community."

Source: Cohen, B., Andrews, M., and Kantor, L.S. *Community Food Security Assessment Toolkit.* ERS E-FAN No. 02-013, July 2002. Available at: http://agmarketing.extension.psu.edu/Retail/PDFs/CommFdScurtyAssesTlKit.pdf. Accessed August 24, 2006.

12.1.3.1 Community Food Security Assessment in Sacramento

In 1999–2000, the Sacramento Hunger Commission conducted a food access study in 2 low-income neighborhoods in Sacramento County, CA. Their subsequent report, *Breaking Barriers: A Road to Improved Food Access,* outlined recommendations made by low-income residents about how to improve food access in their community. The assessment identified a need for improved public transportation to markets supplying fresh, nutritious, affordable food.[18] In response, the commission received funding to implement some of the recommendations in the report. The group's research and advocacy helped implement a neighborhood shuttle and generated a new bus route connecting under-served neighborhoods to a grocery store on the opposite side of a freeway.

Access Denied (1995)[19] describes a neighborhood food system and how it failed to meet community needs. The analysis revealed that access to nutritious affordable food was difficult for much of the community. At the time of the study, these shopping realities limited consumer selection and increased the cost of food for people who could least afford it. The area studied had just 2 supermarkets — both smaller and one more expensive than similar stores in other parts of the town. Securing transportation to these food outlets was often difficult; for many, hiring a taxi was the only way to buy food at the supermarket. As a result of being unable to access supermarkets, many low-income shoppers relied on expensive corner convenience stores. Wholesale grocery companies rarely served these smaller stores, which forced owners to charge higher prices and offer limited selections. There were 38 convenience stores in the community, but only 5 stocked the ingredients for a balanced meal. All of the convenience stores stocked alcoholic beverages, but only 18 carried milk. There were 20 agencies that distributed emergency food in the area studied.

This assessment of food resource accessibility and availability demonstrated that the resources did exist to improve the food system and to overcome obstacles to getting good food. The report suggests community resources and solutions in access, store quality, alternative retail formats, local food production, and food education. The authors of the report list such options as forming grocer cooperatives that could take advantage of group purchasing and shared warehousing for small store owners; forming neighborhood food-buying clubs; initiating shopper shuttles, reduced fares, and other transportation solutions to help people get to stores; support for farmers' markets and produce stands; and local food production through community gardening programs and urban farms.

In the fall of 2003, the Sacramento Hunger Commission proposed a community food security assessment of Avondale/Glen Elder, a low-income neighborhood in the southern part of the city. Avondale/Glen Elder was chosen because of its manageable size and relatively effective organization. Nonetheless, it proved a difficult area to assess because of its diversity of cultures and languages.[20]

A VISTA (Volunteer in Service to America) volunteer and a Hunger Commission intern developed a comprehensive plan and then gathered a plethora of information on the area's food security and food access status. They surveyed "food closet" clients, senior home-delivered meal recipients, and other community residents and evaluated each food resource in the neighborhood to determine its effectiveness

---

Box 12.7 Recommendations from the Avondale/Glen Elder Assessment

- A closer full-service grocery store
- Shuttle bus route 37 improved to connect individuals with services and food resources
- Increased public transit outreach to immigrant populations
- Grocery carpool system, facilitated through Weed & Seed (George Sim Center)
- Farmers' market carpool and bus field trip
- EBT at farmers' markets
- Food closet services consider alternative hours
- Health education; education about healthy foods and cooking
- Community gardens need to be protected
- Community organized food-buying coop
- Improved outreach for public assistance programs
- More WIC farmers' market vouchers; more WIC staff
- Farm-to-school, school gardens
- Staggered lunch at one local high school; work to shorten serving lines at another
- Set length for elementary school lunch periods
- Other beverage options for lactose intolerant youth
- Teachers need to set a positive example

Source: Salcone, J. The Avondale/Glen Elder community food assessment: food security in a South Sacramento neighborhood. The Sacramento Hunger Commission, 2004. Available at: http://www.targethunger.com/Community-Food-Security/avonglen_01_07.htm. Accessed August 24, 2006.

---

in providing affordable, nutritious, culturally appropriate food. The data were then evaluated and presented in a comprehensive report. A steering committee of active community residents oversaw and contributed to the assessment. Box 12.7 presents the recommendations arising from the assessment.

12.2 CONDUCTING AN ASSESSMENT

Despite varying goals and a somewhat different focus, any community assessment entails many of the same components. This section, based primarily on *What's Cooking in Your Food System?*[8] and the *Community Food Security Assessment Toolkit*[17] highlights some of the steps and resources discussed in these documents that can contribute to an effective assessment.

Box 12.8 Assessment, Planning, Implementation, and Evaluation

Problem-solving can be distilled into four basic tasks: assessment, planning, implementation, and evaluation. It is a lucky break for nutritionists that these sequential tasks can be remembered using the acronym APIE. When faced with a problem, the first action one must take is to analyze the situation. Based on that assessment, the second step consists of planning a course of action. Next, the plan is implemented. Finally, the intervention's effectiveness is evaluated. The process can repeat itself as many times as necessary, with the results of the evaluation determining the plan for the next cycle.

Source: Spark, A. Neologisms and mnemonics: linguistic tools in nutrition education and communication. Presented at the annual meeting of the American Dietetic Association, October 22, 1996.

Box 12.9 Planned Approach to Community Health (PATCH)

The Planned Approach to Community Health (PATCH) was developed in 1983 by the U.S. Centers for Disease Control (CDC) in partnership with state and local health departments and community groups. It was designed to provide a model to assist state and local public health agencies, in their partnerships with local communities, to plan, conduct, and evaluate health promotion and disease prevention programs. PATCH was also intended to serve as a mechanism to improve links both within communities and between communities and state health departments, universities, and other agencies and organizations. PATCH combines the principles of community participation with the diagnostic steps of applied community-level epidemiology. The development of PATCH was influenced by the theoretical assumptions underlying the PRECEDE model, by the literature on community organization and development, and by CDC's tradition of working through state health agencies in the application of health promotion and disease prevention programs.

The PATCH process guides users through five phases: (1) mobilizing the community, (2) collecting and organizing data, (3) choosing health priorities, (4) developing a comprehensive intervention plan, and (5) evaluation. Moving from the initiation to the full implementation of PATCH can take can up to a year or more. Successful implementation depends upon actively engaging community members in the process, having adequate time and resources to gather and interpret data to guide program development, and developing cohesion among stakeholder organizations. PATCH is an example of a model that has not only tested the application of theory, but has also facilitated the link between research and practice in community health education and health promotion.

PATCH is widely recognized as a practical and user-friendly model for community health promotion and disease prevention planning. It has been used in combination with other community-based planning frameworks such as Assessment Protocol for Excellence in Public Health (APEXPH) and Healthy Cities.

Public health staff in over 40 states have received training in the PATCH process and it has been applied in over 300 local communities in the U.S., as well as several communities in Canada, Australia, and in the Panama Canal region by the U.S. military. It has also been applied in a wide variety of settings, including hospitals, managed care organizations, universities, voluntary health agencies, local health departments, agricultural extension services, and work sites. PATCH has also been employed to focus on the health needs of diverse populations to address such topics as cardiovascular disease, injury prevention, HIV/AIDS (human immunodeficiency virus/acquired immunodeficiency syndrome), teen pregnancy, and tobacco use.

Although no longer directly funded by the CDC, the PATCH process continues to be referenced and used by many organizations and agencies for community planning and for the training of new public health and health promotion professionals.

Source: Breckon, D., Harvey, J., and Lancaster, R.B. *Community Health Education: Settings, Roles, and Skills for the 21st Century, Fourth Edition.* Rockville, MD: Aspen Publishers, 1998.

12.2.1 ORGANIZE A TEAM

A community assessment is envisioned, planned, conducted, and used by people living and working in the community. Representation from different segments of a community increases access to data, improves the likelihood of participation by their constituencies, ensures a focus on community concerns and goals, and can lead to positive and lasting change. In addition to community representation, assessment participants should provide diversity, expertise and experience, availability, and a capacity for decision making.[8,17]

A team should have 8 to 12 members to be comprehensive without becoming unwieldy. Team members can be recruited from local government agencies, educational institutions, community- and faith-based organizations, health providers, food retailers, residents, and farmers. It is imperative to convince potential members of the importance of the assessment's goals, the need for that indi- vidual's particular skills or knowledge, the clarity of the assessment plan, and the intention to implement change based on results.[8,17]

A review of the literature indicates that health outcomes are improved through community empowerment, with "empowerment domains" defined to include participation, community-based organizations, local leadership, resource mobilization, assessment of problems, links with other people and organizations, and program management. Those with power or with access to it (for example, a health practitioner) and those who desire it (for example, a client) must work together to create the necessary conditions to achieve empowerment, as in a community assessment.[21]

Once a team is gathered, it needs to work together to:

- Clarify goals and interests
- Agree on a planning and decision-making process
- Define the community to be assessed
- Identify funds and other resources
- Plan and conduct the research
- Prepare and disseminate findings
- Evaluate the findings
- Implement follow-up actions in response to the findings[8]

12.2.2 DEFINE THE COMMUNITY AND THE SCOPE OF THE ASSESSMENT

Defining the geographical boundaries of the community to be assessed is fundamental to a com- munity food assessment. Will you be assessing an entire county as in the Missoula County, MT, FoodShed study (see Section 12.1.2.2) or smaller urban neighborhoods as done by the Hunger Commission in Sacramento (see Section 12.1.3.1)?

If conducting a community food assessment or food security assessment, consider the parts of the food system to be examined. Is the study wide-ranging, linking aspects of the food system to health or sustainability? Or is it more narrowly focused on food access in a particular low-income neighborhood? Knowing what and whom you are going to assess helps to refine planning and the development of tools, such as surveys and questionnaires.

12.2.3 DATA COLLECTION

Data collection is vital to the assessment process. Evaluation of results must be based on accurate and reliable information. When selecting data sources or developing questions for surveys, bear the goals of the assessment in mind. Not all data that can be gathered will be pertinent to a particular assessment; conversely, it is important not to overlook useful data sources or replicate research.

Data collection methods commonly used in community assessments include:

- Informal, survey, semistructured, standardize open-ended, focus group, or key informant interviews
- Community meeting/hearing
- Direct or participant observation
- Document analysis
- Photo documentation or novella
- Community asset/problem mapping

Some of these methods are discussed in the following sections. Each has its strengths and weak- nesses; the method to be used depends on an assessment's particular goals and the resources available.

Box 12.10 Components of a Demographic Profile of a Community

Total Population ___

Gender

Number of people   Male___ Female___

Household Structure

Total number of households___   Persons per household___

Family Households (*number of households*) ___

Number of married-couple families ___

Number of single-parent families with a male head of household ___

Number of single-parent families with a female head of household ___

Nonfamily Households (*total number*)___

Number of people who live alone ___

Number of people in households who are ≥ 65 years___

Race/ethnicity

Number of people

White___   Asian/Pacific Islander___   Hispanic origin (of any race)___

American Indian ___   African American___   Other___

Age (in years)

Number of people

< 5	18–21	36–49	65–74
5–12	22–25	50–54	75–84
13–17	26–35	55–64	≥ 85

Median Household Income___

Poverty Status

Number of:

People of all ages below poverty level___

Related children under < 18 years of age in poverty___

Related children ages 5 to 17 years in families in poverty

Employment Status

Number of people ≥ 16 years of age

In labor force___   Civilian___   Not employed___

In armed forces___   Employed___   Not in labor force___

Source: Cohen, B., Andrews, M., and Kantor, L.S. *Community Food Security Assessment Toolkit.* ERS E-FAN No. 02-013, July 2002. Available at: http://agmarketing.extension.psu.edu/Retail/PDFs/CommFdScurtyAssesTlKit.pdf. Accessed May 15, 2005.

12.2.3.1 General Community Characteristics

Community characteristics provide a socioeconomic and demographic profile of the people in the community (see Box 12.10). It includes total population, age, race/ethnicity, citizenship, household structure, employment status, income, and poverty status. Demographic and socioeconomic data such as these are some of the easiest to collect because they are assembled by federal, state, or county agencies. Because these data have been systematically collected, they are almost always reliable and valid. Most are available on the Internet, in the local public library, or from the state

TABLE 12.2
Demographic and Socioeconomic Data

Data	Description	Notes on Usage	Source of Data
Population characteristics	Census data	Estimates from noncensus years, Total of people in county categorized by racial/ethnic group and sex	Department of Health Center for Health Statistics http://www.census.gov
Per capita income	Census data	Per household and family type	Census data
Employment/unemployment rate	Census data		Bureau of Research and Statistics
Occupations/major employers	County statistics		County planning office, Department of Labor
Housing		Kitchen facilities, low income housing available	Census data
Poverty data	Census data	Percent below poverty level by household	Census data
Education literacy rate	Census data	Educational attainment	Census data
Languages spoken other than English	Census data		Census data
Geographic characteristics	County statistics	Community types (urban, suburban, rural), pockets of poverty	County planning office
Public transportation	County statistics	Type and availability	County planning office

Source: Washington State Community Nutrition Education Project. Tables of Potential Data Sources: Demographic and Socioeconomic data. Available at: http://depts.washington.edu/commnutr/assess/dsource-tables.htm. Accessed August 24, 2006.

or county agency. Relying on existing information for the community profile is the least expensive way to gather statistics and provides consistent data that can be used easily for comparative purposes.

The Washington State Community Nutrition Education Project Web site provides tables of potential data sources, such as the demographic and socioeconomic data listed in Table 12.2, as well as health statistics, nutrition program data, and community resources. See http://depts.washington.edu/commnutr/assess/dsource-tables.htm.

12.2.3.1.1 Focus Groups

Focus groups are an effective means of gaining additional insight into a community and for developing appropriate survey questions to be administered to a larger audience. One study conducted a series of focus groups involving specifically targeted segments within a multicultural community. Despite differences in ethnicity, age, and length of residence, community members voiced similar concerns about the advantages and difficulties of living in a multiethnic, multilingual neighborhood; about housing and other environmental issues; and about problems accessing healthcare. In addition, participation in the focus group increased participation in other community endeavors.[22]

Members of each focus group should be fairly homogeneous and be familiar with the topic under discussion. A number of focus groups may need to be convened so that all subgroups within the defined community are represented. Focus groups are conducted by a trained facilitator using a focus group guide.[17]

12.2.3.1.2 Surveys, Questionnaires, and Observation

Surveys aid data gathering from larger numbers of people than possible through focus groups and thus help ensure representativeness. Survey responses are collected by interview, written response, or observation. Questions can be close-ended as in multiple-choice, or scaled answers or open-ended, allowing the respondent or observer to answer freely.

The Food Store Survey provided in the USDA Community Food Security Assessment Toolkit (http://www.ers.usda.gov/Publications/efan02013) is an example of an observational survey. The observer can complete this survey at a store without direct contact with other people.

Many surveys can be administered by nonprofessional volunteers, trained only in data collection. Questionnaires used in nutritional assessment of individuals are generally, though not always, administered one-on-one by trained personnel and are thus more costly and more time-consuming. These include 24-h recalls, food diaries, and food frequency questionnaires (see Box 12.11 and Section 4.2 Dietary Assessment).

To the extent possible, communities need to be helped in identifying assessment methods that are comparable with other surveys.[23] For example, when food frequency and food security questionnaires are used, asking the same questions as are used in national surveys can help make local survey results comparable with national data.

Box 12.11 Dietary Collection and Analysis

There are a variety of techniques to assess dietary intake, each with their own strengths and weaknesses. All dietary assessment methods are limited and absolute validity is difficult to determine. However, this limits all researchers and it sometimes makes sense to collect dietary intake data, even if the information is flawed. Keep in mind that collection and assessment of dietary intake is burdensome to subjects, staff, and is very costly. Carefully consider how you will use the data and if it is really essential for your study.

Twenty-Four Hour Recall

A retrospective detailed interview conducted by a registered dietitian to determine a subject's dietary intake from the preceding 24-h period. The burden to the volunteer is low but you have to collect serial recalls to adequately characterize usual intake. A quantitative assessment is possible with 24-h recalls.

Multiple-Day Food Diary

Volunteers are asked to measure or weigh everything they eat for a specified number of days. Subject burden is high but food diaries are useful for motivating people in intervention studies and are considered the gold standard in dietary assessment. A quantitative assessment is possible with food diaries.

Diet History

An in-depth interview conducted by a registered dietitian to determine the volunteer's usual meal patterns and other details of dietary intake. Diet histories typically provide qualitative rather than quantitative information. The type of information collected can be tailored to meet the needs of your study.

Food Frequency Questionnaires (FFQ)

FFQs are standardized forms inquiring about the frequency of intake of different foods or food groups. They are not as accurate as other measures but are useful in large population studies or when studying the association of a specific food and a disease. Several validated questionnaires exist and the most appropriate one will depend on your study. Some questionnaires can be scanned and quantitatively assessed.

Source: Adapted from the University of Vermont, College of Medicine, General Clinical Research Center, Bionutrition Services. Dietary data collection and analysis. Available at: http://www.uvm.edu/~gcrc/dietintake.htm. Accessed August 24, 2006.

12.2.3.2 Food Resource Availability, Accessibility, and Affordability

Sustained economic and social adversity in low-income neighborhoods often makes it difficult for residents to obtain nutritious, affordable food. A community food resource assessment determines how well equipped the community is to meet the food-related needs of its residents. A profile of all existing resources must be created to determine the adequacy of the extant community food resources, pinpoint possible barriers to food security, and increase access to nutritious food in the community.

Community food resources include retail food stores, farmers' markets, food cooperatives, and food assistance programs. Access to these resources depends on both their presence at reasonable distances from home and the ability to physically get to these resources using a private vehicle or public transportation. Four key areas are investigated in an assessment of food resource accessibility and food availability:

- Identifying retail stores and other places to purchase food in order to determine: availability of authorized food stamp retailers; number, type, and location of retail food stores; number and location of consumer food cooperatives; and number and location of farmers' markets.
- Identifying the number and location of schools that participate in the National School Lunch (NSLP) and School Breakfast Program (SBP); Child and Adult Care Food Program (CACFP) providers; Summer Food Service Program (SFSP) sites; WIC Farmers' Market Nutrition Program (FMNP) sites; and WIC clinics.
- Identifying the community's emergency food assistance providers, including the number, location, and times of operation of food banks, food pantries, emergency kitchens, TEFAP and Commodity Supplemental Food Program (CSFP) distribution sites, and Food Distribution Program on Indian Reservations (FDPIR) sites.
- Describing the rate of participation in Federal Food Assistance Programs: WIC, Food Stamps, NSLP and SBP, CACFP, SFSP, TEFAP Distribution, WIC FMNP, CSFP, FDPIR, Meals on Wheels Program, and Nutrition Services Incentives Program (NSIP).

Defining the spatial relationship between housing and food outlets is an important part of a community food assessment. Groups undertaking an assessment frequently prepare maps of the community to visualize the physical connection or disconnection between residents and various types of food sources (see Section 12.3). Marc Schlossberg at the University of Oregon has done this for the city of Eugene. His series of maps can be seen at http://www-personal.umich.edu/~copyrght/image/solstice/sum04/schlossberg/. In addition, Section 5.2.2.1 provides information on the Community Nutrition Research Group's (CNRG's) Community Mapping Project.

12.2.3.3 Household Food Security

Accurate measurement of household food security can help public officials, policymakers, service providers, and community groups assess the need for assistance, judge the effectiveness of existing programs designed to help such households, and identify population subgroups with unusually severe levels of food insecurity. One main question drives this assessment: Is household food insecurity a problem directly or personally experienced by a significant number of people in the community?

One way to collect household food security data is to conduct a representative household food security survey, as described in the USDA's *Guide to Measuring Household Food Security, Revised 2000*.[24] The assessment is predicated on the Core Module, a measurement tool developed to gather data on household food security.

12.2.3.3.1 CPS-FSS and the Core Module

The Core Module has been used both in national surveys, such as the Current Population Survey Food Security Supplement (CPS-FSS) and in community food security assessments conducted on the local level.[25] The module can form the basis for a sophisticated measurement of the severity of food insecurity as experienced and reported by household members. Local studies using either the 18-question Core Module or the standard abbreviated 6-item subset can document the extent and severity of hunger in the community (see Box 12.12 and Box 12.13).

Box 12.12 U.S. Household Food-Security/Hunger Survey Module: Three-Stage Design

Questionnaire Transition into Module (Administer to all households):
These next questions are about the food eaten in your household in the last 12 months, since (current month) of last year, and whether you were able to afford the food you need.

General Food Sufficiency Questions/Screener: Questions 1, 1a, 1b (Optional: These questions are NOT used in calculating the food-security/hunger scale.)
Question 1 may be used as a screener: (1) in conjunction with income as a *preliminary* screen to reduce respondent burden for higher income households only; and/or (2) in conjunction with the first-stage internal screen to make that screen "more open," i.e., provide another route through it.

1. Which of these statements best describes the food eaten in your household in the last 12 months?

   - Enough of the kinds of food (I/we) want to eat
   - Enough, but not always the kinds of food (I/we) want
   - Sometimes not enough to eat
   - Often not enough to eat

   [1] Enough of the kinds of food we want to eat [SKIP 1a and 1b]
   [2] Enough but not always the kinds of food we want [SKIP 1a; ask 1b]
   [3] Sometimes not enough to eat [Ask 1a; SKIP 1b]
   [4] Often not enough [Ask 1a; SKIP 1b]
   [ ] DK or Refused (SKIP 1a and 1b)

   1a. [IF OPTION 3 OR 4 SELECTED, ASK the following.] Here are some reasons why people don't always have enough to eat. For each one, please tell me if that is a reason why YOU don't always have enough to eat. [READ LIST. MARK ALL THAT APPLY.]
   Yes   NO   DK
               Not enough money for food
               Not enough time for shopping or cooking
               Too hard to get to the store
               On a diet
               No working stove available
               Not able to cook or eat because of health problems

   1b. [IF OPTION 2 SELECTED, ASK the following.] Here are some reasons why people don't always have the quality or variety of food they want. For each one, please tell me if that is a reason why YOU don't always have the kinds of food you want to eat. [READ LIST. MARK ALL THAT APPLY.]
   Yes   NO   DK
               Not enough money for food
               Kinds of food (I/we) want not available
               Not enough time for shopping or cooking
               Too hard to get to the store
               On a special diet

[Begin food-security core module (i.e., scale items)]
Stage 1: Questions 2–6 — Ask all households:

2. Now I'm going to read you several statements that people have made about their food situation. For these statements, please tell me whether the statement was often true, sometimes true, or never true for (you/your household) in the last 12 months, that is, since last [name of current month]. The first statement is "(I/We) worried whether (my/our) food would run out before (I/we) got money to buy more." Was that often true, sometimes true, or never true for (you/your household) in the last 12 months?

[ ] Often true [ ] Sometimes true [ ] Never true [ ] Don't know (DK) or refused (R)

3. "The food that (I/we) bought just didn't last, and (I/we) didn't have money to get more." Was that often, sometimes, or never true for (you/your household) in the last 12 months?
[ ] Often true [ ] Sometimes true [ ] Never true [ ] DK or R

4. "(I/we) couldn't afford to eat balanced meals." Was that often, sometimes, or never true for (you/your household) in the last 12 months?
[ ] Often true [ ] Sometimes true [ ] Never true [ ] DK or R
[IF CHILDREN UNDER 18 IN HOUSEHOLD, ASK Q5–Q6; OTHERWISE SKIP TO FIRST-LEVEL SCREEN.]

5. "(I/we) relied on only a few kinds of low-cost food to feed (my/our) child/the children) because (I was/we were) running out of money to buy food." Was that often, sometimes, or never true for (you/your household) in the last 12 months?
[ ] Often true [ ] Sometimes true [ ] Never true [ ] DK or R

6. "(I/We) couldn't feed (my/our) child/the children) a balanced meal, because (I/we) couldn't afford that." Was that often, sometimes, or never true for (you/your household) in the last 12 months? [ ] Often true [ ] Sometimes true [ ] Never true [ ] DK or R
First-level Screen (screener for Stage 2):
If AFFIRMATIVE RESPONSE to ANY ONE of Question 2 to Question 6 (i.e., "often true" or "sometimes true") OR response [3] or [4] to Question 1 (if administered), then continue to Stage 2; otherwise, skip to end.
Question 7 to Question 11 — Ask households passing the first-level Screen: (estimated 40% of households < 185% poverty; 5.5% of households > 185% poverty; 19% of all households).
[IF CHILDREN UNDER 18 IN HOUSEHOLD, ASK Q7; OTHERWISE SKIP TO Q8]

7. "(My/Our child was/The children were) not eating enough because (I/we) just couldn't afford enough food." Was that often, sometimes, or never true for (you/your household) in the last 12 months? [ ] Often true [ ] Sometimes true [ ] Never true [ ] DK or R

8. In the last 12 months, since last (name of current month), did (you/you or other adults in your household) ever cut the size of your meals or skip meals because there wasn't enough money for food? [ ] Yes [ ] No (SKIP 8a) [ ] DK or R (SKIP 8a)

8a. [IF YES ABOVE, ASK] How often did this happen—almost every month, some months but not every month, or in only 1 or 2 months? [ ] Almost every month [ ] Some months but not every month [ ] Only 1 or 2 months [ ] DK or R

9. In the last 12 months, did you ever eat less than you felt you should because there wasn't enough money to buy food? [ ] Yes [ ] No [ ] DK or R

10. In the last 12 months, were you every hungry but didn't eat because you couldn't afford enough food? [ ] Yes [ ] No [ ] DK or R

11. In the last 12 months, did you lose weight because you didn't have enough money for food? [ ] Yes [ ] No [ ] DK or R
Second-level Screen (screener for Stage 3):
If AFFIRMATIVE RESPONSE to ANY ONE of Questions 7 through 11, then continue to Stage 3; otherwise, skip to end.
Stage 3: Question 12 to Question 16 — Ask households passing the second-level Screen: (esti-mated 7–8% of households < 185% poverty; 1–1.5% of households > 185% poverty; 3–4% of all households).

12. In the last 12 months, did (you/you or other adults in your household) ever not eat for a whole day because there wasn't enough money for food?
[ ] Yes [ ] No (SKIP 12a) [ ] DK or R (SKIP 12a)

12a. [IF YES ABOVE, ASK] How often did this happen—almost every month, some months but not every month, or in only 1 or 2 months? [ ] Almost every month [ ] Some months but not every month [ ] Only 1 or 2 months [ ] DK or R
[IF CHILDREN UNDER 18 IN HOUSEHOLD, ASK 13–16; OTHERWISE SKIP TO END.]

13. The next questions are about children living in the household who are under 18 years old. In the last 12 months, since (current month) of last year, did you ever cut the size of (your child's/any of the children's) meals because there wasn't enough money for food? [ ] Yes [ ] No [ ] DK or R

14. In the last 12 months, did (Child's name/any of the children) ever skip meals because there wasn't enough money for food?
    [ ] Yes [ ] No (SKIP 14a) [ ] DK or R (SKIP 14a)

14a. [IF "YES" ABOVE, ASK the following.] How often did this happen — almost every month, some months but not every month, or in only 1 or 2 months? [ ] Almost every month [ ] Some months but not every month [ ] Only 1 or 2 months [ ] DK or R

15. In the last 12 months, (was your child/ were the children) ever hungry but you just couldn't afford more food? [ ] Yes [ ] No [ ] DK or R

16. In the last 12 months, did (your child/any of the children) ever not eat for a whole day because there wasn't enough money for food?
    [ ] Yes [ ] No [ ] DK or R

Source: Bickel, G., Nord, M., Price, C., Hamilton, W., Cook, J. Measuring Food Security in the United States. *Guide to Measuring Household Food Security Revised 2000.* Alexandria, VA: Food and Nutrition Service, U.S. Department of Agriculture, March 2000. Available at: http://www.fns.usda.gov/FSEC/FILES/FSGuide.pdf. Accessed August 25, 2006.

Box 12.13 Short Form of the Food-Security/Hunger Survey

Short Form of the Food-Security/Hunger Survey

[LEAD] These next questions are about the food eaten in your household in the last 12 months and whether you were able to afford the food you need.

Q3. I'm going to read you two statements that people have made about their food situation. Please tell me whether the statement was OFTEN, SOMETIMES, or NEVER true for (you/you and the other members of your household) in the last 12 months.

The first statement is, "The food that (I/we) bought just didn't last, and (I/we) didn't have money to get more." Was that often, sometimes, or never true for (you/your household) in the last 12 months? [1] Often true [2] Sometimes true [3] Never true [Don't know, Refused] ____

Q4. "(I/we) couldn't afford to eat balanced meals." Was that often, sometimes, or never true for (you/your household) in the last 12 months?
[1] Often true [2] Sometimes true [3] Never true [DK, R] ____

Q8. In the last 12 months, since (date 12 months ago) did (you/you or other adults in your household) ever cut the size of your meals or skip meals because there wasn't enough money for food? [1] Yes [2] No (GO TO 5) [DK, R] (GO TO 5) _____

Optional Screener: If any of the first 3 questions are answered affirmatively (i.e., if either Q2 or Q3 are "often true" or "sometimes true" or Q8 is "yes"), proceed to the next question. Otherwise, skip to end.

Q8a. **[Ask only if Q8 = YES]** How often did this happen?
[1] Almost every month [2] Some months, but not every month [3] In only 1 or 2 months [DK, R] [or X (i.e., Question not asked because of negative or missing response to Q8).]

Q9. In the last 12 months, did you ever eat less than you felt you should because there wasn't enough money to buy food? [1] Yes [2] No [DK, R]

Q10. In the last 12 months, were you ever hungry but didn't eat because you couldn't afford enough food? [1] Yes [2] No [DK, R]

Source: Bickel, G., Nord, M., Price, C., Hamilton, W., Cook, J. Measuring Food Security in the United States. *Guide to Measuring Household Food Security Revised 2000.* Alexandria, VA: Food and Nutrition Service, U.S. Department of Agriculture, March 2000. Available at: http://www.fns.usda.gov/FSEC/FILES/FSGuide.pdf. Accessed August 25, 2006.

The CPS-FSS is the source of national and state-level statistics on food insecurity and hunger used in the USDA's annual reports on household food security. The CPS is a monthly labor force survey of about 50,000 households conducted by the Census Bureau for the Bureau of Labor Statistics. Once each year, after answering the labor force questions, the same households are asked a series of questions (the Food Security Supplement) about food security, food expenditures, and use of food and nutrition assistance programs. Food security data have been collected by the CPS-FSS annually since 1995.[26] The survey consists of questions about several general types of household food conditions, events, and behaviors. They include:

- Anxiety that the household food budget or food supply may be insufficient to meet basic needs.
- Perceptions that the food eaten by household members is inadequate in quality or quantity.
- Reported instances of reduced food intake or consequences of reduced food intake (such as the physical sensation of hunger or reported weight loss) for adults in the household (omitted in the 6-question subset).
- Reported instances of reduced food intake or its consequences for children in the household.

When used to collect data on a periodic basis, the questionnaire can provide systematic monitoring of the community's progress in addressing hunger and other food security needs in the community.

12.2.3.4 Assessment of Food Production Resources

A community's agricultural system can boost the effectiveness of federal food assistance and education programs. Local agriculture can play a role in community food security when implemented together with a strong federal nutrition safety net and emergency food assistance programs. This can increase the availability of high-quality, affordable food within a community, offering small farmers an opportunity to maintain economic viability by supplying the local market with fresh foods, strengthening economic and social ties between farms and urban residents, and channeling a larger share of residents' food spending back into the local economy. Several key questions might be asked in an assessment of food production resources:

- Does the community have food production or food distribution resources?
- Do low-income households have the opportunity to participate in community gardens or other food production activities?
- Are there any school-based gardening programs?
- Are locally produced foods sold through local food retailers and restaurants?
- Does the local school district purchase foods from local producers?
- Are locally produced foods used by other institutional food service outlets, such as colleges, prisons, and hospitals?

12.2.4 Funding and Budgets

Unfortunately, the scope and scale of an assessment is often determined by the available budget. Although volunteers and in-kind resources can reduce the actual cash outlay needed to conduct an assessment, some expenses must be met directly. Below are some assessment expenses to consider:

- Site and refreshments for meetings
- Reimbursement for participation in community outreach
- Support staff
- Research personnel
- Office space, phones, photocopying
- Fund-raising
- Printed materials such as flyers and survey forms

Funding for community assessments is difficult to obtain at the federal level, although the Community Food and Nutrition Program (CFNP) has funded some projects, as has the Community

Food Projects Competitive Grants Program. Community development block grants and food stamp nutrition education funds might prove a fruitful source. Locally, government agencies dedicated to nutrition, health, or community development, for example, may provide some assistance. Community and other private foundations, if you frame your assessment goals to match their interests, may also help with funding.[8] Chapter 16 offers help in writing grants for funding.

12.2.5 ANALYZE AND PRESENT DATA

Analysis of data is both quantitative (such as demographic data) and qualitative (from interviews and focus groups). In addition, the approach used depends on the assessment's goals, whether to compare your community to national data or to develop an action plan to improve food access. Presenting this data to stakeholders, policymakers, and the general public is integral to the assessment process.[17]

The presentation should be easy to understand, with graphic displays such as maps and tables used whenever possible to clarify and amplify narrative presentations. Table 12.3 provides the

TABLE 12.3
Demographic Profile of Power County, ID, and Idaho State

People QuickFacts	Power County	Idaho
Population, 2005 estimate	7,753	1,429,096
Population, percent change, April 1, 2000 to July 1, 2005	2.9%	10.4%
Population, 2000	7,538	1,293,953
Population, percent change, 1990 to 2000	6.4%	28.5%
Persons under 5 years old, percent, 2004	7.2%	7.4%
Persons under 18 years old, percent, 2004	29.9%	26.7%
Persons 65 years old and over, percent, 2004	11.0%	11.4%
Female persons, percent, 2004	50.1%	49.9%
White persons, percent, 2004 (a)	95.5%	95.5%
Black persons, percent, 2004 (a)	0.2%	0.6%
American Indian and Alaska Native persons, percent, 2004 (a)	3.6%	1.4%
Asian persons, percent, 2004 (a)	0.5%	1.0%
Native Hawaiian and Other Pacific Islander, percent, 2004 (a)	0.0%	0.1%
Persons reporting two or more races, percent, 2004	0.2%	1.3%
Persons of Hispanic or Latino origin, percent, 2004 (b)	23.9%	8.9%
White persons, not Hispanic, percent, 2004	72.3%	87.2%
Living in same house in 1995 and 2000, pct age 5+, 2000	61.1%	49.6%
Foreign born persons, percent, 2000	10.5%	5.0%
Language other than English spoken at home, pct age 5+, 2000	21.1%	9.3%
High school graduates, percent of persons age 25+, 2000	74.7%	84.7%
Bachelor's degree or higher, pct of persons age 25+, 2000	14.3%	21.7%
Persons with a disability, age 5+, 2000	1,332	200,498
Mean travel time to work (minutes), workers age 16+, 2000	17.6	20.0
Housing units, 2004	2,936	578,774
Homeownership rate, 2000	74.6%	72.4%
Housing units in multi-unit structures, percent, 2000	9.2%	14.4%
Median value of owner-occupied housing units, 2000	$89,000	$106,300
Households, 2000	2,560	469,645
Persons per household, 2000	2.92	2.69
Per capita money income, 1999	$14,007	$17,841
Median household income, 2003	$32,937	$39,859
Persons below poverty, percent, 2003	14.5%	11.8%

Source: U.S. Census Bureau: State & County Quick Facts. Power County, Idaho. Available at: http://quickfacts.census.gov/qfd/states/16/16077.html. Accessed August 25, 2006.

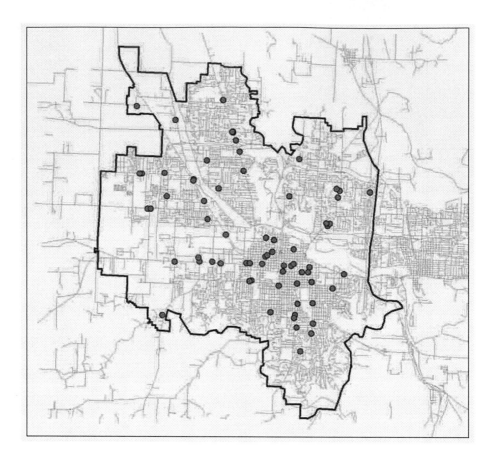

FIGURE 12.1 Visualizing accessibility: Stores and streets. (From Schlossberg, M. Visualizing accessibility II: Access to food. Available at: http://www-personal.umich.edu/~copyrght/image/solstice/sum04/schlossberg/. Accessed August 25, 2006.)

demographic profile of Power County, ID, and that of the state as a whole, courtesy of the U.S. Census. Figure 12.1 plots the location of food markets on a map of Eugene, OR (see Section 12.3, Geographic Information Systems).

An assessment report that incorporates the data analysis can assume many identities other than that of a written report: a series of newsletter articles, a media or policy brief, a research or professional paper, resources guides or databases, a community presentation, or a study guide. Regardless of the form the report takes, it should include an overview of the community and its food system (if applicable), a description of your assessment process, highlights and discussion of key findings, and recommendations for change.[8]

12.2.6 IMPLEMENT FINDINGS

Of course, the ultimate purpose of an assessment is to make positive change. Once an assessment is complete, the same general process, although focused on change, called for by the assessment, will need to be repeated. Types of action might include, for example, community mobilization through door-to-door canvassing, community education through media coverage or bilingual brochures, program or activity development, and public policy advocacy. A recent, innovative instrument for advocacy is the food policy council (see Box 12.14). Refer to Table 12.1 for examples of some outcomes arising from community food assessments done across the country.

Box 12.14 Food Policy Councils

What is a food policy council?
A food policy council is a coalition of food system stakeholders who advise a city, county, or state government on policies related to agriculture, food distribution, hunger, food access, and nutrition. Most governments take actions that affect their local food system, such as zoning laws that affect grocery store placement and school nutrition policies. These policies are often fragmented, however. Food policy councils exist to examine these issues in a more holistic fashion, obtaining previously unknown information about the food system and also developing projects and policies to improve it. Current councils serve as advisory commissions to state and city governments, within departments of health, and as nonprofit organizations. Members may be appointed by the council or by government officials and often include farmers, food processors, wholesalers, distributors, grocers, restauranteurs, anti-hunger advocates, community leaders, representatives of government departments, co-operative extension agents, and concerned citizens. These diverse coalitions often must educate themselves about their members' specialties and overcome their stereotypes in order to be effective.

Why are food policy councils created?
Food policy councils address a variety of issues. They are often created in response to a pressing need. For instance, the Sustainable Food Center's study revealed that the low-income neighborhoods of East Austin, TX, had fewer grocery stores with less variety and higher prices than other areas of the city. The Austin City Council responded by studying the issue further and creating the Austin Food Policy Council to find ways to address this issue and related ones.

What kinds of things do food policy councils do?
Food policy councils perform a variety of tasks, from researching food production, food access, and nutrition in their area to designing and implementing projects and policies to address those issues. Some examples include:

- Creating bus routes that connect low-income neighborhoods to supermarkets
- Developing the nation's first municipal food policies
- Supporting school nutrition programs, including supporting kitchen renovations to allow kitchens to process fresh foods, determining how to use of locally-grown foods in school meals, and advising teachers and administrators on school breakfast implementation
- Publishing a state road map that includes most farms and other sources of locally-grown foods in the state with small descriptions of each site
- Mobilizing farmland preservation efforts
- Monitoring grocery store prices and discouraging differential pricing that disadvantages low-income neighborhoods
- Educating the public and policymakers about food, nutrition, hunger, and agriculture issues through discussion groups and position papers

Source: Willamette Farm and Food Coalition. Food policy councils fact sheet. Available at: www.lanefood.org/pdf/food_ policy_councils/food_policy_council_fact_sheet.pdf. Accessed August 25, 2006.

12.3 GEOGRAPHIC INFORMATION SYSTEMS

Geographic information systems (GIS) are computerized systems for the storage, retrieval, manipulation, analysis, and display of geographically referenced data. This technology provides a useful way to map and display spatial and temporal relationships. Geomapping is a valuable tool for conducting needs assessments, targeting specific populations for outreach, and examining program outcomes. See Section 5.2.2 for information on the Community Nutrition Research Group's (CNRG's) Community Nutrition Mapping project (CNMap).

Box 12.15 Definitions

Geocode — A code which represents the spatial characteristics of an *entity*. For example, a *co-ordinate point* or a *postcode*. A Geocode may be a 5- or a 9-digit zipcode, area code, county, state or health-service area; census block or tract, global positioning system (GPS) reading, or a set of longitudinal-latitudinal coordinates.

Geocoding — The cross-referencing between specifically recorded x,y co-ordinates of a location, relative to a standard reference grid such as the U.S. National Grid (USNG), and non-geographic data such as addresses or post-codes. In this way the accessing of the non-geographic data allows locations to be accurately mapped. Geocoding refers to collecting information to enable GIS presentation of data.

Georeference — To establish the relationship between page co-ordinates on a planar map and known real-world coordinates. Georeferenced data can be tied to a specific location or place, such as an area code, street address, or other census and political boundaries.

Source: Sommer, S. and Wade, T, Eds. *A to Z GIS: An Illustrated Dictionary of Geographic Information Systems.* Redlands, CA: ESRI Press, 2006

As GIS can include physical, biological, cultural, demographic, or economic information, it is a valuable tool in the natural, social, medical, and engineering sciences as well as in business and planning. Researchers, public health professionals, policymakers, and others use GIS to better understand geographic relationships that affect health outcomes, public health risks, disease transmission, access to healthcare, and other public health concerns. GIS is being used with greater frequency to address neighborhood, local, state, national, and international public health issues. For example, the Centers for Disease Control and Prevention (CDC) uses GIS to provide maps and data on public health issues in the U.S. Many of the CDC's efforts are based on online maps provided by the U.S. Census Bureau. These maps can be manipulated in many different ways.

Although a young field that began in the 1960s, the antecedents of GIS go back hundreds of years in the fields of cartography and mapping. The history of GIS parallels that of computation in general, with mapping and geographic studies being early beneficiaries of the increasing power of computers.[27] In 2003, the U.S. National Library of Medicine (NLM) added the term *geographic information systems* to its controlled vocabulary thesaurus known as MeSH (medical subject headings), reflecting the importance and growing use of GIS in health and healthcare research and practice.[28] Today, GIS is a multibillion-dollar-per-year high technology industry. Worldwide spending on GIS software in 2004 was $1.8 billion, of which $ 544 million was spent by U.S. federal, state, and local government agencies.[29]

The geographic data in a GIS consist of a series of map layers that contain information about features located in specific locations. GIS links multiple sets of geospatial data and graphically displays that information as maps, with potentially many different layers of information. Assuming that all the information is at the same scale and has been formatted according to the same standards, users can overlay spatial information about any number of specific topics to examine how the layers interrelate. Each layer of a GIS map represents a particular "theme" or feature, and one layer could be derived from a data source completely different from the other layers.

As illustrated in Figure 12.2, one layer or "theme" could represent all the streets in a specified area. Another could correspond to all the buildings in the same area, and others could show vegetation or water resources. Additional themes could be census tract boundaries with sociodemographic variables collected by the U.S. Census, WIC clinic locations and associated information,

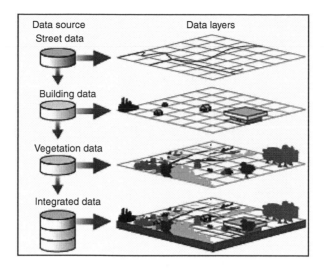

FIGURE 12.2 GIS Layers or Themes. (From Figure 1: GIS Layers or Themes, in GAO-04-703: Geospatial Information — Better Coordination Needed to Identify Reduce Duplicative Investments, June 2004. Available at: www.gao.gov/new.items/d04703.pdf. Accessed August 25, 2006.)

such as hours of operation or capacity, or ZIP code boundaries with data on low-birth-weight or Medicaid-eligible populations. As long as standard processes and formats have been arranged to facilitate integration, each of these themes could be based on data originally collected and maintained by a separate organization. Analyzing this layered information as an integrated whole can significantly aid decision makers in considering complex choices, such as where to locate a WIC center to best serve the greatest number of eligible people.[30] Table 12.4 describes the data themes for the lead agencies that engage in nutrition-related mapping activities.

Use of geocoding in health data systems provides the basis for cost-effective disease surveillance and intervention. *Healthy People 2010* (Objective 23.3) calls for doubling the proportion of all major national, state, and local health data systems that use geocoding in order to promote nationwide use of GIS at all levels.[31] In 1999, data was geocoded by less than half of the major health data systems.[32] The GAO recommends that the U.S. develop a comprehensive, national geospatial strategic plan for coordinating federal GIS activities.[33]

12.3.1 EXAMPLES OF GIS IN FOOD AND NUTRITION PROGRAMS

A community assessment project in Hinds County, MS, used GIS to select survey centers for a target population, evaluate sample representation, and perform geography-based community health assessment. Survey centers focused on either a general population or a specific group within the population. Potential survey centers (such as local grocery stores or large discount stores) were overlaid on block groups to verify their location as a center. Only after the center for a target population had been identified were in-person surveys conducted. Geographic representation involved address geocoding of participants' residences and analysis of the geographic distribution samples in relation to the selected survey centers, demographics, and economic characteristics of the county. Finally, maps were created to depict the geographic distribution of variables such as health status, healthcare access, availability of transportation, and types of healthcare facilities available.[34]

The authors of the study concluded that traditional methods of surveying may disproportionately collect samples from a few, nonrepresentative areas, whereas using GIS to determine survey centers results in better representation of the study center. They also noted that a major disadvantage of GIS in community assessment is the lack of GIS infrastructure.[34] However, as GIS becomes more mainstream, this should change. For example, the California Nutrition Network mapping application

TABLE 12.4
Data Themes, Descriptions, and Lead Agencies for Food and Nutrition-Related Mapping Activities

Data Theme	Lead Agency	Description
Governmental units	DOC/ USCB	These data describe the official boundary of federal, state, local, and tribal governments as reported to the Census Bureau for purposes of reporting the nation's official statistics.
Geographic data	HUD	Geographic data on homeownership rates, location of various forms of housing assistance, underserved areas, and race.
Public health	HHS	Public health themes relate to the protection, improvement, and promotion of the health and safety of all people. For example, public health databases include spatial data on deaths and births, infectious and notifiable diseases, incident cancer cases, behavioral risk factor and tuberculosis surveillance, hazardous substance releases, and health effects, hospital statistics, and similar data.
Buildings and facilities	GSA	Includes federal sites or entities with a geospatial location deliberately established for designated activities; a facility database might describe a factory, military base, college, hospital, power plant, fishery, national park, office building, space command center, or prison.
Transportation	DOT	Transportation data are used to model the geographic locations, interconnectedness, and characteristics of the transportation system within the U.S. The transportation system includes both physical and nonphysical components representing all modes of travel that allow the movement of goods and people between locations.

Source: Adapted from Table 4: OMB Circular A-16 Data Themes, Descriptions, and Lead Agencies, in GAO-04-703: Geospatial Information — Better Coordination Needed to Identify Reduce Duplicative Investments, June 2004. Available at: www.gao.gov/new.items/d04703.pdf. Accessed August 25, 2006.

is an interactive, Internet-based GIS that allows users to view and query mapped nutrition data.[35] The application offers a wide range of nutrition and other health-related data, including:

- Nutrition and school health programs
- WIC grocery stores and other local nutrition resources
- Demographics (race and spoken language) of general and at-risk populations
- Various Department of Health Services regions
- Political (senate and assembly) districts

12.4 CONCLUSION

Conducting a community assessment, whether it focuses on nutritional status, food access, or food security involves a tremendous commitment of time, energy, and resources, yet there is significant payback in terms of heightened understanding of the assets and barriers that exist within a community. It is important to approach an assessment with clearly defined goals, to seek active participation from the diverse groups within the community, and to plan to create positive change.

Numerous tools are available to collect, analyze, and present data; however, the tools selected depend on the goals of the assessment as well as available funding. Most significantly, the information and knowledge attained through an assessment is only as useful as the change it impels.

12.5 ACRONYMS

CACF	Child and Adult Care Program
CDC	Centers for Disease Control and Prevention
CFNP	Community Food and Nutrition Program
CNMap	Community Nutrition Mapping Project
CNRG	Community Nutrition Research Group
CPS-FSS	Current Population Survey–Food Security Supplement
CSFP	Commodity Supplemental Food Program
FDIR	Food Distribution on Indian Reservations
GIS	Geographic Information System
MeSH	Medical Subject Headings
NLM	National Library of Medicine
NSIP	Nutrition Services Incentive Program
NSP	Nutrition Surveillance Program
PATCH	Planned Approach to Community Health
SNAP	Supplemental Nutrition Assistance Program
TEFAP	The Emergency Food Assistance Program
USDA	United States Department of Agriculture
VISTA	Volunteers in Service to America
WIC	Supplemental Program for Women, Infants, and Children

REFERENCES

1. The Committee for the Study of the Future of Public Health. *The Future of Public Health.* Division of HealthCare Services. Institute of Medicine. Washington, D.C.: National Academy Press, 1988.
2. Institute of Medicine, Stoto, M.A., Abel, C., and Dievler, A., Eds. *Healthy Communities: New Partnerships for the Future of Public Health.* Washington, D.C.: National Academy Press, 1996. Available at: http://www.nap.edu/books/030905625X/html/. Accessed May 12, 2005.
3. The Washington State Community Nutrition Assessment Education Project. Available at: http:// depts.washington.edu/commnutr/home/index.htm. Accessed July 14, 2004. [The 12-step approach was developed by Carolyn Gleason, MS, RD, Regional Nutrition Consultant, DHHS/HRSA Seattle Field Office. 206-615-2486, Fax 206-615-2500, cgleason@hrsa.dhhs.gov.]
4. Kretzmann, J.P. and McKnight, J.L. *Building Communities from the Inside Out: A Path Toward Finding and Mobilizing a Community's Assets.* Chicago, IL: ACTA Publications, 1993.
5. Byers, T. Nutrition monitoring and surveillance. In Willett, W., *Nutritional Epidemiology,* 2nd ed. New York: Oxford University Press, 1998, chap. 14.
6. Dodds, J.M. and Melnik, T.A. Development of the New York State Nutrition Surveillance Program. *Public Health Rep.* 106(2), 230–240, 1993.
7. Community Food Security Coalition. Available at: http://www.foodsecurity.org/cfa_home.html. Accessed July 14, 2004.
8. Pothukuchi, K., Joseph, H., Burton, H., and Fisher, A. *What's Cooking in Your Food System? A Guide to Community Food Assessment.* Venice, CA: Community Food Security Coalition, 2002. Available at: http://www.foodsecurity.org/CFAguide-whatscookin.pdf. Accessed October 9, 2005.
9. Community Food Security Coalition. *Community Food Security Programs: What Do They Look Like?* Venice, CA: Community Food Security Coalition, nd. Available at: http://www.foodsecurity. org/CFS_projects.pdf. Accessed May 15, 2005.
10. Pothukuchi, K., Joseph, H., Burton, H., and Fisher, A. *What's Cooking in Your Food System? A Guide to Community Food Assessment.* Venice, CA: Community Food Security Coalition, 2002. Available at: http://www.foodsecurity.org/CFAguide-whatscookin.pdf. Accessed May 11, 2005.
11. Pothukuchi, K. Community food assessment: a first step in planning for community food security. *J Plan. Edn Rsch.* 23, 356–377, 2004.
12. Pothukuchi, K., Joseph, H., Burton, H., and Fisher, A. *What's Cooking in Your Food System? A Guide to Community Food Assessment.* Venice, CA: Community Food Security Coalition, 2002. Available, in part, at: http://www.foodsecurity.org/CFAguide-whatscookin.pdf. Accessed May 11, 2005.

13. *Missoula County Community Food Assessment*, 2004. Available at: http://www.umt.edu/cfa/history.htm. Accessed May 21, 2005.
14. *Our Foodshed in Focus: Missoula County Food and Agriculture by the Numbers.* Available at: www.umt.edu/cfa/indicator.htm. Accessed August 23, 2006.
15. *Grow, Eat, Know: A Resource Guide to Food and Farming in Missoula County.* Available at: http://www.umt.edu/cfa/county.htm. Accessed May 23, 2005.
16. *Food Matters: Farm Viability and Food Consumption in Missoula County.* Available at: http://www.umt.edu/cfa/research.htm. Accessed May 23, 2005.
17. Cohen, B., Andrews, M., and Kantor, L.S. *Community Food Security Assessment Toolkit.* ERS E-FAN No. 02-013, July 2002. Available at: http://agmarketing.extension.psu.edu/Retail/PDFs/CommFd-ScurtyAssesTlKit.pdf. Accessed August 24, 2006.
18. Sacramento Hunger Commission. *Breaking the Barriers: A Road to Improved Food Access.* Available at: http://www.targethunger.com/Community-Food-Security/fdaccess.htm. Accessed May 21, 2005.
19. Sustainable Food Center. *Access Denied,* 1995. East Austin, TX. Available at: http://www.sustainable-foodcenter.org/publications_access_denied.asp. Accessed May 22, 2005.
20. Avondale/Glen Elder Update. Sacramento Hunger Commission. Available at: www.targethunger.org/Community-Food-Security/agonglen_update.htm. Accessed August 23, 2006.
21. Laverack, G. Improving health outcomes through community empowerment: a review of the literature. *J Health Popul Nutr.* 24(1), 113–120, 2006.
22. Clark, M.J., Cary, S., Diemert, G., et al. Involving communities in community assessment. *Pub Health Nurs.* 20(6), 456–463, 2003.
23. Byers, T., Serdula, M., Kuester, S., Mendlein, J., Ballew, C., and McPherson, R.S. Dietary surveillance for states and communities. *Am J Clin Nutr.* 65(4 S), 1210S–1214S, 1997.
24. Bickel, G., Nord, M., Price, C., Hamilton, W., and Cook, J. Measuring Food Security in the United States. *Guide to Measuring Household Food Security Revised 2000.* Alexandria, VA: Food and Nutrition Service, U.S. Department of Agriculture, March 2000.
25. Carlson, S.J., Andrews, M.S., and Bickel, G.W. Measuring food insecurity and hunger in the United States: development of a national benchmark measure and prevalence estimates. *J Nutr.* 129, 510S–516S, 1999.
26. USDA Economic Research Service. *Food Security in the United States: CPS Food Security Supplement.* Available at: http://www.ers.usda.gov/data/FoodSecurity/CPS/. Accessed May 17, 2005.
27. Ricketts, T.C. Geographic information systems and public health. *Annu Rev Public Health.* 24, 1–6, 2003.
28. Boulos, M.N. Towards evidence-based, GIS-driven national spatial health information infrastructure and surveillance services in the United Kingdom. *Int J Health Geogr.* 3(1), 1, January 28, 2004.
29. Welsh, W. Location, location, location. *Washington Technology.* 20, (April 18), 2005. Available at: http://www.washingtontechnology.com/news/20_8/cover-stories/25991-1.html. Accessed May 25, 2005.
30. Koontz, L.D. *Geographic Information Systems. Challenges to Effective Data Sharing.* GAO-03-874T, June 10, 2003. Available at: http://www.gao.gov/new.items/d03874t.pdf. Accessed May 25, 2005.
31. U.S. Department of Health and Human Services. *Healthy People 2010: Understanding and Improving Health,* 2nd ed. Washington, D.C., November 2000. Available at: http://www.healthypeople.gov/document/tableofcontents.htm. Accessed September 1, 2006.
32. A *major* data source is defined as a data system responsible for tracking five or more *Healthy People 2010* objectives. There are 23 data systems that meet these criteria. More than 60% of the objectives are tracked with data from these sources. Included among the data sources that track five or more *Healthy People 2010* objectives are the National Health Interview Survey, National Health and Nutrition Examination Survey, Youth Risk Behavior Surveillance System, and Behavioral Risk Factor Surveillance System.
33. Koontz, L.D. *Geospatial Information. Better Coordination Needed to Identify and Reduce Duplicative Investments.* GAO-04-703, June 2004. Available at: http://www.iwar.org.uk/news-archive/gao/geospatial-info/d04824t.pdf. Accessed May 25, 2005.
34. Faruque, F.S., Lofton, S.P., Doddato, T.M., et al. Utilizing geographic information systems in community assessment and nursing research. *J Comm Health Nurs.* 20(3), 179–191, 2003.
35. California Nutrition Network: GIS map viewer. Available at: http://www.cnngis.org/. Accessed August 25, 2006.

13 Promoting Food Security

> The trouble with being poor is that it takes up all your time.
>
> **William de Kooning (1904–1997)**

At the household level, food security means that all family members have access at all times to enough food for an active, healthy life. Certain groups of Americans are more at risk of material hardship than others. These groups, which include low-income families, children, the elderly, and rural populations, are often the focus of the nation's domestic food and nutrition assistance programs that promote food for an active, healthy life. People living in poverty are at risk of having inadequate resources for food and other necessities. Children account for about 40% of poor people. Although less than 10% of the elderly are poor, poverty rates for older women who live alone are much higher than the average for older people. Programs in the public and private sectors exist to assure the presence of a nutrition safety net to protect individuals and families from malnutrition, hunger, and food insecurity.

13.1 PARSING "FOOD SECURITY"

Over the years "food security" has referred variously to (1) price supports that ensure the continued ability of farmers to produce a food supply adequate to feed the nation, (2) protection of our food supply from both unintentional and intentional contamination (see Chapter 15), and (3) access at all times to enough food for an active, healthy life.

Using the phrase "food security" to describe farm supports has gone out of favor. The 1985 Farm Bill (P.L. 99–198), also known as the *Food Safety Act of 1985*, was the last bill introduced in Congress with "food security" in the title.

Today public health practitioners speak of food security at the household, community, and world levels:

- *Household food security* is defined as access, at all times, to enough food for an active, healthy life for all household members. The U.S. Department of Agriculture (USDA) monitors food security through an annual survey of some 40,000 U.S. households, conducted as a supplement to the U.S. Census Bureau's nationally representative Current Population Survey. As the survey is sent to homes, the USDA is monitoring food security at the household (not individual) level. According to the Economic Research Service (ERS), 89% of American households were food secure throughout the entire year 2004. The remaining households were food insecure at least some time during that year, meaning that these households were uncertain of having (or they were unable to acquire) enough food to meet the basic needs of all their household members because they had insufficient money or other resources. The prevalence of food insecurity rose from 11.2% of households in 2003 to 11.9% in 2004, whereas the prevalence of food insecurity with hunger rose from 3.5 to 3.9%.[1]
- *Community food security* is a relatively new concept with roots in community nutrition, nutrition education, public health, sustainable agriculture, and antihunger and community development (see also Chapter 12). There is no universally accepted definition of community food security. In the broadest terms, it describes a prevention-oriented approach that

supports the development and enhancement of sustainable, community-based strategies to improve access of low-income households to healthful nutritious food supplies, to increase the self-reliance of communities in providing for their own food needs, and to promote comprehensive responses to local food, farm, and nutrition issues.[2] Community food security is also described as a community in which all residents obtain a safe, culturally acceptable, nutritionally adequate diet through a sustainable food system that maximizes self-reliance and social justice,[3] and a sustainable community food system that improves the health of the community, environment, and individuals over time, involving a collaborative effort to build locally based, self-reliant food systems.[4]

- *World food security* describes the universal right of everyone to have access to safe and nutritious food, consistent with the right to adequate food and the fundamental right of everyone to be free from hunger. Signers of the Rome Declaration on World Food Security pledged their common commitment to achieving food security for all and to an ongoing effort to eradicate hunger in all countries, with an immediate view to reducing the number of undernourished people to half their present level no later than 2015.[5]

13.2 POVERTY IN THE U.S.

The source of official poverty estimates is the Current Population Survey, Annual Social and Economic Supplement, a sample survey of approximately 100,000 households nationwide.

Historically, poverty rates have differed, depending on race and Hispanic origin, age, type of household, and residence. For example, blacks and Hispanics have poverty rates that greatly exceed the national average. The poverty rate for all blacks and Hispanics remained near 30% during the

TABLE 13.1
Poverty Among Individuals in the U.S., 2004

Description	Percent	Number (in Millions)
All	12.7	37
Age (in years)		
Under 18	17.8	13
18–64	12.3	20.5
65 and over	9.8	3.5
Race/Ethnicity		
Black	24.3	9
Hispanic origin	21.9	9.1
Asian	9.8	1.21
White, not Hispanic	8.6	16.9
Region		
South	14.1	14.8
West	12.6	8.4
Midwest	11.6	7.5
Northeast	11.6	6.2

Source: From DeNavas–Walt, C., Proctor, B.D., Lee, C.H., U.S. Census Bureau. Current Population Reports, P60-229, *Income, Poverty, and Health Insurance Coverage in the United States: 2004*. Washington, D.C., 2005. Available at: http://www.census. gov/prod/2005pubs/p60-229.pdf. Accessed July 22, 2006.

1980s and mid-1990s, and thereafter began to fall. In 2000, the rate for blacks dropped to 22.1% and for Hispanics to 21.2% — the lowest rate for both groups since the U.S. began measuring poverty in 1959. In contrast, the poverty rate for whites who were not Hispanic has always been below the overall poverty rate. Poverty rates among black and Hispanic children are much higher than among white children and have been so since at least 1977 when the Census Bureau began making separate estimates. In 1979, the average central city poverty rate was 15.7%; at its highest point, in 1993, it was 21.5%.

As indicated in Table 13.1, the official poverty rate in 2004 was 12.7% (up from 12.5% in 2003); 37.0 million people were in poverty (1.1 million more than in 2003). Those who defined themselves as black only or as black and some other race had the highest rates (24.3%), followed by those of Hispanic origin (21.9%), who can be of any race, Asians (9.8%), and whites who were not Hispanic (8.6%). Among children under 18 years of age, 17.8% (13 million) lived in poverty, contrasted with 9.8% of those over 65 years. Of all family groups, poverty is highest among those headed by single women. Poverty rates also depend on where people live. The average poverty rates are greatest in central cities, followed by rural areas, and lowest in the suburbs. The poverty rate is greatest in the South and lowest in the Midwest.

Table 13.2 displays 3-year averages of the poverty rate and the number in poverty for 6 racial and Hispanic origin groups in the U.S., from 2002–2004. To reduce the chances of misinterpreting the poverty rate and the number in poverty, the Census Bureau uses 3-year-average medians for

TABLE 13.2
Poverty Rates and Number in Poverty by Race and Hispanic Origin Using 3-Year Averages, 2002–2004

| Race[a] and Hispanic Origin | 3-Year Average, 2002–2004 | | | |
Description	Percentage (Estimate)	90% Confidence Interval (+ or)[b]	Number in Thousands (Estimate)	90% Confidence Interval (+ or)[b]
All races	12.4	0.2	35,809	489
White	10.5	0.2	24,346	395
White, not Hispanic	8.3	0.2	16,113	326
Black	24.4	0.6	8,794	242
American Indian and Alaska Native	24.3	2.5	554	64
Asian	10.6	0.8	1,257	97
Native Hawaiian and other Pacific Islander	13.2	3.6	92	27
Hispanic origin (any race)	22.1	0.6	8,913	249

[a] Federal surveys give respondents the option of reporting more than one race. Therefore, two basic ways of defining a race group are possible. A group such as Asian may be defined as those who reported Asian and no other race (the race-alone or single-race concept) or as those who reported Asian regardless of whether they also reported another race (the race-alone-or-in-combination concept). Whereas this table shows data using the race-alone approach, note that about 2.6% of people reported more than one race in Census 2000. Information on people who reported more than one race, such as white, American Indian, Alaska Native or Asian, and Black or African American, is available from Census 2000 through American FactFinder.

[b] A 90% confidence interval is a measure of an estimate's variability. The larger the confidence interval in relation to the size of the estimate, the less reliable the estimate.

Source: From DeNavas–Walt, C., Proctor, B.D., Lee, C.H., U.S. Census Bureau. Current Population Reports, P60-229, *Income, Poverty, and Health Insurance Coverage in the United States: 2004.* Table 4. Washington, D.C.: U.S. Government Printing Office, 2005.

presenting data for American Indian, Alaska Natives, Native Hawaiian, and other Pacific Islanders. Because of the relatively small populations of these racial groups, the sampling variability of their data is larger than for other groups and may cause single-year estimates to fluctuate more widely. Using the 3-year averages for poverty rates produced no statistical differences between the rates for blacks (24.4%), American Indians, Alaska Natives (24.3%), and Hispanics (22.1%). There were no statistical differences between the 3-year-average poverty rates for Native Hawaiians and other Pacific Islanders (13.2%) and Asians (10.6%). As expected, the rates for all whites (10.5%) and non-Hispanic whites (8.3%) were lower than for other racial groups.[6]

13.3 NUTRITION AND HEALTH CHARACTERISTICS OF LOW-INCOME POPULATIONS

In 2004, the USDA published the four-volume *Nutrition and Health Outcomes Study*. The study contains analyses of data from National Health and Nutritional Examination Survey or NHANES III (1988–1994), comparing the nutrition and health characteristics of Food Stamp Program (FSP) and Special Supplemental Nutrition Program for Women, Infants, and Children (WIC) participants with their higher-income counterparts and with people who were eligible but did not participate in FSP and WIC. The study also examines low-income school-age children and older Americans, comparing them with their higher-income counterparts.

Specifically, data from NHANES-III (1988–1994) were used to compare the nutrition and health characteristics of FSP participants along with a group of nonparticipants with higher incomes (income above 130% of poverty).[7] This research was designed to establish a baseline from which to monitor over time the nutritional and health characteristics of FSP participants and nonparticipants.

Selected findings from the *Nutrition and Health Outcomes Study* appear in Box 13.1. FSP participants and their higher-income nonparticipant counterparts are compared on the basis of diet quality (based on Healthy Eating Index (HEI) scores), Body Mass Index or BMI, nutritional biochemistries, bone density, infant feeding practices, physical activity, and chronic health conditions. Significant disparities exist between the two groups for all nutrition and health characteristics cited. In essence, the study highlights the health characteristics of low-income people (less than 130% of the poverty level) by comparing them with their counterparts who have more money (more than 130% of the poverty level).

13.4 HUNGER AND FOOD INSECURITY IN THE U.S.

The USDA monitors food security in the nation's households through an annual, nationally representative survey conducted by the Census Bureau. Information about households' food expenditures is also collected.

The physiological phenomenon of hunger is defined as an uneasy or painful sensation caused by not having access to enough food.[8] In 2002 and 2003, one or more family members in an estimated 3.5% of American households did not have enough food to eat at least some time during the year.[9] Unlike the situation in some developing nations where famine is widespread among young children, and hunger manifests itself as *kwashiorkor* and *marasmus*, hunger generally manifests itself in a less severe form in the U.S. This is in part because the USDA food assistance programs help to provide a food safety net for many low-income individuals and families. Whereas starvation seldom occurs in the U.S., children and adults do go hungry and chronic mild undernutrition occurs when financial resources are low.

Food insecurity describes widespread but less severe hunger problems. Food insecurity means that a household had limited or uncertain availability of food, or limited or uncertain ability to acquire foods in socially acceptable ways (in other words, without resorting to emergency food

Box 13.1 Nutrition and Health Characteristics of FSP Participants: Selected Findings From the Nutrition and Health Outcomes Study

Healthy Eating Index Scores
- FSP participants were more likely than higher-income nonparticipants to consume poor diets (24% vs. 15%) and less likely to consume good diets (6% vs. 12%).

Dietary Intake
- FSP participants consumed more food energy than income-eligible nonparticipants (95% of the 1989 Recommended Energy Allowance vs. 91%).
- FSP participants were less likely than higher-income nonparticipants to consume adequate amounts of iron (91% vs. 95%), zinc (80% vs. 88%), and calcium (73% vs. 83%).

Body Weight
- Adult and teenage female FSP participants had significantly greater BMIs than high-income nonparticipants (28.3% vs. 26.4% and 19.8% vs. 19.2%, respectively). Women FSP participants were less likely to be at a healthy weight (28% vs. 49%) and more likely to be obese (42% vs. 22%) than higher-income nonparticipants.

Bone Density
- FSP participants over 80 years were almost twice as likely to have severely reduced bone density than higher-income nonparticipants (42% vs. 24%).

Nutritional Biochemistries
- Female FSP participants were more likely than higher-income nonparticipants to be iron deficient (14% vs. 6% for 20- to 29-year-olds and 20% vs. 9% for 30- to 39-year-olds).
- FSP participants were less likely than higher-income nonparticipants to have low red blood cell (RBC) folate levels (11% vs. 6%).
- Overall, the prevalence of anemia among FSP participants was double that of higher-income nonparticipants (4% vs. 2%).

Infant Feeding Practices
- FSP participants were less likely than higher-income nonparticipants to have breastfed their infants (45% vs. 63%). Among those who breastfed, fewer FSP participants breastfed for at least 6 months (36% vs. 44%). More FSP participants than higher-income nonparticipants started their infants on solid food earlier than 4 months (20% vs. 24%).

Physical Activity
- In comparison with higher-income nonparticipating children, FSP children were less likely to: engage in vigorous physical activity (mean times per week: 4.4% vs. 4.8%), engage in physical activity at least 3 times per week (74% vs. 81%), and be involved in team sports or other organized exercise programs (50% vs. 68%).
- Fewer FSP children than higher-income nonparticipating children 5–16 years of age limited television watching to no more than 2 h/d (55% vs. 68%).
- Fewer FSP adults than higher-income nonparticipating adults were physically active 3 or more times per week (37% vs. 60%) or 5 or more times per week (28% vs. 46%).

Chronic Health Conditions
- FSP participants were more likely than higher-income nonparticipants to report having diabetes (10% vs. 5%), having had a heart attack (5% vs. 3%) or a stroke (4% vs. 2%), and to actually have high blood pressure, based on physician assessment (23% vs. 18%).

Source: Lin, B.-H., Frazao, E., Ralston, K. *Nutrition and Health Characteristics of Low-Income Populations.* Agriculture Information Bulletin No. (AIB796), February 2005. Available at: http://www.ers.usda.gov/Publications/AIB796/. Accessed July 4, 2005.

supplies, scavenging, stealing, or other unusual coping strategies). Through 2006 the USDA recognized two levels of food insecurity (see Box 13.2):

- *Food insecurity without hunger.* At a minimum, food-insecure households worry that they cannot afford to eat balanced meals. The ultimate concern is whether their food will run out and they won't have enough money for more.
- *Food insecurity with hunger.* In addition to being food insecure, adults in the households that are food insecure with hunger ate less than they felt they should and cut the size of meals or skipped meals in three or more months during the year.

State prevalence rates for food insecurity and hunger appear in Table 13.3. Based on these data, 88.6% of American households were food secure in 2002–2004, with 11.6% food insecure without hunger, and 3.6% food insecure with hunger. From 1996 to 2004, food insecurity increased the most — by 3.0 to 4.5% points — in Utah (4.5), South Carolina (3.5), Rhode Island (3.4), Idaho (3.3), Mississippi (3.2), and Alaska (3.0). In 2002–2004, the rates of food insecurity were the highest — 14.6 to 16.4% of the population — in Texas (16.4), Mississippi and New Mexico (15.8), Oklahoma (15.2), Arizona, South Carolina, and Utah (14.8), and Idaho (14.6).

The prevalence of food insecurity follows a discernible geographic pattern; states with the highest rates border the Pacific Ocean, Mexico, and the Gulf of Mexico. During 2002 to 2004, 4.2 to 5.6% of the population in 14 states experienced food insecurity with hunger. The rates were highest in Oklahoma (5.6), South Carolina (5.5), and Arizona (5.3). Young children in U.S. households do not

---

Box 13.2   Low and Very Low Food Security

Prior to 2006, reports on food security used the following general classifications: *food secure, food insecure without hunger,* and *food insecure with hunger.* Households with low food security were described as "food insecure without hunger" and households with very low food security were described as "food insecure with hunger." However, in 2006, the National Research Council's Committee on National Statistics (CNSTAT) recommended that USDA make a clear and explicit distinction between *food insecurity* and *hunger.*

CNSTAT stated in its final report that food insecurity is a household-level economic and social condition of limited or uncertain access to adequate food. Hunger, on the other hand, is an individual level physiological condition that may result from food insecurity. The word "hunger" refers to a potential consequence of food insecurity that, because of prolonged, involuntary lack of food, results in discomfort, illness, weakness, or pain that goes beyond the usual uneasy sensation. CNSTAT advised that the food security survey does not measure hunger, which would require collecting detailed and extensive information on physiological experiences of individual household members.

In response to CSTAT's recommendations, therefore, USDA introduced new language to describe ranges of severity of food insecurity, as depicted in the chart below. The labels "food insecurity without hunger" and "food insecurity with hunger" were replaced by *low food security* and *very low food security,* respectively. The defining characteristic of very low food security is that, at times during the year, the food intake of household members was reduced and their normal eating patterns were disrupted because the household lacked money and other resources for food. (Because the criteria used to classify households did not change, statistics reported since 2006 are directly comparable with those for earlier years for the corresponding categories.)

General categories (old and new labels are the same)	Detailed Categories		
	Old Label	New Label	Description of conditions in the household
Food Security	Food security	High food security	No reported indications of food-access problems or limitations
		Marginal food security	1 or 2 reported indications—typically of anxiety over food sufficiency or shortage of food in the house. Little or no indication of changes in diets or food intake.
Food Insecurity	Food insecurity *without hunger*	Low food security	Reports of reduced quality, variety, or desirability of diet. Little or no indication of reduced food intake.
	Food insecurity with hunger	Very low food security	Reports of multiple indications of disrupted eating patterns reduced food intake.

Sources:

Panel to Review U.S. Department of Agriculture's Measurement of Food Insecurity and Hunger, National Research Council. Wunderlich, G.S. and Norwood, J.L., *Eds., Food Insecurity and Hunger in the United States: An Assessment of the Measure.* Washington, D.C.: The National Academies Press, 2006. Washington, D.C. Available at: http://books.nap.edu/catalog/11578.html#toc. Accessed February 16, 2007.

Nord, M., Andrews, M., and Carlson, S. *Household Food Security in the United States, 2005.* U.S. Department of Agriculture. Economic Research Report No. (ERR-29), November 2006. Available at: http://www.ers.usda.gov/Publications/ERR29/ERR29.pdf. Accessed February 16, 2007.

---

usually experience hunger unless hunger among adults reaches severe levels. Nevertheless, about 0.5 to 0.7% of households with children reported hunger among children at some time during 2004. The mental and physical changes that accompany inadequate food intake can have harmful effects on a child's learning, physical and psychological health, and overall quality of life.[10,11,12]

13.4.1 FOOD-INSECURE HOUSEHOLDS SPEND LESS FOR FOOD THAN FOOD-SECURE HOUSEHOLDS

An indicator of how adequately households meet their food needs is the amount of money spent on food. In 2004, the median U.S. household spent $40 per person for food each week, about 25% higher than the cost of the USDA's Thrifty Food Plan, a low-cost food "market basket" that meets dietary standards, taking into account household size and the age and sex of household members. The name *Thrifty Food Plan* refers to the diet required to feed a family of 4 persons (a man and a woman aged 20–50, a child aged 6–8, and a child aged 9–11). The typical food-insecure household spent 2% less than suggested by the Thrifty Food Plan, whereas the typical food-secure household spent 28% more than the cost of the plan (or almost one-third more than the typical food-insecure household).[13]

TABLE 13.3

Average Prevalence Rates of Food Insecurity and Food Insecurity with Hunger by State, 1996–1998, 1999–2001, and 2002–2004

Prevalence of Food Security, Food Insecurity, and Food Insecurity with Hunger, by Year

| Unit | Total[a] | Food Secure | | Food Insecure | | | | | |
| | | | | All | | Without Hunger | | With Hunger | |
	1,000	1,000	Percent	1,000	Percent	1,000	Percent	1,000	Percent
Households:									
1998	103,309	91,121	88.2	12,188	11.8	8,353	8.1	3,835	3.7
1999	104,684	94,154	89.9	10,529	10.1	7,420	7.1	3,109	3.0
2000	106,043	94,942	89.5	11,101	10.5	7,786	7.3	3,315	3.1
2001	107,824	96,303	89.3	11,521	10.7	8,010	7.4	3,511	3.3
2002	108,601	96,543	89.9	12,058	11.1	8,259	7.6	3,799	3.5
2003	112,214	99,631	89.8	12,583	11.2	8,663	7.7	3,920	3.5
2004	112,967	99,473	88.1	13,494	11.9	9,045	8.0	4,449	3.9
All individual (by food security status of household):[b]									
1998	268,366	232,219	85.5	36,147	13.5	26,290	9.8	9,857	3.7
1999	270,318	239,304	88.5	31,015	11.5	23,237	8.6	7,779	2.9
2000	273,685	240,454	87.9	33,231	12.1	24,708	9.0	8,523	3.1
2001	276,661	243,019	87.8	33,642	12.2	24,628	8.9	9,014	3.3
2002	279,035	244,133	87.5	34,902	12.5	25,517	9.1	9,385	3.4
2003	286,410	250,155	87.3	36,255	12.7	26,622	9.3	9,633	3.4
2004	288,603	250,407	86.8	38,196	13.2	27,535	9.5	10,661	3.7
Adults (by food security status of household):[b]									
1998	197,084	174,964	89.8	22,120	11.2	15,632	7.9	6,488	3.8
1999	198,900	179,960	90.5	18,941	9.5	13,869	7.0	5,072	2.5
2000	201,922	181,586	89.9	20,336	10.1	14,763	7.3	5,573	2.8
2001	204,340	183,398	89.8	20,942	10.2	14,879	7.3	6,063	3.0
2002	206,493	184,718	89.5	21,775	10.5	15,486	7.5	6,289	3.0
2003	213,441	190,451	89.2	22,990	10.8	16,358	7.7	6,682	3.1
2004	215,564	191,236	88.7	24,328	11.3	16,946	7.9	7,382	3.4

(continued)

TABLE 13.3 (Continued)
Average Prevalence Rates of Food Insecurity and Food Insecurity with Hunger by State, 1996–1998, 1999–2001, and 2002–2004

Prevalence of Food Security, Food Insecurity, and Food Insecurity with Hunger, by Year

Unit	Total[a]	Food Secure		Food Insecure					
				All		Without Hunger		With Hunger	
	1,000	1,000	Percent	1,000	Percent	1,000	Percent	1,000	Percent
Households with children:									
1998	38,036	31,335	82.4	6,701	17.6	6,370	16.7	331	0.9
1999	37,884	32,290	85.2	5,594	14.8	5,375	14.2	219	0.6
2000	38,113	31,942	83.8	6,171	16.2	5,916	15.5	255	0.7
2001	38,330	32,141	83.9	6,189	16.1	5,978	15.6	211	0.6
2002	38,647	32,267	83.5	6,380	16.5	6,115	15.8	265	0.7
2003	40,286	33,575	83.3	6,711	16.7	6,504	16.1	207	0.5
2004	39,990	32,967	82.4	7,023	17.6	6,749	16.9	274	0.7
Children (by food security status of household):[b]									
1998	71,282	57,255	80.3	14,027	19.7	13,311	18.7	716	1.0
1999	71,418	59,344	83.1	12,074	16.9	11,563	16.2	511	0.7
2000	71,763	58,867	82.0	12,896	18.0	12,334	17.2	562	0.8
2001	72,321	59,620	82.4	12,701	17.6	12,234	16.9	467	0.6
2002	72,542	59,415	81.9	13,127	18.1	12,560	17.3	567	0.8
2003	72,969	59,704	81.8	13,265	18.2	12,845	17.6	420	0.6
2004	73,039	59,171	81.0	13,868	19.0	13,328	18.2	545	0.7

[a] Totals exclude households whose food security status is unknown because they did not give a valid response to any of the questions in the food security scale. In 2003, these represented 404,000 households (0.4 percent of all households.)

[b] The food security survey measures food security status at the household level. Not all individuals residing in food-insecure households are appropriately characterized as food insecure. Similarly, not all individuals in households classified as food insecure with hunger, nor all children in households classified as food insecure with hunger among children, were subject to reductions in food in take or experienced resource-constrained hunger.

Source: Calculated by ERS using data from the August 1998, April 1999, September 2000, December 2001, December 2002, December 2003, and December 2004 Current Population Survey Food Security Supplements.

Nord, M., Andrews, M., Carlson, S. *Household Food Security in the United States, 2004.* U.S. Department of Agriculture, Economic Research Service Food Assistance and Nutrition Research Report Number 11. 2005. Available at: http://www.ers.usda.gov/publications/err11/err11.pdf. Accessed July 23, 2006.

13.5 NUTRITION ASSISTANCE PROGRAMS

Federal nutrition assistance programs increase food security and reduce hunger by providing children and low-income people access to food, a healthful diet, and nutrition education. The majority of the government's food assistance programs are administered by the Food and Nutrition Service (FNS) within the USDA. There exists 15 such programs, including FSP, WIC, and the child nutrition programs. In addition to tax-supported efforts to help feed low-income people, the private sector also plays a part in reducing hunger in the U.S.

The proposed budget for FY 2007, which began in October 1, 2006, includes almost $56.8 billion for programs aimed at promoting food security and preventing hunger, allocated as follows:

- $37.912 billion for the FSP
- $13.67 billion for child nutrition programs, including the National School Lunch Program (NSLP), School Breakfast Program (SBP), Summer Food Service, Special Milk, and Child and Adult Care Food Programs (CACFP)
- $5.2 billion for WIC[14]

13.5.1 FEDERAL FOOD AND NUTRITION PROGRAMS

The USDA was created by congressional acts in 1862 and 1889, and made an executive department in the federal government under the supervision and control of the Secretary of Agriculture (7 U.S.C. 2201, 2202, 2204).[15] The department has the vast majority of responsibility for providing food assistance programs in the U.S. In addition to the USDA, at least three other cabinet-level departments are charged with the responsibility for administering food assistance programs in the U.S. They are:

- The Department of Health and Human Services (HHS) administers Head Start, which provides meals and snacks to infants and preschool-age children. HHS is also home to the Administration on Aging (AoA), which administers the Nutrition Services Incentive Program (NSIP), the food assistance program for the elderly, although it receives commodity foods and financial support from the USDA's FNS.
- The Department of Defense (DoD) and USDA maintain a partnership that takes advantage of the Defense Department's large-scale buying power to provide fresh fruit and vegetables to the NSLP.
- The Department of Homeland Security (DHS) and USDA work together as part of the efforts to protect America's food supply.

All federal departments are required to prepare five-year strategic plans that identify their key goals and objectives, their strategies for attaining them, and measures of progress. One of the USDA's five strategic goals is to improve the nation's nutrition and health by improving access to nutritious food.[16,17] By 2007, the USDA aims to reduce to 7.4% the number of low-income households that report hunger, increase to 68% the eligible people who participate in the FSP, and increase to 55% the proportion of children enrolled in public and private schools who receive school lunches.[18]*

As indicated in the USDA's organization chart in Figure 13.1, the department maintains seven offices, each administered by its own Under Secretary. FNS is one of the two agencies in the office of Food, Nutrition, and Consumer Services (FNCS).[19] It has the responsibility for administering the USDA's programs. The other agency within FNCS is the Center for Nutrition Policy and Promotion (CNPP), created in 1994 as the focal point within the USDA where scientific research is linked with the nutritional needs of the public.

---

* The USDA's remaining four goals are (1) to enhance economic opportunities for agricultural producers, (2) support increased economic opportunities and improved quality of life in rural America, (3) enhance protection and safety of the nation's agriculture and food supply, and (4) protect and enhance the country's natural resource base and environment.

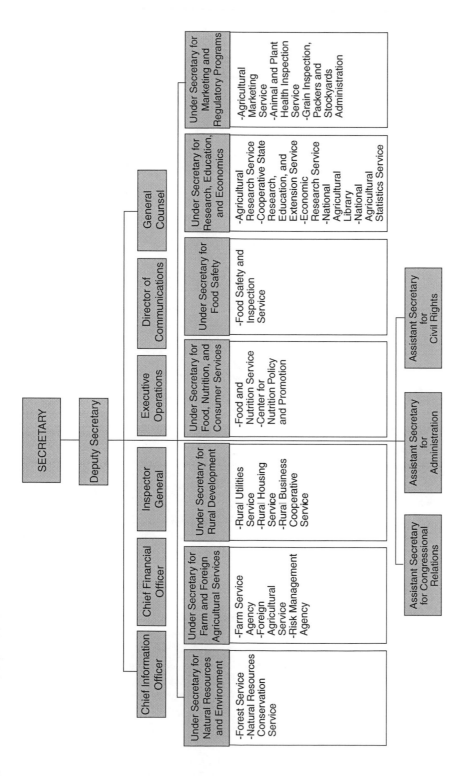

FIGURE 13.1 USDA organization chart. (From United States Department of Agriculture. Department of Agriculture Organization Chart. Available at: http://www.usda.gov/img/content/org_chart_enlarged.jpg. Accessed September 2, 2006.)

13.5.1.1 Food and Nutrition Service (FNS)

FNS has its own strategic plan to support the USDA's goals.[20] It is committed to improving the nutrition and health of low-income Americans and to assisting in meeting the Healthy People 2010 nutrition and related objectives for the nation. This commitment is reflected in the FNS vision — to lead America in ending hunger and improving nutrition and health. FNS's mission is to increase food security and reduce hunger in partnership with cooperating organizations by providing children and low-income people access to food, a healthful diet, and nutrition education in a manner that supports American agriculture and inspires public confidence (see Chapter 9). To that end, FNS administers 15 nutrition assistance programs. These programs touch the lives of one in six Americans each year, with the potential to make an important difference in the lives of children and low-income populations by promoting food security, reducing hunger, and improving nutritional status. Expenditures for the 15 food assistance programs totaled $46 billion in fiscal year (FY) 2004 (October 1, 2003 to September 30, 2004). These programs account for about two-thirds of the USDA's annual budget. Five of the programs alone accounted for 94% of the USDA's total expenditures for food assistance:[21]

- FSP
- NSLP
- WIC
- SBP
- CACFP

For ease of reference, federal food assistance programs with unifying characteristics may be grouped together. There are three broad categories. *Child nutrition programs* encompass the Special Milk Program (SMP) and Summer Food Service Program (SFSP) in addition to the NSLP, SBP, and CACFP. Similarly, the *food distribution programs* include schools/child nutrition commodity programs, the Food Distribution Program on Indian Reservations (FDPIR), the Nutrition Services Incentive Program (NSIP), the Commodity Supplemental Food program (CSFP), and the Emergency Food Assistance Program (TEFAP). *Disaster relief* falls into its own category.[22] Table 13.4 summarizes the major programs.

13.5.1.1.1 Food Stamp Program (FSP)

As the cornerstone of the USDA's nutrition assistance programs, FSP plays a vital role in helping to improve nutrition among low-income individuals. The program provides support to needy households and to those making the transition from welfare to work. It serves as the first line of defense against hunger and enables low-income families to buy nutritious food with Electronic Benefits Transfer (EBT) cards. The program operates in 50 states, the District of Columbia, Guam, and the U.S. Virgin Islands. The federal government oversees the state operation of FSP through state and local welfare offices. In 2005, over 25.5 million individuals in over 11 million households participated in the program.

FSP is an entitlement program; all those who qualify for benefits should receive them. The program provides a monthly benefit amount to eligible low-income families that can be used to purchase food. Eligibility for FSP is based on household income and assets. Many able-bodied, childless, unemployed adults have time limits on their receipt of FSP benefits.

The program traces its origins to the Food Stamp Plan, which began in 1939 to help needy families during the Great Depression (see Box 13.3). The modern program was started as a pilot project in 1961 and authorized as a permanent program in 1964. Expansion of the program occurred most dramatically after 1974, when Congress required all states to offer food stamps to low-income households. The current FSP was enacted in 1977. It is amended regularly, most recently in 2005 through P.L. 108–269.[23] The 1977 Act made significant changes in program regulations, tightening eligibility requirements and administration, and removing the requirement that food stamps be purchased by participants.

The nation's welfare system, including eligibility for food stamps, was radically transformed by P.L. 104–193, the 1996 Personal Responsibility and Work Opportunity Reconciliation Act

TABLE 13.4
Annual Summary of Food and Nutrition Service Programs, FY 2001–2005

	FY 2001	FY 2002	FY 2003	FY 2004	FY 2005
Food Stamp Program[a]					
People participating (thousands)	17,318	19,096	21,259	23,858	25,673
Households participating (thousands)	7,449	8,195	9,154	10,279	11,181
Value of benefits ($ millions)	15,547	18,256	21,404	24,622	28,567
Average monthly benefit per person ($)	74.81	79.67	83.90	86.00	92.73
Average monthly benefit per household ($)	173.93	185.65	194.86	199.62	212.91
Total cost ($ millions)	17,789	20,643	23,821	27,139	31,128
Puerto Rico Grant ($ millions)[b]	**1,296**	**1,351**	**1,395**	**1,413**	**1,495**
National School Lunch Program[c]					
Children participating (thousands)	27,514	28,002	28,392	28,966	29,644
Total lunches Served (millions)	4,585	4,717	4,763	4,842	4,975
Percent free (%)	47.6	48.3	49.0	49.5	49.8
Percent reduced-price (%)	9.3	9.4	9.5	9.6	9.6
Total after-school snacks served (millions)	104	123	139	151	164
Cash payments ($ millions)	5,612	6,050	6,341	6,663	7,054
Commodity costs ($ millions)	863	803	849	963	975
Total cost ($ millions)	6,475	6,853	7,189	7,626	8,028
School Breakfast Program[d]					
Children participating (thousands)	7,794	8,147	8,430	8,905	9,369
Total breakfasts served (millions)	1,335	1,405	1,448	1,525	1,603
Percent free or reduced price (%)	83.2	82.9	82.8	82.4	82.1
Total cost ($ millions)	1,450	1,567	1,652	1,775	1,927
Special Milk Program[e]					
Total half-pints served (millions)	116	113	108	103	100
Total cost ($ millions)	16	16	14	14	17
Child/Adult Care Feeding Program[f]					
Average daily attendance (thousands)	2,726	2,850	2,917	3,010	3,107
Total meals served (millions)	1,680	1,736	1,765	1,800	1,834
Child care centers (millions)	923	984	1,023	1,059	1,106
Day care homes (millions)	717	708	693	687	671
Adult care centers (millions)	40	45	49	54	58
Percent free or reduced price (%)	83.5	83.3	83.2	82.9	82.3
Cash payments ($ millions)	1,548	1,657	1,726	1,812	1,905
Commodity costs ($ millions)	52	57	59	65	71
Total costs ($ millions)	1,737	1,853	1,926	2,019	2,113
Summer Food Service Program[g]					
Average daily attendance (thousands)	2,090	1,923	2,070	1,997	1,956
Total meals served (millions)	131	122	117	117	116
Total cost (millions)	270	263	257	263	267
Child Nutrition State Administration ($ millions)[h]	121	128	130	137	139
WIC (Special Supplemental Food)[i]					
Women, infants, and children participating (thousands)	7,306	7,491	7,631	7,904	8,023
Food cost ($ millions)	3,008	3,130	3,230	3,562	3,603
Average monthly food cost per person ($)	34.31	34.82	35.28	37.55	37.42
Total cost ($ millions)	4,151	4,342	4,526	4,890	4,996
Commodity Supplemental Food Program[j]					
Total participation (thousands)	407	427	456	522	512
Total cost ($ millions)	106	115	122	146	150

(Continued)

TABLE 13.4 (Continued)
Annual Summary of Food and Nutrition Service Programs, FY 2001–2005

	FY 2001	FY 2002	FY 2003	FY 2004	FY 2005
Food Distribution on Indian Reservations					
Total participation (thousands)	113	110	108	104	99
Total cost ($ millions)	72	76	75	77	76
NSIP (Elderly Feeding)					
Total meals served (millions)	253	NA	NA	NA	NA
Total cost ($ millions)	152	150	3	4	4
The Emergency Food Assistance Program					
Total pounds distributed (millions)	549	611	522	533	491
Total food cost ($ millions)	332	380	396	361	314
Total cost ($ millions)	377	435	456	420	372
Other Food Distribution Programs					
Disaster feeding ($ millions)[k]	0.5	0.1	0.4	2.0	7.7
Charitable institutes ($ millions)[l]	7	16	6	10	4

Note: Data as of June 22, 2006.

[a] Participation data are 12-month averages. Total cost includes benefits, the federal share of state administrative expenses, and other federal costs (e.g., printing and processing stamps).

[b] Puerto Rico's Nutrition Assistance Grant provides benefits analogous to the FSP. Smaller outlying areas with similar grants include American Samoa ($5.6 million in FY 2005) and the Northern Marianas ($8.4 million).

[c] NSLP and SBP participation data are 9-month averages (summer months are excluded). They represent average daily meals served adjusted by an attendance factor. School lunch costs include cash payments, entitlement commodities, bonus commodities (surplus foods donated by USDA), and cash-in-lieu of commodities. School breakfast costs are cash payments. Cash payments are federal reimbursements to state agencies based on meals served multiplied by reimbursement rates, which are adjusted annually to reflect changes in food costs. Free and reduced-price meals served to needy children are reimbursed at much higher rates than full-price meals.

[d] NSLP and SBP participation data are 9-month averages (summer months are excluded). They represent average daily meals served adjusted by an attendance factor. School lunch costs include cash payments, entitlement commodities, bonus commodities (surplus foods donated by USDA), and cash-in-lieu of commodities. School breakfast costs are cash payments. Cash payments are federal reimbursements to state agencies based on meals served multiplied by reimbursement rates, which are adjusted annually to reflect changes in food costs. Free and reduced-price meals served to needy children are reimbursed at much higher rates than full-price meals.

[e] Special milk costs are cash payments based on an annually determined reimbursement rate and the actual cost of free milk (a small portion of the total — less than 7% for all years).

[f] Total costs include: cash payments, entitlement and bonus commodities, cash-in-lieu of commodities, sponsor administrative costs, start-up costs, and audits.

[g] Average daily attendance is reported only for July, the peak month of activity. Costs include cash payments, entitlement and bonus commodities, and the federal share of state and sponsor administrative costs. The decline in meals served since FY 2001 is largely attributable to alternative summer meal service in the NSLP and SBP under Seamless Waiver provisions, which eased reporting requirements for sponsors.

[h] The federal share of state administrative costs for the NSLP, SBP, and CAFCP.

[i] Total costs include food benefits, nutrition services and administrative funds, the FMNP, infrastructure, program evaluation, and technical assistance.

[j] Includes commodity distribution costs (entitlement and bonus), the federal share of state administrative expenses, and other costs (such as storage and transportation, food losses and demo. projects — national level only, unavailable prior to FY 1996).

[k] Most disaster relief is provided through FSP.

[l] Includes summer camps.

Box 13.3 URL for Historical Summary

Short historical summaries of the FSP are available on the FSP Web site and in the *Social Security Bulletin* (December 2002) at http://www.findarticles.com/p/articles/mi_m6524/is_2002_Dec/ai_101010917.

(PRWORA). Appropriately, however, many FSP eligibility restrictions were lifted in 2002 with enactment of P.L. 107–171, the Farm Security and Rural Investment Act (FSRIA) informally known as the Farm Bill, which includes, as Title IV, the Food Stamp Reauthorization Act. By means of a number of program enhancements and simplifications, the Farm Bill added $6.4 billion in new funds to the FSP and other nutrition programs through FY 2012. Under this Act, states were provided with options to adopt for improving the accessibility and maintenance of food stamp benefits. The law also gives states new flexibility to improve the FSP for their low-income residents.

Participation generally peaks in periods of high unemployment, inflation, and recession. In 1994, participation reached an all-time high of almost 28 million before declining to about 17.2 million in 2000. By 2004, participation had increased to approximately 23.9 million (see Table 13.5). Currently, approximately 50% of the beneficiaries are children, 40% are adults, and 10% elderly persons (60 years and older).

13.5.1.1.1.1 Eligibility and Benefits

To be eligible to receive FSP benefits, a household must meet certain standards regarding income and resources, work, and citizenship status. The amount of benefits an eligible household receives, called an *allotment*, depends on the age and number of people in the household and on the net monthly household income. Unless someone in the household is over 60 or receiving disability checks, a household may receive food stamps if the gross income (before deductions) is 130% or less of the federal poverty level. To calculate a household's allotment, the household's net monthly income is multiplied by 0.3 (because food stamp households are expected to spend about 30% of their resources on food), and the result is subtracted from the maximum allotment for the household size. Box 13.4 lists the maximum allotments. For example, a household of 3 people with no income can receive up to $393 per month in benefits. The income limits, maximum benefits, and calculation of benefits as well as current standards for eligibility to participate in the program are explained in detail on the FSP Web site at: www.fns.usda.gov/fsp/.

TABLE 13.5
Food Stamp Program Annual Summary, 2002–2005

Fiscal Year	Participation		Benefits Costs (Billions)	Average Monthly Benefit	
	Persons (Millions)	Households (Millions)		Per Person	Per Household
2005	25.7	11.2	$25.567	$92.73	$212.91
2004	23.9	10.3	$24.628	$86.02	$199.67
2003	21.3	9.2	$21.404	$83.90	$194.86
2002	19.1	8.2	$18.256	$79.67	$185.66

Source: From USDA. Food Stamp Program Annual State Level Data, Average Monthly Benefit per Household, and Participation and Costs. Food and Nutrition Service. Available at: http://www.fns.usda.gov/pd/fsmonthly.htm, http://www.fns.usda.gov/pd/fsfybft.htm, http:// www.fns.usda.gov/pd/fssummar.htm. Accessed July 23, 2006.

Box 13.4 Calculating the Maximum Monthly Food Stamp Allotment

The amount of benefits the household receives is known as an allotment. There are two steps for calculating the benefits for a household. First, the net monthly income of the household is multiplied by 0.3 (because food stamp households are expected to spend about 30% of their resources on food). Next, the result is subtracted from the maximum allotment for the household size, according to the following table. For the most recent maximum monthly allotments, go to the Food Stamp fact sheet on resources, income, and benefits at: http://www.fns.usda.gov/fsp/applicant_recipients/fs_Res_Ben_Elig.htm.

People in Household	Maximum Monthly Allotment in 2005
1	$152
2	$278
3	$399
4	$506
5	$601
6	$722
7	$798
8	$912
Each additional person	$114

Source: From USDA Food and Nutrition Service. Food Stamp Program. Fact Sheet on Resources, Income, and Benefits. Available at: http://www.fns.usda.gov/fsp/applicant_recipients/fs_Res_Ben_Elig.htm. Accessed July 23, 2006.

In 2003, the average monthly benefits ranged from a low of $65.57 in Wisconsin to a high of $180.06 in Guam. In addition to Guam, the states and territories with the highest average monthly Food Stamp benefits in 2003 were Hawaii ($129.66), the Virgin Islands ($119.12), Alaska ($108.06), and New York ($97.29).[24] The states and territories with the highest average monthly benefit per household were Guam ($627.42), the Virgin Islands ($350.74), Alaska ($307.77), Louisiana ($228.07), and California ($227.54).[25]

13.5.1.1.1.2 Electronic Benefits Transfer (EBT)
Food stamps and food coupons are no longer issued in paper form, rather food stamp benefits are issued electronically. Benefits are deposited through an electronic accounting system known as *Electronic Benefits Transfer* or *EBT*. Each recipient household receives a plastic EBT card, similar to a bank debit card, which allows withdrawals for food purchases at grocery stores and supermarkets. Funds are transferred from a food stamp benefits account to the retailer's account. No paper coupons change hands.

Each month the household's allotment is added to their EBT card; when benefits are posted, they are immediately available. The recipient can only spend the amount in the account. Households

Box 13.5 Sec. 124 of P.L. 108–265

Sec. 124 of Public Law 108–265, the Child Nutrition and WIC Reauthorization Act of 2004, calls for the implementation and evaluation of a demonstration expansion program in which the income eligibility limit for free school lunches and breakfasts is raised to 185% of the federal poverty income guidelines. This demonstration project is to be carried out in all or part of 5 states, including one largely rural state with a significant Native American population. Activity: *Conduct an Internet search to determine the result of this project.*

Box 13.6 Team Nutrition

Team Nutrition develops messages and materials that can be used consistently throughout the country. It promotes support and training at the state and local levels through infrastructure developed by the NET as well as new Team Nutrition partnerships. The program uses six communication channels (food service initiatives, classroom activities, schoolwide events, home activities, community programs and events, and media events and coverage) to offer a comprehensive network for delivering consistent nutrition messages to children and their caretakers. Team Nutrition is implemented through three behavior-oriented strategies by providing (1) training and technical assistance for food service professionals to help them serve meals that look good, taste good, and meet nutrition standards, (2) multifaceted, integrated nutrition education for children and their parents. This education will build skills and motivation for children to make healthy food and physical activity choices as part of a healthy lifestyle, and (3) support for healthy eating and physical activity by involving school administrators and other school and community partners.

Source: USDA. Evaluation of the School Breakfast Program Pilot Project: Final Report. Report No. CN-04-SBP. Food and Nutrition Service, Office of Analysis, Nutrition and Evaluation. 2004. Available at: http://www.fns.usda. gov/oane/MENU/Published/CNP/FILES/SBPPFinal.pdf. Accessed July 24, 2006.

---

can use their food stamp benefits to buy most foods, and also seeds and plants that produce food for the household members to eat. Excluded items include alcoholic beverages, tobacco, pet foods, soap or paper products, vitamin-mineral supplements, medicines, and hot foods and foods that will be eaten in the store. In some areas, restaurants can be authorized to accept food stamp benefits from qualified homeless, elderly, or disabled people in exchange for low-cost meals.

13.5.1.1.1.3 Food Stamp Quality Control
The EBT has been one of the most promising developments in the fight against food stamp fraud because EBT creates an electronic record of each transaction, making fraud easier to detect. The USDA provides bonus awards to states whose compliance rate exceeds the national average; conversely, states with error rates greatly exceeding the national average pay cash sanctions. Effective management of FSP helps ensure that those families and individuals most in need of nutrition assistance receive it, and the funds intended for this purpose are not diminished by waste or program abuse. To this end, the USDA monitors and works with all states to improve performance and by assuring that the FSP quality control systems remain strong.[26]

A goal of the USDA is to improve food program management and customer service by increasing the Food Stamp payment accuracy rate from 91.3% in 2001 to 94.2% in 2007 and to provide services electronically to increase efficiency, ease-of-use, and benefit delivery within the program.[27] The cost of overpayments, though small as a percentage of all payments (5.04%), amounted to $1.1 billion in 2003. Similarly, the cost of underpayments — the value of benefits that should have been paid to eligible participants but were not — is small as a percentage of payments (1.59%), although still substantial ($340 million). In 2003, the net cost to the government of erroneous payments — the cost of overpayments less the cost of underpayments — was over $700 million.

Virtually all households receiving food stamps are eligible for some benefit. The average overpayment issued to an eligible household was $97, or 37% of the issued benefit. The average underpayment ($78) was about 40% of the average payment. Overpayment errors had little effect on overall household purchasing power. On the other hand, overpayments to ineligible households were larger than to eligible households, averaging $150 in 2003.[28] However, the cost of overpayments is miniscule compared with the money lost to the states for people who are eligible for the FSP but are not enrolled. Of the 37 million individuals who were eligible for food stamp benefits in an average month of 2003, 21 million individuals (56%) chose to participate. In 2003, over 16 million FSP eligible individuals did not participate.[29]

13.5.1.1.1.4 Participation

An important measure of a program's performance is its ability to reach its target population. Each year, FNS estimates the rate of participation in FSP among those eligible for benefits. The participation rate is a ratio of the number of program participants to the number of eligible people. Counts of the number of participants are obtained from administrative records, and counts of the number of people eligible for benefits are estimated based on national survey data and a variety of other sources.

In 2002, participation rates were the highest for Hawaii, West Virginia, and Oregon (more than 70%), whereas the lowest rates (less than 50%) were found in California, Colorado, Florida, Idaho, Kansas, Maryland, Massachusetts, New Hampshire, New Jersey, Nevada, North Carolina, Texas, Utah, and Wyoming.[30] Outreach initiatives are being implemented to increase program participation by making more eligible people aware of food stamps and their nutrition benefits. Although the FSP serves just over half of all eligible individuals, it provides over two-thirds (65%) of the benefits that all eligible individuals could receive. As a result, the FSP appears to be reaching the neediest eligible individuals.[31] Nevertheless, the USDA's goal is to increase the national participation rate to 68% of those eligible to receive program benefits.[32]

The Food Stamp Act of 1977 provides that states have the opportunity to inform low-income households about the availability, eligibility, requirements, application procedures, and benefits of the FSP and receive federal matching funds for such program informational activities.[33] The FSRIA of 2002 resulted in provisions that restore FSP benefits to legal immigrants, a status that must be communicated in a timely fashion to the people who are affected. To that end, FNS funds a national media campaign to promote the program and offers a toll-free food stamp information hotline and a Web site to allow a quick, confidential food stamp eligibility screening. In addition, the 2002 Farm Bill authorized the USDA to award $5 million in grants for projects aimed at simplifying the food stamp application and eligibility systems or improving access to food stamp benefits by eligible households.

In 2003, FNS formed the "Outreach Coalition" to join forces with the hundreds of food banks, community and faith-based groups, and other service organizations nationwide that help members of their community learn about and apply for food stamps. The coalition is comprised of a core group of national antihunger advocacy groups and other groups interested in promoting the health and nutrition benefits of FSP. These organizations work to end hunger and improve nutrition at the national level through both advocacy and outreach to local antihunger projects.[34]

Legal immigrants. Since the inception of the current FSP in 1977, undocumented immigrants and noncitizens who are in the U.S. temporarily, such as students, have not been eligible for benefits. By 2000, a quarter of low-income children in the U.S. had immigrant parents. In the majority of low-income immigrant families, the children were eligible for food stamps because they were citizens, whereas their parents were often barred from eligibility because they were undocumented or ineligible legal noncitizens. Appropriately, the eligibility rules for legal noncitizens change from time to time. Most recently (2002), the FSP was expanded to include noncitizen children, elders, and disabled individuals who entered the U.S. before enactment of the PRWORA in 1996.[35] FSP embarked on a major outreach initiative to publicize this change. Nevertheless, it is estimated that only slightly more than half of eligible individuals/households receive food stamp benefits. Information about food stamp policy for noncitizens who qualify outright or qualify after a certain waiting period is available on the FSP Web site at http://www.fns.usda.gov/fsp/.

Older adults. Although the USDA's FSP has special provisions to facilitate participation by low-income elderly people, fewer than a third of those eligible in this age group receive benefits.[36] As indicated in Table 13.6, as the age of the individual increases, the rate of participation in FSP decreases. In 2003, only a quarter of eligible older adults participated in the program, compared to half of eligible adults under 60 years of age and three-quarters of eligible children under the age of 18 years.[37] Barriers to program participation reported by seniors, interviewed in focus groups, include pride, the perceived stigma of program participation, misinformation, and confusion about

TABLE 13.6
Food Stamp Participation Rates for Individuals by Demographic Characteristics, 2003

Individual Participation Rates by Demographic Characteristics, Fiscal Year 2003			
	Participating (QC)	Eligible (CPS)	Participation Rate (QC/CPS)
Individuals in All Households	20,590,658	37,027,552	55.61
Age of Individual Children Under Age 18	10,456,000	14,172,165	73.78
Preschool	3,480,215	4,560,267	76.32
School-age	6,975,784	9,611,898	72.57
Adults Age 18 to 59	8,369,421	16,437,905	50.92
Elderly Age 60 and Over	1,765,238	6,417,481	27.51
Living Alone	1,263,159	3,611,731	34.97
Living with Others	502,079	2,805,750	17.89
Nondisabled Childless Adults Subject to Work Registration	733,686	2,568,233	28.57
Noncitizens	702,755	1,504,343	46.72
Citizen Children Living with Noncitizen Adults	1,362,096	2,887,621	47.17
Employment Status of Nonelderly Adults Employed	2,340,128	5,459,924	42.86
Not Employed	6,029,293	10,977,981	54.92
Individuals by Race/ Ethnicity of Household Head Black of African American Only	7,053,713	10,175,199	69.32
Hispanic	3,729,579	7,901,295	47.20
White Only	8,957,530	17,383,776	51.53
Not Tabulated Above	849,836	1,567,282	54.22
Individuals by Household Composition Households with Children	16,070,006	23,384,197	68.72
One Adult	9,305,658	9,983,807	93.21
Married Household Head	3,885,099	8,097,562	47.98
Other Multiple Adults	1,805,438	3,873,973	46.60
Children Only	1,073,811	1,428,855	75.15
Households without Children	4,520,652	13,643,355	33.13
Gender of Individual Male	8,465,164	16,043,744	52.76
Female	12,125,495	20,983,778	57.79
Metropolitan Status Urban	15,748,864	28,663,653	54.94
Rural	4,841,794	8,363,899	57.89

Note: These estimates of participants differ from official participant counts. See Appendix C for details.

Source: From Cunnyngham, K. Food Stamp Program Participation Rates: 2003. Mathematica Policy Research, Inc. Table A-3. Available at: http://www.fns.usda.gov/oane/menu/Published/FSP/FILES/Participation/FSPPart 2003.pdf. Accessed July 24, 2006.

the program's eligibility rules, lack of transportation, and language barriers.[38] One measure of the success of the FSP's outreach efforts, such as the Food Stamp Nutrition Education (FSNE) program, will increasingly depend on the program's ability to reach eligible older Americans.

13.5.1.1.1.5 Nutrition Education

Under current regulations (7 CFR 272.2 [d]), states have the option of providing nutrition education to food stamp recipients. The goal of FSNE is to provide educational programs that increase the likelihood of all people eligible to receive food stamp benefits making healthy food choices and choosing active lifestyles consistent with the current edition of the *Dietary Guidelines for Americans*.

From 1992 to 2004, the number of states and territories offering FSNE increased from 7 to 52, including all 50 states, along with the District of Columbia and the Virgin Islands. The USDA reimburses each state 50% of the allowable administrative costs deemed reasonable and necessary to operate FSNE activities. In 2004, the smallest grant was awarded to the Virgin Islands ($68,000) and the largest to California ($86.7 million). State FSP agencies seeking federal funding to implement or to continue providing FSNE must annually submit a plan to FNS for approval.[39] Four "core elements" that form the basic range of educational categories in FSNE must be included in each state's plan. These elements are dietary quality, food security, food safety, and shopping behavior/resource management. Thus, FSNE efforts may be designed to assist food stamp eligible households in:

- Adopting healthy eating and active lifestyles consistent with the *Dietary Guidelines for Americans* (dietary quality).
- Obtaining enough to eat without resorting to emergency food assistance and assuring that people eligible for the FSP but not participating are made aware of its benefits and how to apply for them as part of nutrition education activity (food security).
- Improving safe food handling, preparation, and storage (food safety).
- Enhancing practices related to thrifty shopping and preparation of nutritious foods (shopping behavior/food resource management).

The efforts of FSNE providers are supported by the resource system known as the *Food Stamp Nutrition Connection* (*FSNC*), the result of a collaboration between the USDA's and the National Agricultural Library's Food and Nutrition Information Center, the University of Maryland, and Howard University.[40]

13.5.1.1.1.6 Name Change

In 2004, the USDA requested comments on whether FSP should be renamed. The name FSP remains linked to the original program that was operating in 1939 when benefits were issued to individuals on welfare, in the form of orange and blue stamps. That program ended in 1943 when World War II reduced the nation's widespread unemployment. The program was revived as a pilot program in 1961 and when it was made permanent in 1964, food stamp benefits were issued to recipients in the form of paper coupons. Many stakeholders believe that the archetype "food stamps" is outdated, reflecting neither the current EBT delivery technology nor the program's mission to promote a healthy diet by providing nutrition or food assistance to all who are eligible. Some state agencies have renamed the FSP within their jurisdictions. For example, in Washington, Michigan, and Minnesota, the FSP is known as the Basic Food Program, the Food Assistance program, and the Food Support Program, respectively. Ultimately, Congress will decide whether the FSP should be renamed and, if so, what the name will be.[41] In their annual performance plan for 2007, the USDA reiterated its continuing efforts to rename the FSP to better represent the program's mission of providing nutritional support to low-income families.[42]

13.5.1.1.2 School Food Programs

School food programs encompass the NSLC, the SBP, and after-school and summer feeding programs. Feeding the nation's children is a daunting task, primarily administered by the USDA, with some assistance from the Department of Defense. Many meals are subsidized, based on children's income eligibility, and there is a movement to introduce universal free breakfast in all schools. All meals served through these programs must meet minimum nutrition standards. Team Nutrition within the USDA provides help in improving nutrition and nutrition education, and alternative sources of food, such as locally grown produce are being investigated to aid in the effort to improve food quality.

13.5.1.1.2.1 National School Lunch Program

Although school food service began in the U.S. as long ago as the mid-1850s,[43] it was not until 1946 that the National School Lunch Act (NSLA)[44] authorized the NSLP. The Act asserts that national security depends on encouraging the domestic consumption of nutritious agricultural commodities and safeguarding the health and well-being of the nation's children. Indeed, it has been stated repeatedly that the NSLP legislation came about in response to the claims that many American men had been rejected for World War II military service because of diet-related health problems.[45]

School lunch, the oldest and second largest of the USDA's food assistance programs, is the cornerstone of the largely school-based child nutrition programs. The Act has been amended numerous times. In 2000, the National School Lunch Act of 1946 was renamed the Richard B. Russell National School Lunch Act in recognition of the senator from Georgia who proposed the legislation and played a key role leading to its passage by Congress and ultimate approval by President Truman. The NSLP is celebrated each year during National School Lunch Week on the second Sunday in October.

Public and nonprofit private schools and residential childcare institutions may participate in the NSLP. The program operates in public and nonprofit private schools and residential child care institutions. Nutritionally balanced meals are provided to children each school day. The meals must be available at no cost or for a reduced price for children who meet certain income levels. After-school snacks are also offered in sites that meet eligibility requirements. Schools that offer school lunch receive cash aid and donated goods from the USDA for each meal served that meets federal nutrition requirements. Virtually all public schools and more than 80% of public and private schools combined participate in the program nationwide. Participation in the program varies with income, age, and gender; students certified to receive free or reduced-price meals are more likely to participate than those who are not certified to receive meal benefits; elementary school children participate at a greater rate than secondary school students, and more boys than girls take part in the program.[46]

Students eligible for free lunches and snacks are those from families with incomes at or below 130% of the federal poverty level (see Table 13.7). Those eligible for reduced-price lunches and snacks are from families with incomes between 130 and 185% of poverty. (For SY 2005–2006, 130% of the poverty level was $25,155 for a family of 4; 185% was $35,798.) Children eligible for reduced-price meals cannot be charged more than $0.40 per lunch. All other children pay full price, which is less than the retail value of the meal, because all meal service programs that participate in the NSLP must operate on a nonprofit basis.

The program is administered by the FNS on the national level, by state agencies (usually state departments of education) at the state level, and by school districts at the local level. States receive federal reimbursement and other assistance in establishing, maintaining, and operating the program. State agencies provide local districts with reimbursements and monitor their programs.

13.5.1.1.2.2 Federal Subsidies

Cash reimbursements and commodity food donations are the two types of federal assistance that are available to the participating school food authorities.

Cash reimbursements. The cash reimbursements schools receive are based on the number of lunches and snacks, established reimbursement rates, and poverty level of participating students. A cash subsidy is provided for every program lunch and snack served. Additional cash subsidies are provided for children who qualify for free or reduced-price meal benefits. During SY (school year) 2002–2003, reimbursement rates were $2.14 for free lunches, $1.74 for reduced-price lunches, and $0.20 for children who paid full price for their meals. Snacks were reimbursed at rates of $0.58, $0.29, and $0.05, respectively. Of the 4.7 billion lunches served in FY 2002, 48% were served free and 9% to children who paid a reduced price.

TABLE 13.7
Standards for Determining Eligibility Income Eligibility Guidelines. 48 Contiguous States and the District of Columbia (July 1, 2006 to June 30, 2007)

Household Size	Poverty Level (Annual Income)	125% of Poverty Level Free Meals Food Stamp Program			185% of Poverty Level Reduced Price Meals WIC		
		Year	Month	Week	Year	Month	Week
1	$ 9,800	$12,740	$1,062	$245	$18,130	$1,511	$349
2	$13,200	$17,160	$1,430	$330	$24,420	$2,035	$470
3	$16,600	$21,580	$1,799	$415	$30,710	$2,560	$591
4	$20,000	$26,000	$2,167	$500	$37,000	$3,084	$712
5	$23,400	$30,420	$2,535	$585	$43,290	$3,608	$833
6	$26,800	$34,840	$2,904	$670	$49,580	$4,132	$954
7	$30,200	$39,260	$3,272	$755	$55,870	$4,656	$1,075
8	$33,600	$43,680	$3,640	$840	$62,160	$5,180	$1,196
For each additional family member	$3,400	$4,420	$369	$85	$6,290	$525	$121

Note: This table is revised annually on July 1st. Separate tables are available for Alaska and Hawaii.

Source: From *Federal Register*, 71: 3848–3849, 2006.

Commodities. The commodity program began in the early 1930s as an outgrowth of federal agricultural policies designed to increase the revenue that farmers received from their produce. By buying large quantities of food and, thus, removing large quantities of food from the open market, government was able to keep prices up, whereas making food available to feed people whose jobs were lost during the Depression. Through its commodity programs, the USDA still helps farmers, whereas providing food to people in need. Currently, the USDA supports farmers by purchasing foods that are surplus or in need of price support, then makes these commodities available to schools and other outlets to feed children, the elderly, and the needy.[47] Schools are entitled to receive commodity foods, called *entitlement foods*, at a value of 17.25 cents for each meal served. Schools can also get "bonus" commodities, as they are available from surplus agricultural stocks. *Bonus foods* are considered those over and above entitlement foods. They are offered periodically, but only as they become available through agricultural surpluses. They are then offered to states on a fair-share basis and do not count against a state's regular entitlement dollars. The type and quantity of bonus commodities distributed by the USDA in a given year is dictated by agricultural surpluses and market conditions.

Commodity foods include more than 100 different kinds of products. Entitlement foods available in SY 2005–2006 for the Schools/ Child Nutrition Commodity Programs included fruits and vegetables, meats, dry and canned beans, fruit juices, vegetable shortenings and vegetable oils, peanut products, rice, cheese, pasta products, flour, and other grain products. Bonus products donated in previous years include: applesauce and apple slices, beef roasts, dried fruit products, fresh pears, frozen apricots, nonfat dry milk, orange juice, pork products, salmon, and turkey.[48]

Over the years, the USDA has worked to improve the quality and nutritional content of the products it purchases. In 1980, it required that all fruits be packed in light syrup or natural juices, and also eliminated the use of tropical oils for all its products. Consistent with the School Meals Initiative for Healthy Children, which stipulates that the NSLP meals must not only provide one-third of recommended nutrients but also be consistent with the *Dietary Guidelines for Americans*, beginning in 1985, the department promoted the development of new products that were lower in fat, such as beef patties with a 10–11% fat content and bulk ground beef and bulk ground pork with the fat content lowered from 22–24% to 17–19%, and increased its offerings of poultry products, and added new lower fat items such as ground turkey and turkey sausage, reduced-fat cheddar cheese, "lite" mozzarella cheese, canned salsa, and fully cooked beef patties. In SY 1993–1994, the USDA more than doubled the quantity of a variety of fresh fruits and vegetables distributed to schools.[49]

13.5.1.1.2.3 Nutrition Standards[50]

Meals served under the NSLP must meet specific federal nutrition standards in order to qualify for federal and state cash reimbursements and federal commodities. At a minimum, lunches must provide:

- A third of the Recommended Dietary Allowances (RDAs) for protein, calcium, iron, Vitamin A, and Vitamin C in the appropriate levels for the ages/grades.
- These energy levels, averaged over a week are: 558 calories (3 to 6 years), 667 calories (7 to 10 years), 783 calories (11 to 13 years), and 856 calories (14 or more years).

Additionally, school meals must meet applicable recommendations from the most recent *Dietary Guidelines for Americans* to eat a variety of foods, limit the percentage of calories from total fat and the percent of calories from saturated fat, reduce sodium and cholesterol levels, and increase the level of dietary fiber.

13.5.1.1.2.4 Obesity Prevention

The increase in childhood obesity and reduction in physical activity is leading to a number of health problems for many children. Once they occur, some of these health problems will follow the children into adulthood. Many of these problems can be prevented or alleviated by improved nutrition. The 2004 Child Nutrition and WIC Reauthorization Act calls for a number of initiatives to address childhood obesity prevention.[51] Designed to improve nutrition in school meals programs, the act:

- Requires local school districts to establish a wellness policy that includes nutritional guidelines for food sold in schools and addresses physical activity and nutrition. By SY 2006–2007. Rationale for this legislation. This legislation shifts to the local level, the locus of responsibility for children's health, recognizes the critical role of schools in curbing the epidemic of childhood overweight, and provides an opportunity for school districts to create an environment conducive to healthy lifestyle choices.[52]
- Provides training and technical assistance resources to schools to enhance school nutrition environments consistent with local wellness policies.
- Adds three new states and three new Indian reservations to the USDA's School Fruit and Vegetable Pilot Program (FVPP), targeting high poverty school districts. Background: The Nutrition Title of the 2002 Farm Act provided $6 million to the FVPP for SY 2002–2003 to improve fruit and vegetable consumption among the nation's schoolchildren. The FVPP provided fresh and dried fruits and fresh vegetables free to children in 107 elementary and secondary schools — 100 schools in 4 places (25 schools each in Indiana, Iowa, Michigan, and Ohio) and 7 schools in the Zuni Indian Tribal Organization (ITO) in New Mexico.[53]
- Authorizes a coordinated nutrition education program at federal, state and local levels, Team Nutrition Network, to provide support for a variety of measures to increase students' understanding of healthy eating, increase students' consumption of healthy foods and improve schools' access to healthy local foods. Includes an independent evaluation of Team Nutrition Network. Background: This provision allows for the recreation of state nutrition education coordinators and grants to local districts. At the federal level, it would continue to support Team Nutrition, and at the same time, it provides the resources necessary to deliver Team Nutrition products to schools and children. The formula for allocation of funds is based on $1/_2$ cent per lunch served. (This legislation replaces the Nutrition Education and Training program [NET], which was enacted in 1977 and operated by the FNS to support nutrition education in the child nutrition programs, but had not been funded since the 1990s. The loss of NET funds forced states to eliminate a state level coordinator position that was responsible for working with

school districts in the state to develop and disseminate NET to the local school food service programs. The Team Nutrition Network would combine the best functions of both NET, unfunded for many years, and Team Nutrition, funded at $10 million a year through a line item in the FNS budget.[54,55])

- Authorizes grants for outreach and education on obesity prevention activities to communities with high limited English proficiency populations.
- Increases the variety of milk available to students, including a variety of fat contents, lactose-free milk, and soy milk meeting USDA standards and requested by a medical authority or parent. Background: This section removes the requirement for schools to base their milk offerings on the previous year's milk sales, thus allowing schools to move toward serving more milk with lower fat contents.
- Provides guidance to school food authorities on strategies to increase the availability of foods reflected in the most recent *Dietary Guidelines for Americans* in school menus.
- Promotes school gardens and improving access to local foods from small- and medium-sized farms for use in schools. The "Farm-to-Cafeteria Projects" Act (S 1755 in the Senate and HR 2626 in the House) promotes students eating healthy foods from farms, whereas farmers get to expand their markets. Farm-to-cafeteria projects eligible to receive assistance under this subsection shall be projects designed to (a) procure local foods from small- and medium-sized farms for the provision of foods for school meals; (b) support nutrition education activities or curriculum planning that incorporates the participation of school children in farm and agriculture education projects; and (c) develop a sustained commitment to farm-to-cafeteria projects in the community by linking schools, agricultural producers, parents, and other community stakeholders.[56] This program was merged with a school gardens[57] program when finally approved by Congress. Legislation provides annual grants of up to $100,000 to school districts or nonprofit organizations to create Farm-to-Cafeteria projects, but needs to be funded through the annual appropriations process.

13.5.1.1.2.5 Alternative Sources of School Food

Farm-to-Cafeteria is defined as a program (and movement) to serve locally produced foods from area farmers in institutional cafeterias and educate children, students, adults, and communities about local food and farming.[58] Thus, the movement is not simply about food and nutrition, but also about education and care of the environment. In the mid-1990s, Farm-to-Cafeteria programs began to arise in response to dissatisfaction with the quality of the food provided by the NSLP,[59] the proliferation of "competitive foods" in schools, and a concern about the impact of conventional agricultural practices on the environment. By 2003, 400 school districts in 22 states were operating farm-to-school programs.[60] Selling large amounts of produce to a few local customers reduces labor and transportation costs and, without an intervening wholesaler, allows the farmer to receive a higher percentage of the profits.[61] In addition, local produce in schools and colleges introduces youth — the farmers' future customers — to good taste and to the role of food and farming in the environment.[62]

Benefits of locally and organically grown foods. Taste, nutrition, and protection of the environment are considerations in food service. How foods are grown and how livestock is treated matter. For example, grass-fed lambs have a distinctly different flavor from that of corn-fed lambs raised in feedlots. When buying from local farmers, food service directors and chefs can talk directly to them about their farming practices. In addition, transportation from local venues uses less fossil fuel, and the food remains fresh and flavorful. Quality produce may cost more up front, but with less plate waste, it can end up being less expensive.[63] One Washington State school district found increased consumption of fresh fruits and vegetables by both elementary school students and staff after introducing a salad bar offering locally grown, organic food.[64] Whereas a limited number of studies have found organic and sustainably grown food to be higher in antioxidants,[65] iron, magnesium, and phosphorous than conventionally grown foods, and lower in levels of nitrates and heavy metals,[66] Gussow[67] and Nestle[68] contend that organically grown produce are better. It is not necessarily for

---

Box 13.7 Buy Local Concepts

Sustainability — the ability to provide for the needs of the current population without damaging the ability of future generations to provide for themselves. A sustainable process can be carried out again and again without negative environmental effects or exorbitant cost to anyone involved.

Buy local — a green politics goal of buying locally produced goods and services, paralleling the phrase *think globally, act locally.*

Food miles — the distance food travels from where it is grown or raised to where it is purchased by consumers, an indicator for the environmental impact of the food and its components.

---

nutritional reasons but owing to the fact that organic farming conserves natural resources, whereas reducing pollution of air, water, and soil (see Box 13.7).

Farm-to-school programs. Issues that arise in Farm-to-Cafeteria programs in K–12 schools include serving both breakfast and lunch, meeting USDA dietary requirements, following purchasing guidelines, ensuring food safety, and overcoming limitations of labor costs.[69] The sample programs cited in the following list have each addressed some of these issues in various ways.

- *New North Florida Cooperative Association, Inc.* — begun in 1995 and the granddaddy of the farm-to-school movement, this collective of farmers in Florida, Georgia, and Alabama sells washed, cut, and packaged vegetables to local school districts. In 6 years, the original customer base of 13 schools grew to feed 300,000 students in 15 school districts in 3 states. Farmers provide collard greens, leafy greens, field peas, muscadine grapes, strawberries, and blackberries that are served to students as side dishes or as dessert.
- *Farmers' Market Salad Bar, Santa Monica, CA* — the brainchild of one dissatisfied but energetic parent, the Farmers' Market Salad Bar began at Santa Monica school in 1997. Salad bar offerings include lettuces, beets, zucchini, and oranges from 20 local farms. Every cafeteria in the Santa Monica district (there are 15) offers a fresh fruit and salad bar. At 9 of the schools, a third of the children eating school lunch choose the salad bar. Each school also boasts of a school garden.
- *School Food Plus, New York, NY* — a collaborative, multiagency program committed to improving the eating habits, health, and academic performance of children attending New York City public schools, whereas supporting New York state agriculture. Using foods grown in New York State, 32 recipes have been developed and are served in the schools. Initial focus is on schools in areas that the New York City Department of Health has deemed most at risk for a long list of chronic diseases.

School gardens. Arguably, the jewel in the crown of the farm-to-cafeteria movement, school gardens, provide experiential learning, increased physical activity, and a source of fresh food.[70] A study of first-grade gardeners in California found an increased willingness among children to taste vegetables if they had grown them.[71] A separate study of fourth graders found that students receiving both nutrition education and hands-on gardening retained a preference for more vegetables than those receiving nutrition education only.[72]

- *Edible Schoolyard* — Established in Berkeley, CA, in 1995, this one-acre, asphalt-coated abandoned lot next to a middle school was transformed into an oasis of seasonal produce, herbs, vines, berries, and flowers, surrounded by fruit trees. The garden is wholly integrated into the school's curriculum and lunch program. This approach fosters awareness and appreciation for nourishment, the community, and stewardship of the land.[73]

- The arrival at Yale University of Alice Waters' daughter Fanny (born 1983) meshed perfectly with the student organization Food from the Earth, whose members promoted organic food in the dining halls, a farm, and institutional composting. Out of this relationship emerged, in 2002, the Yale Sustainable Food Project, a joint endeavor of the university's dining services, students, faculty, and administrators. Designed to nourish the interconnected pleasures of growing, cooking, and sharing food, it is the Ivy League, college-level version of the Edible Schoolyard. The dining service actively develops working relationships with local farmers who promote the vitality of soil, seed, and ecosystem; ranchers who care for their livestock using humane and ecological methods; and food distributors who can trace their products to responsible sources.[74]

Farm to college. Farm to college programs are an offshoot of the "buy local" movement, which works to protect the environment by reducing food miles and by supporting family farms. Of the 2,500 colleges and universities in the U.S., about 10% incorporate locally grown food in their dining programs.[75] A Vermont apple grower states he bought his orchard knowing that he could sell some of his crop to the nearby Middlebury College. The college also accounts for 6% of a local dairy's annual sales. In Northfield, MN, almost 20% of St. Olaf College's food purchases are local. They are expecting to double that over the next 2 years.[76] As of 2002, most farmers supplying colleges had been doing so for 6 years or less.[77] Unlike K–12 schools, colleges are more active throughout the year, allowing them to take advantage of the summer growing months. In addition, they are perhaps, among all academic institutions, most receptive to the economic, social, and environmental reasons to use locally and sustainably grown food, most able to meet potentially higher costs, and most likely to have receptive constituents.[78]

Barriers to change and some solutions. A number of barriers exist to Farm-to-Cafeteria programs. These include seasonality, a disjuncture between production capacity and supply requirements of institutions, and a workable payment mechanism. Purchasing locally grown food in the face of prime vendor agreements requires not only dedication to the concept but a solid understanding of the purchasing process. Liability insurance required by vendors can be prohibitive. Further, one-to-one purchasing and ordering take longer, and smaller nearby farms may not be able to offer competitive prices or the quantities needed by large institutions.[79] Solutions to these barriers include menus that take seasonality into account, use produce such as onions and potatoes that have a stable shelf-life and are minimally processed, farm producer cooperatives to enhance efficiency and consistency, farm grower cooperatives to meet volume needs, and educating farmers about purchasing and billing procedures.[80] Overcoming "consumer reluctance" may be a matter of education. A study of 560 K–4 grade students found that after being taught about the history and lore of nutritious, plant-based foods, children in an intervention group ate between 3 and 20 times more new food than children in the control group. The students also proved to be agents of change in their families.[81]

Legislation. Several recent pieces of legislation contain provisions of importance for the farm to cafeteria movement. The 2003 Farm Bill[82] requires that from 2003–2007, the Secretary of Agriculture encourage schools participating in the NSLP and SBP to purchase locally grown food. Section 204 of the Child Nutrition and WIC Reauthorization Act of 2004,[83,84] requires that all school districts participating in the federal school food programs have local wellness policies in place by SY 2006–2007. As a result, innovative policies have been adopted or proposed in an effort to improve school food, such as purchasing food to support local farmers. Section 124 of this act further allows but does not require:

- School garden demonstration projects that allow children to learn about the importance of specialty crops to a healthy diet.
- Improved access to local foods by procuring local foods from small- and medium-sized farms for school meals.

- Support for nutrition education activities or curriculum planning that incorporates the participation of school children in farm and agricultural education activities.
- Development of a sustained commitment to farm-to-cafeteria projects in the community by linking schools, agricultural producers, parents, and other community stakeholders.

13.5.1.1.2.6 School Breakfast Program

The Child Nutrition Act of 1966 established the SBP, a federally assisted meal program that provides nutritionally balanced, low-cost or free breakfasts to children in public and nonprofit private schools and residential child care institutions. The minimum nutrient and calorie levels averaged for over a week are presented in Table 13.8.

SBP is a federally assisted meal program operating in public and nonprofit private schools and residential child care institutions. It began as a pilot project in 1966 and was made permanent in 1975. The program is administered at the federal level by the FNS. At the state level, the program is usually administered by state education agencies, which operate the program through agreements with local school food authorities in nearly 80,000 schools and institutions.

SBP operates in the same manner as the NSLP. Generally, public or nonprofit private schools of high-school grade or under and public or nonprofit private residential childcare institutions may participate. School districts and independent schools that choose to take part receive cash subsidies from USDA for each meal they serve. In return, they must serve breakfasts that meet the federal requirements summarized in Table 13.8, and they must offer free or reduced price breakfasts to eligible children. Children from families with incomes at or below 130% of the federal poverty level are eligible for free meals. Those with incomes between 130% and 185% of the poverty level are eligible for reduced-price meals. Children from families over 185% of poverty pay full price, though their meals are still subsidized to some extent. The Poverty Guidelines are presented in Table 13.9.

Most of the support the USDA provides to schools in the SBP comes in the form of a cash reimbursement for each breakfast served. For SY 2005–2006, the basic cash reimbursement rates were $1.27, $0.97, and $0.23, respectively for free, reduced-price, and paid breakfasts respectively.

TABLE 13.8
Minimum Nutrient and Calorie Levels for School Breakfasts Averaged for a School Week

| | Minimum Requirements | | Optional |
Nutrients and Energy Allowances	Preschool	Grades K–12	Grades 7–12
Energy allowances (calories)	388	554	618
Total fat (as a percentage of actual total food energy)	a	a,b	b
Saturated fat (as a percentage of actual total food energy)	a	a,c	c
RDA for protein (g)	5	10	12
RDA for calcium (mg)	200	257	300
RDA for iron (mg)	2.5	3	3.4
RDA for Vitamin A (RE)	113	197	225
RDA for Vitamin C (mg)	11	13	14

[a] The Dietary Guidelines recommend that after 2 years of age " ... children should gradually adopt a diet that, by about 5 years of age, contains no more than 30% of calories from fat."

[b] Not to exceed 30% over a school week.

[c] Less than 10% over a school week.

Source: From 7 CFR Ch. II Part 220 — *School Breakfast Program.* January 1, 2005. Available at: http://www.fns.usda.gov/cnd/Breakfast/Menu/sbp-planning-approaches.doc. Accessed June 8, 2006.

TABLE 13.9
2006–2007 Poverty Guidelines

Persons in Family or Household	48 Contiguous States and D.C.	Alaska	Hawaii
1	$ 9,800	$12,250	$11,270
2	13,200	16,500	15,180
3	16,600	20,750	19,090
4	20,000	25,000	23,000
5	23,400	29,250	26,910
6	26,800	33,500	30,820
7	30,200	37,750	34,730
8	33,600	42,000	38,640
For each additional person, add:	3,400	4,250	3,910

Source: From *Federal Register*, 71: 3848–3849, 2006.

Schools may qualify for higher "severe need" reimbursements if a specified percentage of their lunches are served free or at a reduced price. Severe need payments are up to 24 cents higher than the normal reimbursements for free and reduced-price breakfasts. About 65% of the breakfasts served in the SBP receive severe need payments. Higher reimbursement rates are in effect for Alaska and Hawaii. Schools may charge no more than 30 cents for a reduced-price breakfast. Schools set their own prices for breakfasts served to students who pay the full meal price (paid), though they must operate their meal services as nonprofit programs. Participation has slowly but steadily grown over the years from half million in 1970 to 7.6 million in 2000. In FY 2002, an average of 8.4 million children participated every day. Of those, 6.9 million received their meals free or at a reduced price. For FY 2003, the program cost $1.63 billion.

Universal free breakfast. Fewer low-income children participate in the SBP than in the NSLP. There is concern that low-income children might be coming to school without eating breakfast and still not be participating in the SBP for a variety of reasons, including a perceived stigma associating school breakfast participation with poverty. One approach to increasing participation in the SBP is to offer free breakfast to all students, regardless of their household income. Some school districts have chosen to provide universal free breakfast, meaning that the program is free for all children in the district, regardless of their ability to pay. In 2003, the New York City Department of Education, which serves almost a million meals a day, started making school breakfasts available to all students "universally" regardless of their ability to pay (see Box 13.8).

13.5.1.1.2.7 Summer Feeding Programs

Summer feeding programs were created to continue providing nutritious meals free of charge to children from low-income areas during periods when schools are closed for vacation. In both the Seamless Summer Feeding Option and the Summer Food Service Program (SFSP), the meals served must conform to the meal pattern requirement standards used in the major child nutrition programs, that is, NSLP and SBP. The programs, which are located in low-income areas, may feed children through 18 years of age. The meals served are reimbursed at the free NSLP/SBP rates. Schools may serve a maximum of 2 meals/d, with a snack counting as a meal option. Allowable meals may include breakfast, morning snack, lunch, afternoon snack, and supper. Up to 2 types of meals per day can be reimbursed (3 for migrant sites and camps).

Summer food service program. The SFSP is authorized under Section 13 of the Richard B. Russell National School Lunch Act (NSLA) (42 U.S.C. 1761). Although millions of children depend on nutritious free and reduced-price meals and snacks at school for 9 months out of the year, just a fraction of that receive the free meals provided by the SFSP. Federal resources are available for local sponsors who want to combine a feeding program with a summer activity program. All

---

Box 13.8 Universal Free Breakfast

Debate

A universal free approach to increasing breakfast participation substantially increases the cost to the federal government. As it is critical to know if such expenditures are warranted, Section 109 of the William F. Goodling Child Nutrition Act of 1998 (P.L. 105–336) authorized the implementation and the evaluation of a study in elementary schools in six school districts representing a range of economic and demographic characteristics. The USDA and FNS conducted the pilot from SY 2000–2001 through SY 2002–2003. Specifically, the pilot study sought to determine if the increase in SBP participation by students in elementary schools offering universal free school breakfast would result in improved dietary intakes and/or measures of academic performance. The study found that the availability of universal free school breakfast significantly increased school breakfast participation but had little impact on other outcomes measured over the course of the evaluation, including academic achievement test scores, attendance, tardiness, health, and discipline. Although treatment school students were more likely to consume a nutritionally substantive breakfast than control school students, there was almost no difference in average food and nutrient intakes at breakfast or over the course of the day. These findings do not negate the importance of eating breakfast but do suggest that simply offering free school breakfast to all elementary school students would not, on average, improve academic or behavioral outcomes beyond what occurs in schools already offering the SBP.

Is a universal free breakfast worth the cost? Present arguments on both sides of this issue.

---

sponsors receive training before starting the program to learn how to plan, operate, and monitor a successful food service program. The payments that sponsors receive are based on the number of meals served and the documented costs of running the program. SFSP sponsors receive payments for serving healthy meals and snacks to children and teenagers, 18 years and younger, at approved sites in low-income areas. Schools, public agencies, and private nonprofit organizations may apply to sponsor the program. They include:

- Public or private nonprofit schools
- Units of local, municipal, county, tribal, or state government
- Private nonprofit organizations
- Public or private nonprofit camps
- Public or private nonprofit universities or colleges

Since 1969, the program has grown from 1,200 sites serving 2.2 million meals at a cost of a third of a million dollars to 2005, with 30,500 sites serving 115.7 million meals at a cost of almost

---

Box 13.9 WIC Legislative Requirements

WIC's legislative requirements are contained in Section 17 of the Child Nutrition Act of 1966, as amended by P.L. 109–85 (October 2005), §17.

Source: U.S. Department of Agriculture. Food and Nutrition Service. WIC Program. Women, Infants, and Children. Laws and Regulations. Available at: http://www.fns.usda.gov/wic/lawsandregulations/default.htm. Accessed February 15, 2007.

Box 13.10 WIC Food Packages URL

The new WIC food packages are described on the program's Web site at http://www.fns.usda.
gov/wic/. benefitsandservices/foodpkg.HTM.

Source: U.S. Department of Agriculture. Food and Nutrition Service. WIC Program. Benefits and Services. WIC
Food Packages. Available at: http://www.fns.usda.gov/wic/benefitsandservices/foodpkg.HTM. Accessed February 15,
2007.

$270 million, which includes cash payments for meals served, sponsor administrative costs, state
administrative expenses, and health inspection costs. In 2005, slightly less than 2 million children
per day were served during the peak month of July. More than a third of the program's daily
attendance was accounted for by 4 states: New York (over 410,000), followed by Pennsylvania
(115,000), Florida (104,000), and California (98,000). Nevertheless, many schools and summer
recreation programs are not aware of the SFSP funds available to provide free meals and snacks
to children in needy areas during the summer months, nor are many parents and guardians aware
of nearby SFSP programs, according to a rudimentary survey conducted in 2004 by the USDA.[85]

Seamless summer feeding option. The Seamless Summer School Option is a permanent option
for school districts participating in the NSLP or SBP. In essence, schools operate SFSP as an
extension of the NSLP. Authorized by the Child Nutrition and WIC Reauthorization Act of 2004,
the option combines features of the NSLP, SBP, and SFSP, whereas streamlining the administrative
and monitoring requirements for operating in the school districts. The option is designed to reduce
paperwork and administrative burden, making it easier for schools to feed children from low-income
areas during the traditional summer vacation periods and for year-round schools, long school
vacation periods (generally exceeding 2–3 weeks). School districts and nonschool settings must
apply to operate a Seamless Summer Feeding Program. The various types of sites allowed to
participate in this option include:

- *Open sites* — all children eat free in communities where at least 50% of the children
  are eligible for free or reduced-price school meals.
- *Restricted open sites* — meet the open site criteria, but are later restricted for safety,
  control, or security reasons.
- *Closed enrolled sites* — may be in any community for an enrolled group of low-income
  children and meets the 50% criteria for open sites. This excludes academic summer
  schools. School districts operating an academic summer school that feeds only those
  children enrolled in the summer school program must extend their NSLP/SBP agreement
  instead of operating under the summer program.
- *Migrant sites* — serving children of migrant families.

The Seamless Summer Feeding Program began as a pilot program in California and Florida.
It expanded to all states in 2002 and was originally set to end in 2004. However, in 2004, this
program became a permanent option for school districts to operate a feeding program during the
summer months.

13.5.1.1.3 Supplemental Nutrition Program for Women,
Infants and Children (WIC)

The WIC serves to safeguard the health of low-income women, infants, and children up to age 5
years who are at nutritional risk by providing: (1) nutritious foods to supplement diets (see Table 13.10),
(2) information on healthy eating, and (3) referrals to healthcare.

TABLE 13.10
WIC Food Package — Maximum Monthly Allowances

Foods	Infants 0–3 Months (I)	Infants 4–12 Months (II)	Children/ Women with Special Dietary Needs (III)	Children 1–5 Years (IV)	Pregnant and Breastfeeding Women (up to 1 Year Postpartum) (V)	Nonbreastfeeding Postpartum Women (up to 6 Months Postpartum) (VI)	Breastfeeding Women Enhanced Package[a] (VII)
Infant formula (concentrated liquid)[b]	403 fl oz	403 fl oz	403 fl oz[c]				
Juice (reconstituted frozen)[d]		96 fl oz[e]	144 fl oz	288 fl oz	288 fl oz	192 fl oz	336 fl oz
Infant cereal		24 oz					
Cereal (hot or cold)			36 oz	36 oz	36 oz	36 oz	36 oz
Milk[f]				24 qt	28 qt	24 qt	28 qt
Cheese[f]							1 lb
Eggs[g]				2–2 $^1/_2$ doz	2–2 $^1/_2$ doz	2–2 $^1/_2$ doz	2–2 $^1/_2$ doz
Dried beans/peas and/or peanut butter				1 lb or 18 oz	1 lb or 18 oz		1 lb and 18 oz
Tuna (canned)							26 oz
Carrots (fresh)[h]							2 lb

[a] Available to breastfeeding women whose infants do not receive formula from the WIC Program.

[b] Powdered or ready-to-feed formula may be substituted at the following rates: 8 lb powdered per 403 fl oz concentrated liquid and 26 fl oz ready-to-feed per 13 fl oz concentrated liquid.

[c] Additional amounts of formula may be approved for nutritional need, up to 52 fl oz concentrated liquid or 1 lb powdered or 104 fl oz ready-to-feed.

[d] Single strength adult juice may be substituted at a rate of 92 fluid oz per 96 fl oz reconstituted frozen.

[e] Infant juice may be substituted for adult juice at the rate of 63 fl oz per 92 fl oz single strength adult juice.

[f] A choice of various forms of milks and cheeses may be available. Cheese may be substituted for fluid whole milk at the rate of 1 lb per 3 qts, with a 4 lb maximum. Additional cheese may be issued in cases of lactose intolerance.

[g] Dried egg mix may be substituted at the rate of 1.5 lb per 2 doz fresh eggs or 2 lb per 2$^1/_2$ doz fresh eggs.

[h] Frozen carrots may be substituted at the rate of 1 lb per 1 lb fresh or canned carrots at the rate of 16–20 oz canned per 1 lb fresh.

Source: From 7 CFR Ch II. (1-1-06 edition), Part 246, Subpart D (Participant benefits), §246.10 (Supplemental foods), pp. 344–352. Available at: http://a257.g.akamaitech.net/7/257/2422/01jan20061500/edocket.access.gpo.gov/cfr_ 2006/ jan-qtr/7cfr246.10.htm. Accessed July 27, 2006.

WIC was launched in 1972 to meet the special nutritional needs of low-income pregnant, breastfeeding, and postpartum nonbreastfeeding women, infants, and children up to 5 years of age who are at nutritional risk. What started as a pilot project has expanded to serve all 50 states, the District of Columbia, Puerto Rico, Guam, American Samoa, the American Virgin Islands, and 34 ITO. These 88 WIC state agencies administer the program through 2,200 local agencies and 9,000 clinic sites. WIC serves nearly half of all newborn infants among the U.S. infants (essentially all the income-eligible U.S. infants) and a quarter of all U.S. children of ages 1 through 4 years, along with many of their mothers.

More than 7.5 million people get WIC benefits each month. In 1974, the first year WIC was permanently authorized, 88,000 people participated. Average monthly participation for FY 2003 was approximately 7.63 million. Children have always been the largest category of WIC participants. Of the 7.63 million people who received WIC benefits each month in FY 2003, approximately half (3.82 million) were children and a quarter each were infants (1.95 million) and women (1.86 million).

WIC's goal is to improve birth outcomes and support the growth and development of infants. WIC provides supplemental foods and nutrition education through payment of cash grants to state agencies that administer the program through local agencies at no cost to eligible persons. The program serves as an adjunct to good healthcare during critical times of growth and development, in order to prevent the occurrence of health problems and to improve the health status of the women, infants, and children identified at risk. WIC is supplementary to FSP and any other any program that distributes foods to needy families, such as soup kitchens, or shelters, or other forms of emergency food assistance.[86]

Supplemental foods are made available monthly in the form of seven different WIC food packages. Most WIC participants access the food packages by redeeming vouchers or food-checks to obtain specific foods at participating retail outlets. WIC also provides nutrition counseling and referrals to health and other social services to participants at no charge.

WIC is not an entitlement program; that is, Congress does not set aside funds to allow every eligible individual to participate in the program. Instead, WIC is a federal grant program for which Congress authorizes a specific amount of funding each year for program operations. FNS, which administers the program at the federal level, provides these funds to WIC state agencies (state health departments or comparable agencies) to pay for WIC foods, nutrition counseling and education, and administrative costs.

Eligible women and their infants and children must meet income guidelines, a state residency requirement, and be individually determined to be at "nutrition risk" by a health professional. To be eligible on the basis of income, applicants' income must fall at or below 185% of the U.S. Poverty Income Guidelines. A person who participates or has family members who participate in certain other benefit programs, such as the FSP, Medicaid, or Temporary Assistance for Needy Families (TANF), automatically meets the income eligibility requirement. Two major types of nutrition risk are recognized for WIC eligibility:

- *Medically based risks* such as anemia, underweight, overweight, history of pregnancy complications, or poor pregnancy outcomes.
- *Dietary risks* such as failure to meet the dietary guidelines or inappropriate nutrition practices.

Nutrition risk is determined by a health professional such as a physician, nutritionist, or nurse and is based on federal guidelines. This health screening is free to program applicants.

13.5.1.1.3.1 WIC Food Benefits

In most WIC state agencies, WIC participants receive checks or vouchers to purchase specific foods each month that are designed to supplement their diets. The foods provided are high in one or more of the following nutrients: protein, calcium, iron, and vitamins A and C. These are the nutrients frequently lacking in the diets of the program's target population. As illustrated in Table 13.10, different food packages are provided for different categories of participants. WIC foods include iron-fortified infant formula and infant cereal, iron-fortified adult cereal, vitamin-C rich fruit or vegetable juice, eggs, milk, cheese, peanut butter, dried beans/peas, tuna fish, and carrots. Special therapeutic infant formulas and medical foods are provided when prescribed by a physician for a specified medical condition.

In 2003, FNS contracted with the Institute of Medicine (IOM) to independently review the WIC food packages. FNS charged IOM with recommending specific changes based on current information about the nutrition needs of WIC participants without affecting the cost of the WIC food packages. The IOM issued two reports: the initial report (2004) describes nutrient needs for the WIC target population and establishes criteria for new food packages; the final report (2005) offers specific recommendations for food package changes.[87]

It was the recommendation of the IOM in 2004 that the new food package should reduce the prevalence of inadequate and excessive nutrient intakes in participants, contribute to an overall dietary pattern that is consistent with the *Dietary Guidelines for Americans* or to a diet that is consistent with dietary recommendations for infants and children younger than 2 years of age, and encourage and support breastfeeding. Foods in the package should be available in forms suitable for low-income persons who may have limited transportation, storage, and cooking facilities; be acceptable, readily available, and commonly consumed; take into account cultural food preferences; and provide incentives for families to participate in the WIC program. Care should be taken to consider the effects on vendors and WIC of changes in the package. The USDA released new rules for the contents of the WIC food packages that reflect these recommendations.[88]

13.5.1.1.3.2 Appropriations and Priorities

Congress appropriated $5.3 billion for WIC in FY 2006. Almost three-quarters of that total was spent on food and the remainder on nutrition services and administration (NSA).[89] Approximately two-thirds of NSA costs are used to provide nutrition education, breastfeeding promotion and support, and linkages to health and other client services (for example, immunization; drug, alcohol and tobacco education; referrals to family and child health social programs). The remaining third is used for traditional management functions. In 2005, the average food benefit per month was $37.42.[90] EBT development has been a key long-term goal of FNS and of the WIC program. The challenge is in finding technological solutions that are both affordable and can meet the functional needs of a relatively complex nutrition program.

WIC cannot serve all eligible people, so a system of priorities has been established for filling program openings. Once a local WIC agency has reached its maximum caseload, vacancies are filled in the order of the following priority levels:

- Pregnant women, breastfeeding women, and infants determined to be at nutrition risk because of a nutrition-related medical condition
- Infants up to 6 months of age whose mothers participated in WIC or could have participated and had a serious medical problem
- Children at nutrition risk because of a nutrition-related medical problem
- Pregnant or breastfeeding women and infants at nutrition risk because of an inadequate dietary pattern
- Children at nutrition risk because of an inadequate dietary pattern
- Nonbreastfeeding, postpartum women with any nutrition risk
- Individuals at nutrition risk only because they are homeless or migrants, and current participants who, without WIC foods, could continue to have medical and/or dietary problems

13.5.1.1.3.3 The WIC Infant Formula Rebate System

Mothers participating in WIC are encouraged to breastfeed their infants if possible, but WIC state agencies provide infant formula for mothers who choose to use this feeding method. WIC state agencies are required by law to have competitively bid infant formula rebate contracts with infant formula manufacturers. This means WIC state agencies agree to provide one brand of infant formula, and in return, the manufacturer gives the state agency a rebate for each can of infant formula purchased by WIC participants. The brand of infant formula provided by WIC varies from one state agency to another, depending on which company has the rebate contract in a particular state. By negotiating rebates with formula manufacturers, states are able to serve more people. For FY 2003, rebate savings were $1.52 billion, supporting an average of 1.9 million participants each month or 25% of the estimated average monthly caseload.

13.5.1.1.3.4 Farmers' Market Nutrition Program (FMNP)

The WIC Farmers' Market Nutrition Program (FMNP) provides fresh, unprepared, locally grown fruits and vegetables from local farmers' markets to WIC recipients (over 4 months of age). The federal food benefit level for FMNP recipients is $10 to $30 per year per recipient, but state agencies may supplement the benefit level. The farmers, farmers' markets, or roadside stands then submit the coupons to the bank or state agency for reimbursement.

A variety of fresh, nutritious, unprepared, locally grown fruits, vegetables and herbs may be purchased with FMNP coupons. Each state agency develops a list of fresh fruits, vegetables, and herbs that can be purchased with FMNP coupons. Nutrition education is provided to FMNP recipients by the state agency, often through an arrangement with the local WIC agency. Other educators and program partners may provide nutrition education and/or educational information to FMNP recipients, such as cooperative extension programs, local chefs, farmers or farmers' markets associations, and various other nonprofit or for-profit organizations. These educational arrangements help to encourage FMNP recipients to improve and expand their diets by adding fresh fruits and vegetables, as well as educate them on how to select, store, and prepare the fresh fruits and vegetables they buy with their FMNP coupons.

During FY 2004, 14,050 farmers, 2,548 farmers' markets, and 1,583 roadside stands were authorized to accept FMNP coupons, which resulted in almost $27 million in revenue to farmers. During FY 2004, 2.5 million WIC participants received benefits. For FY 2006, $19.8 million was appropriated for the program.

13.5.1.1.4   Child and Adult Care Food Program (CACFP)

After an extension of the 1968 Special Food Service Program for Children's 3-year demonstration project, the Child Care Food Program was authorized in 1975, becoming a permanent program in 1978. The name was officially changed to the Child and Adult Care Food Program (CACFP) in 1989 to reflect the adult component of this program. CACFP plays a vital role in improving the quality of day care for children and elderly adults by making care more affordable for many low-income families. CACFP supports nutritious meals and snacks in child care centers, family child care homes, Head Start (see Box 13.11), after-school programs, shelters, and adult day care centers.

Through CACFP, almost 3 million infants and children (birth through age 18 years) and under 100,000 chronically impaired adults or people over age 60 at adult day care centers receive nutritious meals and snacks each day as part of their day care (Table 13.11). CACFP reaches even further to provide meals to children residing in emergency shelters and snacks and suppers to youths participating in eligible after-school care programs. Free meals are provided to: adults who receive food stamps, FDPIR, Social Security Income, or Medicaid; children whose families receive benefits from the FSP, FDPIR, or state programs funded through TANF, or who are income-eligible participants of Head Start or Early Start (more than 900,000 Head Start children in 2005); or children who live in emergency shelters.

CACFP provides reimbursement for food and meal preparation costs, ongoing training in the nutritional needs of children, and onsite assistance in meeting the program's nutritional requirements. Meals served to children are reimbursed at rates based upon a child's eligibility for free, reduced-price, or paid meals.

The USDA's FNS administers CACFP through grants to states. The program is administered within most states by the state educational agency. The child care component and the adult day care component of CACFP may be administered by different agencies within a state, at the discretion

---

Box 13.11 Head Start Child Nutrition Performance Standards

Identification of nutritional needs. Staff and families must work together to identify each child's nutritional needs, taking into account staff and family discussions concerning:

- Any relevant nutrition-related assessment data, such as height, weight, hemoglobin, or hematocrit.
- Information about family eating patterns, including cultural preferences, special dietary requirements for each child with nutrition-related health problems, and the feeding requirements of infants and toddlers and each child with disabilities.
- For infants and toddlers, current feeding schedules and amounts and types of food provided, including whether breast milk or formula and baby food is used, meal patterns, new foods introduced, food intolerances and preferences, voiding patterns, and observations related to developmental changes in feeding and nutrition must be shared with parents and updated regularly.
- Information about major community nutritional issues, as identified through the Community Assessment or by the Health Services Advisory Committee or the local health department.

Nutritional services. Grantee and delegate agencies must design and implement a nutrition program that meets the nutritional needs and feeding requirements of each child, including those with special dietary needs and children with disabilities. Also, the nutrition program must serve a variety of foods, which consider cultural and ethnic preferences and also broaden the child's food experience.

- All Early Head Start and Head Start programs must use funds from the USDA Food and Consumer Services Child Nutrition Programs as the primary source of payment for meal services. Early Head Start and Head Start funds may be used to cover those allowable costs not covered by the USDA.
- Each child in a part-day program must receive meals and snacks that provide at least a third of the child's daily nutritional needs. Each child in a full-day program must receive meals and snacks that provide half to two-thirds of the child's daily nutritional needs, depending on the length of the program day.
- All children in morning programs, who have not received breakfast at the time they arrive at the program, must be served a nourishing breakfast.
- Each infant and toddler must receive food appropriate to their nutritional needs, developmental readiness, and feeding skills, as recommended in the USDA meal pattern or nutrient standard menu planning requirements outlined in 7 CFR parts 210, 220, and 226 (available at: http://www.fns.usda.gov/cnd/Care/Regs-Policy/226-2004%20 Compiled.pdf).
- For 3- to 5-year-olds, foods served must be high in nutrients and low in fat, sugar, and salt. The quantities and kinds of food served must conform to recommended serving sizes and minimum standards for meal patterns recommended in the USDA meal pattern or nutrient standard menu planning requirements outlined in 7 CFR parts 210, 220, and 226 (available at: http://www.fns.usda.gov/cnd/Care/Regs-Policy/226-2004%20 Compiled.pdf).
- Meal and snack periods must be appropriately scheduled and adjusted, where necessary, to ensure that individual needs are met. Infants and young toddlers who need it must be fed "on demand" to the extent possible or at appropriate intervals.
- Staff must promote effective dental hygiene among children in conjunction with meals.
- Parents and appropriate community agencies must be involved in planning, implementing, and evaluating the program's nutritional services.

Meal service. Grantee and delegate agencies must ensure that nutritional services in center-based settings contribute to the development and socialization of enrolled children by providing that:

- A variety of food is served, which broadens each child's food experiences.
- Food is not used as punishment or reward, and that all children are encouraged, but not forced, to eat or taste their food.
- Sufficient time is allowed for each child to eat.
- All toddlers and preschool children and assigned classroom staff, including volunteers, eat together family-style and share the same menu to the extent possible.
- Infants are held while being fed and are not laid down to sleep with a bottle.
- Medically based diets or other dietary requirements are accommodated.
- As developmentally appropriate, opportunity is provided for the involvement of children in food-related activities.

Family assistance with nutrition. Parent education activities must include opportunities to assist individual families with food preparation and nutritional skills.

Food safety and sanitation. Head Start programs must post evidence of compliance with all applicable federal, state, tribal, and local food safety and sanitation laws, including those related to the storage, preparation, and service of food and the health of food handlers. In addition, agencies must contract only with food service vendors that are licensed in accordance with state, tribal, or local laws.

- For programs serving infants and toddlers, facilities must be available for the proper storage and handling of breast milk and formula.

Source: U.S. Department of Health and Human Services. Administration for Children and Families. Head Start Bureau. *Performance Standard. 1304.23 — Child Nutrition.* Available at: http://www.acf.hhs.gov/programs/hsb/performance/130423PS.htm. Accessed April 8, 2005. Also: National Archives and Records Administration. Code of Federal Regulations. Chapter XIII-Office of Human Development Services, Department of Health and Human Services. Performance Standards for the Operation of Head Start Programs by Grantee and Delegate Agencies. 1304.23 — Child nutrition. Revised October 1, 2004. Available at: http://www.access.gpo.gov/nara/cfr/ waisidx_04/45cfr1304_04.html. Accessed April 29, 2005.

---

of the governor. Independent centers and sponsoring organizations enter into agreements with their administering state agencies to assume administrative and financial responsibility for CACFP operations. Participating programs are required to provide meals and snacks according to the nutrition standards set by USDA. The reimbursement rates vary, based on the type of meal (lunches have a higher reimbursement rate than snacks) and the type of institution.

CACFP is an entitlement program. In FY 2005, peak participation in the program reached 3.36 million with a total of 1.8 billion subsidized meals and snacks at a federal cost of $2.13 billion. Average daily attendance in child care centers was 2 million children; approximately 900,000 children were served through family day care homes.

Community-based programs, such as America's Second Harvest Network Kids Cafes, which offer enrichment activities for at-risk children after school, can provide free snacks through CACFP. Programs receiving benefits must be offered in areas where at least 50% of the children are eligible for free and reduced-price meals, based upon school data. Reimbursable meals are also available to children in eligible after-school care programs in 7 states.

To help meet the need for ongoing training of CACFP staff in the nutritional needs of infants, USDA publishes an infant feeding guide. The book contains information about infant development,

TABLE 13.11
CACFP Children's Meal Patterns for Breakfast, Snack, and Lunch/Supper

Breakfast			
Food Components			
Select all three components for a reimbursable breakfast	**Ages 1–2**	**Ages 3–5**	**Ages 6–12**
One serving milk			
Fluid milk	1/2 cup	3/4 cup	1 cup
One serving fruit/vegetable			
Juice,[b] fruit and/or vegetable	1/4 cup	1/2 cup	1/2 cup
One serving grains/bread[c]			
Bread	1/2 slice	1/2 slice	1 slice
Cornbread or biscuit or roll or muffin	1/2 serving	3/4 serving	1 serving
Cold dry cereal	1/4 cup	1/4 cup	3/4 cup
Hot cooked cereal	1/4 cup	1/4 cup	1/2 cup
Pasta or noodles or grains	1/4 cup	1/4 cup	1/2 cup

Snack			
Food Components			
Select two of the four components for a reimbursable snack	**Ages 1–2**	**Ages 3–5**	**Ages 6–12**
One serving milk			
Fluid milk	1/2 cup	1/2 cup	1 cup
1 Serving fruit/vegetable			
Juice,[b] fruit and/or vegetable	1/2 cup	1/2 cup	3/4 cup
One serving grains/bread[c]			
Bread	1/2 slice	1/2 slice	1 slice
Cornbread or biscuit or roll or muffin	1/2 serving	1/2 serving	1/3 serving
Cold dry cereal	1/4 cup	1/3 cup	3/4 cup
Hot cooked cereal	1/4 cup	1/4 cup	1/2 cup
Pasta or noodles or grains	1/4 cup	1/4 cup	1/2 cup
One serving meat/meat alternate			
Meat or poultry or fish[d]	1/2 oz	1/2 oz	1 oz
Alternate protein product	1/2 oz	1/2 oz	1 oz
Cheese	1/2 oz	1/2 oz	1 oz
Egg[e]	1/2 egg	1/2 egg	1/2 egg
Cooked dry beans or peas	1/8 cup	1/8 cup	1/4 cup
Peanut or other nut or seed butters	1 tbsp.	1 tbsp.	2 tbsp
Nuts and/or seeds	1/2 oz	1/2 oz	1 oz
Yogurt[f]	2 oz	2 oz	4 oz

Lunch or Supper			
Food Components	**Ages 1–2**	**Ages 3–5**	**Ages 6–12**
One serving milk			
Fluid milk	1/2 cup	3/4 cup	1 cup
One serving fruits/vegetables			
Juice,[b] fruit and/or vegetable	1/4 cup	1/2 cup	3/4 cup
One serving grains/bread[c]			
Bread	1/2 slice	1/2 slice	1 slice
Cornbread or biscuit or roll or muffin	1/2 serving	1/2 serving	1 serving
Cold dry cereal	1/4 cup	1/3 cup	3/4 cup
Hot cooked cereal	1/4 cup	1/4 cup	1/2 cup
Pasta or noodles or grains	1/4 cup	1/4 cup	1/2 cup

(Continued)

TABLE 13.11 (Continued)
CACFP Children's Meal Patterns for Breakfast, Snack, and Lunch/Supper

Breakfast			

Food Components

Select all three components for a reimbursable breakfast	Ages 1–2	Ages 3–5	Ages 6–12
One serving meat/meat alternate			
Meat or poultry or fish[d]	1 oz	1 1/2 oz	2 oz
Alternate protein product	1 oz	1 1/2 oz	2 oz
Cheese	1 oz	1 1/2 oz	2 oz
Egg[e]	1/2 egg	3/4 egg	1 egg
Cooked dry beans or peas	1/4 cup	3/8 cup	1/2 cup
Peanut or other nut or seed butters	2 tbsp	3 tbsp	4 tbsp
Nuts and/or seeds	1/2 oz	3/4 oz	1 oz
Yogurt[f]	4 oz	6 oz	8 oz

[a] Children age 12 and older may be served larger portions based on their greater food needs. They may not be served less than the minimum quantities listed in this column.

[b] Fruit or vegetable juice must be full strength. Juice cannot be served when milk is the only other snack component.

[c] Breads and grains must be made from whole grain or enriched meal or flour. Cereal must be whole grain or enriched or fortified.

[d] A serving consists of the edible portion of cooked lean meat or poultry or fish.

[e] A half egg meets the required minimum amount (one ounce or less) of meat alternate.

[f] Yogurt may be plain or flavored, unsweetened or sweetened.

Source: U.S. Department of Agriculture. Food and Nutrition Service. Child and Adult Care Food Program. Meal Patterns. Available at: http://www.fns.usda.gov/cnd/care/ProgramBasics/Meals/Meal_Patterns.htm. Accessed February 15, 2007.

Box 13.12 Question

Current events question: Through P.L. 107–76, generally known as the 2002 Farm Bill, Congress authorized $15 million annually for the SFMNP for FY 2003–2007. *What provisions for SFMNP are authorized in the 2007 Farm Bill?*

Box 13.13 USDA Commodity Foods

The USDA makes commodity foods available to state and local agencies, which in turn, distribute the food to eligible recipients participating in food banks and soup kitchens.

Source: U.S. Department of Agriculture. The Emergency Food Assistance Program. Food and Nutrition Service. Food Distribution Fact Sheet. March 2006. The Emergency Food Assistance Program. Available at: http://www. fns.usda.gov/fdd/programs/tefap/pfs-tefap.pdf. Accessed February 15, 2007.

nutrition for infants, breastfeeding and formula feeding, preventing tooth decay, feeding solid foods, drinking from a cup, choking prevention, sanitary food preparation and safe food handling, commercially prepared and home-prepared baby food, the storage and handling of breast milk, and some of the Infant Meal Pattern requirements.[91] Meals served to infants (ages birth through 11 months) must meet the requirements that are outlined in Table 13.12.

13.5.1.1.5 Senior Farmers' Market Nutrition Program (SFMNP)

The Senior Farmers' Market Nutrition Program (SFMNP) was established in FY 2001 to provide low-income seniors with coupons that can be exchanged for eligible foods at farmers' markets, roadside stands, and community supported agriculture programs (CSPs). SFMNP awards grants

TABLE 13.12
CACFP Meal Patterns for Infants through 11 Months of Age

Birth–3 months	4–7 months	8–11 months
Breakfast		
4–6 fl oz formula[a] or breast milk[b,c]	4–8 fl oz formula[a] or breast milk[b,c] and	6–8 fl oz formula[a] or breast milk[b,c] and
	0–3 tbsp infant cereal[a,d]	2–4 tbsp infant cereal[a] and
		1–4 tbsp fruit or vegetable or both
Lunch or Supper		
4–6 fl oz formula[a] or breast milk[b,c]	4–8 fl oz of formula[a] or breast milk[b,c] and	6–8 fl oz formula[a] or breast milk[b,c] and
	0–3 tbsp infant cereal[a,d] and	2–4 tbsp infant cereal[a] and/or
	0–3 tbsp fruit or vegetable or both[d]	1–4 tbsp meat, fish, poultry, egg yolk, cooked dry beans or peas, or $1/_2$–2 oz cheese, or 1–4 oz (volume) cottage cheese, or 1–4 oz (weight) cheese food or cheese spread, and
		1–4 tbsp fruit or vegetable or both
Snack		
4–6 fl oz formula[a] or breast milk[b,c]	4–6 fl oz formula[a] or breast milk[b,c]	2–4 fl oz formula[a] or breast milk,[b,c] or fruit juice[e] and
		0 $1/_2$ bread[d,f] or 0–2 crackers[d,f]

[a] Infant formula and dry infant cereal must be iron-fortified.

[b] Breast milk or formula, or portions of both, may be served; however, it is recommended that breast milk be served in place of formula from birth through 11 months.

[c] For some breast-fed infants who regularly consume less than the minimum amount of breast milk per feeding, a serving of less than the minimum amount of breast milk may be offered, with additional breast milk offered if the infant is still hungry.

[d] A serving of this component is required when the infant is developmentally ready to accept it.

[e] Fruit juice must be full strength.

[f] A serving of this component must be made from whole grain or enriched meal or flour.

Source: From 7 CFR, Volume 4, Revised January 1, 2006. Part 226: Child and Adult Care Food Program. §226.20 Requirements for meals.

Box 13.14 Native Americans' Diets

American Indian families living on reservations are a significant component of the low-income rural population in many of the Western and Plains States. Many Native Americans' diets are based on government-provided commodities — foods that are very different from traditional native fare. Future research could reveal whether there is a difference in blood sugar control between those who consume a diet composed of traditional native foods and those who consume a diet of commodity foods. The University of Arizona's American Indian Studies Program (AISP) administers small grants for research on the food assistance and nutrition needs and problems of American Indians.

Source: RM Bliss. Breaking barriers to American Indian nutrition research. *Agricultural Research*, 2004; 52(July). Available at: http://www.ars.usda.gov/is/AR/archive/jul04/indian0704.htm. Accessed February 15, 2007.

---

to states, U.S. territories, and federally recognized Indian tribal governments to provide low-income seniors with coupons that can be exchanged for eligible foods at farmers' markets, roadside stands, and CSAs. The grant funds may be used only to support the costs of the foods that are provided under the SFMNP; no administrative funding is available. *Low-income seniors* are generally defined as individuals who are at least 60 years old and who have household incomes of not more than 185% of the federal poverty income guidelines. SFMNP benefits are provided to eligible recipients for use during the harvest season. (In some states, the SFMNP season is relatively short, because the growing season in that area is not very long. In other states with longer growing seasons, recipients have a longer period of time in which to use their SFMNP benefits.) In FY 2004, 802,000 low-income seniors received vouchers worth $10 to $20 per year.[92]

Once the SFMNP benefits have been issued to eligible seniors, they can be used to purchase fresh, nutritious, unprepared, locally grown fruits, vegetables, and herbs at authorized farmers' markets, roadside stands, and CSA programs. State agencies may limit SFMNP sales to specific foods that are locally grown, in order to encourage SFMNP recipients to support the farmers in their own states. There are certain foods not eligible for purchase with SFMNP benefits, including dried fruits or vegetables, such as prunes (dried plums), raisins (dried grapes), sun-dried tomatoes or dried chili peppers. Potted fruit or vegetable plants, potted or dried herbs, wild rice, any kind of nuts, honey, maple syrup, cider, and molasses are also not allowed.[93]

For FY 2006, grants were awarded to 46 state agencies and federally recognized Indian tribal governments. Included in the grants were 6 tribal governments (5 Sandoval Pueblos and the San Felipe Pueblo in New Mexico, the Osage Tribal Council in Oklahoma, the Mississippi Band of Choctaw Indians, the Chickasaw Nation in Oklahoma, and the Grand Traverse Indians in Michigan), Puerto Rico, the District of Columbia, and 38 additional states: Alabama, Alaska, Arkansas, California, Colorado, Connecticut, Florida, Hawaii, Illinois, Indiana, Iowa, Kansas, Kentucky, Louisiana, Maine, Maryland, Massachusetts, Michigan, Minnesota, Mississippi, Montana, Nebraska, Nevada, New Hampshire, New Jersey, New York, North Carolina, Ohio, Oregon, Pennsylvania, Rhode Island, South Carolina, Tennessee, Vermont, Virginia, Washington, West Virginia, and Wisconsin.

Box 13.15 Research Question

Research question: Determine the PART rating and OMB's recommendation for improvement for each of the government's major food assistance programs.

According to the Under Secretary of Agriculture in 2005, SFMNP is not likely to have a significant impact on the nutritional health of seniors nor a substantial impact on the market for agricultural commodities, farmers, farmers' markets, CSAs, or roadside stands without additional program funding. An analysis undertaken by FNS indicates that the pilot program has been beneficial in areas where the SFMNP operates; he therefore proposed making the program permanent and increasing the benefit from $20 to $50 per person per year.[94]

13.5.1.1.6 Special Milk Program

The Child Nutrition Act of 1966 authorized the Special Milk Program (SMP), which provides milk free of charge or at a low cost to children in schools and child care institutions that do not participate in other federal child nutrition meal service programs. This federally assisted program reimburses schools for the milk they serve. The federal reimbursement for each half-pint of milk sold to children in SY 2004–2005 was 17.0 cents. For children who receive their milk free, the USDA reimburses schools the net purchase price of the milk. Schools in the NSLP or SBP may also participate in the SMP to provide milk to children in half-day prekindergarten and kindergarten programs where children do not have access to the school meal programs. Expansion of the NSLP and SBP, which include milk, has led to a substantial reduction in the SMP since its peak in the late 1960s. The program served nearly 3 billion half-pints of milk in 1969, 1.8 billion in 1980, and 179 million in 1990. In FY 2003, the program served almost 108 million half-pints of milk at a cost of $14.4 million.

Schools or institutions may choose pasteurized fluid types of unflavored or flavored whole milk, low-fat milk, skim milk, and cultured buttermilk that meet state and local standards. All milk should contain vitamins A and D at levels specified by the Food and Drug Administration (FDA).[95]

13.5.1.1.7 Nutrition Services Incentive Program

The Nutrition Services Incentive Program (NSIP) provides for congregate and home-delivered meals and other nutrition services in a variety of settings, such as senior centers, schools, and in individual homes. Meals served must provide at least a third of the daily recommended intakes, but in practice, participants receive an estimated 40 to 50% of their recommended allowances. The program also provides a range of related services, by some of the aging network's estimated 4,000 nutrition service providers, including nutrition screening, assessment, education, and counseling. These services help older participants to identify their general and special nutrition needs, as they may relate to health concerns such as hypertension and diabetes. There is no means test for participation in the NSIP; services are targeted to older people with the greatest economic or social need, with special attention given to low-income minorities.

People at least 60 years of age, and their spouses (regardless of age), are eligible to receive congregate or home-delivered meals. Additional eligible persons include disabled or handicapped persons, not yet 60, who reside in housing facilities occupied primarily by the elderly and at which congregate meal service for the elderly is provided. Meals are also provided to individuals providing volunteer services during the meals hours.

Formerly the Nutrition Program for the Elderly (NPE), NSIP is administered by the AoA in the Department of HHS, but receives commodity foods (Table 13.13) and financial support from the FNS. NSIP was authorized by § 311 of the Older Americans Act (OAA) of 2000, as amended, and has been authorized in one form or another under the OAA since 1978. Originally, the program was administered by the USDA, which provided cash and/or commodities to supplement meals provided under the authority of the OAA. The Consolidated Appropriations Resolution, 2003, P.L. 108–7, amended the OAA to transfer the NSIP from the USDA to the AoA, which did not result in significant changes to the procedures for administering the program at the state, tribal, and local levels.

13.5.1.1.8 Commodity Distribution Programs

The USDA administers commodity distribution programs that are designed to benefit both agriculture and the low-income population. These programs serve the agricultural community by using

TABLE 13.13
Commodity Supplemental Food Program Commodities, 2005

Food Category	Example
Canned vegetables	Green beans, vegetarian beans, carrots, whole kernel corn, creamed corn, peas, pumpkin, spinach, sliced potatoes, sweet potatoes, tomatoes, and also dehydrated potatoes in boxes
Canned fruits	Applesauce, apricots, fruit cocktail, peaches, pairs, plums
Canned meats	Beef, chicken, pork, tuna
Canned juices	Apple, crabapple, grape, grapefruit, orange, pineapple, tomato
Dairy	Reduced-fat cheese loaves, canned evaporated milk, instant nonfat dry milk packages, powdered infant formula cans
Boxed grains	Rice and oat ready-to-eat cereals, grits, farina, spaghetti, macaroni, oats, rice, infant rice cereal
Packaged dry beans	Blackeye, baby lima, light kidney, great northern, pinto
Oils	Peanut butter in jars
Miscellaneous	Egg mix in packages

Source: From USDA Food and Nutrition Service. *2005 CSFP Commodities.* January 27, 2005. Available at: http://www.fns.usda.gov/fdd/foods/fy05-csfpfoods.pdf. Accessed May 7, 2005.

surplus commodities purchased by the USDA from farmers and other producers. The programs help reduce federal food inventories and storage costs, whereas assisting the needy.

13.5.1.1.8.1 Emergency Food Assistance Program (TEFAP)
The USDA determined that 2.3 million low-income households were food insecure with hunger in 2004. This means that they reported multiple indicators of reduced food intake and disrupted eating patterns due to lack of money or other resources at some point during the year. TEFAP helps supplement the diets of low-income Americans, including elderly people, by providing them with emergency food and nutrition assistance at no cost. State agencies receive the food and supervise overall distribution. Two types of public or private nonprofit groups are eligible to receive assistance from TEFAP. They are:

- Organizations that provide food and nutrition assistance to the needy through the distribution of food for home use or the preparation of meals to be served in a congregate setting. Organizations that distribute food for home use must determine the household's eligibility by applying the income standards that are set by the state.
- Organizations that provide prepared meals are eligible to receive commodities if they can demonstrate that they serve predominately needy persons.

TEFAP is a means-tested program with income eligibility requirements, set by the states, typically between 100 and 155% of the federal poverty threshold. Recipients include some of the vulnerable populations of the elderly, children, working families, and people who are homeless. Regarding households that meet state eligibility criteria, each state sets criteria for determining what households are eligible to receive food for home consumption. Income standards may, at the state's discretion, be met through participation in other existing federal, state, local food, health, or welfare programs for which eligibility is based on income. States can adjust the income criteria in order to ensure that assistance is provided only to those households most in need. However, recipients of prepared meals are considered to be needy and are not subject to a means test.

TEFAP was first authorized as the Temporary Emergency Food Assistance Program in 1981 to distribute surplus commodities to households. The name was changed to the Emergency Food Assistance Program under the 1990 farm bill. Congress appropriated $189.5 million for TEFAP for FY 2006 — $140 million to purchase food and another $49.5 million for administrative support for state and local agencies.

13.5.1.1.8.2 Food Distribution Program on Indian Reservations (FDPIR)

The USDA provides financial assistance to Native Americans via an assortment of programs and services, one of which is the FDPIR, an alternative to the FSP. In 1977, Congress established FDPIR to provide supplemental food to low-income households living on or near rural American Indian reservations as an acceptable alternative to FSP benefits. Because of the remote and geographically dispersed locations of many reservations and other Indian lands, many otherwise eligible American Indian families have been unable to participate in the FSP, as access to food stamp offices and grocery stores has been difficult.

Through FDPIR, commodity foods are provided to low-income households, including the elderly, living on Indian reservations, and to Native American families residing in designated areas near reservations. FDPIR is administered at the federal level by the FNS, and it is administered locally by either ITOs or an agency of a state government. There are approximately 257 tribes receiving benefits under the FDPIR through 97 ITOs and 5 state agencies. The USDA purchases and ships commodities to the ITOs and state agencies based on their orders from a list of available foods. These administering agencies store and distribute the food, determine applicant eligibility, and provide nutrition education to recipients. Each month, participating households receive a food package to help them maintain a nutritionally balanced diet. Participants may select from over 70 products. The USDA provides the administering agencies with funds for program administrative costs.

Average monthly participation for FY 2005 was about 100,000 individuals. In FY 2006, $82.5 million was appropriated for FDPIR, approximately $25 million for the federal share of local level administrative costs (generally, 75% of all allowable administrative costs incurred), and the remainder for food purchases, including no less than $3 million for a special purchase of bison meat. The USDA purchases most foods distributed in the program with FDPIR appropriations; however, some commodities offered through FDPIR may be donated to the program from agricultural surpluses.

Unmet needs. A study conducted by the U.S. Commission on Civil Rights in 2003 examines federal funding of programs intended to assist Native Americans. The commission's report reveals that funding directed to Native Americans through FDPIR, as well as other programs, has not been sufficient to address the basic and urgent needs of indigenous peoples. For example, between 1995 and 1997, 22.2% of Native American households were hungry or on the edge of hunger (food insecure), more than twice the rate of the population as a whole. Recall that the USDA defines "food insecurity" as a shortage of resources leading to outright hunger or to such other serious problems resulting from low incomes as the family being unable to purchase a balanced diet or enough food for the children, or the parents skipping meals so that the children can eat. Overall, 8.6% of the Native American households reported that they were suffering from hunger, also more than double the nationwide rate. The commission found that significant disparities in federal funding exist between Native Americans and other groups in the U.S., as well as the general population. The commission recommends that the USDA and other federal agencies administering Native American programs identify and regularly assess the unmet needs of American Indians. Through laws, treaties, and policies established over hundreds of years, the federal government is obligated to ensure that funding is adequate to meet these needs.[96]

13.5.1.1.9 Food Assistance for Disaster Relief

FNS is responsible for providing nutrition assistance for disaster-affected areas requiring a federal response. In the aftermath of a major disaster or emergency, FNS coordinates with state, local, and voluntary organizations (as well as with other federal agencies) to determine potential nutrition assistance needs of disaster victims.

Agencies of the USDA help in many ways in a disaster, but perhaps the most immediate is to ensure that people have enough to eat. Following a storm, earthquake, civil disturbance, flood or other disaster, it is vital to provide food to people who find themselves suddenly in need. Through its FNS, the USDA assists by providing commodity foods for shelters and other mass-feeding sites, distributing commodity food packages directly to households in need, and issuing emergency food stamps. The Food Distribution Division of the FNS has the primary responsibility of supplying food to disaster relief organizations for mass feeding or household distribution.

In an emergency, disaster relief agencies such as the Red Cross and the Salvation Army request food and nutrition assistance through state agencies that run the USDA's nutrition assistance programs. The state agencies, in turn, notify the USDA of the types and quantities of food needed by the relief organizations for emergency feeding operations. Every state and U.S. territory has on hand stocks of commodity foods that are used for USDA-sponsored food programs. The Child Nutrition Commodity Support Program, which includes the NSLP, TEFAP, and the FDPIR are some of the USDA programs for which states maintain stocks of commodity foods. In an emergency, the USDA can authorize states to release their food stocks to disaster relief organizations to feed people at shelters and mass-feeding sites. If the president declares a disaster, states can distribute commodity foods directly to households that are in need as a result of an emergency, and the USDA can authorize the issuance of emergency food stamps when regular commercial food supply channels have been restored. In order for a disaster FSP to be established, states must request that the USDA allow them to issue emergency food stamps in areas affected by a disaster. The disaster food stamp system operates under a different set of eligibility and benefit delivery requirements than the regular FSP; people who might not ordinarily qualify for food stamps may be eligible under the disaster FSP. In FY 2002, disaster food stamp benefits totaled $21.4 million, and the value of emergency commodities distributed was almost three-quarters of a million dollars.

13.5.1.1.10 Commodity Supplemental Food Program (CSFP)

The Commodity Supplemental Food Program (CSFP) worked to improve the health of low-income pregnant and breastfeeding women, other new mothers up to one year postpartum, infants, children up to age 6, and elderly people at least 60 years of age, by supplementing their diets with nutritious USDA commodity foods. It provided food and administrative funds to states to supplement the diets of low-income women, infants, children, and elderly in selected sites in 32 states, the District of Columbia, and on 2 Indian reservations. The state and tribal grantees operated the program directly or through local agencies. Funding for CSFP (most recently, $107 million in 2006) was eliminated in 2007 because the program duplicated benefits offered by WIC and the FSPs. The 2007 budget provides funding to serve all eligible women, infants, and children who seek services from the WIC program, which is a more effective alternative to CSFP. The budget also funds temporary transitional benefits and outreach to help elderly households transition from CSFP to the FSP.[97] The elimination of CSFP was consistent with the program's low assessment using the Program Assessment Rating Tool (PART). The program's low rating indicated that it was not able to develop acceptable performance goals or collect data to determine whether it was performing.

13.5.1.1.11 Program Assessment Rating Tool

The PART was developed by the U.S. Office of Management and Budget (OMB) to assess and improve program performance so that the U.S. government can achieve better results. A PART review helps identify a program's strengths and weaknesses to inform funding and management decisions aimed at making the program more effective. The PART therefore looks at all factors that affect and reflect program performance, including program purpose and design, performance measurement, evaluations and strategic planning, program management, and program results. Because the PART includes a consistent series of analytical questions, it allows programs to show improvements over time and allows comparisons between similar programs. Programs are evaluated on the basis of performing (effective, moderately effective, or adequate) or not performing (ineffective or results not demonstrated). Nearly 800 PART program assessments are available on ExpectMore.gov, which was launched in 2006 to report on federal program performance and what is being done to improve results.[98]

13.6 NONGOVERNMENT, NONPROFIT ORGANIZATIONS

In addition to the federal food assistance programs administered by the USDA's FNS, hundreds of nongovernmental, nonprofit organizations exist, which work to end hunger in the U.S. America's Second Harvest is the largest charitable hunger-relief organization in the U.S., with a network of more than 200 member food banks and food-rescue organizations serving all 50 states, the District of Columbia, and Puerto Rico. America's Second Harvest Network supports approximately 50,000 local charitable agencies operating more than 94,000 programs, including food pantries, soup kitchens, emergency shelters, and after-school programs (see Box 13.16).

Box 13.16 The First Food Bank

John van Hengel was a soup-kitchen volunteer in 1967 when he founded the first food bank with a truckload of produce gleaned from Arizona farm fields and citrus groves. Soup kitchens and community food pantries have existed for more than a century, but the idea of a food bank took van Hengel's modest local efforts and made them bigger and more reliable. The key was creating a distribution network, convinced corporations that their donated food would be safely handled and would not be resold. In addition, businesses were able to cut the costs of disposing or storing unusable food, take a tax break, and satisfy multiple charities through a single point of contact. His idea grew into a nationwide network of food banks that converts food industry leftovers into meals for the poor. That network, America's Second Harvest, distributes 2 billion pounds of groceries that annually feed 23 million Americans. Currently, the program supports about 50,000 charitable agencies operating more than 94,000 programs, including food pantries, soup kitchens, emergency shelters, and after-school programs.

Working at a soup kitchen in Phoenix, van Hengel often searched in supermarket refuse bins for his own food. van Hengel credited his seminal idea to a woman with 10 children and a husband on death row whom he met while "dumpster diving" for food in refuse bins behind grocery stores. She suggested that what was really needed was a place to both deposit food and check it out — "like a bank." Finding edible, if not salable, food, he persuaded a grocery store manager, and then the manager's boss, to donate surplus food. Soon he and his helpers had more food than they could use, so they started delivering the excess to missions, alcoholism treatment centers, and abused women's shelters. He tried unsuccessfully to persuade several religious and nonprofit organizations in Phoenix to start a warehouse food bank. Finally, a downtown Phoenix church gave him an abandoned bakery, and church members contributed $3,000 for utility bills. St. Mary's Food Bank, which still operates, distributed more than 250,000 lb of food to 36 charities in its first year of operation. In 1975, he accepted a grant to set up 18 food banks; America's Second Harvest incorporated the next year. The timing was auspicious, as the new Tax Reform Act gave corporations tax benefits if they donated inventory to charity.

Source: From Sullivan, P. Obituary. John van Hengel Dies at 83; Founded 1st Food Bank in 1967. *Washington Post.* October 8, 2005, p. B06.

13.7 CONCLUSION

Ensuring food security for at-risk populations, such as the elderly and low-income women and children, has become an enormous undertaking, operating largely under the aegis of the USDA and augmented by nongovernmental organizations such as America's Second Harvest. Programs range from WIC to FSP to Head Start to day care for the elderly. The NSLP alone serves billions of meals each year. As it is not sufficient to provide just any food, programs such as Team Nutrition have been instituted to improve nutrition education in schools receiving assistance from the USDA. In addition, efforts are being made to enhance the quality of the food itself by supporting local farms and delivering fresh fruits and vegetables directly to schools.

13.8 ACRONYMS

AoA	Administration on Aging
BMI	Body Mass Index
CACFP	Child and Adult Care Food Program
CFNP	Community Food and Nutrition Program
CNPP	Center for Nutrition Policy and Promotion
CSA	Community Supported Agriculture
CSFP	Commodity Supplemental Food Program
DHS	Department of Homeland Security
DoD	Department of Defense
EBT	Electronic benefits transfer
EFNEP	Expanded Food and Nutrition Education Program
ERS	Economic Research Service (of USDA)
FDPIR	Food Distribution Program on Indian Reservations
FMNP	Farmers' Market Nutrition Program
FNCS	Food, Nutrition, and Consumer Services
FNS	Food and Nutrition Service (of USDA)
FSNC	Food Stamp Nutrition Connection
FSNE	Food Stamp Nutrition Education
FSP	Food Stamp Program
FSRIA	Farm Security and Rural Investment Act
FY	Fiscal year
HEI	Healthy Eating Index
HHS	Department of Health and Human Services
IOM	Institute of Medicine
ITO	Indian Tribal Organization
NET	Nutrition Education and Training
NHANES	National Health and Nutrition Examination Survey
NPE	Nutrition Program for the Elderly
NSIP	Nutrition Services Incentive Program
NSLA	Richard B. Russell National School Lunch Act
NSLP	National School Lunch Program
PRWORA	Personal Responsibility and Work Opportunity Reconciliation Act
RDA	Recommended Daily Allowance
SBP	School Breakfast Program SBP
SFMNP	Seniors Farmers' Market Nutrition Program
SFSP	School Food Services Program
SMP	Special Milk Program
SY	School year
TANF	Temporary Assistance for Needy Families
TEFAP	The Emergency Food Assistance Program
USDA	United States Department of Agriculture
WIC	Supplemental Nutrition Program for Women, Infants, and Children

REFERENCES

1. Nord, M., Andrews, M., and Carlson, S. *Household Food Security in the United States, 2004.* Economic Research Service, U.S. Department of Agriculture, Economic Research Report No. (ERR11). October 2005. Available at: http://www.ers.usda.gov/Publications/err11/.Accessed July 7, 2006.
2. Kantor, L.S. Community food security programs improve food access. *FoodReview.* 24(1), 20–26, 2001.
3. Hamm, M.W. and Bellows, A.C. Community food security and nutrition educators. *J Nutr Educ Behav.* 35, 37–43, 2003.
4. McCullum, C., Desjardins, E., Kraak, V.I., Ladipo, P., and Costello, H. Evidence-based strategies to build community food security. *J Am Diet Assoc.* 105, 278–283, 2005.
5. Rome Declaration on World Food Security and World Food Summit Plan of Action. November 1996. FAO corporate Document Repository. 1998. Available at: http://www.fao.org/docrep/003/w3613e/w3613e00.HTM. Accessed July 7, 2006.
6. DeNavas-Walt, C., Proctor, B.D., and Lee, C.H., U.S. Census Bureau. Current Population Reports, P60-229, *Income, Poverty, and Health Insurance Coverage in the United States: 2004.* Washington, D.C., 2005.
7. Fox, M.K., Cole, N., with Lin, B.-H. *Nutrition and Health Characteristics of Low-Income Populations: Volume I, Food Stamp Program Participants and Nonparticipants.* USDA Economic Research Service. E-FAN-04014-1, December 2004. Available at: http://www.ers.usda.gov/Publications/efan04014-1/. Accessed April 7, 2005.
8. USDA Economic Research Service. Food Security in the United States: Measuring Household Food Security. Available at: http://www.ers.usda.gov/Briefing/FoodSecurity/measurement/. Accessed April 6, 2005.
9. Nord, M., Andrews, M., and Carlson, S. *Household Food Security in the United States, 2003.* Food Assistance and Nutrition Research Report No. (FANRR42), 2004.
10. Alaimo, K., Olson, C.M., and Frongillo, E.A., Jr. Food insufficiency and American school-aged children's cognitive, academic, and psychosocial development. *Pediatrics.* 108, 44–53, 2001. Erratum in *Pediatrics.* 108, 824b, 2001. Available at: http://pediatrics.aappublications.org/cgi/content/full/108/1/44. Accessed April 6, 2005.
11. Kleinman, R.E., Hall, S., Green, H., Korzec-Ramirez, D., Patton, K., Pagano, M.E., Murphy, J.M. Diet, breakfast, and academic performance in children. *Ann Nutr Metab.* 46(S1), 24–30, 2002. Available at: http://content.karger.com/ProdukteDB/produkte.asp?Aktion=ShowPDF&ArtikelNr=66399&ProduktNr=223977&Ausgabe=228739&filename=66399.pdf. Accessed April 6, 2005.
12. Casey, P.H., Szeto, K.L., Robbins, J.M., Stuff, J.E., Connell, C., Gossett, J.M., and Simpson, P.M. Child health-related quality of life and household food security. *Arch Pediatr Adolesc Med.* 159, 51–56, 2005. Available at: http://archpedi.ama-assn.org/cgi/content/full/159/1/51. Accessed April 6, 2005.
13. Nord, M., Andrews, M., and Carlson, S. *Household Food Security in the United States, 2004.* U.S. Department of Agriculture, Economic Research Service Food Assistance and Nutrition Research Report Number 11. 2005. Available at: http://www.ers.usda.gov/publications/err11/err11.pdf. Accessed July 23, 2006.
14. The Bush Administration's FY 2007 Budget. Available at: http://national.unitedway.org/files/pdf/07budgetsummary.pdf. Accessed July 27, 2006.
15. United States Code. Title 7 — Agriculture. Chapter 55 — Department of Agriculture. Establishment of Department. Available at: http://www.washingtonwatchdog.org/documents/usc/ttl7/ch55/sec 2201.html. Accessed April 18, 2005.
16. USDA. USDA Strategic Plan for FY 2002–2007. September 2002. Available at: http://www.usda.gov/ocfo/usdasp/pdf/sp2002.pdf. Accessed April 17, 2005.
17. USDA. FY 2006 Budget Summary and Annual Performance Plan. Available at: http://www.usda.gov/agency/obpa/Budget-Summary/2006/FY06budsum.pdf. Accessed April 17, 2005.
18. USDA. FY 2004 Annual Performance Plan and Revised Performance Plan for 2003. May 2003. Available at: http://www.usda.gov/ocfo/usdaap/pdf/ap2004.pdf. Accessed April 11, 2005.
19. USDA. Food, Nutrition, and Consumer Services homepage. Available at: http://www.fns.usda.gov/fncs/. Accessed April 17, 2005.
20. USDA. Food and Nutrition Service. Office of Analysis, Nutrition and Evaluation. FNS Strategic Plan. Available at: http://www.fns.usda.gov/oane/menu/gpra/fnsstrategicplan.htm. Accessed April 17, 2005.

21. USDA. Economic Research Service. The Food Assistance Landscape. Food Assistance and Nutrition Research Report Number 28-6, March 2005. Available at: http://www.ers.usda.gov/publications/fanrr 28-6/fanrr28-6.pdf. Accessed April 17, 2005.

22. USDA. Food and Nutrition Service. Nutrition Assistance Programs. Available at: http://www.fns. usda.gov/fns/. Accessed April 17, 2005.

23. http://agriculture.senate.gov/Legislation/Compilations/FNS/FSA77.pdf.

24. USDA Food and Nutrition Service. Food Stamp Program: Average Monthly Benefit per Person. Available at: http://www.fns.usda.gov/pd/fsavgben.htm. Accessed April 11, 2005.

25. USDA Food and Nutrition Service. Food Stamp Program: Average Monthly Benefit per Household. Available at: http://www.fns.usda.gov/pd/fsavghh$.htm. Accessed April 11, 2005.

26. U.S. Department of Agriculture. Food Stamp Program Quality Control Review Handbook. FNS Handbook 310. Alexandria Virginia: Food and Nutrition Service, 2003. Available at: http://www.fns. usda.gov/fsp/qc/pdfs/310_Handbook_2004.pdf. Accessed July 24, 2006.

27. USDA. 2007 Budget Summary and Annual Performance Plan. Available at: http://www.usda. gov/agency/obpa/ Budget-Summary/2007/FY07budsum.pdf. Accessed July 24, 2006.

28. U.S. Department of Agriculture. Impact of Food Stamp Payment Errors on Household Purchasing Power. Food and Nutrition Service. Office of Analysis, Nutrition and Evaluation. 2003. Available at: http://www.fns. usda.gov/oane/MENU/Published/FSP/FILES/ProgramIntegrity/HouseholdWell-Being.pdf. Accessed July 24, 2006.

29. Cunnyngham, K. Food Stamp Program Participation Rates: 2003. Mathematica Policy Research, Inc. Available at: http://www.fns.usda.gov/oane/menu/Published/FSP/FILES/Participation/FSPPart2003.pdf. Accessed July 24, 2006.

30. Cunnyngham, K. Trends in Food Stamp Program Participation Rates: 1999 to 2002. Available at: Accessed April 11, 2005.

31. Cunnyngham, K. Food Stamp Program Participation Rates: 2003. Mathematica Policy Research, Inc. Available at: http://www.fns.usda.gov/oane/menu/Published/FSP/FILES/Participation/FSPPart2003.pdf. Accessed July 24, 2006.

32. USDA. FY 2004 Annual Performance Plan and Revised Performance Plan for 2003. May 2003. Available at: http://www.usda.gov/ocfo/usdaap/pdf/ap2004.pdf. Accessed April 11, 2005.

33. USDA Food and Nutrition Service. *Food Stamp Program State Outreach Plan Guidance*. Available at: http://www.fns.usda.gov/fsp/outreach/pdfs/Outreach_Plan_Guidance.pdf. Accessed April 11, 2005.

34. USDA Food and Nutrition Service. Food Stamp Outreach. Available at: http://www.fns.usda.gov/fsp/ outreach/default.htm. Accessed April 11, 2005.

35. Capps, R., Koralek, R., Lotspeich, K., Fix, M.E., Holcomb, P.A., and Reardon-Anderson, J. Assessing Implementation of the 2002 Farm Bill's Legal Immigrant Food Stamp Restorations: Final Report to the United States Department of Agriculture Food and Nutrition Science. Urban Institute. November 2004. Available at: http://www.urban.org/urlprint.cfm?ID=9158. Accessed April 11, 2005.

36. Wilde, P. and Dagata, E. Food stamp participation by eligible older Americans remains low. *FoodReview*. 25(Summer-Fall), 25–29, 2002. Available at: http://www.ers.usda.gov/publications/FoodReview/ Sep2002/frvol25i2e.pdf. Accessed April 12, 2005.

37. Cunnyngham, K. Food Stamp Program Participation Rates: 2003. Mathematica Policy Research, Inc. Available at: http://www.fns.usda.gov/oane/menu/Published/FSP/FILES/Participation/FSPPart2003.pdf. Accessed July 24, 2006.

38. Gabor, V., Williams, S.S., Bellamy, H., and Hardison, B.L. Seniors' Views of the Food Stamp Program and Ways To Improve Participation — Focus Group Findings in Washington State: Final Report. E-FAN No. (02-012), June 2002. Available at: Accessed April 12, 2005.

39. USDA. Food Stamp Nutrition Education Plan Guidance. Federal Fiscal Year 2006. Food and Nutrition Service. Food Stamp Program. March 2005. Available at: http://www.nal.usda.gov/foodstamp/programplan/ FSNE_Plan_Guidance_06.pdf. Accessed April 12, 2005.

40. USDA National Agricultural Library. Food Stamp Nutrition Connection homepage. Available at: http://www.nal.usda.gov/foodstamp/index.html. Accessed April 12, 2005.

41. USDA. Food and Nutrition Service. Request for comments on whether the Food Stamp Program should be renamed. *Federal Register*. 69(119), June 22, 2004, pp. 34637–34638. Available at: http://www.fns.usda.gov/cga/Federal-Register/2004/062204.pdf. Accessed April 7, 2005.

42. USDA. 2007 Budget Summary and Annual Performance Plan. Available at: http://www.usda.gov/agency/obpa/Budget-Summary/2007/FY07budsum.pdf. Accessed July 24, 2006.

43. Gunderson, G.W. *The National School Lunch Program: Background and Development.* Washington, D.C. 1971 0-429-783. Available at: http://www.cde.state.co.us/cdenutritran/download/pdf/SEC26.pdf. Accessed April 16, 2005.

44. P.L. 79-396, Approved June 4, 1946 (60 Stat. 239). Available at: http://www.ssa.gov/OP_Home/comp2/F079-396.html. Accessed April 16, 2005.

45. Fox, M.K., Hamilton, W., and Lin, B.-H. National School Lunch Program. *Effects of Food Assistance and Nutrition Programs on Nutrition and Health, Vol. 3 Literature Review.* Food Assistance and Nutrition Research Report No. (FANRR19-3), December 2004, chap. 5. Available at: http://www.ers.usda.gov/publications/fanrr19-3/fanrr19-3e.pdf. Accessed April 16, 2005.

46. Fox, M.K., Hamilton, W., and Lin, B.-H. National School Lunch Program. *Effects of Food Assistance and Nutrition Programs on Nutrition and Health, Vol. 3 Literature Review.* Food Assistance and Nutrition Research Report No. (FANRR19-3), December 2004, chap. 5. Available at: http://www.ers.usda.gov/publications/fanrr19-3/fanrr19-3e.pdf. Accessed April 16, 2005.

47. USDA. Food and Nutrition Service. Food Distribution Division. History of the Food Distribution Programs. Available at: Accessed April 18, 2005.

48. USDA. Food and Nutrition Service. Food Distribution Programs. School/Child Nutrition Commodity Programs. Available at: http://www.fns.usda.gov/fdd/faqs/schcnpfaqs.htm. Accessed April 18, 2005.

49. USDA. Farm Service Agency. Agricultural Marketing Service. Food and Consumer Service. *Improving USDA Commodities.* October 1995. Tri-Agency Commodity Specification Review Report. Available at: http://www.fns.usda.gov/fdd/caps/1995impvcomodrpt.PDF. Accessed April 18, 2005.

50. USDA. Food and Nutrition Service. Title 7-Agriculture. What are the nutrition standards and menu planning approaches for lunches and the requirements for afterschool snacks? Sec. 210.10(c) *Code of Federal Regulations.* Title 7, Vol. 4. Chapter II-Food and Nutrition Service. Revised as of January 1, 2003. pp. 21–37. Available at: http://a257.g.akamaitech.net/7/257/2422/14mar20010800/edocket.access.gpo.gov/cfr_2003/pdf/7CFR210.10.pdf. Accessed April 18, 2005.

51. Public Law 108-265. S 2507. HR 3873. Child Nutrition and WIC Reauthorization Act of 2004. June 30, 2004. Available at: http://www.fns.usda.gov/cnd/Governance/Legislation/PL_108-265.pdf. Accessed April 19, 2005.

52. USDA. Food and Nutrition Service. Local Wellness Policy. Team Nutrition. Available at: http://www.fns.usda.gov/tn/Healthy/wellnesspolicy.html. Accessed April 20, 2005.

53. Buzby, J.C., Guthrie, J.F., and Kantor, L.S. Evaluation of the USDA Fruit and Vegetable Pilot Program: Report to Congress. E-FAN No. 03-006. USDA, Economic Research Service. May 2003. Available at: http://www.ers.usda.gov/publications/efan03006/efan03006.pdf. Accessed April 19, 2005.

54. School Nutrition Association. Background Information for 2005 Legislative Issues Paper. Available at: http://www.schoolnutrition.org/uploadedFiles/ASFSA/childnutrition/govtaffairs/2005 issuepaperbg.pdf. Accessed April 20, 2005.

55. Public Law 108–265. S. 2507. H.R. 3873. Child Nutrition and WIC Reauthorization Act of 2004. June 30, 2004. Available at: http://www.fns.usda.gov/cnd/Governance/Legislation/PL_108-265.pdf. Accessed April 19, 2005.

56. HR 2626. Farm-To-Cafeteria Projects Act of 2003. June 26, 2003. Available at: http://thomas.loc.gov/cgi-bin/query/z?c108:H.R.2626.IH. Accessed April 20, 2005.

57. Occidental College. Urban and Environmental Policy Institute. Center for Food and Justice. National Farm to School Program. Available at: http://www.farmtoschool.org/. Accessed April 20, 2005.

58. Sanger, K. and Zenz, L. Farm-to-cafeteria connections: marketing opportunities for small farms in Washington State. Washington State Department of Agriculture, Small Farm and Direct Marketing Program. January 2004. Available at: http://agr.wa.gov/Marketing/SmallFarm/102-FarmToCafeteria Connections_Web.pdf. Accessed October 29, 2005.

59. Okie, S. Eating lessons at school. In *Fed Up! Winning the War against Childhood Obesity.* The National Academies Press, chap. 7. www.nap.edu/books/0309093104/html/183.html. Accessed September 23, 2005.

60. Community Food Security: Innovative Programs for Addressing Common Community Problems. Farm to cafeteria. Available at: www.reinvestinginamerica.org/faqs/ria_064.asp. Accessed October 30, 2005.

61. Sanger, K. and Zenz, L. Farm-to-cafeteria connections: marketing opportunities for small farms in Washington State. Washington State Department of Agriculture, Small Farm and Direct Marketing Program. January 2004. Available at: http://agr.wa.gov/Marketing/SmallFarm/102-FarmToCafeteria Connections_Web.pdf.

62. Sullivan, D. Expanding farm-to-school programs create opportunities for farmers...and children. Available at: www.newfarm.org. Accessed October 30, 2005.

63. Biemiller, L. Fresh from the farm. *Chron Higher Ed.* 52(November 25), A36–A38, 2005.

64. Sanger, K. and Zenz, L. Farm-to-cafeteria connections: marketing opportunities for small farms in Washington State. Washington State Department of Agriculture, Small Farm and Direct Marketing Program. January 2004. Available at: http://agr.wa.gov/Marketing/SmallFarm/102-FarmToCafeteria Connections_Web.pdf.

65. Benbrook, C. Elevating antioxidant levels in food through organic farming and food processing. The Organic Center for Education and Promotion, State of Science Review Number 2, Executive Summary. January 2005. Available at http://www.organic-center.org/science.htm?groupdid=16&articleid=541. Accessed December 5, 2005.

66. Worthington, V. Nutritional quality of organic versus conventional fruits, vegetables, and grains. *J Alternative Complementary Med.* 7, 161–173, 2001.

67. Gussow, J. *Is organic food more nutritious? And, is that the right question?* Available at: http://www.sare. org/sanet-mg/archives/html-home/38-html/0190.html. Accessed July 24, 2006.

68. Nestle, M. *What to Eat.* New York: North Point Press, 2006, p. 55.

69. Sanger, K. and Zenz, L. Farm-to-cafeteria connections: marketing opportunities for small farms in Washington State. Washington State Department of Agriculture, Small Farm and Direct Marketing Program. January 2004. Available at: http://agr.wa.gov/Marketing/SmallFarm/102-FarmToCafeteria Connections_Web.pdf.

70. Gottlieb, R. and Azuma, A. Healthy schools/healthy communities: opportunities and challenges for improving school and community environments. Urban and Environmental Policy Institute, Occidental College. Available at: www.niehs.gov/drept/beaconf/postconf.overview/gottlieb.pdf. Accessed October 30, 2005.

71. Morris, J.L., Neustadter, Zidenbery-Cherr, S. First-Grade Gardeners More Likely to Taste Vegetables. Available at: http://californiaagriculture.ucap.edu/0101JF/pdf/kids.pdf. Accessed September 26, 2005.

72. Morris, J.L. and Zidenberg-Cherr, S. Garden-enhanced nutrition curriculum improves fourth-grade school children's knowledge of nutrition and preferences for some vegetables. *J Am Diet Assoc.* 102, 91–93, 2002.

73. www.edibleschoolyard.org. Accessed December 10, 2005.

74. Yale University. Sustainable Food Project homepage. Available at: www.yale.edu/sustainablefood/overview.html. Accessed February 17, 2007.

75. Martin, A. Students lead charge for local and organic foods. *Chicago Tribune.* April 24, 2004. Available at: www.organicconsumers.org/BTC/students042505.cfn. Accessed November 8, 2005.

76. Biemiller, L. Fresh from the farm. *Chron Higher Ed.* 52(November 25), A36–A38, 2005.

77. Community Food Security Coalition. Farm to College. Available at: www.farmtocollege.org. Accessed October 30, 2005.

78. Sanger, K. and Zenz, L. Farm-to-cafeteria connections: marketing opportunities for small farms in Washington State. Washington State Department of Agriculture, Small Farm and Direct Marketing Program. January 2004. Available at: http://agr.wa.gov/Marketing/SmallFarm/102-FarmTo Cafeteria Connections_Web.pdf.

79. Biemiller, L. Fresh from the farm. *Chron Higher Ed.* 52(November 25), A36–A38, 2005.

80. Sullivan, D. Expanding farm-to-school programs create opportunities for farmers...and children. Available at: www.newfarm.org. Accessed October 30, 2005.

81. Demas, A. Low-fat school lunch programs: achieving acceptance. *Am J Cardiol.* 82, 80T–82T, 1998.

82. Section-by-section summary of provisions affecting special nutrition programs. U.S. Department of Agriculture, Food and Nutrition Service, Newsroom. Available at: www.fns.usda.gov/cga/ 2002_Farm_Bill/special_nutrition.html. Accessed December 11, 2005.

83. Vallianatos, M. Healthy school food policies: a checklist. A working paper of the Center for Food and Justice, Urban and Environmental Policy Institute. June 2005. Version 1.5.

84. PL 108–265, June 30, 2004.

85. Analysis of Summer Food Service Program and food needs of nonparticipating children. Executive Summary. Available at: http://www.fns.usda.gov/OANE/MENU/Published/CNP/FILES/SFSPFood-Needs-ExecSum.htm. Accessed July 27, 2006.

86. *Code of Federal Regulations*. Title 7 (Agriculture), Volume 4, Chapter II (Food and Nutrition Service, Department of Agriculture, Part 246-Special Supplemental Nutrition Program for Women, Infants and Children), Subpart A General), Sec 246.1, p. 305, Washington, D.C.. Revised January 1, 2004.

87. Institute of Medicine. *WIC Food Packages: Time for a Change*. Washington, D.C.: National Academies Press, 2005. Available at: http://www.fns.usda.gov/oane/menu/Published/WIC/FILES/Time4AChange (mainrpt).pdf. Accessed July 27, 2006.

88. Institute of Medicine. *Proposed Criteria for Selecting the WIC Food Packages*. Washington, D.C.: National Academies Press, 20004. Available at: http://www.nap.edu/catalog/11078.html. Accessed July 27, 2006.

89. U.S. Department of Agriculture. Summary of FY2006 Grants WIC. Food and Nutrition Services. Available at: http://www.fns.usda.gov/wic/fundingandprogramdata/grants2006.htm. Accessed July 27, 2006.

90. WIC monthly program data, 2003–2006. Available at: http://www.fns.usda.gov/pd/WIC_Monthly.htm. Accessed July 28, 2006.

91. U.S. Department of Agriculture. *Feeding Infants: A Guide for Use in the Child Nutrition Programs*. Food and Nutrition Service. FNS 258. 2002. Available at: http://www.fns.usda.gov/tn/Resources/feeding_infants.pdf. Accessed July 27, 2006.

92. 7 CFR Ch. II (1-1-06 Edition). § 248.10.

93. U.S. Department of Agriculture. Senior Farmers' Market Nutrition Program. Available at: http://www.fns.usda.gov/wic/SeniorFMNP/SFMNPmenu.htm. Accessed July 28, 2006.

94. U.S. Department of Agriculture. 7 CFR Part 249. Senior Farmers' Market Nutrition Program Regulations: Proposed Rule. May 26, 2006. Available at: http://www.fns.usda.gov/wic/regspublished/SFMNPproposedrule249.pdf. Accessed July 28, 2006.

95. U.S. Department of Agriculture. Special Milk Program. Available at: http://www.fns.usda.gov/cnd/milk. Accessed July 28, 2006.

96. U.S. Commission on Civil Rights. Federal Funding and Unmet Needs in Indian Country. July 2003. Available at: http://www.usccr.gov/pubs/na0703/na0204.pdf. Accessed July 28, 2006.

97. *Budget of the United States Government. Fiscal Year 2007* Available at: http://www.whitehouse.gov/omb/budget/fy2007/agriculture.html. Accessed July 27, 2006.

98. Office of Budget and Management. ExpectMore.gov. Accessed July 27, 2007.

14 Social Marketing and Other Mass Communication Techniques

Health communication contributes to improving the public's health through public education campaigns that create awareness, alter the social climate, change attitudes, and motivate individuals to adopt recommended behaviors. Campaigns traditionally have relied on mass communication (such as public service announcements on billboards, radio, and television) and in the form of printed educational materials such as pamphlets and fact sheets. Other campaigns have integrated mass media with community-based programs. Health communication supports community-centered prevention, which shifts attention from individual to group-level change and emphasizes the ability of communities and the individuals comprising those communities to effect change on multiple levels. Increasingly, health promotion activities take advantage of digital technologies, such as the World Wide Web to target audiences, tailor messages, and engage people in interactive, ongoing exchanges about health. The fairly new technique of tailored health communication offers individuals health information and behavior change tips based on their unique characteristics. An entire chapter of *Healthy People 2010* is devoted to examining the role of health communication for individuals and for the community. As for individuals, health communication determines relations between patients and health professionals; affects exposure to, search for, and use of health information; and influences adherence to clinical recommendations. In terms of communities, health communication shapes the construction of public health messages and compaigns and the dissemination of population risk communication messages. Health communication in the community can be used to influence the public health agenda, advocate for policies and programs, promote desirable changes in the socioeconomic and physical environment, and encourage social norms that benefit health and quality of life.[1]

14.1 SOCIAL MARKETING

Many health campaigns have turned to social marketing techniques to effect change. Coined in 1971,[2] the term *social marketing* describes the application and adaptation of commercial marketing concepts to the design, implementation, and control of programs designed to increase the acceptability of a social idea or bring about behavior change to improve the welfare of targeted individuals or their society. It is, in essence, marketing for societal benefit rather than commercial profit.

At the heart of health promotion is the need to influence consumers, program developers, policymakers, and others. Our ability to change people's lifestyles through improved diets and increased physical activity is intimately connected to our ability to influence behavior supporting good nutrition.

Communication experts posit a conceptual framework for approaching public health and social behaviors, a continuum of options through which to pursue goals of population-based behavior change. This framework assumes that a recommended behavior is a freely available option (an assumption that is only partly true, as for example, in the case of access to fresh fruits and vegetables and other healthy foods or to opportunities for physical activity). Table 14.1 presents a behavior-change continuum. At one end of the continuum we find people who are motivated to act on the basis of information. Those people are likely to adopt a recommended behavior because they are able to see it as in their best interest. Educational campaigns alone may suffice to create behavior change among populations at this end of the continuum. On the other hand, populations at the opposite end of the

TABLE 14.1
Continuum of Activities to Promote Desirable Changes in Food Handling, Nutrient Intake, and Diet

Desirable Consumer Behavior	Information Educational approaches may be used to manage behavior. *Use education if knowing is enough.*	Social Marketing Social marketing approaches may be used to manage behavior *Use social marketing when people need to be convinced.*	Policy or Law Law-based approaches may be used to manage behavior. *Use the law when people refuse to change.*
Increase physical activity	Dietary Guidelines for Americans;[1] MyPyramid[2]	VERB![TM;3] We Can![4]	Some school districts are requiring a minimum amount of physical activity per week
Practice safe food-handling	National Food Safety Education Month[5] Dietary Guidelines	Fight BAC!®[6] Thermy™[7] Food Safety Mobile[8]	HAACP (1999)[9]
Consume-adequate calcium	Dietary Guidelines; MyPyramid	Powerful Bones. Powerful Girls.™[10]	Regulations for most Child Nutrition Programs require that fluid milk be offered at each breakfast, lunch, or supper
Consume adequate folic acid	National Folic Acid Awareness Week;[11] Birth Defects Prevention Month[12]	National Folic Acid Campaign[13]	The U.S. requires folic acid enrichment of grains (1997)[14]
Obtain adequate vitamins A and D	Dietary Guidelines	Global vitamin A fortification and supplementation programs[15]	The U.S. requires fortification of milk with Vitamins D (in the 1930s) and A (1940s);[16] global vitamin A fortification and supplementation programs
Consume less total fat	Dietary Guidelines; MyPyramid	1% or Less Campaign[17]	Reimbursable school lunch programs provide students fluid milk with a variety of fat contents (2004).[18]
Provide healthy school food	Team Nutrition[19]	California Project Lean[20]	Local School Wellness Policy[21]
Consume a healthful diet	Dietary Guidelines; MyPyramid;	We Can!	Food Stamp Nutrition Education[22]
Prevent, or manage, diabetes	National Diabetes Education Program[23]	Small Steps. Big Rewards. Prevent Type 2 Diabetes[24]	Medicare coverage of diabetes-related supplies and services[25]
Breastfeed	CDC Guide To Breastfeeding Interventions[26]	National WIC Breastfeeding Promotion Project	Breastfeeding legislation[27]
Consume adequate iodine	Network for Sustained Elimination of Iodine Deficiency[28]	Network for Sustained Elimination of Iodine Deficiency	Iodized salt introduced in US (1924); Network for Sustained Elimination of Iodine Deficiency

[1] *Dietary Guidelines for Americans.* 6th edition: http://www.health.gov/dietaryguidelines/dga2005/document/pdf/DGA2005.pdf

[2] MyPyramid: http://www.mypyramid.gov/

[3] VERB!™: http://www.cdc.gov/youthcampaign/.

[4] *We Can*!: http://www.nhlbi.nih.gov/health/public/heart/obesity/wecan/

[5] National Food Safety Education Month: http://www.nraef.org/nfsem/

[6] FightBAC ® http://www.fightbac.org/main.cfm.

[7] Thermy™: http://www.fsis.usda.gov/food safety education/thermy/index.asp.

TABLE 14.1
Continuum of Activities to Promote Desirable Changes in Food Handling, Nutrient Intake, and Diet (Continued)

[8] USDA Food Safety Mobile: http://www.fsis.usda.gov/Food Safety Education/Food Safety Mobile/index.asp.

[9] Hazard Analysis and Critical Control Point (HACCP): http://vm.cfsan.fda.gov/~comm/nacmcfp.html#execsum

[10] Powerful Bones. Powerful Girls™: http://www.cdc.gov/nccdphp/dnpa/bonehealth/

[11] National Council on Folic Acid: http://www.folicacidinfo.org.

[12] March of Dimes: http://www.marchofdimes.com.

[13] National Folic Acid Campaign: http://www.cdc.gov/doc.do/id/0900f3ec8000d60c

[14] Folic acid final rule: http://www.foodrisk.org/Doc/FR/1996/FR_V61_N44_P8781–8797.htm.

[15] Global Vitamin A deficiency eradication programs: http://www.fao.org/docrep/X5244E/X5244e03.htm

[16] Milk fortification with vitamins A and D: http://jds.fass.org/cgi/reprint/84/12/2813.pdf.

[17] .1% or Less Campaigns: http://www.cspinet.org/nutrition/1less.htm.

[18] PL 108 265 (Jun 30, 2004): http://www.fns.usda.gov/cnd/Governance/Legislation/PL_108–265.pdf

[19] Team Nutrition: http://teamnutrition.usda.gov/

[20] California Project Lean: http://www.californiaprojectlean.org/

[21] Local School Wellness Policy. PL 108–265 §204: http:///www.fns.usda.gov/TN/Healthy/108–265.pdf

[22] Under Food Stamp regulations at 7 CFR 272.2(d), State agencies have the option to provide nutrition education.

[23] National Diabetes Education Program: http://ndep.nih.gov/

[24] Small Steps. Big Rewards. Prevent Type 2 Diabetes: http://www.ndep.nih.gov/campaigns/SmallSteps_overview.htm

[25] Medicare Diabetes Screening, Supplies, and Self-Management Training: http://www.medicare.gov/Health/Diabetes.asp

[26] CDC Guide to Breastfeeding Interventions: http://www.cdc.gov/breastfeeding/resources/guide.htm

[27] State Breastfeeding Legislation: http://www.usbreastfeeding.org/Issue-Papers/Legislation.pdf

[28] Network for Sustained Elimination of Iodine Deficiency: http://206.191.51.240/index.html

continuum are resistant to the recommended behavior. They may not see a change in behavior as in their self-interest or making the change may be too much trouble. Law- or policy-based approaches such as the fortification of milk with vitamin D in the 1930s and with vitamin A in the 1940s[3] may be required to assure these people receive the nutrition they need.[4,5]

In the middle of the continuum are populations who are neither inclined nor resistant to the recommended behavior. Social marketing may be used to bring about behavior change in this population by increasing the perceived benefits, reducing the perceived barriers, or in other ways improving opportunities and thus enhancing the perceived value of adopting the recommend behavior.

Through market research techniques, such as the use of focus groups, social marketers seek to identify and understand the intended audience and discover the factors that prevent them from adopting a health behavior. People are more likely to adopt a desired behavior if we first assess and then attempt to change their attitudes toward the behavior, their perceptions of the benefits of the new behavior, and their perceptions of how their peers will view that behavior. Social marketers develop, monitor, and constantly adjust a program to stimulate appropriate behavior change. Social marketing programs can address any or all of the traditional marketing mix variables: product, price, place, or promotion.[6] (See Box 14.1.)

14.1.1 WHAT A SOCIAL MARKETING COMMUNICATIONS PROGRAM CAN DO

A strong communications program will both target a specific audience with a prevention message and increase the general public's awareness of prevention-related issues. Raising public awareness can also frequently result in a change in social policies and practices. In addition, effective social marketing and communications can increase knowledge; influence attitudes; show benefits of behavior change; reinforce the desired knowledge, attitudes, and behavior; demonstrate skills; increase demand for services; refute myths and misconceptions; and influence norms.

Every year, new public health mass media campaigns attempting to change health behavior and improve health outcomes are launched. These campaigns enter a crowded media arena flooded with messages from competing sources. Public health practitioners must not only capture the

---

Box 14.1 Focus Groups

A focus group is a gathering of individuals who have been chosen as representatives of a target audience to discuss a specific topic, usually for several hours and in great detail. A focus group generally consists of 6 to 12 participants, with the focus provided by a trained moderator. A focus group study is often used in the development of product concepts or in the first phase of an exploratory investigation of a problem. Qualitative data collected in focus groups provide in-depth information necessary to understanding attitudes and motivations that influence consumers' decisions and behavior. Focus groups give participants an opportunity to describe their experiences and preferences without the limitation of preset response categories.

Source: Burroughs, E., et al. Using focus groups in the consumer research phase of a social marketing program to promote moderate-intensity physical activity and walking trail use in Sumter County, SC. *Prev Chronic Dis.* 3(1), A08, January 2006. Published online December 15, 2005.

---

attention of the public amid this competition but also motivate communities to change entrenched health behaviors or initiate habits that may be new or difficult.

The public health approach to prevention acknowledges that problems arise through the interaction of a host(s), an agent, and the environment. Prevention programs that focus exclusively on the host may overlook influences in the environment or community such as advertisements for foods of high energy but low nutritional value, which promote nutrition-related problems including obesity, type 2 diabetes, heart disease, osteoporosis, and eating disorders. Effective programs take a comprehensive, ecological approach, addressing not only individual risk factors, but also community norms, local policies, the built environment, mass media, and other factors. (See Box 14.2 Ecological Approach.)

14.1.2 How Social Marketing Works

Every social marketing campaign starts with an extensive formative evaluation process that includes focus groups. For example, the formative research that was conducted prior to the development of VERB™ included primary audience research with "tweens," parents, and other influencers (educators and youth leaders);[7] expert consultants; local, state, and national organizations; and lessons learned from other large-scale national media campaigns.[8] Section 14.1.5.1.1 VERB™ It's What You Do describes this program in detail (Figure 14.1).

The fundamental elements of every social marketing program, examples of which are detailed in the sections that follow, are the *product* being promoted; its *price* to the target audience; the strategy to *promote* the product; and the *place* or channel through which the product is communicated to the intended audience. These factors — product, price, promotion, and place — are often referred to as "the four P's" of social marketing. Additional P's included in the social marketing mix are the *public*,

---

Box 14.2 Ecological Approach

The ecological approach assumes that an individual's health is shaped by multiple interacting environmental subsystems, including family, community, workplace, cultural beliefs and traditions, economics, the physical world, and web of social relationships. Therefore, health promotion efforts should be comprehensive, addressing those systems that adversely affect the person's capacity for living a healthy life.

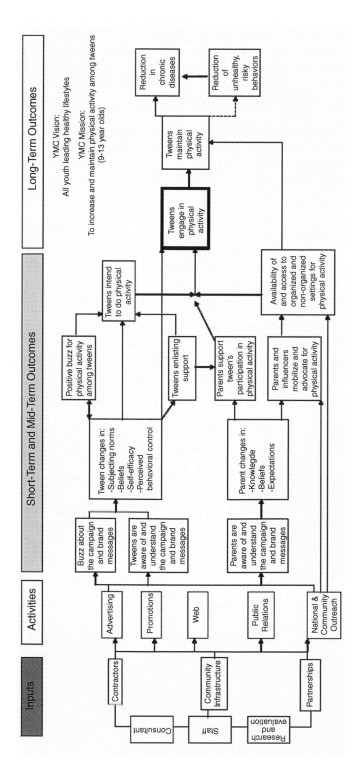

FIGURE 14.1 VERB™ logic model. (From Huhman, M., Heitzler, C., Wong, F. The VERB™ campaign logic model: a tool for planning and evaluation. *Prev Chronic Dis.* [serial online] July 2004. Available at http://www. cdc.gov/pcd/issues/2004/jul/04_0033.htm. Accessed August 28, 2005.)

Box 14.3 Formative Research

The content, tone, and execution of a campaign is determined by formative research, which includes reviews of existing and new research; discussions with expert consultants who conducted similar projects in nongovernmental and state, local and national organizations; and primary audience research with a small group of representatives from the target audiences in order to understand their interests, attributes, and needs. Formative research occurs before a program is designed and implemented. It can help define and understand target populations, help in the creation of programs that are specific to the needs of the target populations, ensure that programs and materials are acceptable and feasible to clients before launching the program, and even improve relationships between clients and agencies. Formative research should be an integral part of developing programs or adapting programs.

Source: Centers for Disease Control and Prevention. Youth Media Campaign. "Formative Research." Available at: http://www.cdc.gov/youthcampaign/research/formative.htm. Accessed February 12, 2007.

or intended audience for the product promotion; *partners*, or alliances in the campaign; *purse* strings or budget; and *policy*[9] and *politics,* or the rules, systems, and environmental change factors that influence voluntary behavior change, not policies that punish undesired behavior.[10]

14.1.2.1 Product (Social Proposition)

Product refers to the knowledge, attitudes, or behavior social marketers want the target audience to adopt. In addition to a desired behavior change, such as drinking low-fat milk, the product may be an actual commodity, such as flavored low-fat milk varieties. A continuum of products exists, ranging from tangible, physical products (low-fat milk), to services (a nutrition education module that promotes low-fat milk), to practices (eating low-fat dairy products). The social marketing product may also be a policy (a regulation addressing the types of milk served in a school district). Other examples of social marketing products include breastfeeding and physical activity. The WIC Breastfeeding Promotion Project promotes breastfeeding as a means toward mother–child bonding rather than as a way to confer passive immunity on the infant.[11] Similarly, the VERB™ campaign[12] presents physical activity as a way to have fun, spend time with friends, and gain recognition from peers and adults rather than to prevent obesity or chronic disease later in life.

Whatever the product, the marketer must develop an enticing package with which it is associated. A viable product helps the target audience first understand that they have a genuine problem, and then recognize the product being offered as a good solution to that problem. One role of social market research is to discover the audience's perceptions of the problem and the product, and to determine how important they feel it is to resolve the problem.

In contrast to commercial exchanges where consumers receive a product or service in exchange for a cash outlay, public health markets rarely exchange an immediate, explicit payback for adoption of healthy behavior. Social marketers distinguish between the *core product* (what people will gain when they perform the behavior) and the *actual product* (the desired behavior). To succeed, the product must provide a solution to problems consumers consider important and/or that offer them a benefit they truly value. For this reason, social marketers conduct research to help them understand the target audience's aspirations, preferences, and other desires (in addition to their health needs) and to identify the benefits most appealing to consumers. The marketing objective is to discover which benefits have the greatest appeal to the target audience and design a product that provides those benefits. In some cases, public health professionals must change their recommendations or modify their programs to provide benefits that consumers value.[13]

14.1.2.2   Price (Cost)

Price describes what the consumer must do or pay to obtain the social marketing product. Specifically, it refers to the money or, more often, intangibles such as time, effort, social approval, lost opportunities, or embarrassment involved in a person's changing his or her behavior. In social marketing, price might be the perceived cost of giving up the rich taste of whole milk or the discomfort associated with behaving differently from one's peers. If the costs outweigh the benefits for an individual, the perceived value of the offering will be low and it is unlikely that it will be adopted. However, if the benefits are perceived as greater than their costs, the chance of trial and adoption of the product is much greater. Price, therefore, represents a balance of the product's benefits with its cost to members of the target audience.

To reduce the perceived costs of behavior change and make the change easy to adopt, social marketers recommend removing social and environmental obstacles. Enacting policy change can help address these barriers by minimizing the price the target audience believes it must pay in the exchange. There are many issues to consider in setting the price: if the product is priced too low or provided free of charge, the consumer may perceive it as being low in quality; if the price is too high, some will be unable to afford it. Social marketers must balance these considerations, while also conferring a sense of dignity on the transaction. Perceptions of costs and benefits can be determined through research and used in positioning the product.

What is the price to the target audience for changing their behavior? The VERB™ campaign proposes a voluntary exchange: tweens who take up physical activity, presumably in place of watching television or just sitting around, will derive the benefits of fun and social engagement.[14]

14.1.2.3   Place (Accessibility)

Place is where the target audience either performs the desired behavior or accesses programs and services. Place also describes how the product reaches the intended audience. For a tangible product, place refers to the distribution system — including the warehouse, trucks, sales force, and retail outlets where it is sold — or locations where it is distributed for free. For an intangible product, place is less clear-cut but refers to the channels through which consumers are provided with information or training. These may include doctors' offices, shopping malls, mass media outlets, schools, houses of worship, or in-home demonstrations.

Place affects price. For instance, if the message to drink more low-fat milk is promoted through the school lunch program, the price of peer pressure may be reduced. The exchange and its opportunities should be made available in places that reach the audience and fit its lifestyles. Another consideration of place is deciding how to ensure accessibility of the offering and quality of the service delivery.

By determining the activities and habits of the target audience, as well as their experience and satisfaction with the present delivery system, researchers can pinpoint the most ideal means of distribution for the offering, such as where the behaviors should or should not occur or what barriers or opportunities exist for the behavior's occurrence. Place should be readily available. To ease access, social marketers should be prepared to move programs or products to places the intended audience frequents. According to the VERB™ campaign, a VERB™ place is where tweens can be physically active in a safe environment.

14.1.2.4   Promotion (Communication)

Because of its visibility, promotion is often mistakenly assumed to comprise the whole of social marketing, although it is only one component. Promotion focuses on creating and sustaining demand for a product through the integrated use of advertising, public relations, media advocacy, personal selling, and entertainment vehicles to convince the target audience that the product is worth its price. It may include publicity campaigns through the mass media, such as news stories and advertisements on television, radio, and in newspapers; public service advertisements and paid advertising; coupons; editorials; food demonstrations and taste tests at a variety of community sites; and supermarket shelf labeling initiatives to draw attention to the program's message.

Research is crucial to determine the most effective and efficient vehicles to reach the target audience and increase demand. Research helps determine the communications that should occur, from what sources to whom, and through what channels of influence. For example, trusted healthcare providers and clergy from communities of various faiths can deliver messages in-person about the benefits of physical activity, changing one's diet, and screening for diabetes. The exchange should be promoted creatively and through channels and tactics that maximize desired responses. Promotion includes multiple ways to reach the target audience to advocate the benefits of the behavior change, including product, price, and place components. Some of the promotion strategies and tactics employed by the VERB™ campaign include paid media advertising, community-based events, contests and sweepstakes, community and corporate partnerships, and Web sites.

14.1.2.5 Publics (Target Audiences)

To be successful, the programs social marketers promote must often reach multiple audiences. These publics include external and internal groups involved in or affected by the program. External publics encompass the target audience, as well as secondary and tertiary audiences, policymakers, and gatekeepers. The primary audience might be children ages 9 through 13, with a secondary audience of the people who influence their decisions — such as parents, teachers, clergy, and physicians — and a tertiary audience of policymakers and directors at local radio stations. Internal publics encompass those involved in some capacity with approval or implementation of the program, such as board of directors and office staff.

The VERB™ program initially segmented its target population by age (youth aged 9–13 and parents/influencers). It then conducted research that identified important differences among specific segments within the tween audience on the basis of activity level, receptivity to physical activity, ethnicity, and gender.[13]

14.1.2.6 Policy (Environmental Supports)

Social marketing programs can inspire individual behavior change, but sustaining that change is difficult unless it is supported in the long run by environmental components. Often, policy change is needed to bring about lasting behavior change. For example, policy efforts of the 1% or Less campaign might focus on increasing milk choices available in the school cafeteria to include low-fat, fat free, and low-fat flavored milk in addition to whole milk. Similarly, the policy component of the VERB™ campaign might focus on increasing the number of bicycle paths in a community and increasing the availability of after-school programs that appeal to the targeted age group.

14.1.2.7 Partnerships (Alliances)

Health issues are often so complex that one agency cannot make a dent by itself. Partnerships or alliances should be cultivated with local or national groups, corporate sponsors, medical organizations, service clubs, or media outlets that have goals similar to those of the social marketing campaign. Partnerships can increase the likelihood for success by creating buy-in throughout the community, enhancing credibility of the program through connections with well-known partners, increasing available financial and human resources, and gaining access to a greater area of expertise in health, social service and business fields. Keeping VERB™ a "cool brand for tweens" is a critically important goal for partners (parks, schools, youth-serving organizations) as they collaborate on the campaign.

Strategic alliances offer many important benefits to the social organization, including improved delivery of their message, heightened influence, and broader reach. However, there are risks involved in the strategic alliance process, such as conflicts of interest. Consider these guidelines[15] when contemplating working with for-profit partners:

- Carefully review each partnership proposal and do not enter into any collaboration that endorses a specific commercial product, service, or enterprise. Only allow your program's logo to be used in conjunction with approved projects and only with your written permission. Retain the right to review all copy such as advertising or publicity prior to the partner's using your program's name or logo.
- Prior to partnership negotiations, confirm that a partnership with this company will not create tensions or conflicts with another partner for your program. Ensure that the company has no unresolved disputes with or is not currently in negotiation for a grant or contract from your organization; that it conforms to standards of health, medical care, and labor practices; and that its products, services, or promotional messages do not conflict with your organization's policies or programs.

14.1.2.8 Purse Strings (Budget)

Purse strings refer to the funding component of strategy development. Most organizations that develop social marketing programs operate with funds provided by foundations, government grants, or donations. When planning and allocating funds, consider how long the funding will last, how strategic partnerships can foster more resources, and whether products or services must be offered for a cost.

14.1.3 THE SOCIAL MARKETING CAMPAIGN

A social marketing campaign consists of six stages: planning the approach, defining the program's messages and channels, developing and pretesting program materials, implementing the program, evaluating the program, and using feedback to refine the program. Each of these components of a health communication campaign can be viewed as a self-contained project of its own and are further defined in the following sections.

14.1.3.1 Plan the Approach

Planning establishes the foundation for the entire campaign. Before moving ahead, an assessment of the problem is undertaken and available resources are identified. During this stage, the target audience is identified and should become increasingly segmented, for example, into groups with common risk behaviors, motivations, or information channel preferences to aid in developing appropriate messages. Goals and objectives are developed during planning. Formative evaluation also begins during the planning stage and continues through the development of materials to be used in the program.

The following should be undertaken during the planning stage:

1. *Perform literature review.* This defines the scope of the problem and identifies the types of programs that have already been developed to address the situation.
2. *Define the audience.* A social marketing program may need to address more than one audience to accomplish its objectives. Planners often differentiate among primary, secondary, and tertiary audiences to pinpoint whom they are trying to reach. The *primary audience* is the specific group or groups the program is designed to influence. Even small, apparently homogeneous communities contain various subgroups within their populations. Personal, environmental, and geographic differences can help define subgroups. Personal factors include age, gender, ethnicity and cultural background, socioeconomic level, literacy or educational level, occupation, or gang membership. Environmental factors include stress, social support, access and barriers, and exposure to harmful agents. The geographic area is where people live.

A primary audience may consist of one subgroup (adolescent males) or a combination of groups (adolescent males and their parents). A *secondary audience* includes individuals who influence the primary audience, such as peers, parents, teachers, clergy, and role models. The *tertiary audience* comprises community decision makers who influence policy and offer financial and logistical support to community-based prevention programs. The support of this group is critical to any prevention program. These individuals may actually comprise the primary audience in some social marketing programs.

3. *Analyze the community*: A community analysis helps identify its driving (positive) and restraining (negative) forces. Your action plan should build on the driving forces and diminish the restraining forces to strengthen a community's prevention efforts. *Social asset mapping* creates an in-depth understanding of a community by identifying local resources, networks, places of importance, prevalent issues, current connections, and where potential new connections might be made. Such an understanding creates numerous possibilities for new and innovative approaches to community empowerment that are compatible with maintaining healthy environments. All communities have assets that can be used as building blocks for economic and social development. Some researchers use geographic information systems (GIS, see Chapter 12) to literally map these assets. Sometimes physically locating assets on a grid renders them less abstract and enables social marketers to better see the relationships between assets across and within communities.

4. *Develop the concept.* State the issue or broad goal the campaign is trying to address, for example, to promote physical activity.

5. *Set goals and objectives.* Determine what you are trying to achieve and what behaviors, if changed, would have the greatest difference. State the desired attributes and expected benefits of each targeted behavior. For example, for physical activity, the desired attributes and anticipated benefits might include burning fat to lose weight, look better, and be sexier; producing endorphins to reduce stress and feel more energy; and building muscle strength to become stronger and thus more independent in daily activities. Describe the specific behaviors the campaign intends to change, how much change is anticipated, who is expected to change, and by when. For example, by July, 2008, the percentage of adults in Peoria who engage in regular physical activity will increase by 30%.

6. *Identify core components or strategies.* This includes deciding how to communicate challenging messages about the desired behaviors, making the desired behaviors more rewarding or attractive, making the desired behaviors easier to achieve or of lower cost, improving peoples' abilities to adopt the behavior change, and decreasing the attractiveness of competing behaviors.

7. *Outline basic principles.* As previously discussed, the principles of a social marketing campaign include product, price, public, place, promotion, policies, and the development of a budget.

14.1.3.2 Select Channels and Materials

The second step in a social marketing campaign is to identify the message or messages to be delivered and choose appropriate and effective channels of communications. It is also important to identify the environments, situations, or settings in which the targeted behavior should or should not occur, such as schools, homes, parks, or other public places.

Typical communication channels include television, radio, newspapers and other print media, and bulletin boards in supermarkets, churches, neighborhood centers, and other places where people congregate. Using multiple channels ensures greater coverage of the issues and improved chances of reaching the target population. A multiple-outlet or a limited-outlet approach may be used.

A *multiple outlet approach* uses as many available resources as possible including television and radio stations, newspapers, and billboards. The community is inundated with information from these outlets. A *limited-outlet approach* concentrates a significant commitment of time and resources on one or two outlets only, resulting in a campaign that becomes very closely tied to the chosen outlet. When choosing communications channels, consider the channel's credibility, cost, reach (the number of people or households exposed to a specific message during a set period of time), and the average number of times an audience is exposed to the message.

The messages the program sends must be meaningful and appealing to the target audience. An effective message stimulates the target audience to think about and discuss the issues. The message should be based on facts and tied to the present, because Americans value instant gratification. The campaign should develop and convey clear, concrete suggestions and model alternative behaviors or ways of doing things without resorting to scare tactics and negativism. The threat of osteoporosis in 30 or 40 years poses little incentive to a 15-year-old to drink milk. Consider, instead, stressing the convenience of a single-serve milk bottle, cheese stick, or yogurt drink that fits easily into a backpack, book bag, or bicycle rack.

The program's ultimate outcome should be to establish social norms that promote and sustain healthy, safe behaviors. The message should minimize the psychological or physical cost of the product to the target audience. For example, if an adolescent assumes that drinking low-fat milk will lower his or her status among peers, the message might minimize this cost by highlighting popular celebrities who drink milk.

14.1.3.3   Develop and Pretest Materials and Methods

Develop a draft of all marketing materials for pretesting with an audience similar to or a subset of your target audience. Ask this group if these materials produce the intended results. Revise them based on their criticism and suggestions. Repeat this process until all stakeholders are satisfied with the end-product. A focus group can greatly facilitate the process of preparing materials that appeal to your audience.

14.1.3.4   Logic Models

Logic models are often developed for public health programs and campaigns. A logic model links campaign inputs and activities with campaign outcomes. It describes the sequence of events for bringing about behavior change and presents the relationship between campaign inputs (research and consultation), campaign activities (marketing and partnership tactics), the impact on outputs (number of people exposed), and outcomes (knowledge, attitude, and behavior change).

A logic model can be used as a tool to:

1. Identify the short-term, intermediate, and long-term outcomes for the campaign.
2. Link those outcomes to each other and to campaign activities.
3. Select outcomes to measure depending on the stage of the campaign's development.
4. Demonstrate how it may take time before long-term outcomes can be associated with the campaign.

An actual logic model (from the VERB™ campaign) is discussed in Section 14.1.5.1.1.1.

14.1.3.5   Implement the Program

Before launching the campaign, all communication materials should be ready and available in sufficient quantities. A method to track and evaluate the program must also be in place. Tracking allows the program planners to determine where the program is succeeding and identify areas where changes are needed. The most successful programs are constantly being updated with current information about the program and the target audience. The process evaluation, which essentially reviews those tasks involved in implementing the program, is appropriate for use during the implementation phase of the program.

14.1.3.6   Evaluate the Program

Assessing a program's effectiveness goes beyond the process evaluation of the planning, defining, and development stages of a campaign. Program evaluation measures if and how much the program affects beliefs, attitudes, and behaviors of the target audience. While outcome and impact evaluation should be designed during the planning stage, it is not conducted until the evaluation stage. When designing a program evaluation, include key questions such as what are our success indicators and how will we know if we have achieved them.

The type of evaluation conducted depends upon several factors, including money, time, policies affecting the ability to gather information, the level of support for evaluation, and the overall design of the program. *Outcome evaluation* is used to gather descriptive information about knowledge and attitude changes, expressed intentions of the target audience, and the initiation of policy changes. *Impact evaluation,* the most comprehensive evaluation, focuses on the long-term outcomes of the program. It measures factors such as changes in morbidity and mortality, long-term maintenance of behavior change, and changes in absenteeism from work or school. Impact evaluation is most often used in multifaceted health education programs that include awareness, education, training, and communication components.

The evaluation should involve all stakeholders including members of the target audience, program implementers, and grant makers. It must identify indicators of success, document evidence of success, and determine how the overall campaign can be improved.

14.1.3.7   Refine the Program and Plan for Sustainability

Use evaluation feedback to make adjustments in campaign components as needed. If, for instance, no change in behavior is seen with a particular subgroup, modify components or intensify exposure to them.

Always be sure to celebrate successes. Group celebrations of accomplishments, such as successfully establishing a supportive policy change, help maintain morale and enthusiasm for the program. Focus attention on improvements in desired behavior and outcomes and honor the individuals who have contributed to those improvements. This may be a simple awards ceremony to acknowledge community champions.

Strategies to sustain the effort long enough to make a difference are vital. These might include:

- Using process evaluation information to help secure sustained support from grant makers and other funding sources.
- Securing media coverage of the issue or goal and successful implementation of relevant components. Hold a news conference and pitch feature stories as part of a media advocacy campaign to promote continued awareness and enhance public support for attempts to address it.
- Promoting adoption of effective campaign components or advocating for changes that contribute to improvement.
- Promoting ongoing implementation through collaborating partners.

14.1.4   Ethics in Social Marketing

Social marketers must pay careful attention to ethical standards and practices if the field is to mature as a profession. Most social marketing and health communications projects give rise to ethical dilemmas related to either the ends being pursued or the strategies and tactics used to achieve them. During the course of a project, issues might be raised by managers, colleagues, audience members, community groups, partners, the media, or opponents to the cause. During the planning stages one might ask if the goals of the program are truly in the public's interest and whether the primary beneficiaries of the program are the targeted groups and subgroups — not the change agents. Social alliances — in other words, partnerships between for-profit and nonprofit organizations — can present ethical challenges for one or both partners. It is thus incumbent upon both companies and nonprofits to give considerable

---

Box 14.4 Ethics Scenario

Social marketing is being adopted by a growing number of government and nonprofit organizations because of its power to bring about social changes. An array of commercial marketing concepts and techniques has been applied to problems ranging from child abuse to teen smoking to environmental neglect. However, in crafting these programs, organizations may face complex ethical challenges, such as:

- Is it acceptable to exaggerate risk and heighten fear if doing so saves more lives or at least reduces morbidity?
- When is it acceptable to improve the lives of people in one group at the expense of another?
- Does a marketing campaign respect a group's culture if it calls for fundamental change within it?

Examine the questions above with regard to the following scenario:

When the Ad Council proposed a campaign that focused on "the risks associated with not breastfeeding" and included statistics from studies that have found that babies fed formula have a higher risk of developing asthma, diabetes, leukemia, and other illnesses, federal officials pulled the ads after two formula companies complained that claims made in the government's campaign were not based on solid science and that the overall approach was like a scare tactic.[1,2,3]

Sources:

[1] Petersen, M. Breastfeeding ads delayed by a dispute over content. *New York Times*, December 4, 2003, C1.

[2] Editorial. About breast-feeding. *New York Times*, July 2, 2006, D9.

[3] Rabin, R. Breast-feed or else. *New York Times*, June 3, 2006, F1,

---

attention to developing ethical standards and procedures for addressing ethical issues when they arise.[16] During the evaluation phase one might want to determine if the strategies and components of the program were implemented responsibly; if potential negative side effects were avoided or minimized, and if the benefits of the program outweighed the risks. (See Box 14.4.)

14.1.5   FOOD AND NUTRITION SOCIAL MARKETING CAMPAIGNS

In the U.S., the most extensive nutrition-related social marketing campaigns are operated by the U.S. Department of Agriculture (USDA) and the Department of Health and Human Services (DHHS). These campaigns include VERB™; Food Stamp Nutrition Education; *Sisters Together: Move More, Eat Better;* National WIC Breastfeeding Promotion Project; and Food Safety Education — Improving Public Health. Smaller programs have been conducted by, among others, the Center for Science in the Pubic Interest (CSPI) and the Partnership for Food Safety Education. The goals and objectives of all these programs support the *Healthy People 2010* health objectives for reducing the burden of disease by 2010.

14.1.5.1   Campaigns to Prevent Overweight and Obesity

In the last 30 years, the prevalence of obesity in the U.S. has seen a rapid rise that shows little sign of abating.[17] Presently, more than 50% of Americans are either overweight or obese.[18] Because of the strong correlation between overweight/obesity and the risk factors for morbidity and mortality, confronting the obesity epidemic is an urgent public health priority.

Overweight and obesity are defined in relation to body mass index (BMI), which is weight in kilograms divided by the square of height in meters. In adults, a BMI of 25.0–29.9 is overweight, of 30.0–39.9 is obese, and over 40.0 is extremely obese.[17] Children are considered *at risk* of being overweight if their BMI is between the 85th and 95th percentiles for age and gender and are overweight with a BMI above the 95th percentile.

Overweight and obesity are known risk factors for cardiovascular disease (CVD), diabetes, metabolic syndrome, high blood pressure, high cholesterol levels, asthma, arthritis, and poor health status as well as physiological ailments such as orthopedic abnormalities and premature menarche.[19,20,21]

14.1.5.1.1 VERB™ It's What You Do

Lack of physical activity is a contributing factor to the increase in childhood overweight as well as the emergence of type 2 diabetes among youth. In 2001, there was little or no physical education in schools, and many youth lead sedentary home lives as well, spending hours of their free time watching television or computer screens. In addition, youth participate in risky activities such as smoking, drinking, and violence. In response to these unhealthy behaviors, in 2001 Congress appropriated $125 million to the Centers for Disease Control and Prevention (CDC) for 5 years to change children's health behaviors. The CDC's response to this sweeping mandate was to focus on the sedentary lifestyle of young adolescents. The VERB™ Youth Media Campaign, launched in 2002, is a 5-year, multiethnic, demonstration media campaign designed to increase and maintain physical activity among tweens, children aged 9 to 13 years.[22] VERB's secondary audience includes parents and influencers such as educators and youth leaders.

The campaign's goals are to increase knowledge and improve attitudes and beliefs about tweens' regular participation in physical activity; increase parental and influencer support for and encouragement of their participation; heighten awareness of options and opportunities for participation; facilitate opportunities for participation; and increase and maintain the number of tweens who regularly participate in physical activity.

Media components available include Web sites for professional (www.cdc.gov/verb), youth (www.VERBnow.com), and parent audiences (www.VERBparents.com); paid traditional media such as television, radio, print, outdoor advertising, and advertorials; targeted distribution of posters, book covers, murals, and school materials. Marketing promotions, such as contests, events, and sweepstakes; and VERB™ 365 promotions, including the Longest Day of Play (June 21), Extra Hour to VERB™ (fall time change), and Extra Day to VERB™ (leap day) have also been implemented. Although it is important to promote this campaign year-round, there is particular emphasis on wintertime, low-activity months.[23]

14.1.5.1.1.1 VERB's Logic Model

The VERB™ logic model (Figure 14.1) illustrates the campaign's vision — all youth leading healthy lifestyles — and mission: to increase and maintain physical activity among tweens.[12] The *inputs* of the campaign are its consultants, staff, contractors, partnerships, the community infrastructure, and the program's research and evaluation. All of these inputs contribute to the campaign activities, which include advertising, promotions, Web sites, public relations, and outreach nationally and into particular communities.

The short-term outcome for the campaign is tween and parent awareness as well as "buzz" about the campaign brand and its messages. Awareness and buzz lead to *mid-term outcomes* that include changes in subjective norms, beliefs, self-efficacy, and perceived behavioral control. The logic model indicates that if these changes occur, there will be a positive "buzz" among tweens about physical activity, and these responses will lead to tweens enlisting support from their parents to participate in physical activity. Awareness and understanding of the campaign and brand messages by parents leads to changes for parents in knowledge, beliefs, and expectations.

Campaign planners hypothesize that as parents internalize changes in knowledge, beliefs, and expectations, they will support tween participation in physical activity, reciprocally enhanced by tweens requesting support from them. As depicted in the model, planners also expect that as parents prioritize their child's physical activity needs, the parents, as well as other influencers of tweens will mobilize to advocate for physical activity. This mobilization as well as national and community outreach will lead to the availability of and access to organized and nonorganized settings for physical activity. Tweens' behavioral intentions as well as available and accessible settings are likely to encourage them to engage in physical activity.

The campaign's *long-term outcomes* include tweens engaging in and maintaining physical activity, thereby reducing chronic diseases. The model indicates that there is a possible displacement strategy that tweens who participate in physical activity may also have fewer unhealthy, risky behaviors.

14.1.5.1.1.2 Evaluating VERB™

Rigorous multiyear evaluation of the campaign is designed to determine its effectiveness in motivating young adolescents to be more active. Specifically, VERB™'s outcome evaluation assesses changes in the target audiences' awareness, knowledge, attitudes, and behaviors related to physical activity and measures how these changes can be attributed to campaign exposure. Campaign effects are assessed in two ways: through a longitudinal survey at the national level (6000 youth and their parents), and through surveys of the high-dose markets of Los Angeles, CA; Miami, FL; Columbus, OH; Greenville, SC; Houston, TX; and Green Bay, WI, where concentrated campaign activities such as community-level partnership development, increased media buys, and local events have been conducted.

A telephone survey was conducted in 2002 and repeated among the same families prior to launching the VERB™ campaign in 2003, and again in 2004. Evaluation results show that after 1 year of the campaign, three-quarters (74%) of the children surveyed were aware of VERB™, and levels of reported sessions of free-time physical activity increased for subgroups of children aged 9 to 13 years.[24]

14.1.5.1.2 We Can!

Analysis of the National Heart Lung and Blood Institute (NHLBI)-supported Dietary Intervention Study in Children (DISC) data indicates that children and their parents can be taught to make lifestyle changes that result in a diet low in saturated fat and dietary cholesterol.[25] DISC demonstrates that children and their families can learn to enjoy healthy foods, be selective in their food choices, and maintain these healthy habits for up to 3 years. The children in the DISC experimental group reported consuming more servings per day of "go" grains, dairy, meats, and vegetables compared with children in the usual-care group, although intake of fruits and vegetables remained below recommended levels in both groups. ("go" vs. "whoa" foods are depicted in Figure 14.2.) The DISC study also suggests that children and their families need the right tools to help them make positive lifestyle changes. To date, however, no longitudinal studies demonstrate that healthy eating habits engendered in childhood carry over to adolescence or adulthood.

Nevertheless, emboldened by the positive results of the DISC analysis, in 2005 the DHHS launched *We Can!* (Ways to Enhance Children's Activity and Nutrition), a national education program from the National Institutes of Health (NIH) to help prevent overweight and obesity among youth ages 8 through 13 years.[26] *We Can!* provides resources and community-based programs for parents, caregivers, and youth to encourage healthy eating, increase physical activity, and reduce sedentary time. Developed by the NHLBI, the program is promoted in collaboration with the National Institute of Diabetes and Digestive and Kidney Diseases (NIDDK), the National Institute of Child Health and Human Development (NICHHD), and the National Cancer Institute (NCI), along with several national private sector organizations.[27] It provides print and online educational materials to help parents teach their children to:

- Eat a sufficient amount of a variety of fruits and vegetables per day
- Choose small portions at home and at restaurants
- Eat fewer high-fat, energy-dense foods such as french fries, bacon, and doughnuts that are low in nutrient value
- Substitute water or fat-free or low-fat milk for sweetened beverages such as sodas
- Engage in at least 60 min of moderate physical activity on most, preferably all, days of the week
- Reduce recreational screen time to no more than 2 h per day

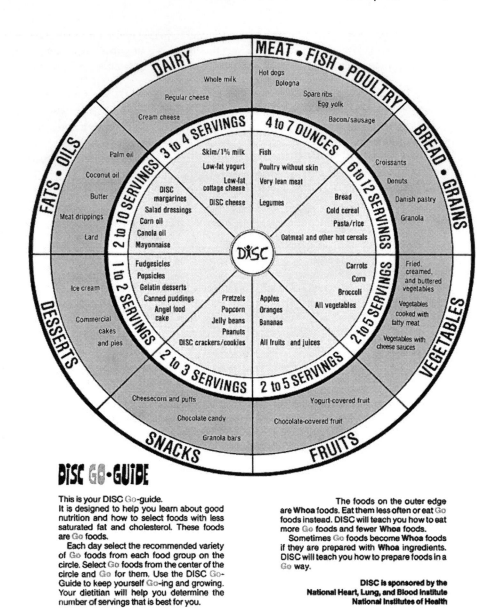

FIGURE 14.2 DISC study. (From Van Horn, L., Obarzanek, E., Aronson Friedman, L., and Barton, B. Children's adaptations to a fat-reduced diet: the dietary intervention study in children (DISC). *Pediatrics*. 2005; 115: 1723–1733. Figure 1 The DISC Go-Guide.)

We Can! tools include a parents' handbook available in Spanish or English as well as a six-lesson curriculum offered through community-based sites. Tested curricula for children are also available for community organizations. In addition, an online resource provides parents, caregivers, communities, national partners, and media with up-to-date health information and tips on maintaining a healthy weight. NIH designed *We Can!* so that local civic groups, parent groups, churches and others can adapt and use the program materials. Thirteen intensive community sites have been selected to receive training and to participate in evaluation of the *We Can!* program.

TABLE 14.2

Strategies for an Expanded Campaign Model Developed for *Sisters Together: Move More, Eat Better*

Stage in the Campaign	Activity
Formative research	Include members of the target population in the planning component of the program
Campaign design	Build a campaign that supports community development
Promotion	Highlight action steps for key public health messages. Promote existing community resources
Demonstration	Design activities that can be adapted for existing community groups
Transfer	Share evaluation findings, skills, and materials with existing community organizations
Sustainability	Work with local groups to integrate the campaign message with their program focus

14.1.5.1.3 Sisters Together: Move More, Eat Better

The *Sisters Together: Move More, Eat Better* pilot campaign (1995–1998) was designed to increase awareness of the importance of healthy eating and physical activity among young African American women aged 18 to 35 in 3 Boston-area, predominantly black communities. The program's "Move More, Eat Better" message was promoted through educational materials and planned activities such as walking groups, dance classes, and cooking demonstrations; distribution of materials promoting healthy eating and regular exercise; and media outreach. The program combined social marketing strategies with a community development focus. The experience resulted in guidelines for communicators using the expanded campaign model for a community campaign. These guidelines are summarized in Table 14.2: Strategies for an expanded campaign model developed for *Sisters Together: Move More, Eat Better.*[28]

Currently, Sisters Together is an initiative of the Weight-Control Information Network (WIN), a national information service of NIDDK. The program's purpose is to raise awareness about how moving more and eating better improves health, reduces risks for certain diseases, and ultimately, enhances quality of life. A national Sisters Together program will aim to develop and disseminate new, culturally relevant messages based on lifestyle interventions, obesity, and physical activity. Partnerships with new organizations and individuals will be pursued during the program's expansion. The nationwide, media-based component of the program works with national and local newspapers, magazines, radio stations and consumer and professional organizations to further raise awareness among black women about the health benefits of regular physical activity and healthy eating. For the Sisters Together messages and activities to resonate with African American women nationally, WIN nurtures and facilitates partnerships with national, state, and local groups as well as individuals, and develops relationships with nontraditional partners such as hair and nail salons. WIN also develops partnerships with agencies and organizations that encourage and promote healthy lifestyle behaviors for many audiences, particularly African American audiences.[29]

Implementation strategies include publicizing the availability of current Sisters Together age-appropriate and culturally relevant brochures developed by WIN that provide black women, their families, and their friends with strategies to increase physical activity and improve their diet.

In addition, a program guide based on the Boston program offers instructions on designing and implementing Sisters Together activities and events. The guide was developed by NIDDK to assist health educators in initiating a program, building partnerships, working with the media, selecting and implementing activities, and evaluating the program's success.[30] (See Box 14.5.)

A manual prepared by NIDDK based on *Sisters Together: Move More, Eat Better* outlines the social marketing approach used to develop the program. It is available online at http://win.niddk.nih.gov/publications/SisPrmGuide2.pdf.

Box 14.5 *Move More Eat Better*

A manual prepared by NIDDK based on *Sisters Together: Move More, Eat Better* outlines the social marketing approach used to develop the program. It is available online at http://win. niddk.nih.gov/publications/SisPrmGuide2.pdf.

The program's performance measure will assess the increase in awareness among African American women of the health benefits of regular exercise and healthy eating. The outcome measure will be the extent to which the results of this media outreach alters the health behavior of African American women regarding exercise and healthy eating.

14.1.5.2 Campaigns to Prevent Osteoporosis

Osteoporosis is defined as a bone mineral density (BMD) value of more than 2.5 standard deviations below the mean for normal young white women. Based on this definition, it is estimated that in the U.S. roughly 10 million individuals over age 50 have osteoporosis of the hip, and an additional 33.6 million individuals over age 50 have low bone mass (sometimes referred to as *osteopenia*) of the hip. As such, they are at risk of osteoporosis later in life. The low bone mass and architectural abnormalities that characterize osteoporosis contribute to bone fragility and increased fracture risk. Although it is the underlying cause of most fractures in older people, the condition is silent and undetected in the majority of cases until a fracture occurs. A fracture is not a benign event, particularly in older people. The major fracture sites associated with osteoporosis are the hip, the spine, and the wrist. Of all the injury sites, hip fractures have the greatest morbidity and socioeconomic impact. During the first six months following a hip fracture there is a 10 to 20% mortality rate. Fifty percent of those people experiencing a hip fracture will be unable to walk without assistance, and 25% will require long-term care.

Osteoporosis is the most prevalent of the bone diseases that affect Americans,[31] but it does not need to be a consequence of aging. As it is largely preventable, public and private organizations have mounted campaigns to promote bone health through increased intake of calcium and increased physical activity.

14.1.5.2.1 Milk Matters

The mission of NICHHD is to ensure that every person is born healthy and wanted, that women suffer no harmful effects from reproductive processes, and that all children have the chance to achieve their full potential for healthy and productive lives, free from disease or disability, and to ensure the health, productivity, independence, and well-being of all people through optimal rehabilitation. In addition to its considerable research agenda, NICHHD provides a variety of information in brochures, booklets, and other materials related to the health of children, adults, families, and populations. Much of this information is based on NICHHD research into these areas. The NICHHD also supports health education and outreach campaigns.

Milk Matters is an example of a NICHHD nationwide campaign.[32] Its goal is to increase calcium consumption among America's children and teens. The campaign was designed to teach parents, children, and healthcare professionals about the importance of calcium for children and adolescents. Channels of information dissemination include brochures, booklets, coloring books, stickers, posters, public service announcements, and press releases.

14.1.5.2.2 The National Bone Health Campaign

The Office on Women's Health (OWH) of DHHS focuses on the overall health of all women throughout their lifespan. Adolescence represents a dynamic developmental period when young women make important choices about lifestyle behaviors, including diets, physical activity, sexual activity, and use of tobacco, alcohol, and other drugs that can influence their health and well-being throughout adulthood.

OWH along with the CDC and the National Osteoporosis Foundation partnered to promote the National Bone Health Campaign (NBHC),[33] a multiyear (2001–2005) initiative to promote optimal bone health in girls 9–12 years old and thus reduce their risk of osteoporosis later in life. The goal of this public/nonprofit partnership was to educate and encourage young girls to establish lifelong healthy habits, especially increased calcium consumption and physical activity to build and maintain strong bones. In addition to girls 9–12 years old, the campaign targets adult influencers, including parents, teachers, coaches, youth group leaders, and healthcare professionals.

To help extend the reach and impact of its messages, NBHC has created a national partnership network of federal, state, and local government allies and nonprofit and for-profit organizations. The network's goal is to facilitate resource and information sharing among a broad range of partner organizations across the country. Partners are encouraged to incorporate bone health messages and activities into their existing programs and to share lessons learned.

14.1.5.3 Campaigns to Prevent Diabetes, Heart Disease, and Cancer

Cardiovascular disease, diabetes, and cancer account for nearly two-thirds of all deaths in the U.S. Campaigns to reduce the incidence and prevalence of these diseases target their shared risk factors — tobacco use, insufficient physical activity, and poor diet.

Excess body weight is an independent risk factor for cardiovascular diseases as well as causing other risk factors such as hypertension, dyslipidemia, and type 2 diabetes. An estimated 70% of type 2 diabetes risk in the U.S. is attributable to overweight and obesity. Modest weight loss of 10% of initial body weight and increases in physical activity result in reduced cardiovascular risk factors such as hypertension, dyslipidemia, and type 2 diabetes. Weight reduction decreases insulin resistance and improves measures of glycemia and dyslipidemia in diabetics.

Epidemiologic and animal studies indicate that overweight and obesity are associated with increased risk for cancers at numerous sites, including breast (among postmenopausal women), colon, endometrium, esophagus, gallbladder, liver, prostate, ovarian, pancreas, and kidney. Obesity may account for 14% of cancers in men and 20% of cancers in women.[34]

14.1.5.3.1 National Diabetes Education Program

The National Diabetes Education Program (NDEP)[35] was launched in 1997 to improve diabetes management and reduce the morbidity and mortality from diabetes and its complications. It is sponsored by the CDC and NIH and partners with more than 200 other entities at the federal, state, and local levels. The NDEP message is that diabetes is serious, common, costly, and controllable. NDEP aims to change the way diabetes is treated — by the media, by the public, and by the healthcare system.

To help fulfill its mission of changing the way diabetes is treated, NDEP has developed awareness campaigns to disseminate information about diabetes prevention and control. Partners who work with NDEP can adopt the program's messages and tailor them for their members, disseminate information to the media, coordinate education activities, and share resources with other partner organizations. The campaign has developed tools for local organizations to provide motivational messages to members of the community. Clinical practice tools and patient education materials are also available for use by professionals to identify and counsel patients with prediabetes to help prevent the onset of the disease, and to work with patients with diabetes to take control and prevent disease complications. (See Box 14.6 National Diabetes Education Program materials for consumers and professionals.)

14.1.5.3.2 1% or Less

The 1% or Less campaign[36] encourages adults and children over age two to switch from whole and 2% milk to 1%, 1/2%, or skim milk as way to reduce consumption of saturated fat. Developed in the mid-1990s by CSPI, a nonprofit organization dedicated to improving the nation's health

---

**Box 14.6 National Diabetes Education Program Materials
for Consumers and Professionals**

Online access is available to all NDEP's campaign tools, including public service announcements (PSAs), fact sheets, press releases, and feature articles that can be customized,
distributed, and promoted in local markets. These materials are available at www.ndep.nih.gov/
campaigns/tools.htm. Materials for professionals may be accessed at www.ndep.nih.gov/
resources/health.htm.

---

through better nutrition, this 1-month campaign includes news stories and advertisements on
television, radio, billboards, and in newspapers; milk taste tests at a variety of community sites;
supermarket shelf labeling to draw attention to low-fat milk; and school activities. Results of 1%
or Less campaigns conducted in Wheeling, WV[37] (popualtion 34,882) and East Los Angeles,[38]
California (population 124,283) suggest that this social marketing campaign can be effective in
increasing low-fat and overall milk consumption in urban communities.

Milk sales data were collected from supermarkets in Wheeling and from comparison communities for 3 1-month time periods (at baseline, immediately following the campaign, and 6 months
after its completion). In addition, pre- and postintervention telephone surveys were conducted.
Results showed that low-fat milk's market share increased from 18% of overall milk sales at baseline
to 41% of overall milk sales in the month following the end of the campaign, an increase that was
sustained at the 6-month follow-up. In the postintervention telephone survey, 38% of those respondents who reported drinking high-fat milk at baseline reported having switched to low-fat milk.
Although it was not a program goal, overall milk sales increased by 16% in the intervention cities
following the campaign and remained high at follow-up. Similarly, the bilingual (Spanish/English)
Adelante con Leche Semi-descremada 1% Campaign, implemented by California Adolescent Nutrition and Fitness Program (CAN Fit) in East Los Angeles in 2000, resulted in a doubling of 1%
milk sales in Latino communities and a 30% increase in milk purchases overall.

Table 14.3 provides the example of a lowfat milk consumption campaign to illustrate types of
social change, by time and level of society.

TABLE 14.3
**A Low-Fat Milk Consumption Campaign Illustrates Types of Social Change, by Time
and Level of Society**

	Micro Level (Individual Consumer)	Group Level (Group or Organization)	Macro Level (Society)
Short-term change	*Behavior change* Example: Switch to low-fat milk at school	*Change in norms; administrative change* Example: Voluntarily provide low-fat and fat-free milk as part of the school breakfast and school lunch programs	*Policy change* Example: Provide price supports for low-fat and fat-free dairy products so they cost the consumer less than their full-fat counterparts
Long-term change	*Lifestyle change* Example: All dairy products consumed are either low fat or fat free	*Organizational change* Example: Require that all schools provide low-fat and fat-free milk	*Sociocultural evolution* Example: Eradication of nutrition-related diseases, such as heart disease

14.1.5.3.3 5 A Day for Better Health

The 5 A Day for Better Health program is a national initiative to increase consumption of fruits and vegetables by all Americans to 5 to 9 servings a day.[39] Eating 5 to 9 servings of fruits and vegetables a day promotes good health and reduces the risk of many cancers, high blood pressure, heart disease, diabetes, stroke, and other chronic diseases. The program seeks to increase public awareness of the importance of eating 5 to 9 servings of fruits and vegetables every day, providing consumers with specific information about how to include more servings of fruits and vegetables in their daily routines, and to increase the availability of fruits and vegetables at home, school, work, and other places where food is served. The program provides a simple, positive message: Eat 5 or more servings of fruits and vegetables every day for better health.

Founded in 1991 as a partnership between NCI and the Produce for Better Health Foundation, 5 A Day is the nation's largest public/private partnership for nutrition. The program includes federal, state, and local government agencies, and industry and volunteer organizations. The 5 A Day network consists of state coordinators and coalitions in all 50 states and U.S. territories. State coordinators work closely with partnering organizations and are responsible for planning and conducting 5 A Day activities in their state. Program components include state, regional, and community interventions; media communications; environmental and policy change advocacy; point-of-sale advertising; and behavioral research.[40]

The program has been extensively evaluated. People are more aware now of the need to consume fruits and vegetables, but data from the Behavioral Risk Factor Surveillance System (BRFSS) indicate little change in fruit and vegetable consumption between 1994 and 2000.[41,42] However, the program has been instrumental in effecting environmental change, which in turn is expected to increase consumption of fruits and vegetables.

An example of environmental change advocated by 5 A Day is its support of the Fruit and Vegetable Pilot Program proposed by Iowa Sen. Tom Harkin (Democrat), then chairman of the Senate Committee on Agriculture, Nutrition, and Forestry, in 2001 and passed as part of the 2002 Farm Bill. The pilot allocated $6 million to 25 schools in Iowa, Indiana, Michigan, and Ohio, and six schools on an Indian reservation in New Mexico for purchase of fruit and vegetable snacks to be offered free to children throughout the school day. High school, middle school, and elementary schools all participated and distributed fruits and vegetables using a combination of kiosks, vending machines, and in-class methods.

The Fruit and Vegetable Pilot Program was an unqualified success;[43] in 2004, when the Child Nutrition and WIC Reauthorization Act was enacted, it made the Fruit and Vegetable Pilot Program permanent. The act also provides for expanding the program to three other states (Washington, North Carolina, and Pennsylvania) and two Indian reservations (one or more tribes belonging to the Intertribal Council of Arizona and the Ogallala Sioux Tribe of the Pine Ridge Reservation in South Dakota). Effective October 1, 2004, $9 million became available to participating schools to operate the program during the 2004–2005 school year. The USDA and the National 5 A Day Partnership also provide educational materials to participating schools.

14.1.5.3.3.1 Fruits & Veggies — More Matters™

In late 2006, *Fruits & Veggies — More Matters*™ replaced 5 A Day as the brand promoted by the Produce for Better Health (PBH) Foundation, which, together with the National Cancer Institute, was the main sponsors of the 5-A-Day campaign. During focus groups, PBH discovered that women preferred the term "veggies."

14.1.5.4 Campaigns to Prevent Foodborne Illness

The CDC estimates that foodborne diseases cause approximately 76 million illnesses, 325,000 hospitalizations, and 5,000 deaths in the U.S. each year. Known pathogens account for an estimated 14 million illnesses, 60,000 hospitalizations, and 1,800 deaths. Three pathogens — *Salmonella, Listeria, Toxoplasma* — are responsible for 1,500 deaths annually or more than 75% of those caused by known pathogens. Unknown agents account for the remaining 62 million illnesses, 265,000 hospitalizations, and 3,200 deaths. Overall, foodborne diseases appear to cause more illnesses (but fewer deaths) than previously estimated.[44,45] Several factors explain why the incidence of food borne illnesses has increased: fewer meals are prepared at home; one quarter of the U.S. population is composed of people with weakened immune systems — the elderly, pregnant women, the very young, and people with HIV/AIDS; and diets include more fresh, often imported, produce.[46] The number of documented outbreaks of human infections associated with the consumption of raw fruits, vegetables, and unpasteurized fruit juices has increased in recent years. In the U.S., the number of reported produce-related outbreaks per year doubled between the periods 1973–1987 and 1988–1992.[47,48]

Using a four-round Delphi technique, food safety educators, food microbiologists, food safety policy specialists, and epidemiologists were asked to rank food-handling and consumption behaviors associated with 13 food borne illnesses. Assessment of their collective opinions indicates the extent to which various food borne illnesses could be prevented by such behaviors as keeping foods at safe temperatures, using a thermometer to cook foods adequately, protecting food and equipment from cross-contamination, hand washing, and avoiding high-risk foods.[49] The results of this study are summarized in Table 14.4.

14.1.5.4.1   Food Safety Education

Food handling observations show that food-handling errors are made by consumers during home food preparation,[50] by food service employees at the retail level, and to a lesser extent in hospitals and schools.[51] Four broad categories of risk factors contributing to food borne illness were identified in consumers' homes. These include improper cleaning (inadequately washing hands and food preparation surfaces), cross-contamination, improper refrigeration, and cooking foods to less than the proper temperature. Similarly, five broad categories of risk factors contributing to food borne illness were identified in institutional food service establishments, restaurants, retail food stores,

TABLE 14.4
Food-Handling Behaviors and Prevention of Food-Borne Illness

Behavior	Relative Importance in Preventing Food-Borne Illness	
	First-Degree Importance	Second-Degree Importance
Keeping foods at safe temperatures	*Bacillus cereus* *Clostridium perfingens*	*Staphyloccus aureus*
The use of a thermometer to cook foods adequately	*Campylobacter jejuni* Salmonella species *E. coli* O157:H7 *Toxoplasma gondii* *Yersinia enterocolitica*	
Avoiding cross contamination		*Campylobacter jejuni* Salmonella species *E. coli* O157:H7 *Toxoplasma gondii* *Yersinia enterocolitica*
Handwashing Avoiding specific contaminated foods	Shigellosis *Listeria monocytogenes* Noroviruses *Vibrio* species	

Source: From Hillers, V.N., Medeiros, L., Kendall, P., Chen, G., and DiMascola, S. Consumer food-handling behaviors associated with prevention of 13 foodborne illnesses. *J Food Prot.* 66, 1893–1899, 2003.

schools, and hospitals: food from unsafe sources, inadequate cooking, improper holding temperatures, contaminated equipment, and poor personal hygiene.

The Food Safety Inspection Service (FSIS) is the public health agency within the USDA responsible for ensuring that the nation's commercial supply of meat, poultry, and egg products is safe, wholesome, and correctly labeled and packaged. FSIS works with FDA and state and local authorities to improve food safety practices at the retail level. It also works with other government agencies, the food industry, and others to educate consumers on safe food handling practices. FSIS consumer education programs are modeled on the concept of integrated marketing, a management concept designed to make all aspects of marketing communication such as advertising, sales promotion, public relations, and direct marketing work together as a unified force, rather than permitting each to work in isolation. The three components of the FSIS integrated marketing model each support the other:

- *Mass media* — reaching out to the broad public
- *Cluster targeting* — using demographic, geographic, and sociodemographic information to target communications to segmented audiences
- *One-on-one interactions* — such as through the USDA's Food Safety Mobile used in the Is It DONE Yet? campaign, which expands outreach programs to include new services and partnerships for minorities and underserved populations

Each component of the integrated marketing program is developed based on risk research, delivered via social marketing concepts, and assessed through evaluative research. Ongoing nationwide surveys and consumer focus group studies are used to evaluate and ensure the continuing effectiveness of the initiative and to continue to track the documented changes in consumer behavior.

FSIS is committed to communicating with all food handlers, especially those who serve others in large-scale food operations or are personally at-risk for food borne illness. The agency has made great strides in reaching out to citizens who may not speak English. Food safety publications for both industry and consumers have been translated into several languages including Spanish, Korean, and Mandarin Chinese. The agency employs national television, cable networks, educational television, radio, magazines, newspapers, and Web sites to enhance public education efforts. Four major food safety education campaigns operate under the aegis of FSIS: Fight BAC!, Thermy, National Food Safety Education Month, and the Food Safety Mobile.

The FDA/USDA Food Safety Survey (FSS) is a random-digit, dial survey of a nationally representative sample of American consumers conducted by FDA. The FSS obtains information FDA uses for risk assessments, regulatory and policy matters, and consumer education purposes. Surveys have been conducted in 1988, 1993, 1998, and 2001, with sample sizes of 3200, 1620, 2001, and 4482, respectively. The 2001 questionnaire is available online at: http://www.food-safety.gov/~fsg/fs01surv.html. In each survey conducted through 2001, the key factor influencing consumer behavior was individual perception of risk. Survey questions regarding behavior and risk were the most likely to yield a strong link to good food safety practices.[52] The 2005 survey included a random, nationally representative sample of 4,000 adults in households: Hispanics were over sampled and a sample of initial nonrespondents participated in a short version of the survey to conduct a nonresponse analysis. The majority of the survey questions are identical to those in the 2001 survey. However, it is expected that consumer knowledge and attitudes regarding food safety have changed due to consumer education campaigns, such as those discussed in this chapter.

A survey of representatives of 48 U.S. states and 20 nations attending an international conference for food safety educators (2002) sponsored by the USDA and DHHS in cooperation with the Partnership for Food Safety Education revealed what these experts deemed essential regarding target audiences and food safety education priorities. Food service workers are the highest priority target audience, followed by the general pubic, children, the school community, parents of young children, and the elderly. Understandably, participants representing the food industry were most concerned about food safety education of a culturally diverse audience, while participants representing

TABLE 14.5
Food Safety Recommendations in the 2005 *Dietary Guidelines for Americans*

To avoid microbial foodborne illness:

    Clean hands, food contact surfaces, and fruits and vegetables. Meat and poultry should not be washed or rinsed

    Separate raw, cooked, and ready-to-eat foods while shopping, preparing, or storing foods

    Cook foods to a safe temperature to kill microorganisms

    Chill (refrigerate) perishable food promptly and defrost foods properly

Avoid raw (unpasteurized) milk or any products made from unpasteurized milk, raw or partially cooked eggs or foods

    containing raw eggs, raw or undercooked meat and poultry, unpasteurized juices, and raw sprouts

---

federal agencies selected food biosecurity as their top priority (see Chapter 15 for additional information on biosecurity). Other food safety education priorities rank ordered by the conference participants include encouraging hand washing, educating children, and promoting the principles expressed in Fight BAC!®.[53]

The 2005 *Dietary Guidelines for Americans*[54] contains recommendations for food safety (see Table 14.5). Those recommendations reflect the key food-handling messages promulgated by the campaigns discussed in the following sections.

14.1.5.4.1.1   Fight BAC!

The public/private Partnership for Food Safety Education (PFSE) is a nonprofit organization dedicated to educating the public about safe food handling to help reduce food borne illness. PFSE was formed as a direct response to a 1996 independent panel report, *Putting the Food Handling Issue on the Table: The Pressing Need for Food Safety Education,*[55] which specifically called for a public/private partnership to educate the public about safe food handling and preparation. PFSE uses a social marketing model to decrease food borne illness by educating consumers on simple steps they can take to reduce or eliminate food borne pathogens. Scientific and technical experts reviewed extant public opinion research to develop campaign concepts, messages, and graphics materials that are accurate, understandable, and persuasive. The PFSE campaign is named Fight BAC! Its key message can be summarized in just four words: *clean, separate, chill,* and *cook.*

The food safety steps of the Fight BAC! campaign are to *clean* by washing hands and food preparation surfaces often, *separate* to prevent cross-contamination, *chill* by refrigerating foods at 40° or less, and *cook* to the proper temperature (see Section 14.1.5.4.1.2). Fight BAC! combines the resources of the federal government, industry, and several consumer organizations to implement a broad-based food safety education campaign designed to reach men, women, and children of all ages. The campaign uses multiple information channels, such as the mass media, public service announcements, the Internet, point-of-purchase materials, and school and community outreach to a broad constituency of educators, media groups, and consumers to bring Americans face-to-face with the problem of foodborne illness and to motivate them to take action. The campaign enlists a national network of public health, nutrition, food science, education and special constituency groups to support the campaign and greatly extend its reach. Initially, the campaign was funded by the contributions of industry trade associations with technical assistance and in-kind support provided by government agencies and consumer organizations. To date, Fight BAC! has reached millions of consumers through government outreach, private industry initiatives, school education programs, and media placements.

PFSE was charged with keeping the Fight BAC! campaign fresh and providing ongoing value-added products to keep the target audiences engaged and advance the four basic safe food handling messages. Encouraged by the success of Fight BAC!, in 2004 PFSE launched the Produce Handling Education Campaign, which focuses on safe handling of fresh fruits and vegetables. As part of the produce education campaign, additional recommendations highlight the consumer's need to *check*

TABLE 14.6
Fight BAC!® Food Safety Guidelines

Clean hands often by washing them thoroughly with soap and water; air dry or use a clean towel. Be sure there are plenty of clean utensils and platters for food preparation and serving. Clean food thermometer after use

Separate raw and cooked/ready-to-eat food to prevent cross-contamination

Cook to a safe internal temperature. Ground beef should be cooked to 160° F

Chill leftovers in the refrigerator or freezer within 2 h of taking food off the grill. On hot days above 90° F refrigerate or freeze within 1 h. Make sure the temperature is 40° F or below and 0° F or below in the freezer. Check the temperature occasionally with a refrigerator/freezer thermometer

Check fresh fruits and vegetables for bruising and damage, and refrigeration, if cut

Throw away fresh fruits and vegetables under certain conditions that may render them unsafe

produce for bruising or damage and to make sure the products have been refrigerated if fresh cut and to *throw away* fresh produce under certain conditions that render them unsafe.[56] The Fight BAC! food safety guidelines are summarized in Table 14.6. The logos for four campaigns are presented in Figure 14.3.

14.1.5.4.1.2 National Food Thermometer Education Campaign

Prior to1997, consumers who did not use a food thermometer had been advised by FSIS to cook ground beef patties until the center and the cooked-out juices were no longer pink. In 1998, the USDA concluded that the internal temperature and therefore the safety of cooked hamburgers could not be judged by visual inspection. Data showing that nearly 25% of the hamburgers judged to be thoroughly cooked according to color could still be contaminated with Salmonella and *Eschericia coli* O157:H7[57] demonstrated the need for a meat thermometer. The temperature at which pathogens are killed, 160° F, is considered the threshold for safe consumption of ground beef.[58] For this reason, the Food Safety Education Staff (FSES) of FSIS undertook a campaign to promote the use of food thermometers. Initial focus groups found that consumer food safety knowledge was lacking, particularly with regard to thermometer use to gauge doneness of cooked meat. Key recommendations from these groups suggested that the FSES promote food thermometer use for everyday meals and as a means to improve taste as well as safety. They further suggested FSES should target parents of young children.

In 2000, FSIS launched a national food safety education campaign, employing the best of social marketing concepts, to promote the use of food thermometers. The campaign theme "It's safe to bite when the temperature is right!"[59] delivered by Thermy™, a cartoon food thermometer, is designed to encourage consumers to use a food thermometer when cooking meat, poultry, and egg products. PFSE, the Food Temperature Indicator Association, and a number of grocery chains and thermometer companies around the country are cooperating with FSIS in the Thermy™ campaign.[60] The campaign's goal is to increase the use of food thermometers by American consumers in their homes and by food service workers in institutional settings. Fight BAC!'s cook to the proper temperature message is reinforced by the Thermy™ campaign.

The campaign was expanded to institutional settings in 2002. Soon thereafter, a social marketing approach was developed to increase the impact of the national food thermometer education program.[61] Goals of the social marketing project were to refine and define appropriate audience segments; identify appropriate desired behaviors of those segments; identify barriers to behavior change and ways to overcome them; identify opportunities and strategies for education; identify setting, time and delivery systems for implementation; and recommend evaluation techniques for the campaign.[62]

In 2004, FSIS partnered with Michigan State University's National Food Safety and Toxicology Center, Department of Food Science and Human Nutrition, and Extension service in an effort to increase consumers' use of food thermometers. The "Is It DONE Yet?" initiative again used social marketing principles to promote positive behavior change among parents of children under 10 years

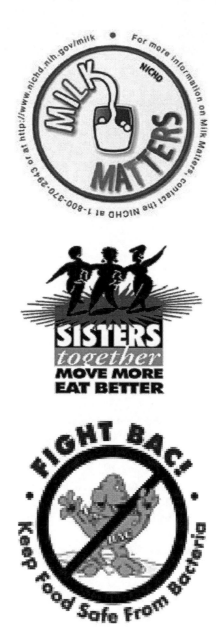

FIGURE 14.3 Logos for social marketing campaigns. (From Milk Matters: http://www.nichd.nih.gov/publications/pubs_details.cfm?from=milk&pubs_id=44; Sisters Together: http://win.niddk.nih.gov/publications/SisPrmGuide2.pdf; Fight Bac! http://www.fightbac.org/images/download/BAC_1clr_words.tif.)

of age, chosen as those most likely to change behavior. The campaign included carnival games, a full media and advertising plan, construction of a pre-/posttest survey technique, and development of strategies to attract target audiences. Researchers studied how to field test social-marketing tactics, develop skills in determining target audiences, identify strategies that can change consumers' behavior, and recognize styles for communicating with different audiences. This pilot is expected to be a role model for other states and serve as the basis for the national launch of this program in 2005.[63] When available, results of the pilot program will be posted on the FSIS food thermometer research page: www.fsis.usda.gov/education/food_thermometer_research/index.asp.

14.1.5.4.1.3 Mobile Food Safety Van

From 2003 through 2005, FSIS sponsored a Food Safety Mobile, a grassroots education campaign designed to reach millions of consumers with food safety messages.[64] The mobile was a 35-foot, recreational-type vehicle emblazoned with bold, eye-catching graphics and prominent food safety messages, including PFSE's four Fight BAC!® messages. It served as a "rolling billboard" for food safety messages and as an attention-getting backdrop for educational exhibits and events appealing to adults and children alike. The graphic nature of the mobile was designed to attract diverse groups including children, parents, seniors, and various ethnic, low-literacy, and non-English speaking audiences. It was stocked with materials for general audiences, for specific audiences just listed, and for food service personnel and included materials in Spanish. When available, a food safety or public affairs specialist with knowledge of specific audience needs or Spanish language skills will accompany the mobile. The goals of the Food Safety Mobile programs were to:

- Increase awareness of food safety and promote the use of the four key food safety behaviors: clean, separate, refrigerate, and cook
- Meet the needs of local food safety educators and organizations by generating positive media attention for food safety education and reaching specific audiences
- Provide food safety education information to consumers at a grassroots level by personally interacting with them
- Target under-served populations
- Strengthen existing partnerships and create new ones through enhanced communication, thereby fostering increased collaboration in food safety education and food security outreach to localities nationwide
- Educate consumers on new food safety technologies, such as irradiation
- Inform the public about its role in food safety and security, and ask consumers to do their part in homeland security
- Increase familiarity among the general public with the role of the USDA and FSIS in protecting public health

14.1.5.4.1.4 National Food Safety Education Month

The National Restaurant Association Educational Foundation's International Food Safety Council designated September as National Food Safety Education Month[SM] (NFSEM) to heighten awareness of the importance of food safety education throughout the restaurant and food service industry. Goals of NFSEM are to reinforce food safety education and training among restaurant and foodservice workers, and to educate the public on how to handle and prepare food properly at home, whether cooking from scratch or serving take-out meals and restaurant leftovers. Restaurants and food service operations; hospitality associations; colleges and universities; federal, state, and local government agencies; and consumer organizations across the country participate in NFSEM in a variety of ways each year. Each year FDA and FSIS develop a kit of consumer education materials for NFSEM in support of the four key food safety practices. These kits reach more than 40,000 health educators, including FDA and USDA field staff, State and local health department personnel, school food service directors, and school nurses are involved in a variety of local educational activities.[65] Each year a new theme and training activities are created for the restaurant and food service industry to reinforce proper food safety practices and procedures. Themes for previous NFSEM are summarized in Table 14.7.

14.1.5.5 Campaigns to Promote Health through Nutrition

In addition to preventing disease, nationwide efforts are made to actively promote health through nutrition, beginning with conception. These efforts provide target audiences such as women of child-bearing age, nursing mothers, and low-income individuals with the supportive environment needed to make healthy choices that will circumvent the onset of disease. As seen by the programs discussed in this section, environment can be interpreted to mean the nature of the food available

TABLE 14.7
Themes Used for National Food Safety Education Month:
1998–2004

1998	Keep It Clean — The First Step to Food Safety
1999	Cook it Safely — It's a Matter of Degrees
2000	Be Smart. Keep Foods Apart — Don't Cross Contaminate
2001	Be Cool. Chill Out. Refrigerate Promptly
2002 (retail)	CHECK IT OUT before You Check It In
2002 (consumer)	Four Steps to Food Safety
2003	Store It. Don't Ignore It
2004	Be Aware When You Prepare

for purchase (folate fortification), emotional support (WIC peer counseling), financial assistance (food stamps), or enhanced nutrition knowledge through education and outreach.

14.1.5.5.1 National Folic Acid Education Campaign

Studies have shown that folate supplements taken around the time of conception significantly reduce occurrence of neural tube defects (NTDs) in infants. To lower the risk of NTDs, women are advised to consume 400 micrograms a day of folate prior to conception and 600 micrograms during the first trimester of pregnancy. However, only 30% of women of child-bearing age consume sufficient folic acid to prevent spina bifida and anencephaly. Because folic acid alone or in a vitamin supplement has been proven to reduce the risk of an NTD-affected pregnancy by 50–70%, as of 1999, all refined grain products — bread, cereal, corn meal, farina, flour, pasta, rice — are fortified with folate. Folate in fortified foods and supplements is absorbed almost twice as well as folate naturally available in green leafy vegetables, citrus fruits, whole grain breads, or legumes.[66,67]

According to the CDC, half of all pregnancies are unplanned.[68] Therefore, the CDC's National Folic Acid Education Campaign targets *all* women of childbearing age, both those who are thinking about becoming pregnant and those who are not planning a pregnancy now or in the future. Other audience segments include healthcare providers and other health professionals who care for women, Hispanic women, and adolescent girls.

The campaign's goals are to:

- Increase awareness of the need for women who can become pregnant to consume folic acid every day.
- Increase the knowledge that folic acid taken daily before and during early pregnancy can prevent some serious birth defects.
- Change behavior of all women who are capable of becoming pregnant to consume 400 micrograms of folic acid daily.
- Educate the influencers of women (such as healthcare providers) to conduct information sessions about folic acid. Policymakers also need to be influenced to include folic acid in programs.[67]

The campaign provides free educational materials in English and Spanish to concerned organizations, including radio public-service announcement scripts, posters, and downloadable fact sheets.

14.1.5.5.2 National WIC Breastfeeding Promotion Project

Research confirms that breast milk is the best food for a baby's first year of life. Breastfeeding provides many health, nutritional, economical, and emotional benefits to both mother and child. Because a major goal of the WIC program is to improve the nutritional status of infants, WIC mothers are encouraged to breastfeed their infants unless medically contraindicated.

The Breastfeeding Promotion Project offers the following:

- WIC mothers choosing to breastfeed are provided information through counseling and breastfeeding educational materials.
- Breastfeeding mothers receive follow-up support through peer counselors.
- Breastfeeding mothers are eligible to participate in WIC longer than nonbreastfeeding mothers.
- Mothers who exclusively breastfeed their infants receive an enhanced food package.
- Breastfeeding mothers can receive breast pumps, breast shells, or nursing supplements to help support the initiation and continuation of breastfeeding.[69]

14.1.5.5.3 Food Stamp Nutrition Education Program

The Food Stamp Program enables low-income families to buy nutritious food with Electronic Benefits Transfer (EBT) cards and serves as a first line of defense against hunger. Food stamp recipients spend their benefits to buy eligible food in authorized retail food stores.[70]

In 1995 and 1996, the USDA's Food Stamp Program stimulated the development of 22 state-based nutrition education social marketing networks. Housed principally in land grant universities, cooperative extensions, and state health departments, the networks moved ahead independently to develop an array of innovative interventions for low-income population groups ranging from preschoolers to senior citizens, based on state priorities. Programs varied widely in focus, scope, complexity, and funding levels.

In 2003, the USDA conducted a series of networking sessions with state representatives from the various nutrition assistance programs to strengthen collaboration on nutrition education and promotion efforts. Over 300 representatives from programs in 49 states met to identify a common nutrition goal and begin formulating a plan for working together to achieve that goal. Over 90% of the states identified their common goal — for example, Iowa's goal is to promote fruit and vegetable consumption, whereas that for Texas is to promote healthy eating and active lifestyles — and began developing a state wide nutrition plan with objectives, strategies, and tactics for achieving that single goal. The State Nutrition Action Plan (SNAP) was the outcome of this process. the USDA's SNAP Web site supports state committees by providing funding and program participation data, links to state-specific data sources, and other resources. This site also provides a mechanism for sharing state-based SNAP activities and connects people involved in this process.[71]

Currently, Food Stamp Nutrition Education is the largest adult-oriented nutrition promotion effort in the U.S. As such, the lessons being learned from the program may inform the development of other initiatives to prevent chronic diseases, including those aimed at eliminating health disparities and reversing the nation's obesity epidemic.

14.2 TAILORED HEALTH COMMUNICATION

Since the late 1990s, tailored health communication has emerged as a promising, innovative approach to addressing public health issues. Defined as "any combination of information and behavior change strategies intended to reach one specific person, based on characteristics that are unique to that person, related to the outcome of interest, and derived from an individual assessment,"[72] tailored communications are created especially for an individual based on knowledge of that person. This information may be gathered through a survey or a brief personal interview with a professional. The results of these questions are entered into a computer, which draws from a "library" of possible messages to create materials that directly address the individual's needs, interests, or concerns. Once a program has been developed for a certain health issue, it can be used to produce tailored print materials with the potential to reach large populations. Thus, tailored communications are a promising and innovative approach that can be used to address a variety of public health issues.

A subset of the larger field of health communications, tailored communications are distinct from more familiar, but less personalized, methods of developing *targeted* materials — messages prepared using information about population segments — or *personalized* materials — a person's name draws attention to a generic message. Because they can address cognitive and behavioral patterns as well as individual demographic characteristics, tailored materials are more sophisticated than targeted ones.

According to the first scientific review of tailoring research, "tailored print communications have demonstrated an enhanced ability to attract notice and readership ... are more effective than nontailored communications for influencing health behavior change ... (and) can be an important adjunct to other intervention components."[73] Although the field is still in its infancy, empirical research shows that tailored print materials are more effective than nontailored ones in helping people change health behaviors, such as physical activity and diet,[74] although tailored materials have not been equally effective for all individuals.[75] Tailored weight loss materials are more effective in bringing about more positive thoughts about the materials, personal connections to the materials, self-assessment thoughts, and thoughts indicating behavioral intention than nontailored materials.[76] Thus, the tailoring of health information can significantly improve the chances the information will be considered and can stimulate prebehavioral changes such as self-assessment and intention.

NCI maintains an online guide that coaches the user to create a simple tailored letter using Microsoft Word™.[77] The topics covered in the demonstration program include creating a sample database, creating a master letter, linking the main document to the database, inserting merge fields and word fields into the master document, adding a tailored illustration, and performing the merge. A study of NCI's tailored print materials to increase fruit and vegetable consumption found a significant mean serving difference between those receiving untailored and tailored materials.[78]

14.3 ACRONYMS

BMD	Bone mineral density
BMI	Body mass index
CDC	Centers for Disease Control and Prevention
CSPI	Center for Science in the Public Interest
CVD	Cardiovascular disease
DHHS	Department of Health and Human Services
DISC	Dietary Intervention Study in Children
EBT	Electronic benefits transfer
FDA	Food and Drug Administration
FSES	Food Safety Education Staff
FSIS	Food Safety Inspection Service
FSS	Food Safety Survey
NBHC	National Bone Health Campaign
NCI	National Cancer Institute
NDEP	National Diabetes Education Program
NFSEM	National Food Safety Education Month
NHLBI	National Heart, Lung, and Blood Institute
NICHHD	National Institute of Child Health and Human Development
NIDDK	National Institute for Diabetes and Digestive and Kidney Disease
NIH	National Institutes of Health
NTD	Neural tube defect
OWH	Office of Women's Health
PFSE	Partnership for Food Safety Education
USDA	United States Department of Agriculture
WIC	Special Supplemental Nutrition Program for Women, Infants, and Children
WIN	Weight-Control Information Network

REFERENCES

1. U.S. Department of Health and Human Services. Healthy People 2010: Understanding and Improving Health. 2nd ed. Washington. DC: U.S. Government Printing Office. November 2000. Available at: http://www.healthypeople.gov/document/Word/Volume1/11 HealthCom.doc. Accessed February 12, 2007.

2. Kotler, P. and Zaltman, G. Social marketing: an approach to planned social change. *JF Marketing*. 35(July), 3–12, 1971.

3. Murphy, S.C., Whited, L.J., Rosenberry, L.C., Hammond, B.H., Bandler, D.K., and Boor, K.J. Fluid milk vitamin fortification compliance in New York State. *J Dairy Sci.* 84, 2113–2820, 2001. Available at: http://jds.fass.org/cgi/reprint/84/12/2813.pdf. Accessed June 24, 2006.

4. Rothschild, M. Carrots, sticks, and promises: a conceptual framework for the management of pubic health and social behaviors. *J Mark.* 63, 24–37, 1999.

5. Maibach, E.W., Rothschild, M.L., and Novelli, W.D. Social marketing. In Glanz, K., Rimer, B.K., and Lewis, F.M., eds. *Health Behavior and Health Education: Theory, Research, and Practice*, 3rd ed. San Francisco, CA: Jossey-Bass, 2002, chap. 19.

6. Montazeri, A. Social marketing: a tool not a solution. *J R Soc Health.* 117, 115–118, 1997.

7. Message Strategy Research to Support Development of the Youth Media Campaign (YMC). Revealing Target Audience Receptiveness to Potential YMC Message Concepts. Prepared for the CDC by Aeffect, Inc., Lake Forest, IL., January 2001. Available at: www.health.gov/communication/db/FileDownload. asp?ID=20. Accessed June 26, 2006.

8. Anon. Life's First Great Crossroad: Tweens Make Choices that Affect Their Lives Forever. Available at: www.tweensafety.org/_docs/Tween%20Booklet.pdf. Accessed June 26, 2006.

9. Weinreich, N.K. The social marketing mix. In *Hands-On Social Marketing: A Step-by-Step Guide*. Thousand Oaks, CA: Sage Publishing, 1999, chap. 3.

10. The Social Marketing Collaborative. *Social Marketing: A Resource Guide*. 2002. Available at: www.turningpointprogram.org/Pages/social_marketing_101.pdf. Accessed January 23, 2005.

11. Lindenberger, J.H. and Bryant, C.A. Promoting breastfeeding in the WIC Program: a social marketing case study. *Am J Health Behav.* 24, 53–60, 2000. Available at: https://www.extenza-eps.com/ extenza/loadPDF?objectIDValue=32255. Accessed January 20, 2005.

12. Wong, F., Huhman, M., Heitzler, C., Asbury, L., Bretthauer-Mueller, R., McCarthy, S., et al. VERB™ — a social marketing campaign to increase physical activity among youth. *Prev Chronic Dis.* [serial online] July 2004. Available at URL: http://www.cdc.gov/pcd/issues/2004/jul/04_0043.htm. Accessed January 20, 2005.

13. Grier, S. and Bryant, C.A. Social marketing in pubic health. *Ann Rev Public Health.* 26, 319–339, 2005.

14. Bauman, A. Commentary on the VERB™ campaign — perspectives on social marketing to encourage physical activity among youth. *Prev Chronic Dis.* [serial online] July 2004. Available at: http://www. cdc.gov/pcd/issues/2004/jul/04_0054.htm. Accessed September 4, 3005.

15. Adapted from: U.S. Department of Health and Human Services. National Institutes of Health. National Cancer Institute. *Making Health Communication Programs Work*, 1989, rev. 2001. Available at: http://cancer.gov/pinkbook. Accessed January 19, 2005.

16. Andreasen, A.R. and Drumwright, M.E. Alliances and ethics in social marketing. In Andreasen, A.R., ed. *Ethics in Social Marketing*. Washington, DC: Georgtown University Press, 2000, chap. 5. Available at: http://press.georgetown.edu/excerpt.html?session=e08858323f715ef52a76906e137763e0&cat=4&id =0878408207 & expid=230. Accessed August 28, 2005.

17. Hedley, A.A., Ogden, C.L., Johnson, C.L., Carroll, M.D., Curtin, L.R., and Flegal, K.M. Prevalence of overweight and obesity among U.S. children, adolescents, and adults, 1999–2002. *JAMA.* 291(23), 2847–2850, 2004.

18. Finkelstein, E.A., Fiebelkorn, I.C., and Wang, G. National medical spending attributable to overweight and obesity: how much, and who's paying? *Health Aff.* W3, 219–226, 2003.

19. Mokdad, A.H., Ford, E.S., Bowman, B.A., Dietz, W.H., Vinicor, F., Bales, V.S., and Marks, J.S. Prevalence of obesity, diabetes, and obesity-related health risk factors, 2001. *JAMA.* 289(1), 76–79, 2003.

20. Hardy, L.R., Harrell, J.S. and Bell, R.A. Overweight in children: definitions, measurements, confounding factors, and health consequences. *J Pediatr Nurs.* 19(6), 376–384, 2004.

21. Eckel, R.H., Grundy, S.M., and Zimmet, P.Z. The metabolic syndrome. *The Lancet.* 365, 1415–1428, 2005.

22. Bauman, A. Commentary on the VERB™ campaign — perspectives on social marketing to encourage physical activity among youth. *Prev Chronic Dis.* [serial online] 2004. Available at: http://www.c. Accessed August 28, 2005.

23. U.S. Department of Health and Human Services. Centers for Disease Control and Prevention. Campaigns and Programs At-A-Glance. Available at: http://www.cdc.gov/communication/campaigns/verb.htm. Accessed January 9, 2005.

24. Huhman, M., Potter, L.D., Wong, F.L., Banspach, S.W., Duke, J.C., and Heitzler, C.D. Effects of a mass media campaign to increase physical activity among children: year-1 results of the VERB campaign. *Pediatrics.* 116, e277–e284, 2005. Available at: http://pediatrics.aappublications.org/cgi/content/full/116/2/e277. Accessed August 28, 2005.

25. Van Horn, L., Obarzanek, E., Friedman, L.A., Gernhofer, N., and Barton, B. Children's adaptations to a fat-reduced diet: the Dietary Intervention Study in Children (DISC). *Pediatrics.* 115, 1723–1733, 2005. Available at: http://pediatrics.aappublications.org/cgi/content/full/115/6/1723. Accessed August 27, 2005.

26. National Institutes of Health. National heart, Lung, and Blood Institute. *We Can*! homepage. Available at: http://www.nhlbi.nih.gov/health/public/heart/obesity/wecan/. Accessed August 27, 2005.

27. Founding partners for *We Can*! include Action for Healthy Kids, the American Academy of Family Physicians, the Association for State and Territorial Public Health Nutrition Directors, Black Entertainment Television (BET) Foundation, the International Food Information Council Foundation, North American Association for the Study of Obesity, Parents' Action for Children, the President's Council on Physical Fitness and Sports, and Univision; supporting organizations include the American College of Sports Medicine, the Produce for Better Health Foundation, and the University of Michigan Health System.

28. Goldberg, J., Rudd, R.E., and Dietz, W. Using 3 data sources and methods to shape a nutrition campaign. *J Am Diet Assoc.* 99, 717–722, 1999.

29. Eyre, H., Kahn, R., and Robertson, R.M. The ACS/ADA/AHA Collaborative Writing Committee. Preventing cancer, cardiovascular disease, and diabetes: a common agenda for the American Cancer Society, the American Diabetes Association, and the American Heart Association. *CA Cancer J Clin.* 54, 190–207, 2004. Available at: http://caonline.amcancersoc.org/cgi/content/full/54/4/190. Accessed September 5, 2005.

30. NIDDK Strategic Plan on Minority Health Disparities, 2003. Available at: http://www.niddk.nih.gov/federal/planning/mstrathealthplan.htm. Accessed August 29, 2005.

31. Department of Health and Human Services. National Institutes of Health. *Sisters Together: Move, More Eat Better Program Guide.* National Institute of Diabetes and Digestive and Kidney Diseases. NIH Publication No. 99-3329. January 1999. Available at: http://win.niddk.nih.gov/publications/SisPrm Guide2.pdf. Accessed August 29, 2005.

32. U.S. Department of Health and Human Services. *Bone Health and Osteoporosis: A Report of the Surgeon General.* Rockville, MD: U.S. Department of Health and Human Services, Office of the Surgeon General, 2004. Available at: http://www.surgeongeneral.gov/library/bonehealth/content.html. Accessed September 5, 2005.

33. National Institutes of Health: National Institute of Child Health and Human Development. Milk Matters. Tweens and teens need calcium now more than ever! Available at www.nichd.nih.gov/milk/milk.cfm. Accessed June 26, 2006.

34. Center for Disease Control and Prevention. Powerful Girls Have Powerful Bones. Available at: www.cdc.gov/powerfulbones/. Accessed June 26, 2006.

35. U.S. Department of Health and Human Services. Centers for Disease Control and Prevention. National Center for Chronic Disease Prevention and Health Promotion. National Diabetes Education Program homepage. Available at: http://www.cdc.gov/diabetes/ndep/about.htm. Accessed January 11, 2005.

36. 1% or Less Campaign. Center for Science in the Public Interest. http://www.cspinet.org/nutrition/1less.htm. Accessed January 7, 2005.

37. Reger, B., Wootan, M.G., Booth-Butterfield, S., and Smith, H. 1% or Less: a community-based nutrition campaign. *Public Health Rep.* 113, 410–419, 1998.

38. *Connection* (The Quarterly Newsletter of the California Adolescent Nutrition and Fitness Program). Fall 2000. Available at: http://www.canfit.org/pdf/newsletter_fall_2000.pdf. Accessed January 7, 2005.

39. Eat 5 to 9 A Day. Available at: www.5aday.gov/index.html. Accessed June 26, 2006.

40. National Cancer Institute. Monograph. Five-a-Day for Better Health Program. National Institutes of Health. NIH Publication 01-5019. September 2001. Available at: http://www.5aday.gov/about/pdf/masimaxmonograph.pdf. Accessed September 3, 2005.

41. 5 A Day for Better Health Program Evaluation Report. 2000. Available at: http://www.cancercontrol.cancer.gov/5aday_12-4-00.pdf. Accessed September 3, 2005.

42. Serdula, M.K., Gillespie, C., Kettel-Khan, L., Farris, R., Seymour, J., and Denny, C. Trends in fruit and vegetable consumption among adults in the United States: behavioral risk factor surveillance system, 1994–2000. *Am J Pub Health.* 94, 1014–1918, 2004. Available at: http://www.ajph.org/cgi/content/full/94/6/1014. Accessed September 3, 2005.

43. Buzby, J.C., Guthrie, J.F., and Kantor, L.S. Evaluation of the USDA Fruit and Vegetable Pilot Program: Report to Congress. Food Assistance and Nutrition Research Program, Food and Rural Economics Division, Economic Research Service, U.S. Department of Agriculture. E-FAN No. (03-006), April 2003. Available at: http://www.ers.usda.gov/publications/efan03006/. Accessed September 3, 2005.

44. Nestle, M. *Safe Food: Bacteria, Biotechnology, and Bioterrorism.* Berkeley, CA: University of California Press, 2003.

45. Mead, P.S., Slutsker, L., Dietz, V., McCaig, L.F., Bresee, J.S., Shapiro, C., Griffin, P.M., and Tauxe, R.V. Food-related illness and death in the United States. *Emerging Infect Dis.* [serial on the Internet]. September–October 1999. Available at: http://www.cdc.gov/ncidod/EID/vol5no5/mead.htm. Accessed January 22, 2005.

46. McCabe-Sellers, B.J. and Beattie, S.E. Food safety: emerging trends in foodborne illness surveillance and prevention. *J Am Diet Assoc.* 104, 1708–1717, 2004.

47. Buck, J.W., Walcott, R.R., and Beuchat, L.R. Recent trends in microbiological safety of fruits and vegetables. Plant Health Progress. 2003. Available at: http://www.apsnet.org/online/feature/safety/. Accessed January 28, 2005.

48. U.S. Food and Drug Administration, Center for Food Safety and Applied Nutrition. Analysis and Evaluation of Preventive Control Measures for the Control and Reduction/Elimination of Microbial Hazards on Fresh and Fresh-Cut Produce. A Report of the Institute of Food Technologists for the Food and Drug Administration of the United States Department of Health and Human Services. September 21, 2001. Available at: http://www.cfsan.fda.gov/~comm/ift3-toc.html. Accessed January 28, 2005.

49. Hillers, V.N., Medeiros, L., Kendall, P., Chen, G., and DiMascola, S. Consumer food-handling behaviors associated with prevention of 13 foodborne illnesses. *J Food Prot.* 66, 1893–1899, 2003.

50. Anderson, J.B., Shuster, T.A. Hansen, K.E., Levy, A.S., and Volk, A. A camera's view of consumer food-handling behaviors. *J Am Diet Assoc.* 104, 186–191, 2004.

51. U.S. Department of Health and Human Services. U. S. Food and Drug Administration. Center for Food Safety and Applied Nutrition. Report of the FDA Retail Food Program Database of Foodborne Illness Risk Factors. Prepared by the FDA Retail Food Program Steering Committee. August 10, 2000. Available at: http://vm.cfsan.fda.gov/~dms/retrsk.html. Accessed January 27, 2005.

52. U.S. Department of Health and Human Services. Food and Drug Administration, Center for Food Safety and Applied Nutrition, Consumer Studies Branch. Food Safety Survey: Summary of Major Trends in Food Handling Practices and Consumption of Potentially Risky Foods. August 27, 2002. Available at: http://vm.cfsan.fda.gov/~dms/fssurvey.html. Accessed January 28, 2005.

53. *Proceedings: Thinking Globally-Working Globally: A Conference for Food Safety Educators.* September 18–20, 2002. Orlando, FL. Available at: http://www.fsis.usda.gov/Orlando2002/Proceedings.pdf. Accessed January 28, 2005.

54. U.S. Department of Health and Human Services, U.S. Department of Agriculture. *Dietary Guidelines for Americans 2005.* HHS Publication number HHS-ODPHP-2005-01-DGA-A. USDA Publication number: Home and Garden Bulletin No. 232. Available at: http://www.health.gov/dietaryguidelines/dga2005/document/pdf/DGA2005.pdf. Accessed January 30, 2005.

55. U.S. Department of Agriculture. Food Safety and Inspection Service The Final Rule on Pathogen Reduction and Hazard Analysis and Critical Control Point (HACCP) Systems, July 1996. Available at: http://www.fsis.usda.gov/OA/background/finalrul.htm. Accessed January 27, 2005.

56. BAC Fighters News and Tools — Welcome. Available at: http://portal.fightbac.org/pfse/. Accessed January 28, 2005.

57. USDA-ARS/FSIS. 1998. Premature Browning of Cooked Ground Beef. Food Safety and Inspection Service Public Meeting on Premature Browning of Ground Beef. May 27, 1998. USDA, Washington, D.C.

58. U.S. Department of Agriculture. Food Safety and Inspection Service. Food Safety Education. Food Safety Education Staff. Color of Cooked Ground Beef as It Relates to Doneness. Slightly Revised April 2003. Available at: http://www.fsis.usda.gov/Frame/FrameRedirect.asp?main=http://www.fsis.usda.gov/oa/thermy/researchfs.htm. Accessed January 10, 2005.

59. U.S. Department of Agriculture. Food Safety and Inspection Service. Consumer Education and Information/ Consumer Research and Focus Group Testing. Final Research Report: A Project to Apply Theories of Social Marketing to the Challenge of Food Thermometer Education in the United States. 2001 (updated 2002). Available at: http://www.fsis.usda.gov/Frame/FrameRedirect.asp?main=/oa/research/research.htm. Accessed January 10, 2005.

60. Food and Drug Administration, Food Safety and Inspection Service, Centers for Disease Control and Prevention. *Healthy People 2010* Food Safety Data Progress Review. Food Safety Education Examples. May 11, 2004. Available at: http://www.foodsafety.gov/~dms/hp2010ed.html. Accessed January 27, 2005.

61. U.S. Department of Agriculture. Food Safety and Inspection Service. Food Safety Education. Thermy™ web page. Available at: http://www.fsis.usda.gov/food_safety_education/Thermy/index.asp. Accessed January 10, 2005.

62. U.S. Department of Agriculture. Food Safety and Inspection Service. Consumer Education and Information/Consumer Research and Focus Group Testing. Final Research Report. A Project to Apply Theories of Social Marketing to the Challenge of Food Thermometer Education in the United States. Report Provided by the Baldwin Group, Inc. December 21, 2001. Available at: http://www.fsis.usda.gov/oa/research/thermom_edu.pdf. Accessed January 26, 2005.

63. U.S. Department of Agriculture and Michigan State University Join Forces to Promote Food Thermometer Use. Available at: http://www.fsis.usda.gov/news_&_events/Const_Update_080604/ index.asp. Accessed January 27, 2005.

64. U.S. Department of Health and Human Services. Food and Drug Administration, Food Safety and Inspection Service, Centers for Disease Control and Prevention. *Healthy People 2010* Food Safety Data Progress Review. Food Safety Education Examples. May 11, 2004. Available at: http://www.foodsafety.gov/~dms/hp2010ed.html. Accessed January 27, 2005.

65. Boyle, M.A. *Community Nutrition in Action: An Entrepreneurial Approach*, 3rd ed. Thomson Wadsworth. Belmont, CA. 2003.

66. CDC. Communication at CDC, National Folic Acid Education Campaign. Available at: www.cdc.gov/communication/campaigns/folic.htm and http://www.cdc.gov/ncbddd/folicacid. Accessed June 25, 2006.

67. CDC Foundation. Birth defects: good nutrition a good defense. Available at: www.cdcfoundation.org/healththreats/birthdefects.aspx. Accessed June 27, 2006.

68. U.S. Department of Agriculture: Food and Nutrition Service: breastfeeding promotion and support in WIC. Available at: http://www.fns.usda.gov/wic/Breastfeeding/breastfeedingmainpage.HTM. Accessed June 26, 2006.

69. U.S. Departmenbt of Agriculture, Food and Nutrition Service. Food Stamp Program. Available at: http://www.fns.usda.gov/fsp/. Accessed June 26, 2006.

70. U.S. Department of Agriculture, Food and Nutrition Service, State Action Plans. Available at: http://www.fns.usda.gov/oane/SNAP/SNAP.htm. Accessed June 26, 2006.

71. Kreuter, M., Farrell, D., Olevitch, L., and Brennan, L. *Tailored Health Messages: Customizing Communication with Computer Technology.* Mahwah, NJ: Lawrence Erlbaum Associates, 2000.

72. Skinner, C.S., Campbell, M.K., Rimer, B.K., Curry, S., and Prochaska, J.O. How effective is tailored print communication? *Ann Behav Med.* 21, 290–298, 1999.

73. Patrick, K., Sallis, J.F., Prochaska, J.J., Lydston, D.D., Calfas, K.J., Zabinski, M.F., Wilfley, D.E., Saelens, B.E., and Brown, D.R. A multicomponent program for nutrition and physical activity change in primary care: PACE+ for adolescents. *Arch Pediatr Adolesc Med.* 155, 940–946, 2001.

74. Holt, C.L., Clark, E.M., Kreuter, M.W., and Scharff, D.P. Does locus of control moderate the effects of tailored health education materials? *Health Educ Res.* 15, 393–403, 2000.

75. Kreuter, M.W., Bull, F.C., Clark, E.M., and Oswald, D.L. Understanding how people process health information: a comparison of tailored and nontailored weight-loss materials. *Health Psychol.* 18, 487–494, 1999.

76. U.S. Department of Health and Human Services. National Institutes of Health. National Cancer Institute. Cancer Control and Population Sciences. Health Communication and Informatics Research. Health Message Tailoring. Available at: http://cancercontrol.cancer.gov/messagetailoring/guide.html. Accessed January 19, 2005.
77. Heimendinger, J., O'Neill, C., Marcus, A.C., Wolfe, P., Julesburg, K., Morra, M., et al. Multiple tailored messages are effective in increasing fruit and vegetable consumption among callers to the Cancer Information Service. *J Health Commun.* 10(Suppl. 1), 65–82, 2005.
78. U.S. Department of Health and Human Services. Food and Drug Administration, Food Safety and Inspection Service, Centers for Disease Control and Prevention. *Healthy People 2010* Food Safety Data Progress Review. Food Safety Education Examples. May 11, 2004. Available at: http://www.food-safety.gov/~dms/hp2010ed.html. Accessed January 27, 2005.

15 Food Safety and Defense

I prefer butter to margarine, because I trust cows more than chemists.

Joan Dye Gussow, 2001[1]

The terms *food safety* and *food security* are often used interchangeably and are thus confused. Within this text, food safety refers to protecting food from biological and other sources of contamination, whereas food security refers to access to food and issues of hunger as discussed in Chapter 13. Food supplies in the U.S. are generally maintained at high levels of safety — protected from accidental or deliberate contamination — so that citizens seldom give much thought to the subject. Food safety rarely becomes a public issue, except on occasions when outbreaks of foodborne illness or malicious threats make headline news. The following discussion of food safety reviews federal, state, and local roles in regulation, surveillance, emergency preparedness and response to disasters resulting from either natural or human causes, as well as the safety education of both responders and the general public (see also Chapter 14, Section 14.1.5.4.1 Food safety education).

The safety and quality of the U.S. food supply are governed by a complex system administered by the 15 agencies listed in Table 15.1. The U.S. Department of Agriculture (USDA) and the Food and Drug Administration (FDA) within the Department of Health and Human Services (HHS) have primary responsibility for food safety. The Web site www.Food-Safety.gov is self-described as the *gateway* to food safety information from the federal government.

15.1 SAFETY, WHOLESOMENESS, AND LABELING

Although most experts agree that the U.S. food supply is among the safest in the world, foodborne illness is nevertheless recognized as a significant public health problem. Foodborne pathogens sicken many people in the U.S. every year. The Centers for Disease Control and Prevention (CDC) attributes 76 million illnesses, 325,000 hospitalizations, and 5,000 deaths to foodborne pathogens annually. It is likely that these numbers may underestimate the magnitude of the problem as many people do not seek medical help for foodborne illness, thus occurrences are not officially reported. Known pathogens are estimated to cause one-third of deaths, whereas the remaining two thirds are caused by unknown agents. Most vulnerable to foodborne diseases are children, pregnant women, the elderly, and people who are immune compromised[2]. As a large proportion of prisoners are HIV positive, they are also a particularly vulnerable population[3] (see also Section 8.5). Box 15.1 summarizes the common foodborne pathogens. For more information, see the *Foodborne Pathogenic Microorganisms and Natural Toxins Handbook* (a.k.a. the *Bad Bug Book*) at: http://vm.cfsan.fda.gov/~mow/intro.html.

TABLE 15.1
U.S. Federal Agencies' Food Safety Responsibilities

	Agency	Responsible For
U.S. Department of Agriculture	Food Safety and Inspection Service	All domestic and imported meat, poultry, and processed egg products
	Animal and Plant Health Inspection Service	Protecting the health and value of U.S. agricultural resources (e.g., animals and plants)
	Grain Inspection, Packers, and Stockyards Administration	Establishing quality standards, inspection procedures, and marketing of grain and other related products
	Agricultural Marketing Service (AMS)[a]	Establishing quality and condition standards for dairy, fruit, vegetable, livestock, meat, poultry, and egg products
	Agricultural Research Service	Conducting food safety research
	Economic Research Service	Providing analyses of the economic issues affecting the safety of the U.S. food supply
	Natural Agricultural Statistics Service	Providing statistical data, including agricultural chemical usage data, related to the safety of the food supply
	Cooperative State Research, Education, and Extension Service	Supporting food safety research, education, and extension programs in the land-grant university system and other partner organizations
Department of Health and Human Services	Food and Drug Administration	All domestic and imported food products, except meat, poultry, and processed egg products
	Centers for Disease Control and Prevention	Protecting the nation's public health, including foodborne illness surveillance
Department of Commerce	National Marine Fisheries Service	Voluntary, fee-for-service examinations of seafood for safety and quality
Environmental Protection Agency		Regulating the use of pesticides and maximum allowable residue levels on food commodities and animal feed
Department of the Treasury		Enforcing laws covering the production, use, and distribution of alcoholic beverages
Department of Homeland Security[b]		Coordinating various agencies' food security[c] activities
Federal Trade Commission		Prohibiting false advertisements for food

[a] According to the USDA, AMS has no statutory authority in the area of food safety. However, AMS performs some functions related to food safety for several foods. For example, AMS graders monitor a shell egg surveillance program that identifies cracked and dirty eggs. In addition, AMS performs functions related to food safety for the National School Lunch Program.
[b] In 2001, by an executive order, President Bush stated that the then Office of Homeland Security, as part of its efforts to protect critical infrastructures, should coordinate efforts to protect livestock, agriculture, and food systems from terrorist attacks. In 2002, Congress enacted the Homeland Security Act of 2002, P.L. 107–296, 116 Stat. 2135 (2002), setting out the department's responsibility to protect and secure critical infrastructures and transferring several food safety related responsibilities to the DHS. As a result of the executive order, the Homeland Security Act of 2002 established the DHS, and subsequent to presidential directives, the DHS provides overall direction on how to protect the U.S. food supply from deliberate contamination.
[c] Food security refers to the vulnerability of a nation's food supply to deliberate actions that contaminate food or reduce the available quantity of food.

Source: United States Government Accountability Office. Food Safety -- Experiences of Seven Countries in Consolidating Their Food Safety Systems. GAO-05-212. February 2005. Washington, DC: Government Accountability Office. Available at: http://www.gao.gov/new.items/d05212.pdf. Accessed February 16, 2007.

Box 15.1 Common FoodBorne Pathogens[1]

Norovirus is the leading cause of diarrhea in the U.S. Any food can be contaminated with norovirus if handled by someone who is infected with this virus. Common names of the illness caused by the Norwalk and Norwalk-like viruses are viral gastroenteritis, acute nonbacterial gastroenteritis, food poisoning, and food infection.

Campylobacter, according to CDC, is the most common bacterial cause of diarrhea in the U.S., resulting in 1 to 6 million illnesses each year. Sources include raw and undercooked meat and poultry, raw milk, and untreated water.

Clostridium botulinum produces a toxin which causes botulism, a life-threatening illness that can prevent the breathing muscles from moving air in and out of the lungs. Sources: home-prepared foods and herbal oils; honey should not be fed to children less than 12 months old.

E. coli **O157:H7** can produce a deadly toxin. Since 1982, *E. coli* O157:H7 has emerged as an important cause of foodborne illness, causing 20,000 to 70,000 cases of foodborne illness each year. Sources: meat, especially undercooked or raw hamburger, produce, and raw milk.

Listeria monocytogenes causes listeriosis, a serious disease for pregnant women, newborns, and adults with a weakened immune system. Sources of the pathogen include unpasteurized dairy products and soft cheeses, raw and undercooked meat, poultry, seafood, and produce, as well as soil and water. Foodborne *L. monocytogenes* is rare and declining but potentially life threatening when illness occurs. Foodborne illness caused by listeriosis in pregnant women can result in miscarriage, fetal death, and severe illness or death of a newborn infant. Others at risk for severe illness or death are older adults and those with weakened immune systems.[2,3] CDC's FoodNet indicates that *L. monocytogenes* caused 1500 serious illnesses in 2002, more than 38% decrease in the incidence of foodborne *L. monocytogenes* infections since 1996.[4] Nevertheless, due to its high fatality rate (20%), ongoing efforts are needed to continue to reduce the public health impact of this disease.

Salmonella, the most common cause of foodborne deaths, is responsible for 2 to 4 million cases of foodborne illness annually. Sources of infection include raw and undercooked eggs, undercooked poultry and meat, dairy products, seafood, fruits, and vegetables. Illnesses occur each year in the U.S. from the more than 2000 strains of salmonella.

Staphylococcus aureus is a bacterium that produces a toxin that causes vomiting soon after eating contaminated food. Sources: cooked foods that are rich sources of protein, such as cooked ham, salads, bakery products, and dairy products.

Shigella causes an estimated 300,000 cases of diarrheal illnesses annually in the U.S. Shigella may be passed from person to person due to poor hygiene. Sources: salads, milk and dairy products, and unclean water.

Toxoplasma gondii are parasites that cause toxoplasmosis, a disease that can produce central nervous system disorders particularly mental retardation and visual impairment in children. Pregnant women and people with weakened immune systems are at higher risk. Sources: meat (primarily pork).

Vibrio vulnificus causes gastroenteritis or a syndrome known as *primary septicemia*. People with liver diseases are especially at high risk. Sources: raw or undercooked seafood.

Sources:

[1] Food and Drug Administration. *Foodborne Pathogenic Microorganisms and Natural Toxins Handbook. Center for Food Safety and Applied Nutrition.* 1992. Available at: http://www.cfsan.fda.gov/~mow/intro.html. Accessed February 18, 2005.

[2] FDA Press Release. Risk Assessment Reinforces That Keeping Ready-To-Eat Foods Cold May be the Key to Reducing Listeriosis. October 21, 2003. Available at: http://www.fda.gov/bbs/topics/NEWS/2003/NEW00963.html. Accessed February 18, 2005.

[3] Centers for Disease Control and Prevention. Preliminary FoodNet data on the incidence of infection with pathogens transmitted commonly through food — Selected sites, United States, 2003. *MMWR* 53: 338, 340–343, 2004. Available at: http://www.cdc.gov/mmwr/PDF/wk/mm5316.pdf. Accessed Febrary 18, 2005.

[4] Walls, I. Achieving continuous improvement in reductions in foodborne Listeriosis — A risk based approach. A Report from the ILSI Risk Science Institute Expert Panel on *Listeria monocytogenes* in Foods. Available at: http://www.ilsi.org/file/ccfhsummary-final.pdf. Accessed February 18, 2005.

15.1.1 FEDERAL AUTHORITY

Federal, state, and local authorities play complementary and interdependent roles in regulating food and food processing facilities. Under the current federal system, the responsibility for assuring the safety, wholesomeness, and proper labeling of all foods lies with two departments, the USDA and the HHS, and one independent agency, the Environmental Protection Agency (EPA). The Food Safety and Inspection Service (FSIS) of the USDA ensures that meat, poultry, eggs, poultry-based foods, and some egg-based products are safe, wholesome, and accurately labeled. The FDA, an agency within HHS, is charged with protecting consumers from impure, unsafe, and fraudulently labeled domestic and imported foods, other than those regulated by the FSIS. It is also responsible for ensuring that all animal drugs and feeds produce no risk to human health when used in livestock. No food or feed item may be marketed legally in the U.S. if it contains a food additive or drug residue not permitted by the FDA. The CDC, another agency within HHS, tracks foodborne illness outbreaks. The EPA's mission includes protecting public health and the environment from risks posed by pesticides. It establishes tolerances for pesticide residues in foods and ensures the safety of drinking water. All these agencies use existing food safety and environmental laws to also regulate plants, animals, and foods developed through biotechnology.

In 2005, the food safety budgets requested for the FSIS and the FDA were $824.7 million and $556.2 million, respectively. These allowances include support for food safety and counterterrorism initiatives in the FDA, as well as funds for the USDA's Office of Food Security and Emergency Preparedness that coordinates the development of infrastructure to prevent, prepare for, and respond to an intentional attack on the U.S. food supply.[4,5]

15.1.1.1 Legislation

The earliest enacted food legislation was associated with safety. The Federal Food, Drug, and Cosmetic Act (FFDCA) was enacted in 1906 to prevent the manufacture, sale, or transportation of adulterated, misbranded, poisonous, or deleterious foods, drugs, medicines, and liquors. The Federal Import Milk Act of 1927 stipulates that milk and cream must meet defined minimum safety standards in order to be imported into the U.S. The Public Health Service Act of 1944 was enacted to protect consumers from communicable diseases and other illness through the licensing of clinical laboratories.

15.1.1.2 Food and Drug Administration (FDA)

Regulatory authority for food is conferred on the FDA by the FFDCA; the Federal Import Milk Act; the FFDCA of 1938, as amended; the Public Health Service Act; the Fair Packaging and Labeling Act of 1966; the Infant Formula Act of 1980, as amended; the Nutrition Labeling and Education Act of 1990; and the Dietary Supplement Health and Education Act (DSHEA) of 1994.

15.1.1.2.1 Food Packaging and Labeling

Only after food safety had been addressed did legislation address food packaging and labeling. Food labeling in the U.S. is mandated under two federal agencies, the FDA and the FSIS. The FDA is responsible for food labeling regulations on all food products, except meat and poultry items, which are regulated under the FSIS. The FFDCA prohibits the entry into interstate commerce of adulterated or misbranded foods. Under this authority, the FDA has established guidance and regulatory requirements for manufacturers to assure that food is safe and unadulterated. The Fair Packaging and Labeling Act was passed to help consumers make informed decisions about the products they were purchasing and established general and specific principles for food labeling.

The Nutrition Labeling and Education Act passed by Congress in 1990 amended the FFDCA, allowing regulations to be expressed on food labels. This act mandated nutrition labeling on most packaged food products and instructed the FDA to control and set standards for the content and format of the nutrition label. Food labeling laws apply to all retail sales including mail orders.

In passing the DSHEA in 1994, Congress amended the FFDCA to include several provisions, exempting dietary supplements and their dietary ingredients from the premarket safety evaluations required of other new food ingredients, or for new uses of old food ingredients. Dietary supplements must still meet the requirements of other safety provisions.

15.1.1.2.1.1   Genetic Modification

Genetically modified foods, though extremely controversial, are similarly exempt from information labeling in the U.S. Genetic modification transfers specific traits, or genes, from one organism to a different plant or animal. Desirable traits include pesticide and herbicide resistance, improved hardiness, and increased content of specific nutrients. A gene is a specific sequence of bases that creates proteins that confer a trait to a plant or animal. That the vast majority of genes do not code for a unique protein, as was previously believed, undermines the foundations of genetic engineering of food crops. Foreign genes have the potential to create unintended proteins with unpredictable effects on the ecosystem and human health.

Genes are inserted into DNA using either a gene gun or bacterial vectors (for transport). The gene gun fires microscopic pellets coated with DNA into a host cell, and some of this DNA coating is left within the cell as the pellet passes through — an imprecise and unstable form of insertion, rather than the precise, predictable, and safe method its advocates claim. Mutation could occur during insertion, accidentally affecting the levels of toxins a plant produces or otherwise impacting a plant's normal metabolism. Key experiments to assess both the environmental risks and benefits of gene insertion have not been undertaken.

Despite these concerns, genetic engineering has enjoyed considerable success. Approximately 70% of foods on supermarket shelves in the U.S. have GM ingredients. However, many of the anticipated benefits — decreased input dependence, increased nutritional quality, and feeding hunger — have not materialized. The Genetic Engineering Action Network recommends four major areas of reform:

- *Prior informed choice*: a labeling regime must be created
- *Assessment*: better oversight, and raising and apportioning resources for an effective system
- *Protection*: ending exposure of farmers and consumers to unchecked industry power
- *Liability*: accountability for harm caused to humans and the environment

Box 15.2 lists arguments for and against the pursuit of genetic modification, whereas Box 15.3 presents a timeline that encompasses labeling-related issues. Box 15.4 contains a discussion about genetically modified food from a legal perspective.

Box 15.2 For and Against Genetically Modified Organisms (GMOs)

Claims for:

- Reduces pesticide use[1,2]
- Improves crop yield[1,2,3]
- Reduces famine due to crop failure[4]

- Improves weed control and reducing fuel use and soil erosion[2]
- Enhances nutritional quality,[1,5,3] for example, in rice enhanced with vitamin A
- Eliminates allergens, for example, the P34 gene in soy[6]
- Incorporates vaccines that can eliminate disease[5]
- Expands agriculture to inhospitable land, for example, in sub-Saharan Africa[1,5,7] and to resource-poor farmers[5,7]

Arguments against:

- Introduces new allergens into the food supply[8,9,10,11]
- Antibiotic resistance to marker genes[12]
- Reduces nutrient quality such as loss of phytoestrogens[8,11]
- Reduces usefulness of Bt as an insecticide[8,9,13,14] and harms nontarget organisms[5,8,13]
- Introduces superweeds through gene flow from herbicide resistant crops to wild relatives[8,9,13]
- Impacts animals, such as the medaka fish, where genetic manipulation for size affected reproductive fitness[9]
- Possible long-term side effects of ingesting genetically modified foods[6]
- Lack of the promised yields in GM crops,[8] possibly from conflict with other selection criteria[9,14]
- Reduces the nonedible fiber portion of grain, reducing availability of fiber for weaving, impacting local handicrafts[14]
- Contaminates due to cross-pollination (inevitable and hard to detect)[2]
- Lack of adequate testing for environmental and human impact before release[8,13]

Sources:

[1] Timmer, C.P. Biotechnology and food systems in developing countries. *J Nutr.* 133: 3319–3322, 2003.

[2] Harlander, S.K. Safety assessments and public concern for genetically modified food products: the American view. *Toxicol Pathol.* 30(1): 132–134, 2002.

[3] Atherton, K.T. Safety assessment of genetically modified crops. *Toxicology.* 181–182, 421–426, 2002.

[4] Borlaug, N.E. Ending world hunger: the promise of biotechnology and the threat of antiscience zealotry. *Plant Physiology.* 124: 487–490, 2000.

[5] McGloughlin, M. Ten reasons why biotechnology will be important to the developing world. *AgBioForum.* 2(3&4): 163–174, 1999.

[6] Bren, L. Genetic engineering: the future of foods? *FDA Consumer Magazine.* November–December 2003. www.fda.gov/fdac/features/2003/603_food.html. Accessed July 13, 2006.

[7] Borlaug, N.E. Ending world hunger: the promise of biotechnology and the threat of antiscience zealotry. *Plant Physiology.* 124: 487–490, 2000.

[8] Altieri, M.A., Rosset, P. Ten reasons why biotechnology will not ensure food security, protect the environment and reduce poverty in the developing world. *AgBioForum.* 2(3&4): 155–162, 1999.

[9] McCullum, C. Food biotechnology in the new millennium: promises, realities, and challenges. *J Am Diet Assoc.* 100(11): 1311–1315, 2000.

[10] Atherton, K.T. Safety assessment of genetically modified crops. *Toxicology.* 181–182, 421–426, 2002.

[11] Fagan, J.B. Assessing the safety and nutritional quality of genetically engineered foods. www.psrast.org/jfassess.htm. Accessed July 13, 2006.

[12] Bakshi, A. Potential adverse health effects of genetically modified crops. *J Toxicol Environ Health.* 6(3): 211–225, 2003.

[13] Altieri, M.A., Rosset, P. Strengthening the case for why biotechnology will not help the developing world: a response to McGoughlin. *AgBioForum.* 2(3&4): 226–236, 1999.

[14] Babcock, B.C., Francis, C.A. Solving global nutrition challenges requires more than new biotechnologies. *J Am Diet Assoc.* 100(11): 1308–1311, 2000.

Box 15.3 GMOs and Labeling: A Timeline

1953

Watson and Crick discover the structure of DNA.

1970s

Scientists isolate genes that code for specific proteins.[1]

1972

Paul Berg creates the first genetically modified DNA molecule.[2,3]

1973

Stanley Cohen, Annie Chang, and Herbert Boyer develop recombinant DNA (rDNA) technology (i.e., DNA segments containing a desirable gene are inserted [recombined] into the DNA of a distinct organism).[4,5]

1974

Stanford University files the first patent applications to cover rDNA technology.[6]

NIH convenes an rDNA Advisory Committee (RAC) to oversee genetic research.

1975

At the Asilomar Conference in California, scientists agree to draft and abide by a set of research guidelines for the safe use of the technology.[7]

1976

NIH releases a comprehensive set of rules governing the practice of rDNA technology and banning the release of GMOs into the environment.[8]

1980s

Monsanto lobbies the proderegulation Reagan/Bush administration to regulate biotechnology in order to limit its liability if sued (in response to its tarnished public image from the harm caused by Agent Orange and PCBs).[9] The administration finally concedes and Monsanto begins developing recombinant bovine somatotropin (rBST), a bovine growth hormone that increases milk production.

1980

The landmark case *Diamond v. Chakrabarty*[10] is decided by the U.S. Supreme Court.

1982

The NIH ban on the release of GMOs into the environments is lifted, as insulin, produced through genetic modification, is approved for sale by the FDA.

1983

Four independent groups of scientists working on transgenic plants announce successful results. Three have inserted bacterial genes into plants; the fourth has inserted a bean gene into a sunflower plant.

1985

Transgenic plants are field-tested for the first time.[11]

1986

The USDA issues a policy statement: The Coordinated Framework for Regulation of Biotechnology,[12] authored essentially by Monsanto lawyers.[9] It becomes the cornerstone of U.S. biotechnology policy but does not establish any new regulatory or legal requirements.

1991

Researchers develop an experimental, genetically engineered (GE) tomato that expresses a cold-resistant gene from an Arctic flounder; experiment is a failure and never makes it to market.[13]

1992

The FDA issues official Statement of Policy on Foods Derived from New Plant Varieties,[14] described by Vice President Quayle to mean that: "biotech products will receive the same oversight as other products, instead of being hampered by unnecessary regulation."[15] In its statement, the FDA embraces the substantial equivalence doctrine (focus on product rather than process; a food product that is substantially equivalent to an existing food need not be put through further regulatory requirements) developed by an OECD Working Group earlier that year.[16] Most of the remaining countries, including the European Union countries, and Japan, adopt the *precautionary principle* (government may impose restrictions on activities that pose potential risks to human health or to the environment without scientific proof pertaining to the nature and seriousness of those risks).

1992

Term *Frankenfood* is coined by Paul Lewis, English professor at Boston College, in an article on the FDA's decision to allow corporations to market genetically modified food.[17]

Mid-1990s

Pioneer Hi-Bred voluntarily removes from market a GE soybean, intended for poultry feed, containing a sulfur gene from a Brazil nut that when tested induced allergic reactions in humans having Brazil nut allergies. Though not intended for direct human consumption, the company could not see how the GE beans could be kept out of the human food supply.[15]

1994

The FDA approves sale of Monsanto's controversial recombinant bovine growth hormone (rBGH) that increases levels of insulinlike growth factor-I (IGF-I) in cow's milk, a possible cancer stimulant in adults.[18]

1995

Genetically modified foods appear in grocery stores[19]; incidences of food allergies rise significantly in the ensuing decade. However, the FDA's position that GE foods are no different from traditional foods and the lack of labeling leaves no practical way to learn if increase in food allergies is associated with GE foods.[20]

1996

Dairy manufacturers challenge the constitutionality of a Vermont statute requiring identification of products that were, or might have been, derived from dairy cows treated with rBST.[21] The Vermont Court of Appeals agrees with the dairy manufacturers that such labeling infringes on their constitutional right not to speak, which is not outweighed by the state's interest in informing its citizens; the legislation is based on the public's right to know rather than on any health or safety concerns. The court notes that it is unaware of any case where consumer interest alone is sufficient to justify a requirement that is the functional equivalent of a warning.

1998

The Alliance for Bio-Integrity leads a coalition of scientists, health professionals, religious leaders, and consumers in filing a lawsuit against the FDA, alleging that the agency's policy permitting GE foods to be marketed without testing and labels violates the agency's mandate to protect the national food supply.[22]

The judge rules against the plaintiffs on every claim in the complaint, holding that the FDA's right to set policy trumps consumers' right to know. However, a major result of the discovery phase of the lawsuit was the revelation of the FDA internal documents that indicated their own scientists had safety concerns about GM foods.[23]

1992–2000

Under the Clinton Administration, the FDA holds public hearings on GE foods in response to public criticism of regulatory policies. In May, 2000, the FDA proposes a rule to make premarket consultation with the agency mandatory.[24]

1999

Rep. Dennis Kucinich (D-OH) introduces HR 3377, Genetically Engineered Food Right-to-Know Act, which would require mandatory labeling for all foods containing at least 0.1% ingredients of GMOs.[25] It was subsequently introduced to the House a number of times, most recently in 2006.

2000

Senator Barbara Boxer (D-CA) introduces S 2080 Genetically Engineered Food Right-to-Know Act, which requires mandatory labeling for all bioengineered food.[25]

2000

Following the 2000 presidential elections, the new Bush administration requests that all executive agencies withdraw all proposed and final regulations submitted to the Office of the Federal Register that remain unpublished. The proposed FDA rule and both bills disappear from the agendas of Congress and the FDA.

2000

StarLink, a GE corn developed by Aventis Corp. but not approved by the EPA for human consumption, is detected in Taco Bell's taco shells distributed by Kraft Foods Inc., and voluntarily recalled.[18] StarLink is subsequently detected in a plethora of corn products. Although only 1% of the year's corn crop, StarLink may have contaminated up to 50% of the year's total corn harvest. After testing only 18 to 20 people, the CDC and the FDA conclude that there is insufficient evidence that sensitivity to the inserted protein caused an allergic reaction.[26]

Sources:

[1] Biotechnology Research and Education Initiative (BREI) Cooperative Extension Service. University of Kentucky. College of Agriculture. *Food Biotechnology Teaching Guide*. Available at: http://www.ca.uky.edu/agc/pubs/brei/ brei3tg/ brei3tg.htm.

[2] http://www.accessexcellence.org/RC/AB/BC/1953-1976.html.

[3] Mallery, C. *Modern History of Biotechnology*, prepared for Introductory Biology for Majors at the University of Miami, College of Arts and Sciences, Coral Gables, Florida. Available at: http://fig.cox.miami.edu/~cmallery/150/gene/ hisbiotech/hisbiotech.htm.

[4] 2001 Thinkquest Internet Challenge. BioTechnology: The Technical and Ethical Sides Uncovered: Timeline of Genetics Research. Available at: http://library.thinkquest.org/C0111983/timeline.html.

[5] Biotechnology Industry Organization. Guide to Biotechnology: Timeline. Available at: http://www.bio.org/speeches/ pubs/er/timeline.asp.

[6] Wright, S. *Molecular Politics: Developing American and British Regulatory Policy for Genetic Engineering, 1972–1982*. University of Chicago Press. 1994. pp. 73–78.

[7] Fish, A.C., Rudenko, L. Guide to U.S. Regulation of Genetically Modified Food and Agricultural Biotechnology Products. Washington, D.C. Pew Initiative on Food and Biotechnology, September 2001:4. Available at: http://pewagbiotech. org/resources/issuebriefs/1-regguide.pdf. Accessed May 22, 2006.

[8] Douglas A. Kysar, Preferences for processes: the process/product distinction and the regulation of consumer choice, 118 *Harv. L. Rev.* 525, 559 (Dec. 2004).

[9] Walgate, R. Genetically Modified Food: The American Experience. Summary of a conference organised by the Danish Centre for Bioethics and Risk Assessment and the BioTIK Secretariat, Copenhagen. June 11–12, 2003: 24. Available at: http://www.bioethics.kvl.dk/gmexperience/GM%20Food.pdf.

[10] 447 US 303 (1980).

[11] Biotechnology Industry Organization. Guide to Biotechnology: Timeline. Available at: http://www.bio.org/speeches/ pubs/er/timeline.asp.

[12] 51 Fed. Reg. 23,302 (June 26, 1986).

[13] Cornell Cooperative Extension. Genetically Engineered Organisms — Public Issue Education Project (GEO-PIE). Available at: http://www.geo-pie.cornell.edu/gmo.html. Accessed May 21, 2006.

[14] 57 Fed. Reg. 22, 984 (May 29, 1992).

[15] Smith, J.M. *Seeds of Deception: Exposing Industry and Government Lies About the Safety of the Genetically Engineered Foods You're Eating*. Yes! Books, Fairfield, IA, 2003.

[16] McGarity, T.O., Hansen, P.I. Breeding Distrust: An Assessment and Recommendations for Improving the Regulation of Plant Derived Genetically Modified Foods. Prepared for the Food Policy Institute of the Consumer Federation of America, January 11, 2001. Available at: http://www.mindfully.org/GE/Breeding-Distrust-2.htm. p. 5.

[17] Wikipedia. Frankenfood definition. Available at: http://en.wikipedia.org/wiki/Frankenfood. Accessed May 21, 2006.

[18] Nestle M. *Safe Food: Bacteria, Biotechnology and Bioterrorism*. University of California Press, Berkeley, CA, 2003, p. 199.

[19] Biotechnology Industry Organization. Guide to Biotechnology: Timeline. Available at: http://www.bio.org/speeches/ pubs/er/timeline.asp.

[20] Van Tassel, K. The introduction of biotech foods to the tort system: creating a new duty to identify. *U Cin L Rev* 72, 1645, 1662, 2004.

[21] *International Dairy Foods Assn v. Amestoy*, 92 F. 3d 67 (1996).

[22] Alliance for Bio-Integrity. Landmark Lawsuit Challenges FDA Policy on Genetically Engineered Food. Available at: http://www.biointegrity.org/Lawsuit.html.

[23] *Alliance for Bio-Integrity v. Shalala*, 116 F. Supp. 2d 166, D.D.C., September 29, 2000.

[24] 66 FR 4706 Proposed Rule.

[25] Congressional Research Service Reports. Available at: http://www.ncseonline.org/NLE/CRSreports/Agriculture/6. Accessed May 22, 2006.

[26] Bratspies, R.M. Myths of voluntary compliance: lessons from the Starlink corn fiasco. 27 *Wm. and Mary Envtl. L. and Policy Rev.* 593.

Box 15.4 The Courts and Genetically Modified Food

The course of events since the landmark case of *Diamond v. Chakrabarty*, 447 U.S. 303 (1980), demonstrates the impact the U.S. legal system has on the development of U.S. food policy related to genetically modified food plants. Chakrabarty, a genetic engineer employed by General Electric Co., developed a GE bacterium capable of breaking down crude oil.[1] The microorganism had the potential to be used to control oil spills.[1] The first order of business, however, for Chakrabarty and GE was to apply for a patent for the bacterium. Although the patent was initially rejected on the basis that the law had never extended patents to living things,[2] the Supreme Court eventually held that the scientist was entitled to a patent on the microorganism because it was synthetic, did not occur naturally in any other bacterium, and therefore qualified as "a manufacture or composition of matter"[3] or, in other words, "patentable subject matter."[4]

The 1980 ruling made it possible for Stanford University to receive the patent it had applied for in November 1974 on behalf of scientists Stanley Cohen and Herbert Boyer to cover the technology they developed for rDNA.[5] In 1973, Cohen, his lab assistant, Annie Chang, and Boyer perfected techniques to cut and paste DNA (using restriction enzymes and ligases) and reproduce the new DNA in bacteria.[6,7] The patent (actually three separate patents)[8] covered not only the processes developed in the experiments but also the cells containing the new DNA.[7,9] The patent, which may be the most successful patent in university licensing, generated $139 million in royalties in the first 15 years that it was held.[10]

The Supreme Court decision spurred a boom for the creation of "dedicated biotechnology companies (DBCs)"; in the 4-year period, 1980 to 1984, funding surged for companies dedicated to biotechnology.[11] Approximately 60% of the DBCs in existence in the 1990s were founded between 1980 and 1984.[11,12]

The legal precedent set in *Diamond v. Chakrabarty* was extended by the California Supreme Court in 1990 in the to date leading case[*] on the issue of gene patenting: *Moore v. the Regents of the University of California.*[13] In this case, a leukemia patient at the UCLA Medical Center sued his physician, who, after excising Mr. Moore's spleen and collecting numerous additional tissue samples from him over the years following the surgery, patented a cell line developed entirely from Moore's tissue.[14] Mr. Moore's suit focused on the appropriation of property rights over his body parts without his informed consent.[14] Although the court agreed that the patient had a cause of action against the doctor's breach of his duty to receive the patient's informed consent, the patient had no rights over the tissue samples voluntarily given.[14]

These two cases taken together have tremendous implications for property rights over genetic materials. In light of these rulings, biotechnology companies can confidently develop patentable technologies relating to cell genetic material, from animal or plant sources, regardless of how the original tissues were obtained. Over the last two decades, major agrochemical companies have been racing to buy up seed companies and patent their seeds.[15] In fact, Monsanto alone amassed over 11,000 seed patents since 1978.[15] The market share strategy combined with a careful regulatory strategy were part of a larger plan (created in the 1980s and leaked to the press in 2001)[16] to transform the food industry and make GE food more acceptable to the public. However, although the Center for Food Safety estimates that as much as 60% of processed foods on supermarket shelves contain GE ingredients,[17] the revenues derived from the planting of genetically modified crops are actually falling.[18] This is due, in part, to the consumer backlash against genetically modified foods, resulting from media coverage of inconsistencies in regulatory practices and safety testing,[19] as well as highly publicized trials concerning consumer's right to know which foods contain genetically modified ingredients.[20] The courts are being used to silence and bully small farmers who have rejected the technology,[21] and the public outrage that these tactics have generated has further contributed to consumer backlash.

---

[*] The case is considered a leading case, but is not controlling; when the Supreme Court of the U.S. decides an issue, all other courts must adhere to its ruling; but, when the supreme court of a state rules (in this case, California, a highly influential state), other states may choose to rule accordingly, or may issue a completely independent ruling. Courts tend to give substantial weight to decisions issued by influential state courts.

Questions:

1. Why does the ability to patent biotechnology make it potentially more profitable? Does increased profitability ensure that research dollars will be devoted to the technology, or does it create too large an incentive to take shortcuts that may have serious safety consequences?
2. How can a court simultaneously rule that a patient has a right to informed consent, and that a physician has a property right in any discoveries that a physician made during the course of the patient's treatment? Are not the two parts of the decision incompatible?

3. Contrast how scientists have used the court system to establish their intellectual property rights with how some large corporations have used the courts to silence critics. Is either or both of these legal tactics an abuse of process? How can the rules of the game be amended to avoid such abuses?

Source:

[1] 447 US 303, at 305.

[2] 447 US 303, at 306.

[3] 447 US 303, at 308.

[4] 447 US 303, at 303.

[5] Wright, Susan. *Molecular Politics: Developing American and British Regulatory Policy for Genetic Engineering, 1972–1982.* University of Chicago Press, 1994, pp. 73–78.

[6] 2001 Thinkquest Internet Challenge. BioTechnology: The Technical and Ethical Sides Uncovered: Timeline of Genetics Research. http://library.thinkquest.org/C011983/timeline.html.

[7] Biotechnology Industry Organization. Guide to Biotechnology: Timeline. Available at: http://www.bio.org/speeches/pubs/er/timeline.asp.

[8] http://www.nap.edu/readingroom/books/property/5.html.

[9] 2001 Thinkquest Internet Challenge. BioTechnology: The Technical and Ethical Sides Uncovered: Timeline of Genetics Research. http://library.thinkquest.org/C011983/timeline.html.

[10] http://www.nap.edu/readingroom/books/property/5.html.

[11] http://www.acephale.org/bio-safety/IoC-intr.htm.

[12] U.S. Congress, Office of Technology Assessment. *Biotechnology in a Global Economy,* OTA-BA-494 (Washington, D.C.: U.S. Government Printing Office, October 1991), p. 45.

[13] 51 Cal. 3d 120, 793 P. 2d 479, 271 Cal. Rptr. 146 (1990), *reh'g denied, Moore v. The Regents of the University of California,* No. S006987 (Cal. Supreme Ct. Aug. 30, 1990) (1990 CAL. LEXIS 3975, States library, Cal file).

[14] Dorney, M.S. *Moore v. The Regents of the University of California*: Balancing the Need for Biotechnology Innovation Against the Right of Informed Consent. *Berkeley Technology Law Journal.* Fall 1990 at 339. Available at: http://btlj.boalt.org/data/articles/5-2_fall-1990_dorney.pdf.

[15] Garcia, D.K. The Future of Food (documentary film). Lily Films, 2004.

[16] Eichenwald K. Redesigning nature: hard lessons learned; biotechnology food: from the lab to a debacle. *New York Times,* January 25, 2001.Sec. A, column 2.

[17] http://www.centerforfoodsafety.org/geneticall2.cfm.

[18] See Nestle, M. *Safe Food: Bacteria, Biotechnology and Bioterrorism.* University of California Press, Berkeley, CA, 2003, pp. 245, 246. Nestle points out that in the late 1990s, because conventionally grown seed was fetching a premium price and because domestic and foreign sales outlets for genetically modified crops were shrinking, the acreage of land revenue from genetically modified corn and soybean plants was falling.

[19] See the Starlink Corn Affair, described in detail in *Safe Food.*

[20] See *International Dairy Foods Assn v. Amestoy,* 92 F. 3d 67 (1996).

[21] See *Monsanto Inc. v. Oakhurst Dairy; Monsanto v. Percy Schmeiser* (featured in The Future of Food).

15.1.1.2.2 Infant Formula

Prior to 1980, infant formula was regulated under 21 CFR (Code of Federal Regulations) 105.65, Infant Foods. This regulation specified minimum levels of certain nutrients for infant formulas, including protein, fat, and some vitamins and minerals, but a level for chloride was not specified.

In 1978, a major manufacturer of infant formula reformulated two of its soy products by discontinuing the addition of salt. This resulted in infant formula products containing an inadequate amount of chloride, an essential nutrient for infant growth and development. By mid-1979, a cluster of infants had been diagnosed with hypochloremic metabolic alkalosis, a syndrome associated with chloride deficiency, which was eventually associated with prolonged and exclusive use of the chloride-deficient soy formulas. Chloride deficiency can result in growth retardation or manifest central nervous system effects such as cerebral dysfunction or impaired cognitive function. This outbreak highlights two critically important elements of public health practice: First, developing and using appropriate case definitions for both surveillance and for the investigation of outbreaks of both infectious and noninfectious origin enables local and state health departments and the Public Health Service to respond rapidly. Second, clinicians play a significant role in identifying and resolving public health emergencies.[6]

After reviewing the matter, Congress determined that to improve protection of infants using infant formula products, greater regulatory control over the formulation and production of infant formula was needed, including modification of industry and the FDA's recall procedures. Thus was born the Infant Formula Act of 1980 (P.L. 96–359). This law amended FFDCA to include Section 412 (21 U.S.C. 350a). The FDA, in turn, adopted regulations implementing the act, including regulations on recall procedures, quality control procedures, labeling, and nutrient requirements.[7]

The Infant Formula Act was designed to ensure the safety and nutrition of infant formulas, including minimum and, in some cases, maximum levels of specified nutrients. One of the most specific and detailed acts ever passed by Congress, the act gives the FDA authority to regulate the labeling of infant formula and to establish quality control rules and regulations governing formula manufacturing. The act establishes minimum nutrient requirements, defines adulteration, provides for establishing nutrient and quality control procedures, prescribes recall procedures, and specifies inspection requirements. It addresses three related requirements for the manufacturer of the formula: (1) notifying the FDA before processing an infant formula, (2) notifying the FDA after a change in formulation or processing, and (3) meeting testing requirements based on regulations with regard to major and minor changes in the formula. In 1985, the act was revised to include minimum concentrations of 29 nutrients and maximum concentrations of 9 nutrients in infant formula. Recently, the FDA requested more explicit guidelines for assessing safety of new ingredients added to infant formula.[8] A key limitation of the current approach is the lack of explicit guidelines to help formula manufacturers and their outside expert reviewers determine what safety data are needed on a proposed ingredient, and how they should be gathered.

In passing the 1980 Infant Formula Act and its amendments, Congress recognized infant formulas as a special category of foods that, because there is no margin for error in ensuring the healthy growth and development of infants, requires more regulation than other types of foods. Regulation of infant formulas involves both general safety provisions of the act and additional requirements specific to infant formulas (e.g., CGMPs, quality control procedures, nutrient levels and analysis, and quality factors). For most of the requirements specific to infant formula, manufacturers must provide assurances that the requirements have been met for each new product (including marketed products in which a major change has occurred) prior to marketing.

15.1.1.2.3 Food Allergies

Some foods can cause severe illness and, in extreme cases, a life-threatening allergic reaction. In the U.S., approximately 1.5% of adults and up to 6% of children under the age of 3 — about 4 million people — have a true food allergy. An estimated 150 Americans die each year from severe allergic reactions to food. It is critical for people with food allergies to identify them and avoid foods that cause allergic reactions.[9] In children, milk, egg, peanuts, wheat, soy, and tree nuts (e.g., walnuts and pecans) account for 90% of food allergy reactions. In adults, peanuts, tree nuts, fish, and shellfish account for 90% of allergic reactions.[10] Proteins have been identified as major allergens in foods. These include casein and whey in cow's milk, ovomucoid in egg whites, and tropomycin in shellfish.

Currently, the only way to treat a food allergy is to avoid the triggering food. However, diligent label reading does not suffice. Allergy alerts on packaging are purely voluntary and are not required by law. If a food allergen, such as peanuts, is not cited in an ingredient list, or if there is no food allergy alert printed on the packaging, many food allergic people mistakenly assume the food is safe to eat. Even if a company uses allergy alerts, it is difficult to be absolutely certain that their employees will always observe the safety precautions put in place. Food products made in the U.S. can have potential food allergens masked by nonspecific terms, such as natural flavors, seasonings, and spices, in the ingredients list.[11]

Since 2000, the FDA has presented information on food allergies at over a dozen public meetings. It is working with food manufacturers and consumer groups to increase consumer awareness about the seriousness of food allergies and to ensure proper labeling. The National Food Products Association (now known as the National Food Processors Association) has called for a voluntary listing on labels of the eight most common food allergens in plain language, for example, using the word *milk* in addition to the word *caseinate*. Whereas the FDA requires food processors to label foods with all ingredients, there are gaps due to, for example, practices such as shared manufacturing equipment. The Food Allergen Labeling and Consumer Protection Act of 2004,[12] enacted in 2006, mandates labeling of the top eight allergens in plain language, rather than relegating it to voluntary cooperation.

15.1.1.3 Food Safety and Inspection Service (FSIS)

The FSIS is the public health agency within the USDA responsible for ensuring that the nation's commercial supply of meat, poultry, and egg products is safe, wholesome, and correctly labeled and packaged. This responsibility encompasses the commercial supply of meat, poultry, and egg products in interstate commerce, as well as products imported from other countries. The FSIS relies on state-of-the-art, comprehensive, science-based initiatives to understand, predict, and prevent microbiological contamination of meat, poultry, and egg products, thereby improving health outcomes for Americans.

15.1.1.4 Centers for Disease Control and Prevention (CDC)

The CDC's role in the area of food safety includes investigating outbreaks and establishing both short-term control measures and long-term improvements to prevent similar outbreaks in the future. The CDC works with state and local health departments to investigate foodborne outbreaks and make information available to the public. Outbreak data maintained by the CDC are derived primarily from the Foodborne Diseases Active Surveillance Network (FoodNet), detailed in Section 15.6 Surveillance Systems in this chapter.

15.1.1.5 Environmental Protection Agency (EPA)

Laboratory studies show that pesticides can cause health problems, such as birth defects, nerve damage, cancer, and other effects, that might develop over a long period of time. These effects depend on the pesticide's toxicity and how much of it is consumed. Some pesticides also pose unique health risks to children. For these reasons, the EPA, in cooperation with the individual states, regulates pesticides to ensure that their use does not pose unreasonable risks to infants, children, and adults, or the environment.

The EPA regulates pesticides under two major federal statutes. The Federal Insecticide, Fungicide, and Rodenticide Act (FIFRA) of 1947 authorizes the EPA to register pesticides for use in the U.S. and prescribe labeling and other regulatory requirements to prevent unreasonable adverse effects on health or the environment. Under the FFDCA, the EPA establishes tolerances (maximum legally permissible levels) for pesticide residues in food. Tolerances are enforced by the FDA for most foods; by the FSIS for meat, poultry, and some egg products; and by the USDA's Office of Pest Management Policy.

In 1996, Congress passed landmark legislation amending both laws to establish a more consistent, protective regulatory scheme. It mandates a single, health-based standard for all pesticides in all foods; provides special protection for infants and children; expedites approval of safer pesticides; creates incentives for the development and maintenance of effective crop protection tools for American farmers; and requires periodic reevaluation of pesticide registrations and tolerances to ensure that the scientific data supporting pesticide registrations will remain current in the future.[13]

15.2 STATES AND TERRITORIES

In addition to inspections conducted by the federal government, states and territories also oversee inspection and regulation activities that help ensure the safety of foods produced, processed, or sold within their jurisdictions. State and local authorities — not federal agencies — are responsible

Box 15.5 The Food Code

The Food Code is a reference document for regulatory agencies responsible for overseeing food safety in retail outlets such as restaurants and grocery stores, and institutions such as nursing homes and child care centers. It is neither federal law nor federal regulation and is not preemptive, but may be adopted and used by agencies at all levels of government that have responsibility for managing food safety risks at retail. The Food Code is a model for safeguarding public health, and ensuring food is unadulterated and honestly presented when offered to the consumer. It represents advice for a uniform system of provisions that address the safety and protection of food offered at retail and in food service. This model is made available for adoption within local, state, and federal governmental jurisdictions for administration by the various departments, agencies, bureaus, divisions, and other units within each jurisdiction that have been delegated compliance responsibilities for food service, retail food stores, or food vending operations. The Food Code is available online in both HTML and PDF versions, and may also be purchased in a printed version or on CD-ROM through the National Technical Information Service in the Technology Administration of the U.S. Department of Commerce.

Source: National Technical Information Service homepage. Available at: http://www.ntis.gov/index.asp? Accessed February 19, 2005.

for licensing and inspecting the 600,000 restaurants, nursing homes, child care agencies, and other institutional food service establishments; the 235,000 supermarkets, grocery stores, and other food establishments operated in the U.S.

To help these jurisdictions achieve uniform national food safety standards, the federal government developed a voluntary Food Code (see Box 15.5) that provides practical, science-based guidance and manageable, enforceable provisions for mitigating risk factors known to cause foodborne illness. The code is a reference document for regulatory agencies that oversee food safety in food service establishments, retail food stores, other food establishments at the retail level, and institutions such as nursing homes and child care centers. Adoption of the code is endorsed by HHS and the USDA as a strategy for the local jurisdictions to attain at least minimum national food safety standards and to enhance the efficiency and effectiveness of the nation's food safety system.

First published in 1993, the code had been revised and updated every two years through 2001, when it started a 4-year revision cycle. The 2005 edition was developed collaboratively by the FDA, the CDC, and the FSIS. In 2004, the code had been adopted by 86% of the 56 states and territories in the U.S., representing 80% of the population.

15.3 CRITIQUE OF THE FOOD SAFETY REGULATORY APPARATUS

For many years, analysts in the Government Accountability Office (GAO) have questioned the organizational efficiency and jurisdictional responsibilities of the current food safety regulatory structure. It is their unequivocal position that enhancing the safety of the nation's food supply will remain spotty until the department and the other agencies that share this responsibility are brought together in a single food safety focus.[14,15,16,17,18] GAO proponents of a streamlined federal food inspection system claim that the current system is ill equipped to meet the challenges of emerging pathogens, an aging population, an increasing number of food imports, and potential terrorist threats to our food supply. GAO representatives have testified many times that oversight and inspection resources, as well as differences in state and local laws and regulations, leave the U.S. system fragmented, inconsistent, and lacking in a strategic design intended to protect the public.

Under the current system, meat and poultry production receive continuous inspection, whereas fish, shellfish, produce, and other foods are inspected sporadically, if at all, and most food that is recalled is never recovered.[19] In addition, many industry sectors must respond to multiple — often conflicting — requirements. The GAO has recommended that the several different federal agencies currently responsible for food safety be consolidated into a single entity.[20] Bills introduced into the 107th Congress (2001–2002) would have placed the FSIS, the Center for Food Safety and Applied Nutrition (CFSAN), the Center for Veterinary Medicine (CVM), and the Department of Commerce's National Marine Fisheries Service into a single independent food safety agency.[21]

In 2004, GAO suggested that Congress consider enacting a comprehensive, uniform, and risk-based food safety legislation and establish a single food safety agency or, if Congress does not opt for an entire reorganization, that it consider modifying existing laws to designate a lead agency for food safety inspection matters.[22] Those who support the *status quo* maintain that centralizing the responsibility for food safety would not necessarily result in reduced cost or a safer food supply.[23]

15.4 EPIDEMIOLOGY

The epidemiology of foodborne illness is changing.[24] During the 20th century, for example, substantial progress was made in preventing typhoid fever, now almost completely eradicated by the disinfection of drinking water, milk pasteurization, and shellfish bed sanitation. However, since the mid-1970s, more than a dozen microorganisms have been newly identified as human pathogens associated with foodborne transmission. These pathogens are listed in Table 15.2.

As detailed in the list below, factors contributing to the emergence of foodborne diseases are complex and not entirely understood. They include changes in human demographics, food consumption, industry and technology, travel and commerce, microbial adaptation, economic development and land use, and the breakdown of the public health infrastructure.[25,26]

1. The proportion of the U.S. population with heightened susceptibility to foodborne disease has increased both due to the increased proportion of the population with the human immunodeficiency virus (HIV) and to the increasing median age of the population. Similarly, advances in medical technology have extended the life expectancy of people with organ transplants and those who are undergoing cancer therapy, heightening their susceptibility to severe foodborne illness.

TABLE 15.2
Pathogens That Are FoodBorne and Newly Recognized in the U.S. in the Last 30 Years

Campylobacter jejuni
C. fetus subsp. Fetus
Cryptosporidium cayetanensis
Escherichia coli O157:H7 and related *E. coli*
Listeria monocytogenes
Norwalk-like viruses
Nitzchia pungens
Salmonella enteritidis
S. typhimurium DT 104
Vibrio cholerae O1
V. vulnificus
V. parahaemolyticus
Yersinia enterocolitica

Source: From Tauxe, R.V. Emerging foodborne diseases: an evolving public health challenge. *Emerg Infect Dis.* 3: 425–434, 1997. Available at: http://www.cdc.gov/ncidod/EID/vol3no4/tauxe.htm. Accessed February 17, 2005.

---

2. Changes in food consumption have resulted in the identification of microbial foodborne hazards. For example, increased consumption of fresh fruit and vegetables has resulted in outbreaks associated with fresh produce, unpasteurized cider, sliced tomatoes, fresh squeezed orange juice, frozen strawberries, green onions, alfalfa sprouts, raspberries, and lettuce. Additionally, the increase in the number of meals eaten away from home has increased exposure to outbreaks, predominantly the result of improper food handling practices.
3. The centralization of the food industry has increased dispersion of outbreaks, which affect large numbers of people.
4. International travel raises the risk of travelers returning to the U.S. infected with foodborne pathogens, which may be carried home to affect nontravelers. Additionally, imported food may harbor pathogens.
5. Antimicrobial resistant strains of salmonella have become increasingly prominent in the U.S. Other resistant pathogens have been identified as well.
6. Manure from farm animals serves as a reservoir for salmonella, *C. jejuni*, and other farm pathogens. It is becoming increasingly difficult in the U.S. to dispose of the 1.6 billion tons of manure it generates annually.
7. Limited budgets in public health agencies have resulted in underreporting of foodborne infections. When the infrastructure for disease surveillance is limited, recognition of outbreaks is jeopardized.

15.5 PREVENTION

In 1998, the FDA, in consultation with the USDA, published the *Guide to Minimize Microbial Food Safety Hazards for Fresh Fruits and Vegetables,* which is available in four languages. This provides guidelines for growers and packers of fresh fruits and vegetables on reducing associated microbiological hazards by addressing key areas such as water quality, worker hygiene, field and facility sanitation, manure management, and transportation. The two agencies work together to educate the agricultural industry about these guidelines.[27]

In 1999, following outbreaks traced to sprouts, the FDA issued *Reducing Microbial Food Safety Hazards for Sprouted Seeds and Sampling and Microbial Testing of Spent Irrigation Water During Sprout Production* for distribution to the sprouts industry. In 2000, in conjunction with the California Department of Health, the agency produced and distributed an educational video for sprout producers. It also assessed the sprout industry's adherence to good agricultural practices (GAPs) by inspecting 150 sprout producers.[27]

In response to growing worries about bovine spongiform encephalopathy (BSE), in January 2001 HHS formed the Interdepartmental Steering Committee for BSE/TSE Affairs with representatives from the FDA, the CDC, National Institutes of Health (NIH), the USDA, and numerous other federal and state agencies. This committee assures coordination, integrated contingency planning, and communication of risk plans among all involved agencies.[27]

15.6 SURVEILLANCE SYSTEMS

Enhanced surveillance and investigation are integral to developing and evaluating new prevention and control strategies, which can improve the safety of our food and the public's health. Ongoing surveillance is necessary to document the effectiveness of new food safety control measures, such as Hazard Analysis and Critical Control Point (HACCP), in decreasing the number of cases of foodborne diseases that occur in the U.S. each year; to monitor the number and extent of outbreaks; to track the causes of outbreaks; and to aid in case detection and intervention. This section introduces the primary surveillance systems that monitor the incidence of foodborne illness in the U.S.

TABLE 15.3
The Pathogens under Surveillance by FoodNet

Campylobacter
Escherichia coli O157
Listeria monocytogenes
Salmonella
Shigella
Vibrio
Yersinia enterocolitica
Cyclospora
Cryptosporidium

Source: From Centers for Disease Control and Prevention. Preliminary FoodNet data on the incidence of infection with pathogens transmitted commonly through food —selected sites, United States, 2003. *MMWR* 53: 338–43, 2004. Available at: http://www.cdc.gov/mmwr/preview/mmwrhtml/mm5316a2.htm. Accessed February 16, 2005.

15.6.1 FOODNET (CDC)

The Foodborne Diseases Active Surveillance Network (FoodNet) is a sentinel network that produces national estimates of the burden and sources of foodborne diseases in the U.S. It is the principal foodborne disease component of the CDC's Emerging Infections Program (EIP). FoodNet is a collaborative project that collects data on diseases caused by enteric pathogens, transmitted commonly through food in 10 states (Connecticut, Georgia, Maryland, Minnesota, New Mexico, Oregon, Tennessee, and selected counties in California, Colorado, and New York), which represent 15% of the U.S. population.[28] FoodNet quantifies and monitors the incidence of 9 pathogens by conducting active surveillance for laboratory diagnosed illness. The network, established in 1996, augments long-standing activities at the CDC, the USDA, the FDA, and at the state level, identify, control, and prevent foodborne disease hazards. The pathogens under surveillance in FoodNet are listed in Table 15.3. FoodNet data are subject to at least four limitations, summarized in Table 15.4.

15.6.2 PULSENET (CDC)

PulseNet, the National Molecular Subtyping Network for Foodborne Disease Surveillance, is the CDC's network of public health laboratories, which perform a DNA "fingerprinting" method known as *pulsed field gel electrophoresis* (PFGE) on foodborne bacteria. The network permits rapid

TABLE 15.4
Limitations of FoodNet Data

Although the majority of foodborne illnesses are not laboratory diagnosed, FoodNet data are limited to laboratory diagnosed illnesses and are thus biased by factors that affect the probability of an illness being reported.

Illnesses reported to FoodNet might be acquired through nonfood-borne sources (e.g., contaminated water, person-to-person contact, and direct animal exposure); reported incidences do not represent foodborne sources exclusively.

Although FoodNet data provide the most detailed information available for these infections, the findings might not be generalizable to the entire U.S. population.

Year-to-year changes in incidence might reflect either annual variation or sustained trends; further data are needed to discern trends clearly.

Source: From Centers for Disease Control and Prevention. Preliminary FoodNet data on the incidence of infection with pathogens transmitted commonly through food —selected sites, United States, 2003. *MMWR* 53: 338–43, 2004. Available at: http://www.cdc.gov/mmwr/preview/mmwrhtml/mm5316a2.htm. Accessed February 16, 2005.

comparison of these fingerprint patterns through an electronic database. PulseNet provides critical data for the early recognition and timely investigation of outbreaks, thus reducing the burden of foodborne disease. PulseNet began in 1996 with ten laboratories typing a single pathogen (*Escherichia coli* O157:H7). Now PulseNet subtypes five foodborne pathogens (*E. coli* O157:H7, salmonella serotypes, *Listeria monocytogenes*, *Shigella*, and *Campylobacter*); other bacterial, viral, and parasitic organisms are expected to be added.

The network has increased to encompass all 50 state public health laboratories — the public health laboratories in Washington D.C.; Houston, TX; Los Angeles County, CA; Milwaukee, WI; New York City, Orange County, CA; Philadelphia, PA; San Diego County, CA; Santa Clara County, CA; and Tarrant County, TX; USDA-FSIS Laboratory, Agricultural Research Service (USDA-ARS), and Agricultural Marketing Service (USDA-AMS); and the FDA laboratories in CFSAN and CVM. Recently, PulseNet expanded internationally. PulseNet Canada consists of six provincial Canadian laboratories and the Canadian national laboratory, which joined the consortium in 1999–2000. Both PulseNet Europe and PulseNet Asia-Pacific came aboard in 2002, and PulseNet Latin America joined in 2004. PulseNet has achieved its goal of becoming a global network of public health laboratories working with food regulatory agencies and industry to improve food safety worldwide.[29]

15.6.2.1 Role of PulseNet in Outbreak Investigations

In 1996, epidemiologists in Washington State health departments traced outbreak of *E. coli* O157:H7 infections in four states and one Canadian province to commercial unpasteurized apple juice. Of 70 persons identified as part of this outbreak, 25 required hospitalizations, 14 had hemolytic uremic syndrome, and 1 died. DNA fingerprinting by PFGE at the Washington State Public Health Laboratory, a PulseNet area laboratory, showed that isolates from patients and the apple juice were the same strain. Prompt recognition of the apple juice as the source of this outbreak resulted in rapid recall of the widely distributed product. This outbreak demonstrated that unpasteurized juices must be considered a potentially hazardous food. The magnitude and severity of this outbreak ultimately led the FDA to propose two new regulations and led to widespread changes in the fresh juice industry.[30] By the end of 1999, it was determined that unpasteurized fruit and vegetable juices must carry a label stating, "WARNING: This product has not been pasteurized and therefore may contain harmful bacteria that can cause serious illness in children, the elderly, and persons with weakened immune systems."[31] and effective early 2002, HACCP principles must be applied to the processing of fruit and vegetable juices.[32] (See Box 15.6: The Hazard Analysis and Critical Control Point (HACCP).)

Box 15.6 The Hazard Analysis and Critical Control Point (HACCP)

HACCP is a food safety program developed by NASA to prevent foodborne illnesses among astronauts. The program uses a systematic approach to the identification and assessment of the risk of biological, chemical, and physical hazards from a particular food production process or practice and the control of those hazards. Manufacturers using HACCP systems conduct science-based analyses of food production processes, locate where the hazards can occur, take steps to prevent problems, and respond rapidly to problems. The FDA inspectors will do spot-checks to ensure that the processors' HACCP systems are working.

HACCP is a preventive system of hazard control that places the responsibility for identifying safety problems with the manufacturer. Use of the HACCP system means that a firm is engaged in continuous problem prevention and problem solving, rather than relying on facility inspections by regulatory agencies or consumer complaints to detect a loss of control. HACCP provides for real-time monitoring to assess the effectiveness of control. A HACCP system put in place by a manufacturer for a particular facility is unique and reflects the type of food product, method of processing and packaging, the facility in which it is prepared, and the intended consumers. A preventive system, such as HACCP, appears to offer the most effective way to control the significant microbial hazards, along with other hazards, that have become a problem with food processing.

Source: Food and Drug Administration. HACCP. Available at: http://www.cfsan.fda.gov/~lrd/haccp.html. Accessed September 2, 2006.

15.6.3 FOODBORNE OUTBREAK RESPONSE AND SURVEILLANCE UNIT (CDC)

The Foodborne Outbreak Response and Surveillance Unit is a program of the CDC's Foodborne and Diarrheal Diseases Branch. It works closely with state and local health departments to investigate outbreaks and establish short-term controls and long-term improvements to prevent future outbreaks. Its Web site provides data from three surveillance systems:

- *FoodBorne Disease Outbreaks*: all U.S. foodborne disease outbreaks reported to CDC by the state epidemiologists through the Foodborne Outbreak Reporting System.
- *E. coli* 0157:H7 *Outbreaks*: *E. coli* outbreaks and clusters reported to the CDC by states or regulatory agencies.
- *Salmonella enteritidis Outbreaks*: foodborne salmonella outbreaks reported to the CDC by states or regulatory agencies.

For public health professionals, the site provides an outbreak investigation toolkit, guidelines for reporting an outbreak, and epidemiologic software. Also available are reports and publications on past outbreaks.[33]

15.6.4 ELEXNET (FDA)

The electronic Laboratory Exchange Network, an FDA network of food testing data from federal, state, and local food safety laboratories, facilitates data information sharing and communication. It is being piloted in two federal, four state, and two local laboratories, originally with *E. coli* and presently with the addition of salmonella, listeria, and campylobacter. Its objective is to link the nationwide food testing laboratories, providing an early warning system for potentially hazardous food.[27]

15.6.5 NATIONAL ANTIBIOTIC RESISTANCE MONITORING SYSTEM (FDA, CDC, AND USDA)

The National Antibiotic Resistance Monitoring System (NARMS), a cooperative enterprise of the CDC, the FDA, and the USDA, monitors emerging resistance in foodborne pathogens. Begun in 1995, NARMS facilitated the recognition of *Salmonella typhimurium* DT 104 as highly resistant to antibiotics and prompted the CDC to alert state health departments, provide preventive steps, and minimize its spread.[27]

15.6.6 ADDITIONAL SURVEILLANCE SYSTEMS

- *CaliciNet*: Developed by the CDC and based on the PulseNet model, this system will fingerprint strains of calicivirus (including noroviruses, formerly called *Norwalk-like viruses*).[34]
- *EHS-Net*: A network of environmental health specialists and epidemiologists that facilitates information exchange regarding environmental causes of foodborne illness. The network is a collaboration of the CDC, FoodNet, and the FDA.[35]

15.7 NUMBERS OF OUTBREAKS AND CASES

A study by the Center for Science in the Public Interest (CSPI) found that in the U.S. between 1990 and 2003, a total of 3,023 outbreaks occurred involving 92,304 people (see Table 15.5). Those food vehicles most likely to be implicated in these outbreaks were seafood and seafood dishes; produce and produce dishes; poultry and poultry dishes; beef and beef dishes; and egg and egg dishes. FDA-regulated foods accounted for 67% of the outbreaks, USDA-regulated foods accounted for 26%, and the remaining 7% of the outbreaks were linked to foods regulated by both the FDA and the USDA. The report notes that whereas 67% of outbreaks occur in FDA-regulated food, its budget comprises only one-third of the total federal budget for food safety inspections. In light of these findings, CSPI called for a unified, independent food safety agency.[36]

15.8 EMERGENCY MANAGEMENT

Emergency management, as it is known in the U.S. today, began at the local level with neighbors helping neighbors in time of need. The formal involvement and role of state and federal governments prior to the 20th century was reactionary rather than proactive, resulting in varied responses and a nonstandard use of resources. The expansion of the country and population shifts from the rural settings to urban centers created not only new challenges but also increased risks. Today, emergency management continues to evolve, as risks and threats are reassessed and new legislation is passed. At present, local and state governments share the responsibility for protecting their citizens from disasters, and for helping them to recover when a disaster strikes. In some cases, a disaster is beyond the capabilities of the state or local government to respond.

TABLE 15.5
Foodborne Illness Outbreaks and Cases 1990–2003

Food Category	Outbreaks		Cases		Cases per Outbreak Numbers
	Numbers	Percentage	Numbers	Percentage	
Seafood and seafood dishes	720	23.8	8,044	8.7	11.2
Produce and produce dishes	428	14.2	23,857	25.8	55.7
Poultry and poultry dishes	355	11.7	11,898	12.9	33.5
Beef and beef dishes	338	11.2	10,795	11.7	31.9
Egg and egg dishes	306	10.1	10,449	11.3	34.1
Multi-ingredient foods[a]	591	19.6	17,728	19.2	30.0
Dairy	120	4.0	4,575	5.0	38.1
Breads and baked goods	90	3.0	2,767	3.0	30.7
Beverages	53	1.8	2,035	2.2	38.4
Game	22	0.7	156	0.2	7.1
Total	3023	100.0	92,304	100.0	
Average cases/outbreak					31.1

[a] Specific food not identified, includes ethnic foods, salads, rice or beans, and sandwiches.

Source: Based on data in Center for Science in the Public Interest. *Outbreak Alert! Closing the Gap in Our Federal Food-Safety Net.* Updated and revised March 2004. Available at: http://www.cspinet.org/new/pdf/outbreakalert2004.pdf. Accessed June 28, 2006.

Box 15.7 Online Courses in Preventing and Responding to Terror Strikes

Hundreds of U.S. colleges have created programs to meet the demand of employers for a workforce trained in homeland security. The programs originated with students from the military and National Guard in mind. But, students from other fields, like business and municipal government, have enrolled as well. Government agencies and businesses do not necessarily want to create full-time positions focused on fighting terrorism, but they do want their workers to be more broadly familiar with homeland security so employees can apply it to their day-to-day duties. Students who enroll in the programs learn valuable information about risk assessment.

Some institutions offer certificates; others, undergraduate and graduate degrees. Programs include courses about the history of terrorism, weapons of mass destruction, and how to manage a security team responsible for protecting a large area. Many of the courses have been put online to meet the needs of students working in the field. In 2004, the University of Southern California created an online master's degree program in homeland security, which it piggybacked onto its research program on terrorism. The U.S. Department of Homeland Security awarded the university a 3-year, $12-million grant in 2003 to do research on the economic effects of terrorism and to teach courses on how to protect against it. The university used part of the money to create both online and on-campus master's degree programs. However, one major challenge the new programs face is identifying enough qualified instructors. Universities want instructors with not only a strong academic background but also years of hands-on knowledge.

Source: Carnevale, D. A degree you hope you never need: colleges offer online courses in preventing and responding to terror strikes. *Chron Higher Educ.* February 18, 2005, p. A33. Available at: http://chronicle.com/weekly/v51/i24/2 4a03301. htm. Accessed June 28, 2006.

Within the last two decades, emergency management has undergone a metamorphosis into a respected and professional field. Colleges and universities throughout the U.S. offer individual courses, majors, and entire degree programs (associate to doctoral degrees) in hazard, disaster, and emergency management[37] (see Box 15.7).

15.8.1 STAFFORD ACT

The Robert T. Stafford Disaster Relief and Emergency Assistance Act, Public Law 93–288 (the Stafford Act), was enacted in 1988 to support state and local governments and their citizens when disasters overwhelm them. The act legislates cost-sharing requirements for public assistance programs, provision of funds for states and local governments to manage public assistance programs, funds for hazard mitigation, and authority to the federal government to provide assistance for disasters regardless of cause (see Box 15.8). An amendment, the Disaster Mitigation Act of 2000, focuses on mitigation before and after disasters, and the establishment of a national predisaster mitigation fund to assist with mitigation efforts at the state and local levels.

15.8.2 FEDERAL EMERGENCY MANAGEMENT AGENCY (FEMA)

Prior to 1979, disaster relief efforts were plagued by the many parallel programs and policies that existed at all levels of government. In 1979, FEMA was created by merging over 100 federal agencies involved in some aspect of disasters, hazards, and emergencies. In 2003, FEMA became part of the Department of Homeland Security.

Box 15.8 Classification of Disasters

Disasters are classified as natural, human-caused, or technologic. Human-caused disasters include explosive, biological, or chemical terrorist attacks. Technologic disasters involve hazardous materials incidents and nuclear power plant failures. Natural disasters may be weather related (floods, tornadoes, hurricanes, thunderstorms and lightning, winter storms and extreme cold and heat), geologic (earthquakes, volcanoes, and tsunamis), incendiary (fires and wildfires), and avalanches, landslides, and debris flow (mudslides).

Although headquartered in Washington D.C., FEMA maintains 10 regional offices and 2 area offices. Each region serves several states. Regional staff members work directly with the states to help plan for disasters, develop mitigation programs, and meet needs when major disasters occur. FEMA is staffed by full-time employees, plus standby disaster assistance employees who are available for deployment after disasters. Often, FEMA works in partnership with other organizations that are part of the nation's emergency management system, such as state and local emergency management agencies, other federal agencies, and the American Red Cross.[38]

To understand FEMA's activities consider the life cycle of disasters (see Box 15.9). This cycle describes the steps emergency managers follow in preparing for emergencies and disasters, responding to them when they occur, helping people and institutions recover from them, mitigating their effects, reducing the risk of loss, and preventing disasters from occurring. Prior to the actual occurrence of a disaster, the dominant management activity is *preparedness*. As the event unfolds, disaster management personnel become involved in the *response* phase. There is a period of *recovery* following the response to the disaster event. The *mitigation* phase then occurs as disaster management improvements are made in anticipation of the next disaster event.[39] FEMA is present at every stage of the cycle, building and supporting the nation's emergency management system. The agency's refocus and emphasis on mitigation and initiation of their "Project Impact" mitigation program seeks to address the impacts of disasters in communities before they occur.

15.9 BIOTERROISM

Food terrorism is an act or threat of deliberate contamination of food for human consumption, including animals used for food, with chemical, biological, or radioactive agents for the purpose of causing injury or death to civilian populations and/or disrupting social, economic, or political stability. Theoretically, terrorists could attack livestock, crops, or processed food at any stage of the food supply cycle: production, processing, harvesting, storage, manufacturing, transport, storage, distribution, or service.

"Agroterrorism" targets livestock and crops during the food cycle, deliberately introducing disease intended to generate fear, cause economic losses, and/or undermine stability. With annual revenues of approximately $100 billion,[40] the U.S. livestock industry is a likely target for economic warfare (see Box 15.10).

The term *syndromic surveillance* applies to surveillance using health-related data that precede diagnosis and signal a sufficient probability of a case or an outbreak to warrant further public health response. Though historically syndromic surveillance has been utilized to target investigation of potential cases, its utility for detecting outbreaks associated with bioterrorism is increasingly being explored by public health officials.

Whereas we are experienced in dealing with unintentional foodborne illness outbreaks and their impact on public health, we do not have actual data on the extent an impact from a terrorist event could have. However, epidemiologists have attempted to extrapolate what the impact could be based

Box 15.9 The Disaster Life Cycle: Disaster Response, Recovery, Mitigation, Prevention, and Preparedness

Response activities address the short-term, direct effects of an incident. Response includes immediate actions to save lives, protect property, and meet basic human needs such as food, water, clothing, and shelter. Response may also include activating a public warning, instituting a curfew, executing emergency operation plans such as mobilizing emergency and security personnel and equipment, and generally undertaking incident mitigation activities designed to limit the loss of life, personal injury, property damage, and other unfavorable outcomes.

Recovery is the process of returning to normal. Salvage, resumption of business processes, and repair are typical recovery tasks. It includes the development, coordination, and execution of service- and site-restoration plans for affected communities, and the resumption of government operations and services through individual, private sector, nongovernmental, and public assistance programs that identify needs and define resources; providing housing and promoting restoration; addressing long-term care and treatment of affected individuals; incorporating mitigation measures and techniques; evaluating the incident for lessons learned; and developing initiatives to mitigate the effects of future incidents. Recovery activities might also involve returning vital life-support systems to minimum operating standards; damage insurance/loans and grants; temporary housing; disaster unemployment insurance; public information; health and safety education; reconstruction; counseling programs; and economic impact studies.

Mitigation is the sustained action that reduces or eliminates long-term risk to people and property from natural hazards and their effects. Mitigation activities eliminate or reduce the probability of occurrence of a disaster, or reduce the effects of unavoidable disasters. Mitigation measures include building codes; vulnerability analyses updates; tax incentives and disincentives; zoning and land use management; building use regulations and safety codes; allocations and interstate sharing of resources; preventive healthcare; and public education. Information resources and services important in mitigation activities include Geographic Information System (GIS)-based risk assessment; claims history; facility or resource identification; land use or zoning; and building code information. Use of modeling or prediction tools for trend and risk analysis is also important.

Prevention encompasses the actions taken to avoid an incident or to intervene to stop an incident from occurring in order to protect lives and property.

Preparedness is the range of deliberate, continuous, critical tasks and activities necessary to build, sustain, and improve the ability to prevent, protect against, respond to, and recover from domestic incidents. Government agencies at all levels have an obligation to prepare themselves and the public for emergencies. Community groups, service providers, businesses, and civic and volunteer groups are all partners in this effort as everyone needs to be prepared. During the preparedness phase, responsible parties develop plans to save lives, minimize disaster damage, and enhance disaster response operations. Preparedness measures include preparedness plans; emergency exercises or training; warning systems; emergency communication systems; evacuation plans and training; resource inventories; emergency personnel or contact lists; mutual aid agreements; and public information or education.

on the data from foodborne illness outbreaks. Is the threat of a terrorist event that compromises our food supply real or exaggerated?

On the one hand, the FDA has concluded that there is a possibility for a terrorist event that might affect a large number of people.[41] The recognition of the U.S. as one of the most, if not the most, powerful nation has made an attack on U.S. soil more likely. As demonstrated on September 11, 2001, adversaries that resent America's global dominance, envy its wealth, decry its culture, or fear its military prowess can effectively strike America with unconventional means, especially if they are willing to die for their cause. The threat of foodborne contamination is magnified by a unique feature of uncertainty; officials would not immediately know the course and nature of the outbreak or the potential number of victims. U.S. authorities would be forced to assume the worst and, in attempting to protect as many people as possible, might exacerbate the panic.

On the other hand, the only documented case of food terrorism designed to achieve political goals in the U.S. originated when members of a communal religious sect in Oregon contaminated salad bars with salmonella to prevent local residents from voting on a ballot proposition to which the group objected.[42] Two other incidents involving intentional food poisoning were not motivated by political ideology. In 2003, a supermarket worker was charged with intentionally contaminating 200 lb of meat with a nicotine-containing insecticide,[43] and in 1997, a laboratory worker intentionally contaminated his coworkers' pastries with a strain of shigella.[44] No deaths occurred. Not all public health practitioners consider widespread food terrorism a realistic scenario, see Box 15.11: Is preparing for a bioterrorist attack a misappropriation of our public health resources?

15.9.1 INDUSTRY VULNERABILITY

The agricultural industry consists of both consolidated and highly fragmented sectors. Food safety is an issue across the entire food supply chain. However, vulnerability to agroterrorism is greatest in locations where food storage or processing is centralized, and therefore more susceptible to tampering or contamination. For example, fresh produce is low risk because its production and distribution is highly fragmented among local and regional growers. Meat packing, on the other hand, tends to be dominated by a few large companies (four in the U.S.) with concentrated centers and, thus, is far more vulnerable to contamination. This is particularly true with distribution and transportation companies, which employ centralized facilities. However, tampering at food production centers is a lower risk, because there are thousands of widely dispersed facilities.[45] Additionally, the intentional contamination of animal feed to reduce the availability of animal-derived food or to infect human populations could be a target for bioterrorists.[46]

The combination of inexpensive food from overseas and the consolidation of domestic production compromises America's ability to feed itself safely and sustainably. A food system where control of critical elements is concentrated in a few hands is prone to accidents and is vulnerable to terrorism. A growing number of people believe that many of the world's most pressing problems, including America's vulnerability to terrorism, can be reduced by decentralizing its food supply

---

Box 15.10 Tommy Thompson Quote

For the life of me, I cannot understand, why the terrorists have not attacked our food supply, because it is so easy to do.

Outgoing Agriculture Secretary Tommy Thompson
December 2004

Source: Pear, R. U.S. health chief stepping down, issues warning. *The New York Times.* December 4, 2004.

Box 15.11 Is Preparing for a Bioterrorist Attack a Misappropriation of Our Limited Public Health Resources?

Infectious disease epidemiologist and colleague Philip Alcabes asks if the "bio" in "biosecurity" means that we should turn our public health into a matter of civil defense? He wants to know if it is prudent public policy to rush to protect the country against the threat of attack with germs that could cause an epidemic? Sometimes epidemics have come from foreign enemies. For example, although it is unlikely that the Spaniards deliberately infected the Aztecs with smallpox, the disease so diminished the American natives that Cortés had only to finish the debacle the disease started. However, in the French and Indian War in the early 1760s, smallpox does seem to have been spread deliberately. Lord Jeffrey Amherst, the British commanding general, approved a plan to distribute smallpox-contaminated blankets "to inoculate the Indians" besieging Fort Pitt. Later, during World War I, the German biological warfare program sought to create animal epidemics that would diminish their enemies' ability to fight. More than 200 Argentine mules intended as dray animals for Allied forces died after being inoculated with both glanders (principally an equine disease) and anthrax. During World War II, one report holds that Colorado beetles were dropped by German airplanes on potato crops in southern England.

The best documented, and most successful, deliberately caused human epidemic was set by the infamous Unit 731 of the Japanese Imperial Army, stationed in conquered China during World War II. The unit dropped plague-carrying fleas on 11 Chinese towns. The number of Chinese who died of plague was probably about 700.

There is little evidence that terrorists are more likely, or better able, to use microbes as part of their armamentarium than ever before. In the creation of epidemics, the gap between intention and deed itself is a wide one. Just four communicable diseases — malaria, smallpox, AIDS, and tuberculosis — killed well over half a billion people in the 20th century, or about ten times the combined tolls of World Wars I and II, history's bloodiest conflicts. The black death killed a third of Europe's population in just four years in the mid-1300s. The Spanish flu killed between 20 and 40 million in 16 months in 1918–1919. Pre-vision is of little help against epidemic disasters but neither is pre-science necessary. Each epidemic, even the ones that turned out to be the most terrible, began slowly, percolated a while, and could have been stopped with conventional public health responses had anyone acted in time. It is usually social circumstances that make epidemics possible and public health funding that stops them. If we worry about the germ-bearing foreign enemy, we forego the upkeep of a workaday public health apparatus. Federal grant money, such as the multimillion-dollar Project BioShield program, has been allocated to technologic innovation for bioterrorism prevention. The NIH has funded two new National Biocontainment Laboratories and new facilities at Regional Biocontainment Laboratories, most at major universities, to the tune of $360 million in start-up costs.

The core issue here is that bioterrorism is not a public health problem and will not become one. The biopreparedness campaign discredits the simple logic of public health: lose the distinction between the miniscule risk of dying in an intentional outbreak and the millionfold higher chance of dying in a natural pandemic, it says; ignore the hundredfold higher still chance of dying of cancer or heart disease; defund the prenatal care clinics, the chest clinics, the exercise and cancer screening, and lead abatement programs; ignore the lessons of history, forget that human attempts to create epidemics have almost always failed; and dismiss the repeated ability of a well-funded public health apparatus to control epidemic disease with time-tested measures. The lesson of history that we ignore at our peril is this: nobody can tell us how the next epidemic will happen. Anyone who promises certain protection from the next plague is selling us a bill of goods.

Source: Adapted from Alcabes, P. The bioterrorism scare. *American Scholar.* 73(2): 35–45, 2004.

and relying more on locally produced products.[47] Reinventing community-based food systems to include numerous small farmers raising a diversity of products would make it impossible to intentionally contaminate the food supply on a large scale. Decentralizing the nation's processing, production, and distribution systems, and placing greater reliance on small family farms — key factors in the ability of the U.S. to protect its food supply — is summed up with the maxim — "Think globally, eat locally."[48]

15.9.2 BIOTERRORISM ACT

In the aftermath of the terrorist attacks on the World Trade Center and the Pentagon, and organized anthrax attacks in several American cities, there has been renewed debate on the risks of further biological attacks and reducing vulnerability to terrorism. The events of September 11, 2001, gave rise to concerns about unconventional terrorist attacks, including the threat of attacks on the U.S. food supply. Those events also heightened international awareness that nations could be targets for biological or chemical terrorism, a threat that had long concerned military and public health officials. In the aftermath of those incidents, the FDA took steps to improve its ability to prevent, prepare for, and respond to incidents of food sabotage. Though motivated by concerns about deliberate contamination, those activities built upon and expanded the agency's continuing efforts to protect consumers from foods that have been unintentionally contaminated through processing failures or handling errors.

According to the United Nations' World Health Organization (WHO), plans to mitigate the effects of sabotage of the food supply should be incorporated within existing emergency response systems. Separate systems related to terrorism would in most cases be wasteful of resources, especially as there are many common elements of response to natural or accidental incidents that may threaten public health. Nevertheless, a system for responding to food sabotage possesses some unique aspects. For example, national emergency plans should incorporate laboratory capacity for analyzing uncommon agents in food. It should also have closer links with food tracing and recall systems. In general, national needs and priorities in respect to food terrorism should be considered in order to ensure that the measures are proportional to other public health priorities.[49]

There are many points along the farm-to-table continuum during which infectious agents can arise from or be introduced into the food supply. With the globalization of the world's food supply, an attack on one country's food supply cannot be seen in isolation. Food is a major item of trade for many countries; furthermore, most countries, including developing countries, are both importers and exporters of food, making many incidents international in nature.[50,51] Consequently, the response to a terrorist threat to food will require collaboration with specialized agencies within the United Nations, such as WHO and Food and Agricultural Organization (FAO), and possibly other international organizations. Thus, WHO has warned that "the malicious contamination of food for terrorist purposes is a real and current threat." The CDC similarly concluded that sabotage of food and water is the easiest means of biological or chemical attack, and based on a risk assessment, the FDA concludes a high likelihood exists, over the course of a year, that a significant number of people could be affected by an act of food terrorism that might result in serious foodborne illness.[52]

The Public Health Security and Bioterrorism Preparedness and Response Act of 2002[53] (the Bioterrorism Act), which became fully operational in 2006, was enacted to improve the ability of the U.S. to prevent, prepare for, and respond to bioterrorism and other public health emergencies. The act directed HHS to develop a national preparedness strategy designed to improve communications between state and local governments, and federal agencies. This resulted in the National Response Plan discussed in the following text.

The act contains provisions to ensure safe drinking water by requiring community water suppliers to undertake an assessment of their facilities in order to identify and correct vulnerabilities. *The Agricultural Bioterrorism Protection Act of 2002,* a subpart of the Bioterrorism Act, was designed to improve the ability of the U.S. government to prevent, prepare for, and respond to bioterrorism and other public health emergencies that could threaten American agriculture.

For example, by improving the process by which imported food is inspected, the bill aims to decrease the likelihood that imported food can become a vehicle for bioterrorism through tampering. The act requires (1) all food facilities — domestic and foreign — to register with the FDA; (2) the FDA to maintain records on the sources and recipients of foods; (3) the FDA to receive notice in advance of food shipments being imported into the U.S. with details about the type of food, country of origin, and so on; and (4) businesses involved in the nation's human and animal food supply to maintain records showing where they received food from and where they shipped it. This fourth rule applies to any firms that manufacture, process, pack, transport, distribute, receive, hold, or import food and will help investigators determine the source of contamination after the fact. The FDA is permitted to detain any foods thought to cause harm to humans or animals without court hearings or a specified time frame.

15.9.3 Homeland Security

The Office of Homeland Security was established on October 8, 2001, with the mission to develop and coordinate the implementation of a comprehensive national strategy to secure the U.S. from terrorist threats or attacks. The office coordinates the executive branch's efforts to detect, prepare for, prevent, protect against, respond to, and recover from terrorist attacks within the U.S. These efforts included working with executive departments and agencies, state and local governments, and private entities to ensure the adequacy of the national strategy. In 2003, Homeland Security became a cabinet-level department with the 3-part mission to prevent terrorist attacks within the U.S., reduce America's vulnerability to terrorism, and minimize the damage from attacks and natural disasters.

15.9.3.1 National Response Plan (NRP)

The NRP, originally published in 2004 and updated in May 2006, defines a comprehensive approach to responding to domestic incidents. The plan incorporates best practices and procedures from multiple public entities, including homeland security, emergency management, law enforcement, firefighting, public works, public health, responder and recovery, worker health and safety, emergency medical services, as well as the private sector, integrating them into a unified structure. It forms the basis of how the federal government coordinates with the state, local, and tribal governments, and the private sector during incidents.[54] This comprehensive approach to disaster response clarifies the role of the federal government, reinforces its partnerships with state governments and local communities, and continues to expand the concept of citizen preparedness.

15.9.3.2 Research and Development

The National Center for Food Protection and Defense (NCFPD)[55] is a university-based Homeland Security Center established in 2004 by Homeland Security. The Center is a national consortium of academic, public sector, and industry partners led by the University of Minnesota, whose mission is to advance the security and safety of the nation's food supply through research, education, and outreach. NCFPD expects to achieve its mission by: (1) developing strategies to reduce the likelihood of deliberate contamination at any point along the food chain, from the farm to the consumer; (2) expanding the pool of available personnel with expertise in food biosecurity through interdisciplinary degree programs and specialized training; (3) developing rapid and efficient methods to identify intentional contamination; and (4) enhancing strategies for responding effectively to potential deliberate contamination.

15.9.3.3 Preparing Leaders

The NRP[56] specifies how the resources of the federal government will work in concert with state, local, and tribal governments and the private sector to respond to incidents of national significance. The NRP establishes processes, protocols, and best practices for these entities to work in concert to identify standardized training, organization, and communication procedures for an incident involving multiple jurisdictions. It also identifies local jurisdictions and first responders as the primary entities for handling incidents. The plan provides a comprehensive framework for private and nonprofit institutions to plan and integrate their own preparedness and response activities, nationally and within their own communities. The NRP uses the National Incident Management System (NIMS)[57] to establish standardized training, organization, and communications procedures for multijurisdictional interaction and clearly identifies authority and leadership responsibilities. Individuals must be identified who can be trained in advance to assume leadership when a disaster strikes. Those affected by the incident must be prepared not only to recognize the leaders but also to follow their instructions.

Homeland Security developed NIMS to integrate effective practices in emergency preparedness and response into a comprehensive national framework for an incident management system. NIMS enables responders at all levels to work together more effectively and efficiently to manage domestic incidents no matter what the cause, size, or complexity, including catastrophic acts of terrorism and disasters. Together the NRP and the NIMS provide a nationwide template for working together to prevent or respond to threats and incidents regardless of cause, size, or complexity. The benefits of the NIMS system include standardized organizational structures, processes, and procedures; standards for planning, training, and exercising, and personnel qualification; information management systems; and supporting technologies (voice and data communications systems, and information systems).

15.10 DISASTER RESPONSE

Responding to a disaster is a complex multipronged effort; depending on the nature of the disaster, responders provide basics such as food, water, and shelter, as well as medical care for both acute and chronic conditions, security services, and damage control. An effective response demands advanced planning and a high level of organization.

15.10.1 FOOD AND WATER

The three Emergency Support Function (ESF) areas in which food and water are most heavily involved include mass care, housing, and human services; public health and medical services; and agriculture and natural resources. Each of these areas is a grouping of government and certain private-sector capabilities into an organizational structure to: provide the support, resources, program implementation, and services most likely to be needed to save lives; protect property and the environment; restore essential services and critical infrastructure; and help victims and communities return to normal, when feasible, following domestic incidents. The ESFs serve as the primary operational-level mechanism to provide assistance to state, local, and tribal governments, or to federal departments and agencies conducting missions of primary federal responsibility.

15.10.1.1 Mass Care, Housing, and Human Services

Mass care involves coordinating nonmedical mass care services such as feeding operations. Feeding may be provided to victims through a combination of fixed sites, mobile feeding units, and bulk distribution of food. Feeding operations are based on current dietary guidelines that include meeting requirements of those with special dietary needs. Bulk distribution includes providing relief items to meet the needs of victims through sites established within the affected area. These sites are used to coordinate food, water, and ice requirements, and distribution systems with federal, state, local, and tribal governmental entities and nongovernmental organizations (NGOs), such as the Red Cross.

15.10.1.2 Public Health and Medical Services

Public health and medical services include assessment of public health/medical needs. HHS, in coordination with state health agencies, enhances existing surveillance systems to monitor the health of the general population and special high-risk populations. HHS may ask its components to ensure the safety and security of federally regulated foods; to give advice on protective actions related to indirect exposures through contaminated food and water; to provide information on public health; to assess whether food facilities in the affected area are able to provide safe and secure food; to conduct tracebacks or recalls of contaminated products; to ensure the proper disposal of contaminated products; and to provide support for public health matters for radiological incidents as a member of the Advisory Team for Environment, Food, and Health. The USDA supports a multiagency response to domestic incidents through provision of nutrition assistance and assurance of food safety and security in accordance with other responsible federal agencies. The Joint Information Center is authorized to release general public health response information after consultation with HHS.

15.10.1.3 Role of Food and Nutrition Service (FNS) and USDA

The USDA supports state, local, and tribal authorities, and other federal agency efforts to address the provision of nutrition assistance and the assurance of food safety and food security. Whereas numerous concerns arise following a storm, earthquake, civil disturbance, flood, or other disaster, none is perhaps more important than providing food in areas where people may find themselves suddenly, and often critically, in need.

When a disaster strikes and food assistance is needed, the USDA has three disaster feeding options through FNS: mass feeding, also known as *congregate feeding sites*, distribution of commodity foods directly to households in need, and the Disaster Food Stamp Program (DFSP). As part of the NRP, FNS has primary responsibility for supplying food to disaster relief organizations, such as the Red Cross and the Salvation Army, for both mass feeding and household distribution. Disaster organizations request food and nutrition assistance through state agencies that run the USDA's nutrition assistance programs. These agencies notify the USDA of the types and quantities of food that relief organizations need for emergency feeding operations.[58]

Provision of nutrition assistance by FNS includes determining nutrition assistance needs, obtaining appropriate food supplies, arranging for delivery of the supplies, and authorizing disaster food stamps. The FNS is activated when notified by DHS of the occurrence of a potential or actual incident that warrants a federal response. Actions undertaken are guided by and coordinated with state and local emergency preparedness and response officials, DHS officials, and existing the USDA internal policies and procedures as follows:

- Food supplies that are secured and delivered must be determined to be suitable for household distribution or for congregate meal service.
- Transportation and distribution of food supplies within the affected area will be arranged by federal, state, local, and voluntary organizations. Second Harvest is an example of a voluntary organization that could participate in the transport of food.
- The USDA officials coordinate with and support agencies responsible for mass care, housing, and human services that are involved in mass feeding.
- The USDA officials should encourage the use of congregate feeding arrangements as the primary outlet for disaster and food supplies.
- Priority is given to moving critical supplies of food into areas of acute need and then to areas of moderate need.
- Upon notification that commercial channels of trade have been restored, the USDA officials may authorize the use of disaster food stamp program procedures.
- Assurance of the safety and security of the commercial food supply includes the inspection and verification of food safety aspects of slaughter and processing plants, products, distribution and retail sites, and import facilities at ports of entry; lab analysis of food samples; control of products suspected of being adulterated, plant closures; and foodborne disease surveillance.

Box 15.12 Disaster Help

A part of the Egov initiative (www.egov.gov), the Disaster Help Web site (www.disasterhelp.gov) is aimed at enhancing disaster management on an interagency and intergovernmental basis. The disaster management plan uses information technology to deliver disaster assistance information and services by creating a single Internet-based portal to serve the public's requirement for assistance and the government's requirement to provide disaster information and services. This system is expected to make disaster assistance information easier to find, cut the "red tape" for citizens to apply for disaster assistance, and eliminate redundant agency processes. Disaster services providers should save resources and, potentially, lives. The timely provision of information and services to disaster victims is expected to expedite recovery, reduce government spending, speed up rebuilding, and restore public confidence.

- The public side of the portal consists of a single location, where the public and private businesses can access disaster information and services provided by government agencies and nongovernmental organizations.
- The government side of the portal provides a layered, secure environment that provides access to disaster information made available from government and nongovernmental organizations, and the means to securely exchange sensitive information relating to disaster preparedness, response, mitigation, and recovery. Government emergency managers will be able to use the portal to monitor major disaster and national security events, coordinate federal, state, and private organization responses, and collaborate on damage assessments and summaries.

15.10.1.4 Organization

The USDA's response is coordinated at both headquarters and regional levels. Response information is communicated to the responders and to the public through a number of channels, including DisasterHelp at www.disasterhelp.gov (see Box 15.12).

15.10.1.4.1 Headquarter-Level Response Structure

The USDA coordinator directs all of the department's emergency activities. FNS's National Disaster Coordinator is the point person who coordinates FNS's nutrition assistance response activities with other agencies on behalf of FNS's disaster task force. However, the FSIS assumes primary responsibility for any incident involving food safety. Once the teams are activated at the National Response Coordination Center in Washington, D.C., activities are coordinated through the USDA. The coordinator convenes a conference call with appropriate support agencies and NGO partners to assess the situation and determine appropriate actions. The agency then alerts supporting organizations and requests that they provide representation. The FNS has several functions:

- Determines the availability of the USDA foods, including raw agricultural commodities such as wheat, corn, oats, and rice that can be used for human consumption, and assesses damage to food supplies.
- With state, local, and tribal officials, it determines the nutrition needs of the population in the affected area, based on the following categories: acutely deficient, deficient, self-sufficient, and surplus supplies.
- At the discretion of the FNS administrator and upon request of the state, approves emergency issuance of food stamp benefits to qualifying households within the affected area.

- At the discretion of the FNS administrator, makes emergency food supplies available to households for take-home consumption in lieu of providing food stamp benefits for qualifying households.
- Works with state and voluntary agencies to develop a plan of operation that ensures timely distribution of food in good condition to the proper location, once the need has been determined.

15.10.1.4.2 Regional-Level Response Structure

For nutrition assistance, the point person is the regional FNS disaster coordinator. The coordinator:

- Determines the critical needs of the affected population in terms of numbers of people, their location, and usable food preparation facilities for congregate feeding, and then establishes logistical links with organizations involved in long-term congregate meal services.
- Catalogs available resources of food, transportation, equipment, storage, and distribution facilities, and locates these resources geographically.
- Ensures that all identified the USDA food is fit for human consumption.
- Coordinates shipment of the USDA food to staging areas within the affected area.
- Initiates direct market procurement of critical food supplies that are unavailable from existing inventories.
- If necessary, authorizes the Disaster Food Stamp Program and expedites requests for emergency issuance of food stamp benefits after access to commercial food channels is restored.
- Establishes the need for and effects replacement of food products transferred from existing FNS nutrition assistance program inventories.

The district and field offices nationwide coordinate the field response activities for food supply and safety according to internal policies and procedures. These activities include assessing the operating status of inspected meat, poultry, and egg product processing, distribution, import, and retail facilities in the affected area, and evaluating the adequacy of available inspectors, program investigators, and laboratory services relative to the emergency on a geographical basis.

15.10.1.5 Disaster Food Stamp Program

Each year disasters damage and destroy personal property, cut access to financial resources, disrupt links to human services programs, interrupt employment, or result in sudden medical expenses. Any of these misfortunes may precipitate a crisis for low-income communities. In recognition of the need to assist low-income people in such precarious situations, the Food Stamp Act and the Robert T. Stafford Disaster Relief and Emergency Assistance Act (also called the Disaster Mitigation Act of 2000, P.L. 106–390) grant the president and the USDA FNS broad authority to provide emergency food relief after disasters. The cornerstone of federal nutrition assistance in a disaster scenario is the Disaster Food Stamp Program (DFSP). The federal child nutrition programs and the distribution of commodity foods also play important roles.

The Food Stamp Act of 1977 and the Stafford Act of 1988 give the Secretary of Agriculture authority to issue emergency food stamps during emergencies. The Disaster Food Stamp Benefits Program (DFSBP) provides timely food assistance to households who lose food or have limited access to food as a result of a declared state of emergency. The DFSBP operates under a different set of eligibility and benefit delivery requirements than the regular Food Stamp Program described in Chapter 13. People who might not ordinarily qualify for food stamps may be eligible under the DFSBP if they have had damage to their homes, expenses related to protecting their homes, lost income as a result of the disaster, or have no access to bank accounts or other resources.[58]

Disaster Food Stamps is the FNS's first line of defense when dealing with emergencies, because it is less complex to provide food stamps in areas where retail food stores are still operating than it is to identify and arrange for the transportation of commodity foods.[58]

15.10.1.6 Commodity Donations

Commodities may be taken from local, state, and federal inventories.[60,61] Every state and U.S. territory has on hand stocks of commodity foods used for the USDA-sponsored food programs, such as the National School Lunch Program, the Emergency Food Assistance Program, and the Food Distribution Program on Indian reservations. Local inventories from school kitchens and school district warehouses located close to the emergency are usually the first sources disaster organizations turn to when they want donations of the USDA commodities.[58]

State inventories from within the state, and sometimes from another state, are tapped when local inventories do not contain sufficient resources. In an emergency, the USDA can authorize states to release these food stocks to disaster relief agencies to feed people at shelters and mass feeding sites. If the president declares a disaster, states can also, with the USDA approval, distribute commodity foods directly to households that are in need as a result of an emergency. Such direct distribution takes place when normal commercial food supply channels, such as grocery stores, have been disrupted, damaged, or destroyed, or cannot function for some reason, such as lack of electricity.

If a state does not have enough food on hand to meet emergency needs, the USDA makes arrangements for food to be shipped from other states or from the USDA's own food inventories. The USDA inventories of storage commodities may be immediately available for disaster feeding if state supplies are not sufficient. Stores of the commodity foods purchased by the USDA to distribute in their various programs are maintained in Carthage, MO and Albuquerque, NM.

The Rapid Food Response System was established to supplement, not replace, existing disaster feeding efforts by making a nutritionally balanced commodity offering available for congregate feeding during presidentially-declared disasters. The offering contains five basic categories of the USDA commodity foods that can be used to supplement existing disaster feeding efforts. Under the aegis of the regional FNS offices, seven states (New York, Pennsylvania, North Carolina, Ohio, Okhlahoma, Colorado, and California) will make their currently existing inventory available to any state nationwide.

The Secretary of Agriculture can authorize special funding to buy or replenish the USDA food stocks used in an emergency. Transportation of food donated by the USDA for disaster relief efforts is normally handled by commercial carriers. Shipping arrangements are made by the supplier or, if food is being shipped from program inventories, by the USDA's Kansas City Commodity Office. In some situations, the military or other public and private emergency assistance agencies are called on to assist in transporting food quickly to where it is needed.[58]

15.10.2 PUBLIC NUTRITION

The field of public nutrition has existed for a long time, although not by that name.[62] The term first appeared in 1996 in a letter to the editor of the *American Journal of Clinical Nutrition*.[63] The mission of public nutrition is to anticipate and address the nutritional outcomes of emergencies (malnutrition, mortality, and morbidity) by identifying the causes of malnutrition and mortality in emergency situations, and to identify the broad range of management skills needed in relation to humanitarian response initiatives, including nutrition assessment, policy development, and program design and implementation. Public nutrition has been described as a broad-based, problem-solving approach to addressing nutritional problems of populations or communities. Nutritional problems exist at national, community, and individual levels, and include hunger, childhood malnutrition, famine, suboptimal growth, infection, dietary imbalance or deficiency, and chronic disease.

Public nutrition recognizes that food insecurity is only one of the determinants of malnutrition in emergencies. Interventions need to address both the health and social environment to have an impact on malnutrition. To accomplish its mission, public nutrition uses a wide range of strategies that take into account public policies and programs in food-related fields, like economics, trade, and agriculture, as well as health.[64] Some leaders in the field believe that putting public nutrition under the rubric of health would medicalize the field, whereas putting it under agriculture would marginalize it. Public nutrition has a distinct identity, incorporating the relevant aspects of the variety of disciplines that bear on the nutrition problem, as well as incorporating scientific advances in the understanding of nutritional problems.[62]

15.10.3 PREPARING THE PUBLIC

A primary mandate of Homeland Security is to educate the public on a continuing basis about how to be prepared in case of a national emergency, including a possible terrorist attack. Table 15.6 contains a list of online resources designed for citizen preparedness. The common sense approach of Ready.gov[65] is designed to initiate learning about citizen preparedness and helps fulfill Homeland Security's mandate to educate the public. The America Prepared Campaign (APC), Inc.,[66] is a nonprofit, nonpartisan campaign that employs the expertise and energy of national leaders in emergency preparedness, media, marketing, government, and business to help Americans prepare for emergencies, including a terrorist attack. Similar to the social marketing approach used by the seat belt and recycling public education campaigns, the objective of all APC communications is to build awareness of preparedness as a philosophy, to encourage Americans to integrate thinking about preparedness into their everyday lives, and to provide specific information and direction about actions to take to achieve peace of mind. During an emergency, people should listen to radio or television messages from their local emergency managers, who will inform them whether to shelter in place or when to leave the area, and the location of the nearest volunteer agency facility.

TABLE 15.6
Online Resources for Citizen Preparedness

www.ready.gov	*Ready.gov* is a common sense framework designed to launch a process of learning about citizen preparedness. People are recommended to check back frequently. The information in this site should be adapted to personal circumstances. This site advises people to stay informed about how to react to various situations; in the event of an incident, people are advised to follow instructions received from authorities on the scene.
http://www.fema.gov/pdf/areyou ready/areyouready_full.pdf	*Are You Ready? An In-depth Guide to Citizen Preparedness,* released in 2004 by FEMA, contains chapters on basic preparedness, natural hazards, technological hazards, terrorism, recovery, and provides appendices regarding water conservation, disaster supplies checklist, and a family communication plan.
http://www.homeownership alliance.com/documents/emer gency_final_000.pdf	*The Emergency Preparedness Guide* gives homeowners practical measures they can take to prepare themselves, their families, and homes for possible emergencies. The guide is based on strategies developed for the Ready.gov campaign.
www.americaprepared.org	*The America Prepared Campaign (APC)* is a nonprofit, nonpartisan, social marketing campaign that utilizes the expertise and energy of national leaders in emergency preparedness, media, marketing, government, and business to help Americans to prepare for a terrorist attack and other emergencies. The objective of all APC communications is to build awareness of preparedness as a philosophy, to encourage Americans to integrate thinking about preparedness into their everyday lives, and to provide specific information and direction about actions to take to achieve peace of mind.

Box 15.13 Emergency Water Sources

In an emergency, having an adequate supply of clean water is a top priority. When water supplies run low, emergency sources of water can be obtained either outdoors or indoors. Outdoor sources of water include rainwater; streams, rivers, and other bodies of moving water; ponds and lakes; and natural springs. Indoor sources include ice cubes from freezer compartment of the refrigerator, the hot-water tank, and even the toilet.

- Defrosted ice yields potable water if the water that was used to make the ice cubes was itself drinkable.
- To tap the water supply in a water heater, turn off the power that heats the tank and let it cool. Place a container underneath and open the drain valve at the bottom of the tank.
- As a last resort, water is available from the toilet reservoir tank (not bowl).

Water of uncertain purity should be purified by boiling, disinfection, and/or distillation.

- Heat the water and cook at a full roiling boil for 3–5 min.
- Disinfect the water by adding 16 drops of chlorine bleach per gallon of water, stir, and let stand for 30 min. If the water does not have a slight bleach taste, repeat the dosage, and let stand for an additional 15 min.
- Distill the water by filling a large pot halfway with water. Tie a cup to the handle of the pot cover so that the cup is hanging right side up when the lid is upside down. Do not let the water touch the rim of the suspended cup. Boil the water. The water that drips down from the lid into the cup is the distilled water.

Source: Federal Emergency Management Agency and American Red Cross. Food and Water in an Emergency. November 2004. Available at: www.fema.gov/pdf/library/f&web.pdf. Accessed June 29, 2006.

15.10.3.1 Food SAFE (Shelf Available for Emergencies)

Although the American Red Cross, the Salvation Army, and other volunteer agencies will provide food, water, and clothing, people are advised to keep on hand a manual can opener, eating utensils, and a 3-d supply of water and food. One gallon of water per person per day is required for drinking and sanitation. More water may be needed for children, nursing mothers, sick people, and in warm weather climates. Water should be stored in tightly closed clean plastic containers, such as 2-l soft drink bottles. Box 15.13 contains information about emergency sources of water for people who cannot leave a stricken area.

In addition, a food supply providing each person with 800 cal/d should also be maintained.[65,67] Appropriate foods include nonperishable items that require no refrigeration, preparation or cooking, and little or no water, such as ready-to-eat canned meats, fish, fruits, vegetables; protein or fruit bars; dry cereal or granola; crackers (low sodium or unsalted); canned 100% fruit juices; nonperishable pasteurized milk; high-energy foods like nuts, dried fruits, and peanut butter; vitamin/mineral supplements; tea bags, instant coffee, cocoa mix; table sugar; comfort/stress foods; and — if necessary — food for infants and pets.

15.11 CONCLUSION

Protecting our food supply from accidental or deliberate contamination, ensuring accurate labeling on packaging, and avoiding potentially deadly nutrient deficiencies is a complex enterprise requiring coordination within and between every level of government. A wide array of individuals — from politicians to emergency and healthcare personnel to scientists — must be trained to respond rapidly and appropriately to any number of possible events, whether food poisoning at a local restaurant or providing safe food to thousands of displaced persons. Individual citizens must also be educated to read food labels to avoid allergic reactions, to maintain stores of safe food, and to seek help from the appropriate sources should the need arise.

15.12 ACRONYMS

AMS	Agricultural Marketing Service (USDA)
APC	America Prepared Campaign, Inc.
BSE	Bovine Spongiform Encephalopathy
CDC	Centers for Disease Control and Prevention
CFR	Code of Federal Regulations
CFSAN	Center for Food Safety and Applied Nutrition (FDA)
CGMPs	Current Good Manufacturing Practices
CSPI	Center for Science in the Public Interest
CVM	Center for Veterinary Medicine
DFSBP	Disaster Food Stamp Benefit Program
DSHEA	Dietary Supplement Health and Education Act
EPA	Environmental Protection Agency
ESF	Emergency Support Function
FAO	Food and Agriculture Organization (United Nations)
FDA	Food and Drug Administration (HHS)
FEMA	Federal Emergency Management Agency
FFDCA	Federal Food Drug and Cosmetic Act (1906)
FIFRA	Federal Insecticide, Fungicide, and Rodenticide Act
FNS	Food and Nutrition Service (USDA)
FSIS	Food Safety Inspection Service (USDA)
GAPs	Good Agricultural Practices
GAO	Government Accountability Office
HACCP	Hazard Analysis and Critical Control Point
HHS	Department of Health and Human Services
NARMS	National Antibiotic Resistance Monitoring System
NCFPD	National Center for Food Protection and Defense
NGO	Nongovernmental Organization
NIH	National Institutes of Health
NIMS	National Incident Management System
NRP	National Response Plan
PFGE	Pulse-field gel electrophoresis
TSE	Transmissible spongiform encephalopathy
USDA	U.S. Department of Agriculture
WHO	World Health Organization

REFERENCES

1. Gussow, J.D. *This Organic Life: Confessions of a Suburban Homesteader.* New York: Chelsea Green Publishing Co., 2001.
2. Mead, P.S., Slutsker, L., Dietz, V., McCaig, L.F., Bresee, J.S., Shapiro, C., Griffin, P.M., and Tauxe, R.V. Food-related illness and death in the United States. *Emerging Infect Dis.* 5, 607–625, 1999. Available at: http://www.cdc.gov/ncidod/EID/vol5no5/mead.htm. Accessed January 22, 2005.

3. Cieslak, P.R., Curtis, M.B., Coulombier, D.M., Hathcock, A.L., Bean, N.H., and Tauxe, R.V. Preventable disease in correctional facilities: desmoteric foodborne outbreaks in the United States, 1974–1991. *Arch Intern Med.* 156, 1883–1888, 1996.

4. Food and Drug Administration. Office of Budget and Program Analysis, Budget Formulation and Presentation Division.

5. U.S. Department of Agriculture, Office of Budget and Program Analysis, Budget Control and Analysis Division.

6. Infant metabolic acidosisand soy-based formula — United States. *MMWR.* 28, 358–359, 1979. Republished with 1996 editorial in Landmark articles from the *MMWR* 1961–1996. *MMWR.* 45, 985–988, 1996.

7. Kleinman, R.E., ed. *Pediatric Nutrition Handbook,* 5th ed. American Academy of Pediatrics, 2004.

8. Committee on the Evaluation of the Addition of Ingredients New to Infant Formula. *Infant Formula: Evaluating the Safety of New Ingredients*. Washington, D.C.: National Academies Press, 2004. Available at: http://www.nap.edu/catalog/10935.html?onpi_newsdoc03012004. Accessed February 26, 2005.

9. Formanek, R. Food allergies: When Food becomes the Enemy. U.S. Food and Drug Administration. *FDA Consumer Magazine.* July–August 2001. Available at: www.fda.gov/fdac/features/2001/401_food.html. Accessed June 27, 2006.

10. American Academy of Asthma, Allergy, and Immunology. Patient/Public Education: Fast Facts. Food Allergy. Available at: www.aaaai.org/patients/resources/fastfacts/food_allergy.stm. Accessed June 27, 2006.

11. NuConnexions. Managing food allergies. Available at: www.nuconnexions.com/Allergy/manage.htm. Accessed June 27, 2006.

12. Food Allergen Labeling and Consumer Protection (Public Law 108–282). Available at: www.cfsan.fda.gov/~dms/alrgact.html. Accessed June 27, 2006.

13. U.S. Environmental Protection Agency. The Food Quality Protection Act (FQPA) background. Available at: www.epa.gov/oppfod01/fqpa/backgrnd.htm. Accessed June 27, 2006.

14. Food Safety: Opportunities to Redirect Federal Resources and Funds Can Enhance Effectiveness. GAO/RCED-98-224, August 6, 1998.

15. Food Safety: Fundamental Changes Needed to Improve Food Safety. GAO/RCED-97-249R, September 9, 1997.

16. Food Safety: New Initiatives Would Fundamentally Alter the Existing System. GAO/RCED-96-81, March 27, 1996.

17. Food Safety and Quality: Uniform, Risk-Based Inspection System Needed to Ensure Safe Food Supply. GAO/RCED-92-152, June 26, 1992.

18. Food Safety and Quality: Who Does What in the federal Government. GAO/RCED-90-19A & B, December 21, 1990.

19. Food Safety: USDA and FDA Need to Better Ensure Prompt and Complete Recalls of Potentially Unsafe Food. GAO-05-51, October 2004.

20. U.S. General Accounting Office. Food Safety and Security: Fundamental Changes Needed to Ensure Safe Food. Statement of Robert A. Robinson, Managing Director, Natural Resources and Environment. October 10, 2001; GAO: GAO-02-47T.

21. Vogt, D.U. Food Safety Issues in the 108th Congress. CRS Report for Congress. Congressional Research Service. The Library of Congress. Updated August 16, 2004. Available at: http://www.ncseonline.org/NLE/CRSreports/04Aug/RL31853.pdf. Accessed February 18, 2005.

22. Major Management Challenges at the Department of Agriculture. Available at: Accessed February 19, 2005.

23. Federal Food Safety and Security System: Fundamental Restructuring is Needed to Address Fragmentation and Overlap. GAO-04-588T, March 30, 2004.

24. Tauxe, R.V. Emerging foodborne diseases: an evolving public health challenge. *Emerg Infect Dis.* 3, 425–434, 1997. Available at: http://www.cdc.gov/ncidod/EID/vol3no4/tauxe.htm. Accessed February 17, 2005.

25. Global Microbial Threats in the 1990s. Report of the NSTC Committee on International Science, Engineering, and Technology (CISET) Working Group on Emerging and Re-emerging Infectious Diseases. Available at: http://clinton1.nara.gov/White_House/EOP/OSTP/CISET/html/toc.html. Accessed February 17, 2005.

26. Altekruse, S.F., Cohen, M.I., and Swerdlow, D.L. Emerging foodborne diseases. *Emerging Infect Dis.* 3, 285–293, 1997. Available at: ftp://ftp.cdc.gov/pub/EID/vol3no3/adobe/cohen.pdf. Accessed February 17, 2005.

27. Schwetz, B.A. Statement before the Committee on Governmental Affairs, Subcommittee on Oversight of Government Management, Restructuring and the District of Columbia. U.S. Food and Drug Administration, October 10, 2001. Available at: www.fda.gov/ola/2001/foodsafety1010.html. Accessed June 28, 2006.

28. CDC, Preliminary FoodNet Data on the Incidence of Infection with Pathogens Transmitted Commonly Through Food — 10 States, United States, 2005. *MMWR.* 55(14), 392–395, 2006. Available at: http://www.cdc.gov/mmwr/preview/mmwrhtml/mm5514a2.htm?s_cid=mm5514a2_e. Accessed June 28, 2006.

29. CDC. PulseNet home. National Molecular Subtyping Network for Foodborne Disease Surveillance. Available at: http://www.cdc.gov/pulsenet/. Accessed February 28, 2005.

30. Cody, S.H., Glynn, M.K., Farrar, J.A., Cairns, K.L., Griffin, P.M., Kobayashi, J., Fyfe, M., Hoffman, R., King, A.S., Lewis, J.H., Swaminathan, B., Bryant, R.G., and Vugia, D.J. An outbreak of *Escherichia coli* O157:H7 infection from unpasteurized commercial apple juice. *Ann Intern Med.* 130, 202–209, 1999.

31. FDA. Food labeling: Warning and notice statement; Labeling of juice products. *Federal Register.* 63, 20486–20493, 1998. Available at: http://vm.cfsan.fda.gov/~acrobat/fr98424b.pdf. Accessed February 28, 2005.

32. FDA. Hazard Analysis and Critical Control Point (HACCP) procedures for the safe and sanitary processing and importing of juice. *Federal Register.* 63, 20449–20486, 1998. Available at: http://www.cfsan.fda.gov/~lrd/fr01119a.html. Accessed February 28, 2005.

33. CDC, Foodborne Outbreak and Response Surveillance Unit. Available at: http://www.cdc.gov/food-borneoutbreaks/index.htm. Accessed June 28, 2006.

34. CDC. Norovirus technical fact sheet. Available at: http://www.cdc.gov/Ncidod/dvrd/revb/gastro/norovirus-factsheet.htm. Accessed June 28, 2006.

35. CDC. EHS-net: CDC's Environmental Health Specialist's Network. Available at: www.cdc.gov/nceh/ehs/EHSNet/. Accessed June 28, 2006.

36. Center for Science in the Public Interest. Outbreak Alert! Closing the Gap in Our Federal Food-Safety Net. Updated and revised March 2004. Available at: http://www.cspinet.org/new/pdf/outbreakalert2004.pdf. Accessed June 28, 2006.

37. U.S. Department of Homeland Security. Lessons Learned/Information Sharing. Available at: https://www.llis.dhs.gov/about.cfm. Accessed February 7, 2005.

38. FEMA homepage. Available at: http://www.fema.gov. Accessed February 6, 2005.

39. DisasterHelp. Available at: https://disasterhelp.gov/portal/jhtml/help/instructions.jhtml?community=. Accessed February 10, 2005.

40. First Research. Agriculture Livestock Production Industry Profile Excerpt. Available at: http://www.firstresearch.com/Industry-Research/Agriculture-Livestock-Production.html. Accessed June 28, 2006.

41. U.S. Food and Drug Administration. Center for Food Safety and Applied Nutrition/Office of Regulations and Policy. Risk Assessment for Food Terrorism and Other Food Safety Concerns. October 7, 2003. Available at: http://vm.cfsan.fda.gov/~dms/rabtact.html. Accessed February 9, 2005.

42. Miller, J., Engelberg, S., and Broad, W. *Germs: Biological Weapons and America's Secret War.* New York: Simon and Schuster, 2001.

43. Nicotine Poisoning After Ingestion of Contaminated Ground Beef — Michigan, 2003. *MMWR.* 52, 413–416, 2003.

44. Kolavic, S.A., Kimura, A., Simons, S.L., Slutsker, L., Barth, S., and Haley, C.E. An outbreak of Shigella dysenteriae type 2 among laboratory workers due to intentional food contamination. *JAMA.* 278, 396–398, 1997.

45. Monke, J. Agro-terrorism: Threats and Preparedness. CRS Report for Congress. August 13, 2004. Available at: http://www.fas.org/irp/crs/RL32521.pdf. Accessed February 9, 2005.

46. van Bredow, J., Myers, M., Wagner, D., Valdes, J.J., Loomis, L., and Zamani, K. Agroterrorism: agricultural infrastructure vulnerability. *Ann NY Acad Sci.* 894, 168–180, 1999.

47. Rodale. 2001 Annual Report. Available at: http://www.rodaleinstitute.org/report_2001/taking_steps/home.shtml. Accessed September 2, 2006.

48. Wilkins, J. Think globally, eat locally. *New York Times,* December 18, 2004. Available at: http://www.globalpolicy.org/socecon/hunger/economy/2004/1218localfood.htm. Accessed February 8, 2005.

49. Schlundt, J. Terrorist Threats to Food: WHO Activities and Guidance for Prevention and Response. World Health Organization, October 2003. Available at: http://intlforum.tamu.edu/Schlundt.htm. Accessed February 9, 2005.

50. Knobler, S.L., Mahmoud, A.A.F., and Pray, L.A., eds. Biological Threats and Terrorism: Assessing the Science and Response Capabilities. Workshop Summary. Based on a Workshop of the Forum on Emerging Infections. Washington, D.C.: National Academy Press, 2002.

51. Schlunt, J. Terrorist Threats to Food: WHO Activities and Guidance for Prevention and Response (abstract). Available at: http://intlforum.tamu.edu/Schlundt.htm. Accessed February 9, 2005.

52. Food and Drug Administration. Risk Assessment for Food Terrorism and Other Food Safety Concerns. October 13, 2003. Available at: http://www.cfsan.fda.gov/~dms/rabtact.html. Accessed February 8, 2005.

53. The Public Health Security and Bioterrorism Preparedness and Response Act of 2002. 2002 (June 12). PL 10–188. Available at: http://frwebgate.access.gpo.gov/cgi-bin/getdoc.cgi?dbname=107_cong_ public_ laws&docid=f:publ188.107.pdf. Accessed February 12, 2005.

54. Department of Homeland Security. Emergencies and Disasters: planning and prevention. National Response Plan. Available at: www.dhs.gov/dhspublic/interapp/editorial/editorial_0566.xml. Accessed July 12, 2006.

55. National Center for Food Protection and Defense homepage. Available at: http://www.fpd.umn.edu/. Accessed February 9, 2005.

56. U.S. Department of Homeland Security. National Response Plan. Washington, D.C.: Department of Homeland Security. December 2004. Available at: http://www.dhs.gov/interweb/assetlibrary/NRP_ FullText.pdf. Accessed February 6, 2005.

57. National Incident Management System homepage. Available at: http://www.fema.gov/nims/. Accessed February 6, 2005.

58. United States Department of Agriculture. Food and Nutrition Service. Food Distribution Programs. Available at: http://www.fns.usda.gov/fdd/programs/fd-disasters. Accessed June 21, 2006.

59. Food and Nutrition Service. Food Distribution Division. Disaster Manual. Alexandria, VA: United Stated Department of Agriculture, August 2004. Available at: http://www.fns.usda.gov/fdd/programs/ fd-disasters/CommodityDisasterManual.pdf. February 8, 2005.

60. United States Department of Agriculture. Food and Nutrition Service. Disaster Assistance. Available at: http://www.fns.usda.gov/disasters/response/faq.htm. Accessed February 10, 2005.

61. Food and Nutrition Service. Food Distribution Division. Disaster Manual. Alexandria, VA: United States Department of Agriculture. Available at: http://www.fns.usda.gov/fdd/programs/fd-disasters. Accessed February 10, 2005.

62. Rogers, B. and Schlossman, N. "Public nutrition": the need for cross-disciplinary breadth in the education of applied nutrition professionals. Food and Nutrition Bulletin. 18(2) June 1997. Available at http://www.unu.edu/unupress/food/V182e/begin.htm#Contents. Accessed October 22, 2004.

63. Mason, J., Habicht, J.-P., Greaves, J.P., Jonsson, U., Kevany, J., Martorell, R., Rogers, B. Public nutrition. Letter to the editor. Am J Clin Nutr. 63, 399–400, 1996.

64. Harinarayan, A. What is public nutrition?. ENN (Emergency Nutrition Network) Field Exchange. No. 8, 13, 1999.

65. Ready.gov homepage. Available at: http://www.ready.gov. Accessed February 6, 2005.

66. America Prepared Campaign homepage. Available at: http://www.americaprepared.org/index.html. Accessed February 2, 2005.

67. American Prepared Campaign. Homeland Security Starts at Home. New York Times Magazine. February 6, 2005, pp. 25–29.

16 Grants to Support Initiatives in Public Health Nutrition

Community-based nonprofit organizations fill the gap that is created when the for-profit sector and government systems do not adequately address community needs.

Grants are important to the welfare of many communities. Grants made to community-based organizations help these agencies improve the overall health, education, work skills, and earning power of people in the neighborhood. With greater purchasing power of its citizens, community-based commerce is strengthened. Thus, local businesses as well as individuals profit from funds awarded to organizations charged with improving the community's health, education, and welfare. However, as the number of community-based organizations increases, there is an increase in competition to secure the grant money needed to stimulate and support their work.

It is not surprising, then, that people who have developed grantwriting skills are among the most coveted professionals in the public health workforce. Public health agencies, including community-based organizations, have an insatiable appetite for external support to start new projects and to expand existing ones. Fund-raising is integral to the functioning of these organizations and is particularly important for nonprofit community-based entities that rely heavily on grants.

A grant is an award made to an organization. The grant is earmarked to carry out a specific project proposed by one or more of the organization's members. The grant may be in the form of goods and services as well as money. Occasionally, an award is made to an individual, but most grantors prefer to make awards to the organization itself because the life span of the organization is greater than the expected tenure of an individual employee. Thus, the applicant for a grant is the organization submitting the proposal, not the employee writing the grant application.

The information in this chapter applies to all seekers of funds to support public health nutrition programs. The chapter's particular focus is on obtaining external funding for nonprofit organizations (NPO). *Nonprofit organization* is the legal term that indicates an organization is exempt from federal income tax under section 501(c)(3) of the Internal Revenue Code. Private sector grantors rely on this determination to claim a tax deduction for contributions they make, and government relies on this determination when defining eligibility for certain programs.

All the references in this chapter are available online. This is consistent with the current practice of grantors providing information about their funding opportunities online and with their requirement that applicants submit grant applications electronically.

16.1 FUNDING SOURCES

This section describes the public and private sectors, presents an overview of the two major federal departments that support programs in public health nutrition, and provides examples of the kinds of projects that government supports.

Grants in support of public health initiatives are available from government and from the private sector. It is estimated that the annual total dollar value of assistance from public and private sources is over a quarter trillion dollars ($1 trillion is $1 billion multiplied by 1000). Government supplies $240 billion in the form of project discretionary grants and block grants. Foundations, corporations, and individuals contribute another $10 billion in grant support.

16.1.1 Programs in the Public Sector (Tax-Supported Programs)

The U.S. government is divided into three branches — the executive, the judicial, and the legislative (also referred to as Congress, which is composed of the U.S. House of Representatives and the U.S. Senate). The executive branch of the federal government is composed of the White House offices and agencies. These offices include the cabinet, which helps develop and implement the policies and programs of the president. The cabinet is made up of the vice president and, by law, the heads of 15 executive departments — the secretaries of Agriculture (USDA), Commerce, Defense, Education, Energy, Health and Human Services (HHS), Homeland Security, Housing and Urban Development, Interior, Labor, State, Transportation, Treasury, and Veterans Affairs, and the attorney general. Four additional officials have cabinet-level rank: the administrator of the Environmental Protection Agency, the director of the Office of Management and Budget, the director of National Drug Control Policy, and the U.S. Trade Representative. Each of these departments is appropriated funds each year by Congress.

Agencies in the public sector are supported by taxes paid to the government. HHS and the USDA are the major federal sources of funding for nutrition programs at the state and local levels. More than 90% of government support for nutrition-related research and training is supplied by these two departments. A large percentage of funds from HHS and the USDA are distributed by the states to local governments and community-based organizations to address local public health problems. Some funds are awarded directly from the federal government to community organizations. Box 16.1 contains information about identifying sources of federal funding for programs in public health nutrition.

Box 16.1 Identifying Sources of External Funding

U.S. Government: www.Grants.gov

Department of Health and Human Services: www.hhs.gov
- National Institutes of Health
  - Funding opportunities and notices: http://grants1.nih.gov/grants/guide/index.html
  - Requests for proposals listed by Institute: http://ocm.od.nih.gov/contracts/rfps/mainpage.htm
  - Requests for applications: http://grants.nih.gov/grants/guide/rfa-files/
- Administration for Children and Families: www.acf.gov
- Administration on Aging: www.aoa.dhhs.gov
- Food and Drug Administration: www.fda.gov
- Centers for Disease Control and Prevention: www.cdc.gov
- Indian Health Service: www.ihs.gov

U.S. Department of Agriculture: http://www.usda.gov
- Cooperative State Research, Education, and Extension Service (CSREES): http://www.csrees.usda.gov/
  - Community Food Projects Competitive Grants Program: http://www.csrees.usda.gov/fo/fundview.cfm?fonum=1080
  - National Research Initiative Competitive Grants Program: http://www.csrees.usda.gov/fo/fundview.cfm?fonum=1112
- Food and Nutrition Service: http://www.fns.usda.gov/fns/
- Food Safety and Inspection Service: http://www.fsis.usda.gov

Department of Education: http://www.ed.gov
- Office of Elementary and Secondary Education: http://www.ed.gov/about/ offices/list/oese

---

16.1.1.1 Health and Human Services

The Department of Health and Human Services (HHS) is the cabinet-level department of the federal executive branch most involved with the nation's human concerns. It was created as the Department of Health, Education, and Welfare in 1953 and became the Department of Health and Human Services in 1980.[1] In one way or another, HHS touches the lives of more Americans than any other federal agency because of the wide spectrum of activities it covers. The department is sectioned into more than 300 programs that include such activities as:

- Gathering national health and other data.
- Health and social science research.
- Preventing disease, including immunization services.
- Assuring food and drug safety.
- Medicare (health insurance for elderly and disabled Americans) and Medicaid (health insurance for low-income people). Medicare is the nation's largest health insurer, handling more than 900 million claims per year. Medicare and Medicaid together provide healthcare insurance for one in four Americans.
- Financial assistance and services for low-income families.
- Improving maternal and infant health.
- Head Start (preschool education and services).
- Services for older Americans, including home-delivered meals.
- Comprehensive health services for Native Americans.

HHS represents almost a quarter of all federal outlays and administers more grant dollars than all other federal agencies combined. The department works closely with state and local governments because many HHS-funded services are provided at the local level by state or county agencies, or through private sector grantees.

One of the agencies in HHS is the Office of Public Health and Science.[2] The functions of this office are to ensure that the National Institutes of Health (NIH) conduct broad-based public health assessments designed to anticipate future public health issues and problems, and devise and implement appropriate interventions and evaluations to maintain, sustain, and improve the health of the nation; coordinate population-based health, clinical preventive services, and science initiatives; provide presentations on international health issues; and, through the surgeon general, provide direction and policy oversight for the Public Health Service Commissioned Corps. The corps is a uniformed service of more than 6000 health professionals, including about 80 registered dietitians, who serve in HHS and other federal agencies. More than one-half of the officers in the dietitian category are assigned to the Indian Health Service (49%) and NIH (15%).

In FY 2004 the HHS budget was $548 billion. HHS programs are administered by these operating divisions:

- Administration for Children and Families (ACF)
- Administration on Aging (AoA)
- Agency for Healthcare Research and Quality (AHRQ)
- Agency for Toxic Substances and Disease Registry (ATSDR)
- Centers for Disease Control and Prevention (CDC)
- Centers for Medicare and Medicaid Services (CMS)
- Food and Drug Administration (FDA)
- Health Resources and Services Administration (HRSA)
- Indian Health Service (IHS)
- National Institutes of Health (NIH)
- Office of Public Health and Science (OPHS)
- Program Support Center (PSC)
- Substance Abuse and Mental Health Services Administration (SAMHSA)

HHS is committed to achieving the health promotion and disease prevention objectives of *Healthy People 2010*. All applications for support from HHS must include work plans that address specific appropriate *Healthy People 2010* objectives.

The divisions highlighted in the following text are the HHS agencies most likely to fund programs and research concerned with nutrition in public health.

16.1.1.1.1 Food and Drug Administration (FDA)

FDA[3] assures the safety of foods and cosmetics, and the safety and efficacy of pharmaceuticals, biological products, and medical devices — products that represent almost one-quarter of U.S. consumer spending. The FDA was established in 1906 when the Pure Food and Drugs Act gave regulatory authority to the Bureau of Chemistry. In FY 2004 its budget was $1.7 billion. FDA's Center for Food Safety and Applied Nutrition (CFSAN) supports research that aims to reduce the incidence of foodborne illness and protect the integrity of the nation's foods and the food supply, including additives and dietary supplements. Food safety guidance and policymaking are other areas of research interest.

16.1.1.1.2 Centers for Disease Control and Prevention (CDC)

CDC[4] works with states and other partners to provide a system of health surveillance to monitor and prevent disease outbreaks (including bioterrorism), implements disease prevention strategies, maintains national health statistics, and provides for immunization services, workplace safety, and environmental disease prevention. Working with the World Health Organization, CDC also guards against international disease transmission, with personnel stationed in more than 25 foreign countries. CDC was established in Atlanta in 1946 as the Communicable Disease Center. In FY 2004 its budget was $7 billion.

The CDC's National Center for Chronic Disease Prevention and Health Promotion (NCCD-PHP)[5] administers the Preventive Health and Health Services Block Grant (PHHSBG) program. Block grants are the primary source of funding that provides states the latitude to fund any of the 265 national health objectives in Healthy People 2010. The PHHSBG supports clinical services, preventive screening, laboratory research, outbreak control, workforce training, public education, data surveillance, and program evaluation. A strong emphasis is placed on programs for adolescents, communities with little or poor healthcare services, and disadvantaged populations. The states depend on the block grant to support public health funding where no other adequate resources are available. The PHHSBG is a major source of funding for health promotion and disease prevention in communities across the nation and it funds health programs in heart disease and stroke, health education and promotion, physical activity and nutrition, cancer, oral health and fluoridation, and diabetes. In 2004, NCCDPHP provided about $15 million for coordinated school health programs to promote lifelong healthy behavior patterns, which include a healthy diet. Another $14 million was granted directly to researchers (through RO1 grants) to support projects identifying innovative cost-effective health promotion policies, programs, and activities in the workplace or affecting the workplace.

16.1.1.1.3 Indian Health Service (IHS)

IHS[6] works with tribes to provide health services to 1.6 million American Indians and Alaska Natives representing more than 550 federally recognized tribes. The Indian health system includes 49 hospitals, 236 health centers, 309 health stations, satellite clinics, Alaska Native village clinics, and 34 urban Indian health centers. The IHS was established in 1921 and its mission was transferred from the Interior Department in 1955. In FY 2004, the IHS budget was $3.7 billion.

The IHS's Special Diabetes Program for Indians was created by Congress in 1998. From 2003 to 2008, $100 million in grants will support programs to prevent and treat diabetes among American Indians and Alaska Natives, especially children and teenagers. The grants will go to 318 tribal, urban Indian, and Indian organizations, and IHS health programs to support diabetes prevention and treatment, including efforts to reduce cardiovascular disease associated with diabetes.

16.1.1.1.4 Administration for Children and Families (ACF)

ACF[7] is responsible for some 60 programs that promote the economic and social well-being of children, families, and communities. ACF administers the state and federal welfare programs and the Temporary Assistance for Needy Families (TANF) program, providing assistance to an estimated 5 million persons, including 4 million children. ACF administers the Head Start program, serving more than 900,000 preschool children. It also provides funds to assist low-income families in paying for child care, and supports state programs for foster care. ACF was established in1991 by bringing together several already-existing programs. In FY 2004, its budget was $49 billion.

16.1.1.1.4.1 The Community Services Block Grant Act (CSBG)

CSBG[8] provides states and federal and state-recognized Indian tribes with funds to provide a range of services to address the needs of low-income individuals to ameliorate the causes and conditions of poverty. The CSBG is administered by the Division of State Assistance in the Office of Community Services (OCS), Administration for Children and Families (ACF), in HHS. The AFC funds state, territory, local, and tribal organizations to provide family assistance (welfare), child support, child care, Head Start, child welfare, and other programs relating to children and families. Actual services are provided by state, county, city, and tribal governments, and public and private local agencies. ACF assists these organizations through funding, policy direction, and information services. A minimum of 90% of the grants must be passed from the states to local grantees, who use the funds to run programs to assist with finding and retaining employment, obtaining housing, and providing emergency food services. In FY 2003, $704.2 million was appropriated for Community Services Act programs. Most of these funds ($645.8 million) were provided for the block grant. Other provisions were: $27 million for Community Economic Development, $7.2 million for Rural Community Facilities, $16.9 million for National Youth Sports, and $7.3 million for Community Food and Nutrition. (http://edworkforce.house.gov/issues/108th/education/csbg/3030billsummary.htm)

16.1.1.1.4.2 Community Action Agencies

Working through a network of community action agencies and other neighborhood-based organizations, CSBG provides assistance to states and local communities for the reduction of poverty. The goal of the community action agencies is to revitalize and empower low-income families and individuals in rural and urban areas to become fully self-sufficient through:

- Strengthening community capabilities for planning and coordinating the use of a broad range of federal, state, local, and other assistance (including private resources) for the elimination of poverty, so that this assistance can be used in a manner responsive to local needs and conditions;
- Organization of a range of services related to the needs of low-income families and individuals, so that these services may have a measurable and potentially major impact on the causes of poverty in the community and may help the families and individuals to achieve self-sufficiency;
- Greater use of innovative and effective community-based approaches to attacking the causes and effects of poverty and community breakdown;
- Maximum participation of low-income communities and groups served by programs assisted through the block grants to empower them to respond to the unique problems and needs within their communities; and
- Broadening the resource base of programs for the elimination of poverty, so as to secure a more active role in the provision of services for (1) private, religious, charitable, and neighborhood-based organizations and (2) individual citizens and business, labor, and professional groups, who are able to influence the quantity and quality of opportunities and services for the poor.

States must submit an application for CSBG funds, which in turn make subcontracts to community action agencies and locally based community organizations. CSB legislation and

appropriations by state for FY 2004 are available on the CSBG Web site at http://www.acf.hhs.gov/
programs/ocs/csbg/. An example of the CSBG funding is its assistance for community-based food
and nutrition programs.

The Community Food and Nutrition Program: CSBG authorizes funds for the Community
Food and Nutrition (CFN) program.[9] In FY 2004, over $4 million was allocated in CFN funds to
the 50 states, plus American Samoa, Guam, Northern Mariana Islands, Puerto Rico, and the Virgin
Islands. The purposes of the program are to coordinate existing private and public food assistance
resources to better serve low-income populations, assist low-income communities to identify potential sponsors of child nutrition programs, initiate new programs in underserved or unserved areas,
and to develop innovative approaches at the state and local levels to meet the nutrition needs of
low-income people.

Grants are awarded to states to be used for subgrants to statewide public or private nonprofit
agencies. These agencies must demonstrate that their proposed activities are statewide in scope,
conduct activities which represent a comprehensive and coordinated effort to alleviate hunger within
the state, involve a broad range of organizations within the state also committed to alleviating
hunger, and, preferably, have demonstrated a track record of successfully implementing programs
designed to alleviate hunger. Activities funded through this award must also include outreach and
public education activities designed to inform low-income and unemployed individuals of the
nutrition services available under various federally assisted programs. Projects that expand and
enlarge other outreach activities or that generate additional funds and resources from other sources
to support program purposes are encouraged.

The state must submit a final narrative report that lists and describes the substate recipient
organizations, the goals of the program, the purposes for which the funds were expended, and the
extent to which the objectives of the program were achieved.

16.1.1.1.5 Administration on Aging (AoA)

AoA[10] supports a nationwide aging network, providing services to the elderly, especially to enable
them to remain independent. It also offers some 240 million meals for the elderly each year,
including home-delivered "meals on wheels." AoA helps provide transportation and at-home services. It offers ombudsman services for the elderly and provides policy leadership on aging issues.
In FY 2004, its budget was $1.4 billion.

When the Older Americans Act (OAA)[11] was signed into law in 1965, it created the AoA and
authorized grants to states for community planning and service programs, as well as for research,
demonstration, and training projects in the field of aging. Later amendments to the act added grants
to area agencies on aging for local needs identification, planning, and funding of services, including
nutrition programs in the community as well as for those who are homebound, programs which
serve Native American elders, services targeted at low-income minority elders, health promotion
and disease prevention activities, in-home services for frail elders, and services to protect the rights
of older persons.

Each year, AoA provides grant funding to states and territories, recognized Native American
tribes and Hawaiian Americans, as well as nonprofit organizations, including faith-based and
academic institutions. Individuals are not eligible to apply for AoA funding. Through grants and
cooperative agreements, AoA transfers its appropriated funding resources to the AoA's Aging
Network. Grants are used when AoA has no substantial involvement in the administration of project,
and there is no direct benefit to AoA. If, however, AoA expects to have substantial involvement in
the direction and implementation of a project, it often uses cooperative agreements.

16.1.1.1.5.1 Formula Grants and Discretionary Grants

There are two basic types of federal grants: formula (or mandatory) grants and discretionary grants.
Title III and Title VII of the OAA make funds available to grantees through formula grants. They
are ongoing programs administered by state agencies for which no application or competition is
required. By congressional mandate, however, the funds for these two programs are divided among

individual states and U.S. territories using a population-based formula. In addition, grantees are required to match a percentage of the federal funds received with state-appropriated funds and to administer the total of state and federal program funds in accordance with an AoA-approved state plan.

Through discretionary grants, AoA funds projects under Title IV of the Older Americans Act to encourage projects that develop, test, and disseminate best practices to be used by organizations in the Aging Network (a national coalition of 56 state units and 655 area agencies on aging, 236 tribal and Native organizations, plus thousands of service providers, adult care centers, caregivers, and volunteers). Competitive grants allow AoA to exercise discretion in selecting the projects to be funded and determining the amount to be awarded. Because of the nature of these projects, substantial involvement on the part of the agency is often necessary. As a result, discretionary grants are increasingly being administered as cooperative agreements. In addition, funds that Congress has set aside for specific legislatively defined purposes are used for Title IV projects.

16.1.1.1.6 National Institutes of Health (NIH)

NIH[12] is the world's premier medical research organization, supporting some 35,000 research projects nationwide in diseases including cancer, Alzheimer's, diabetes, arthritis, heart ailments, and AIDS. NIH includes 27 separate health institutes and centers. It was established in 1887 as the Hygienic Laboratory in Staten Island, NY, and now maintains 10 regional offices throughout the U.S., as indicated in Table 16.1. The goal of all the research supported by NIH is to advance

TABLE 16.1
Regional Offices of the Department of Health and Human Services

Region	Areas Covered	Location (City)	Address
1	Connecticut, Massachusetts, Maine, New Hampshire, Rhode Island, Vermont	Boston	Government Center John F. Kennedy Federal Building Boston, MA 02203
2	New Jersey, New York, Puerto Rico, the Virgin Islands	New York City	Jacob K. Javits Federal Building 26 Federal Plaza New York, NY 10278
3	Washington D.C., Delaware, Maryland, Pennsylvania, Virginia, West Virginia	Philadelphia	Public Ledger Building 150 S. Independence Mall West Philadelphia, PA 19106-3499
4	Alabama, Florida, Georgia, Kentucky, Mississippi, North Carolina, South Carolina, Tennessee	Atlanta	Sam Nunn Atlanta Federal Center 61 Forsyth St., SW Atlanta, GA 30303-8909
5	Illinois, Indiana, Michigan, Ohio, Wisconsin	Chicago	1233 N. Michigan Ave. Chicago, IL 60601
6	Arkansas, Louisiana, New Mexico, Oklahoma, Texas	Dallas	1301 Young St. Dallas, TX 75202
7	Iowa, Kansas, Missouri, Nebraska	Kansas City	Bolling Federal Building 601 East 12th St. Kansas City, MO 64106
8	Colorado, Montana, North Dakota, South Dakota, Utah, Wyoming	Denver	Byron G. Rogers Federal Office Building 1961 Stout St. Denver, CO 80294-3538
9	Arizona, California, Hawaii, Nevada, Guam, Trust Territory of the Pacific Islands, American Samoa	San Francisco	Federal Office Building 50 United Nations Plaza San Francisco, CA 94102
10	Alaska, Idaho, Oregon, Washington	Seattle	2201 6th Ave. Seattle, WA 98121

scientific knowledge in order to improve public health. In FY 2004, the NIH budget was $28 billion. NIH funds researchers to undertake a wide spectrum of basic, clinical, and epidemiologic training and other programs in universities, medical schools, and academic health centers (known as "extramural" research). They also employ scientists who conduct research in laboratories on the NIH campus (known as "intramural" research).

CRISP (Computer Retrieval of Information on Scientific Projects)[13] is a searchable database of federally funded biomedical research projects conducted at universities, hospitals, and other research institutions. The database, maintained by the Office of Extramural Research at the NIH, includes projects funded by the NIH, Substance Abuse and Mental Health Services (SAMHSA), Health Resources and Services Administration (HRSA), Food and Drug Administration (FDA), Centers for Disease Control and Prevention (CDC), Agency for HealthCare Research and Quality (AHRQ), and Office of Assistant Secretary of Health (OASH). Users can use the CRISP interface to search for scientific concepts, emerging trends and techniques, or identify specific projects and investigators. In addition, this homepage serves as the gateway to interactive searching of award information.

Introduced here are the institutes that fund most studies in areas related to nutrition in public health.

16.1.1.1.6.1 National Institute of Diabetes and Digestive and Kidney Diseases (NIDDK)
NIDDK[14] supports research programs in the areas of diabetes, digestive diseases, epidemiology, genetic metabolic diseases, obesity, and nutrition. Located across the country are four diabetes research and training centers and four obesity and nutrition research centers, supported by the institute.[15] The institute's Obesity Prevention and Treatment Program[16] supports research that focuses on the prevention and treatment of overweight and obesity. Prevention includes primary and secondary approaches through control of the initial development of overweight or obesity, weight maintenance among those at risk of becoming overweight, and prevention of weight regain, once weight loss has been achieved. This program also includes environmental, and policy- and population-based approaches to the prevention and treatment of obesity.

16.1.1.1.6.2 National Heart, Blood and Lung Institute (NHLBI)
NHLBI[17] provides leadership for a national program in diseases of the heart, blood vessels, lung, and blood; blood resources; and sleep disorders. It plans, conducts, fosters, and supports integrated and coordinated programs of basic research, clinical investigations and trials, observational studies, and demonstration and education projects. Research related to the causes, prevention, diagnosis, and treatment of the diseases and disorders mentioned earlier is conducted in the institute's own laboratories and by institutions supported by research grants and contracts. NHLBI also has administrative responsibility for the NIH Woman's Health Initiative.

16.1.1.1.6.3 National Institute of Aging (NIA)
NIA[18] sponsors research on aging through extramural and intramural programs. The extramural program funds research and training at universities, hospitals, medical centers, and other public and private organizations nationwide; the intramural program conducts basic and clinical research in NIA's own facilities by institutions supported by research grants and contracts.

16.1.1.1.6.4 Trans-NIH Research
Frequently, a Request for Applications (RFA) will be posted by a consortium of NIH agencies. For example, in 2004, nine NIH divisions jointly committed more than $6 million in a trans-NIH RFA that called for research projects to test intervention programs delivered in primary care practices, including dental practices.[19]

- National Institute of Child Health and Human Development (NICHD): $3 million
- National Center for Complementary and Alternative Medicine (NCCAM): $250,000
- National Center on Minority Health and Health Disparities (NCMHD): $250,000

- National Heart, Lung, and Blood Institute (NHLBI): $1 million
- National Institute of Dental and Craniofacial Research (NIDCR): $500,000
- National Institute of Diabetes and Digestive and Kidney Diseases (NIDDK): No set amount; participation based on level of response and scientific merit of applications appropriate to the core mission of NIDDK
- National Institute of Nursing Research (NINR): $500,000
- NIH Office of Behavioral and Social Sciences Research (OBSSR): $250,000
- NIH Office of Disease Prevention (ODP): $100,000

The aim of this research initiative was to improve dietary and physical activity behaviors of pediatric patients in order to prevent excessive weight gain in children at risk for obesity and/or to prevent further weight gain or to promote weight loss in children who are already obese. NIH proposed a number of public health nutrition-related research projects that would be appropriate responses to this RFA.

- Office-based programs providing on-site dietary and/or physical activity interventions designed to prevent weight gain in children at risk for obesity.
- Family-based interventions carried out in a primary care setting to promote weight loss or limit weight gain in overweight children and adolescents.
- Office-based interventions designed to limit sedentary behaviors and to increase physical activity.
- Collaborations between primary healthcare providers or clinics and nonclinic sites, such as hospital-based dietitians, community recreation centers, qualified complementary or alternative practitioners, and commercial weight-loss programs.
- Carefully controlled pharmacological interventions carried out in a primary care setting in combination with lifestyle interventions that are designed to induce or sustain weight loss in obese children.
- Projects designed to detect synergistic interactions between dietary interventions and interventions that involve decreased sedentary behavior or increased physical activity.
- Interventions to address physician, parent, and child barriers to acceptance of weight management interventions and to improve adherence to dietary and physical activity recommendations.
- Studies that evaluate the impact of weight management interventions on the psychosocial well-being of children and families, including quality of life and the development of eating disordered behaviors and/or body dissatisfaction.
- Office-based projects that include components of behavior modification, particularly projects designed to reduce sedentary activities, such as watching television, surfing the Internet, or playing videogames, and those designed to encourage children to be more physically active.
- Studies evaluating complementary or alternative medicine (CAM) approaches to weight maintenance and the prevention and treatment of overweight or obesity in children. Of particular interest are those CAM approaches used by qualified practitioners of CAM (e.g., meditation, naturopathy, and acupuncture) in a primary care setting.

16.1.1.2 United States Department of Agriculture

The USDA was founded by President Abraham Lincoln in 1862 when almost half of the nation's population produced at least some of their own food. Today, the USDA's services focus on all aspects of the U.S. food supply and the effects of diet and nutrition on health. Seven agencies along with their affiliated offices are located within the department: Farm and Foreign Agricultural Services; Natural Resources and Environment; Marketing and Regulatory; Rural Development; Food Safety; Nutrition and Consumer Services; and Research, Education, and Economics.

The USDA offices most likely to fund programs and research concerned with nutrition in public health include the Food Safety and Inspection Service in the division of Food Safety, the Food and Nutrition Service in Nutrition and Consumer Services, and Cooperative State Research Education and Extension Service in Research, Education, and Economics.

16.1.1.2.1 Food Safety and Inspection Service (FSIS)

Research plays an important role in the ability of the FSIS[20] to assure that the foods it regulates continue to be safe. As FSIS does not carry out its own research, it depends on both the public and private research communities to conduct the research vital to its mission. In 2003, several FSIS public health nutrition research priorities included:

- Ongoing and evolving development of validated cooking temperatures for food handlers
- Developing a better understanding of food safety hazards to further develop science-based policies and regulations
- Testing methods to measure the effectiveness of food safety education and risk communication to the consumer
- Studying cross contamination by retail food handlers and consumers in order to generate data to improve the farm-to-table risk assessment

16.1.1.2.2 Food and Nutrition Service (FNS)

FNS[21] administers USDA's nutrition assistance programs:

- Food Stamp Program (FSP)
- Special Supplemental Nutrition Program for Women, Infants and Children (WIC)
- National School Lunch Program (NSLP)
- Summer Food Service Program (SFSP)
- The Emergency Food Assistance Program (TEFAP)
- Child and Adult Care Food Program (CACFP)
- Commodity Supplemental Food Program (CSFP)
- Special Milk Program (SMP)
- Food Distribution Program on Indian Reservations (FDPIR)
- Nutrition Services Incentive Program (formerly Nutrition Program for the Elderly)
- Nutrition assistance program for Puerto Rico, American Samoa, and the Commonwealth of the Northern Mariana Islands
- Nutrition education

FNS provides children and low-income families better access to food and a more healthful diet through its food assistance programs and nutrition education efforts. Although FNS was established in 1969, many of its food assistance programs had their origins much earlier. FSP and NSLP originated during the Depression of the 1930s. FNS works in partnership with the states in all its programs. States determine most administrative details regarding distribution of food benefits and participants' eligibility, whereas FNS provides funding to cover most of the states' administrative costs. Congress appropriated $37.9 billion for FNS programs in FY 2002. In 2003, FNS awarded 150 discretionary grants: 134 through competition open only to government (predominantly state) agencies, 11 to specifically designated organizations, and the remaining 5 through competition open to all types of organizations.

16.1.1.2.3 Cooperative State Research, Education, and Extension Service

The USDA's Cooperative State Research, Education, and Extension Service (CSREES) focuses on critical issues affecting people's daily lives and the nation's future. Nutrition and health research supported by CSREES empowers people in communities to solve problems and improve their lives at the local level. CSREES maintains an extensive network of state, regional, and county extension offices in every U.S. state and territory. These offices have educators and other staff who respond to public inquiries and conduct informal, noncredit workshops and other educational events.

CSREES supports the base programs of state agricultural experiment stations and the cooperative extension system nationwide at land-grant universities.

As the USDA's primary extramural research agency, CSREES provides working funds to researchers at institutions of higher education throughout the U.S. These research programs benefit all Americans. CSREES helps ensure that a high-quality higher education infrastructure will be available at the nation's land-grant universities to address national needs. It uses the scientific expertise from these and other colleges, universities, and public and private laboratories to address national priorities.

Nutrition and health is one of 11 national priority areas CSREES has identified to target for its programs. Through funding opportunities as well as program leadership, CSREES' food, nutrition, and health programs strengthen the nation's capacity to address issues related to food safety and biotechnology, food science and technology, health, hunger and food security, nutrition, and obesity and healthy weight.

16.1.1.2.3.1 Administration of Federal Appropriations

CSREES administers federal appropriations through three basic funding mechanisms:

Competitive funding. Projects supported through competitive programs are funded based upon the recommendations of proposal review panels. CSREES requests proposals from eligible entities, and a panel of subject matter experts reviews each proposal and prioritizes projects for funding. CSREES' competitive programs include the National Research Initiative (NRI), which funds projects in human nutrition and obesity, food safety, and improving human nutrition for optimal health.

Formula programs. CSREES provides support for research and extension activities at land-grant institutions through programs that distribute federal appropriations on the basis of statutory formulas. CSREES' formula-funded programs include the cooperative extension system. In most cases, the states are required to match the federal formula dollars they receive with nonfederal contributions.

Congressionally directed funding. Each year, Congress directs CSREES to fund and administer certain state or commodity-specific programs through the Special Grant and federal administration appropriation accounts. These funds may be awarded to individual investigators at universities or consortia of universities and be further distributed on a competitive basis by the recipient institution. The Community Food Projects Competitive Grant Program (CFPCGP) is an example of congressionally directed funding. Projects funded by CFPCGP are expected to fight food insecurity through developing local food projects that help promote the self-sufficiency of low-income communities.

Community food projects competitive grant program: Community food projects are designed to increase food security in communities by bringing the whole food system together to assess strengths, establish linkages, and create systems that improve self-reliance of the communities for their food needs. The program is designed to meet the needs of low-income people by increasing their access to fresher, more nutritious food supplies, increase the self-reliance of communities for their own food needs, and promote comprehensive responses to local food, farm, and nutrition issues. Additionally, projects should meet specific state, local, or neighborhood food and agricultural needs for infrastructure improvement and development, plan for long-term solutions, and create innovative marketing activities that mutually benefit agricultural producers and low-income consumers.

Preferred projects are also expected to develop linkages between two or more sectors of the food system, support the development of entrepreneurial projects, develop innovative linkages between the for-profit and nonprofit food sectors, encourage long-term planning activities and multisystem, interagency approaches with multistakeholder collaborations. These linkages are expected to build the long-term capacity of communities for addressing their food and agricultural problems with approaches, such as food policy councils and food planning associations. CFPCGP grants are intended to help eligible private nonprofit entities establish and carry out multipurpose community food projects. They range from $10,000 to $300,000 and last from 1 to 3 years. Funds for CFPCGP have been authorized through 2007 at $5 million per year. These grants require a dollar-for-dollar match in resources, meaning that the agency applying for the grant must be able to demonstrate in-kind or other support from other sources. (See Subsection 16.2.2.3.)

16.1.2 THE PRIVATE SECTOR

Although at its core philanthropy represents a direct effort to help others (ideally, without expectations of getting something in return), all corporations and some individuals use charitable giving to decrease their tax burden. The funder's motive for providing grants may be entirely charitable (as it sometimes is for small donors) or the rationale for donating funds may be fiscal exigence (as it always is for large donors). In either case, contributors have the right to provide funds for the causes they value. At the same time, grantwriters have the need to present funders with the most compelling case possible to assure that their organizations benefit from the limited pool of donated resources.

The private sector includes private foundations, corporate grantmakers, grantmaking public charities, and community foundations. Descriptions of private sector donors appear in Box 16.2. Information about identifying private funders is available in the Foundation Center at http://fdncenter.org/funders/. Founded in 1956, the Foundation Center is an authority on philanthropy that serves grantseekers, grantmakers, researchers, policymakers, the media, and the general public. Other resources for identifying nationally and internationally recognized funding organizations are GuideStar (http://www.guidestar.org/) and ePhilanthropyFoundation.org (http://www.ephilanthropy.org/site/PageServer).

Box 16.2 Funding in the Private Sector

Private foundation: Nongovernmental, nonprofit organization with an endowment (usually donated from a single source, such as an individual, family, or corporation) and program managed by its own trustees or directors. These are established to maintain or aid social, educational, religious, or other charitable activities serving the common welfare, primarily through the making of grants. Examples of private foundations with a history of supporting nutrition causes are the Gerber Foundation, Rockefeller Foundation, W.K. Kellogg Foundation, Robert Wood Johnson Foundation, Bill and Melinda Gates Foundation, and the Cooper Institute.

Corporate grant makers: Company-sponsored foundations and corporate giving programs. A company-sponsored foundation (also known as a corporate foundation) is a private foundation whose assets are derived primarily from the contributions of a for-profit business. Although a company-sponsored foundation may maintain close ties with its parent company, it is an independent organization with its own endowment and as such is subject to the same rules and regulations as other private foundations. Corporate giving programs are grant making programs established and administered within a for-profit business organization. Some companies make charitable contributions through both a corporate giving program and a company-sponsored foundation. Examples of corporate grantmakers with a history of supporting nutrition causes are Land O'Lakes Foundation, ConAgra, Inc., Johnson & Johnson, Proctor and Gamble Fund, Burger King Corporation, General Mills, Inc., and Abbott Laboratories Fund.

Grant making public charity: A public foundation is a nongovernmental public charity that operates grant programs benefiting unrelated organizations or individuals as one of its primary purposes. There is no legal or IRS definition of a public foundation, but such a designation is needed to encompass the growing number of grantmaking institutions that are not private foundations. Examples of grantmaking public charities with a history of supporting nutrition causes are the American Dietetic Association Foundation, School Food Service Foundation, International Life Sciences Institute, and Share Our Strength (SOS).

Community foundations: Community foundations are 501(c)(3) organizations that make grants for charitable purposes in a specific community or region. A community foundation is much like a private foundation; its funds, however, are derived from many donors rather than a single source, as is usually the case with private foundations. The funds available to a community foundation are usually held in an endowment that is independently administered; income earned by the endowment is then used to make grants. Although a community foundation may be classified by the IRS as a private foundation, most are classified as public charities and are thus eligible for maximum tax-deductible contributions from the general public.

Community foundations make up one of the fastest growing sectors of philanthropy in the U.S. They build and strengthen communities by making it possible for a wide range of donors to create permanent, named component funds to meet critical needs. There are more than 650 community foundations in the U.S., located in almost every region and state in the country. Community foundations accept gifts of various sizes and types from private citizens, local corporations, other foundations, and government agencies. They hold almost $30 billion in assets. In 2002, community foundations received an estimated $5.6 billion in gifts and gave approximately $3.2 billion to a wide variety of nonprofit activities: urban affairs, the arts, education, environmental projects, health, and disaster relief. Community foundations range in size from the largest community foundation in the U.S., the New York Community Trust (with assets in 2007 totaling more than $1.9 billion), to some with endowments of $100,000 or less. The funds are invested in diverse portfolios and management is a major aspect of each community foundation's work. All share the common goal of serving donors, NPOs and their communities.

The Foundation Center maintains an online directory of Web sites of community foundations arranged by state.

Sources:

Council on Foundations. Fact Sheet—Community Foundations. Available at: http://www.cof.org/Members/content.cfm?ItemNumber=1281. Accessed February 12, 2007.

The New York City Community Trust homepage. Available at: http://www.nycommunitytrust.org. Accessed February 12, 2007.

16.2   GRANT APPLICATION MECHANISMS

There are two mechanisms whereby organizations submit applications for competitive grants. Grant applications may be solicited by the funder (grantmaker), or the applicant (grantseeker) may submit to the funder an unsolicited request for support.

16.2.1   GRANTMAKER-INITIATED REQUESTS FOR PROPOSALS

Some grants are awarded in response to funder-initiated requests for proposals, such as an advertised request for proposal (RFP) or a request for application (RFA). Grantors may also issue a Notice of Funding Availability. This single notice contains announcements of several independent funding streams. The purpose of the notice is to assist potential applicants to better identify the programs for which they can compete and give proposals to the programs most suitable to the issues faced by the target population. It also helps eligible applicants to understand the range of issues that may be supported by various related programs and encourages collaborations among organizations that provide complementary services. Each week the NIH transmits, via the NIH listserv, a table of contents

(TOC) giving that week's funding announcements. The TOC contains links to each RFA, program announcement (PA), and notice published for that week. Instructions for subscribing to NIH's weekly listserv are available at http://grants.nih.gov/grants/guide/listserv.htm. Proposals may be solicited in three ways: program announcements, requests for applications, and requests for proposals.

- Program announcement (PA) is open for 3 years (unless otherwise stated); applications must be postmarked or received at NIH by a specified date
- Request for applications (RFA) is a one-time solicitation, and applications must be *received at NIH* by the mandatory date
- Request for proposals (RFP) is a contract solicitation

16.2.2 Grantseeker-Initiated Requests for Proposals

Other grants are awarded on the basis of unsolicited appeals to potential funders. In this case, the applicant takes the initiative to submit a proposal for funding within the context of the funding organization's requirements.

Examples of investigator-initiated grant mechanisms are the research project grants (RO1) and small research grants used by the NIH, which provide support for health-related research and development consistent with the mission of the particular NIH Institute to which the grant is submitted.

16.2.2.1 NIH RO1

RO1 grants are awarded to all types of organizations (universities, colleges, small businesses, for-profit, foreign and domestic, faith-based, etc.). The RO1 mechanism allows an investigator to define the scientific focus or objective of the research based on a particular area of interest and competence. Almost all institutes and centers at NIH fund RO1 grants. Research grant applications are assigned to an institute or center based on receipt and referral guidelines, and many applications are assigned to multiple institutes and centers as interdisciplinary and multidisciplinary research is encouraged. Each institute and center maintains a Web site with funding opportunities and areas of interest. Allowable costs include salary and fringe benefits for the principal investigator (PI), key personnel, and other essential personnel; equipment and supplies; consultant costs; alterations and renovations; publications and miscellaneous costs; contract services; consortium costs; facilities and administrative costs (indirect costs); and travel expenses. Modular applications are most prevalent with modules of $25,000, up to the limit of $250,000. Grants are generally awarded for 1 to 5 years. The application for an RO1 follows the instructions provided in PHS 398 Grant Application kit. Receipt dates for RO1 grant applications are posted at http://grants.nih.gov/grants/funding/submissionschedule.htm. Those applicants that are not successful the first time may resubmit revisions up to two times.

16.2.2.2 NIH RO3

The small research grant (RO3) offers unsolicited research support, specifically limited in time and amount, providing flexibility for initiating studies that are generally short-term or pilot projects. Furthermore, the time interval from application to funding of RO3 grants is short, thus allowing new ideas to be investigated or pursued in a more expeditious manner. The common characteristic of the small research grant is the provision of limited funding for a short period of time. Examples of the types of projects that NIH Institutes and Centers support with RO3 include the following: pilot or feasibility studies; secondary analysis of existing data; small, self-contained research projects; development of research methodology; and development of new research technology. A project period of up to 2 years and a budget for direct costs of up to two $25,000 or one $50,000 module per year may be requested. One revision of a previously reviewed small grant application may be submitted.

16.2.2.3 In-Kind Support

Although grant awards are usually monetary, they may also include in-kind support for (1) products, supplies, and equipment (furniture, computers, office equipment), (2) use of corporate services/facilities (financial and administrative support services, meeting space, mailing services, computer services, printing and duplicating), and (3) professional services and employee expertise (graphic arts and design, advertising, promotion marketing, advice on taxes, business and finances). Product philanthropy is a key element in many major companies' giving programs. In 1999, product donations made up almost one-third of total contributions of the largest companies in the U.S. Gifts In Kind International (www.giftsinkind.org), a charity that deals exclusively in product philanthropy, maintains a network of more than 450 affiliates that provide nonprofit organizations with access to millions of dollars annually in product and service donations. In 2002, it distributed nearly $800 million in product donations. Operating at less than 1% of the fair market value of products donated, it is one of the most cost-efficient charities in the world.

A glossary of terms used in public health nutrition grants appears in Box 16.3.

Box 16.3 Glossary of Terms for Grants in Public Health Nutrition

- **Audience** — Individual, group, or institution for which the organization's products and services are provided, e.g., children, adults, parents, educators, clinic visitors, or partner institutions. Target audience: individual, group, or institution that is the focus of the project's goals. Characteristics or attributes of target: age, geographic location, number, and job position of the target audience that should be considered when analyzing their needs.
- **Beneficiary** — Immediate: target audience that will experience the project's desired results in the earliest stages of its implementation and whose involvement may be necessary to ensure that the organization's goals are achieved. Intermediate: target audience that will experience the project's desired results within 1 to 2 years of the implementation of the project. Long-term: audience that will experience the project's desired results after the project is concluded.
- **Benefit** — Gain or payoff accruing to the project stakeholders, including target audiences, as a result of the project.
- **Best practices** — Practices that incorporate the best objective information currently available regarding effectiveness and acceptability.
- **Block grant** — An intergovernmental transfer of federal funds to states and local governments for broad purposes such as health, education, or community development in general. A block grant makes few requirements as to how the money is to be spent, instead offering state and local municipalities discretion, within general guidelines established by Congress and the executive branch. Annual program plans or applications are normally required.
- **Budget** — Total estimated cost of the project, including direct costs associated with each of the project's activities, as well as indirect costs.
- **Capacity building** — Activities that assist eligible entities to improve or enhance their overall or specific capability to plan, deliver, manage, and evaluate programs efficiently and effectively to benefit low-income individuals. This may include upgrading internal financial management or computer systems, establishing new external linkages with other organizations, adding or refining a program component or replicating techniques or programs piloted in another local community, or making other cost-effective improvements.
- **Budget period** — The time interval into which a grant period is divided for budgetary and funding purposes.
- **Capital request** — A planned undertaking to purchase, build, or renovate space or building or to acquire equipment.

- **Communication strategy** — Outline of the messages to be conveyed to stakeholders about the project's processes and results the most efficient and effective channels and timing for transmitting the messages, and the means for obtaining feedback.
- **Community** — The people living in the same district, city, state or locale.
- **Community Development Corporation (CDC)** — A private nonprofit corporation that has a board of directors consisting of residents of the community and business and civic leaders, and has as a principal purpose planning, developing, or managing low-income housing or community development activities.
- **Contribution** — A tax-deductible gift, cash, property, equipment, or service from an individual to a nonprofit organization, often given annually.
- **Cost-benefit analysis** — Comparison of the total cost of doing the project with the anticipated value or payoff of the project. A formal analysis involves calculating the ratio of the numerical value of the anticipated benefits to the anticipated costs.
- **Costs** — Direct costs: personnel, material, and service expenses associated with specific project activities. Indirect costs: project expenses, e.g. energy, rent, and insurance, that cannot be directly tied to a specific project activity.
- **Data analysis** — Organization, processing, and presentation of information that is collected for the purpose of making recommendations or drawing conclusions.
- **Desired result** — Goal the project is designed to achieve for its stakeholders. It may be expressed as an outcome or an output.
- **Developmental or research phase** — The time during the project period that precedes the operational phase. Grantees accomplish preliminary activities during this phase, as establishing third-party agreements, mobilizing monetary funds and other resources, assembling, rezoning, and leasing of properties, conducting architectural and engineering studies, constructing facilities, etc.
- **Direct costs** — Personnel, material, and service expenses associated with specific project activities.
- **Dissemination plan** — Strategy for making the project's results, products, processes or benefits accessible through acceptable communication channels so the results of the project will benefit the broader population.
- **Displaced worker** — An individual in the labor market who has been unemployed for 6 months or longer.
- **Distressed community** — A geographic urban neighborhood or rural community of high unemployment and pervasive poverty.
- **DUNS** — Dun and Bradstreet Data Universal Numbering System. A nine-digit number required when applying for federal grants or cooperative agreements. Grantee organizations can verify that they have a DUNS number or take steps needed to obtain one at no cost by calling 1-866-705-5711 or contacting http://www.dunandbradstreet.com. The requirement for a DUNS number applies to all organizations that apply for NIH grants and cooperative agreements. Nonaffiliated individuals who apply for a grant or cooperative agreement are exempt from this requirement.
- **Eligible applicant** — State and local governments, Indian tribes, and public and private nonprofit agencies/organizations, including faith-based and community organizations.
- **Employment education and training program** — A program that provides education and/or training to welfare recipients, at-risk youth, public housing tenants, displaced workers, homeless and low-income individuals and that has organizational experience in education and training for these populations.
- **Empowerment Zone and Enterprise Community Project Areas (EZ/EC)** — Urban neighborhoods and rural areas designated as such by the secretaries of the Department of Housing and Urban Development and Agriculture.
- **Evaluation plan** — Protocol for assessing the extent to which a project has met its goals.

- **Faith-Based Community Development Corporation** — A community development corporation that has a religious character.
- **Formative evaluation** — Gathering information that can be used as a management tool to improve the way a program operates while the program is in progress. It should also identify problems that occurred, how the problems were resolved, and what recommendations are needed for future implementation.
- **Gantt chart** — Bar chart that shows graphically the duration, of the project's activities (the start and end dates), as well as its milestones. It can also show the relationships between the project's activities, e.g., the finish of one task before another begins.
- **Goals** — The broad results the project is expected to accomplish, which guide the development of the project's objectives and activities.
- **General operating support** — Funds, both contributions and grants that support the ongoing services of the organization.
- **Grants** — Usually an allocation from foundations, corporations, or government for special projects or general operating expenses. Grants may be multiyear or annual.
- **Hypothesis** — An assumption made in order to test a theory. It should assert a cause-and-effect relationship between a program intervention and its expected result. Both the intervention and its result must be measured in order to confirm the hypothesis. The following is an example: "Eighty hours of classroom training will be sufficient for participants to prepare a successful loan application." In this hypothesis, data would be obtained on the number of hours of training actually received by participants (the intervention) and the quality of loan applications (the result) to determine the validity of the hypothesis (that eighty hours of training is sufficient to produce the result).
- **Indian Tribe** — A tribe, band, or other organized group of Native American Indians recognized in the state or states in which they reside, or considered by the secretary of the Interior to be an Indian tribe or an Indian organization.
- **Indicator** — Measurable condition or behavior that can show an outcome was achieved. This is usually expressed as a number or percentage of the target audience that demonstrates an observable, measurable sign or characteristic representing the intended outcome.
- **Implementation activities** — Tasks performed to deliver the project's final products or services to the target audience.
- **Indirect costs** — Project expenses that cannot be directly tied to a specific project activity, e.g., energy, rent, and insurance.
- **In-kind support** — A contribution of equipment/materials, time, and services that the donor has placed a monetary value on for tax purposes, and noncash contributions provided by nonfederal third parties. These contributions may be in the form of real property, equipment, supplies, and other expendable property.
- **Innovative project** — One that departs from, or significantly modifies, past program practices and tests a new approach.
- **Intervention** — Any planned activity within a project that is intended to produce changes in the target population and the environment, and that can be formally evaluated. For example, assistance in preparing a business plan is an intervention.
- **Job creation** — New jobs, i.e., jobs not in existence prior to the start of the project. These result from new business startups, business expansion, development of new services industries, and other newly undertaken physical or commercial activities.
- **Job placement** — Placing a person in an existing vacant job of a business, service, or commercial activity not related to the new development or expansion activity.
- **Letter of commitment** — A signed letter or agreement from a third party to the applicant that pledges financial or other support for the grant activities contingent only on OCS accepting the applicant's project proposal.

- **Logic model** — A diagrammatic representation of a program that describes the logical linkages among program resources, conditions, strategies, short-term outcomes, and long-term impact.
- **Matching funds** — Funds which must be supplied by the grantee in an amount equal to or a percentage of the award amount in order to receive the award. In the case of a federal grant, the matching funds must usually come from non-federal sources.
- **Modular application** — A type of grant application in which support is requested in specified increments without the need for detailed supporting information related to separate budget categories. When modular procedures apply, they affect not only application preparation but also review, award, and administration of the application/award.
- **Methodology** — A sequence of activities needed to accomplish the program objectives.
- **Milestone** — Signpost or marker that shows accomplishment of logically related activities, e.g., design and development or achievement of the project's interim or final targets.
- **Mission** — Overall purpose of an organization. It typically identifies key broad audiences and purposes, and often broadly describes the methods by which the organization will achieve its mission.
- **Monitoring** — Steps or processes for continual tracking of current performance in relation to a plan, e.g., schedules and budgets, number of services provided, number of participating institutions or people, and for identification of any corrective steps necessary to improve performance.
- **Need** — Gap between the current condition and the desired condition.
- **Needs analysis** — Systematic process of identifying the gap between what the current state is and what the grantmaker wants to achieve, and determining appropriate solutions to close the gap.
- **Nonprofit organization (NPO)** — An organization, including faith-based and community-based, that provides proof of nonprofit status.
- **Operational phase** — The time interval during the project period when businesses, commercial development or other activities are in operation, and employment, business development assistance, and so forth are provided.
- **Outcomes vs. output** — Outcomes refer to the program's desired effect on its target audience. They are usually specified in terms of: a) learning, including enhancements to knowledge, attitudes, and behaviors, and b) skills. Outcomes are often presented temporally (short-term, intermediate, and long-term). Outputs are usually the tangible results of the major activities of the program. They are usually accounted for by their number, for example, the number of people who were screened for blood pressure, blood sugar, and cholesterol.
- **Outcomes** — The changes in (or benefits achieved by) clients due to their participation in program activities. This may include changes to participants' knowledge, skills, values, behavior, or status.
- **Outcome evaluation** — An assessment of project results as measured by collected data that define the net effects of the interventions applied in the project. An outcome evaluation will produce and interpret findings related to whether the interventions produced desirable changes and their potential for being replicated. It should answer this question: Did the program work?
- **Outcome-based evaluation approach (OBE)** — Set of principles and processes to provide information about the degree to which a project has met its goals in terms of creating benefits for individuals in the form of knowledge, skill, attitude, behavior, status, or life condition.
- **Output-based evaluation approach** — Set of principles and processes to provide information about the degree to which the project's products and services have achieved the desired result; e.g., the quantity or quality of services, the volume of users or participants, or the number of products that met the target audience's expectations.

- **Performance standard** — The number and percentage of clients who are expected to achieve the result. Also called target, they should be set based on professional judgment, past data, research, or professional standards.
- **Pilot test** — Dry run of a process, such as a workshop or training session, on a selected group of people in a realistic setting to obtain feedback and make necessary adjustments before delivery of the final product or service to the target audience.
- **Poverty Income Guidelines** — Guidelines published annually by the U.S. Department of Health and Human Services that establish the level of poverty defined as low income for individuals and their families. The guideline information is posted on the Internet at: http://www.hhs.aspe.gov/poverty/.
- **Predevelopment phase** — The time interval during the project period when an applicant or grantee plans a project, conducts feasibility studies, prepares a business or work plan, and mobilizes nonfederal funding.
- **Principal investigator** (or program director or project director) — An individual designated by the grantee to direct the project or activity being supported by the grant who is responsible for the scientific and technical direction of a project, the day-to-day management of the project or program, and is accountable to the grantee for the proper conduct of the project or activity.
- **Product** — Anything created or obtained as a result of some operation or work.
- **Project director** — Main person responsible for the project; coordinates all project tasks and promotes good relationships and communications among all team members.
- **Process evaluation** — The ongoing examination of the implementation of a program. It focuses on the effectiveness and efficiency of the program's activities and interventions (for example, methods of recruiting participants, quality of training activities, or usefulness of follow-up procedures). It should answer these questions: Who is receiving what services, and are the services being delivered as planned?
- **Program** — An organized set of services designed to achieve specific outcomes for a specified population that will continue beyond the grant period.
- **Project** — A planned undertaking or organized series of related activities that begins and ends within the grant period, and that is designed to achieve specific outcomes for its target audience. A successful project may become an ongoing program.
- **Project period** — The total time for which a project is approved for support, including any approved extensions.
- **Proposal** — A written document prepared to present a problem to a funding organization and to communicate to the proposal reviewers the strategy that the researcher intends to use in search of a solution to that problem. The proposal should set forth the exact nature of the matter to be investigated and a detailed account of the methods to be employed. It must answer the standard research questions: What? Why? How? When? Who? Where? To what effect?
- **Risk** — Potential events or conditions that could have a positive or a negative impact on the project goals.
- **Risk analysis** — Process of identifying risks, analyzing the likelihood that they will occur and the degree of impact that they will have on the project goals, and selecting strategies to eliminate or manage them.
- **Sample** — A representative subgroup of the population that is being studied.
- **Schedule** — The start and finish dates of the project and each of the project activities. It may also include the milestones or markers showing accomplishment of logically related activities or targets, as well as relationships among the activities.
- **Scope** — Boundary of the project described in the project plan. It includes the need that will be addressed, the target audience, the goals that will be achieved within a certain time frame, the main activities that will be performed, the project performers, and the

outcome, product, or service that will result; by implication, anything that is not included in these components is "out of scope."

- **Service** — Activity carried on to provide people with the use of something.
- **Self-sufficiency** — A condition where an individual or family does not need, and is not eligible to receive, TANF assistance under Title I of the Personal Responsibility and Work Opportunity Reconciliation Act of 1996 (Part A of Title IV of the Social Security Act.); the economic status of a person who does not require public assistance to provide for his or her needs and that of immediate family members.
- **Self-employment** — The employment status of an individual who engages in self-directed economic activities.
- **SMART** — Acronym that stands for goals or targets that are specific, measurable, achievable, realistic (and relevant), and time-bound.
- **Summative evaluation** — Provides information on the project's efficacy (its ability to do what it was designed to do).
- **Success story** — An example that illustrates the program's positive or desired effect.
- **Sustainability activities** — Tasks performed to ensure that the project's benefits extend beyond the period of a grant or the "official" conclusion of the project.
- **Target** — Measurable amount of success the proposed project should achieve within a certain time frame. When expressed as an output, it refers to the amount, quality, or volume of use the proposed project should achieve within a certain time frame. When expressed as an outcome, it refers to the measurable amount of success the proposed project should achieve with regard to the target audience's knowledge, skills, attitudes, behaviors, status, or life condition, within a certain period of time.
- **Target audience** — Individuals, groups, or organizations that are the focus or beneficiaries of the products or services of your project.
- **Technical assistance** — A problem-solving event generally using the services of a specialist. Such services may be provided on-site, by telephone, or by other communications. These services address specific problems and are intended to assist with immediate resolution of a given problem or set of problems.
- **Temporary Assistance for Needy Families (TANF)** — The federal block grant program authorized in Title I of the Personal Responsibility and Work Opportunity Reconciliation Act of 1996 (Public Law 104–193). The TANF program transformed welfare into a system that requires work in exchange for time-limited assistance.
- **Third party** — Any individual, organization, or business entity that is not the direct recipient of grant funds.
- **Third party agreement** — A written agreement entered into by the grantee and an organization, individual, or business entity (including a wholly owned subsidiary) by which the grantee makes an equity investment or a loan in support of grant purposes.
- **Underserved area** — A locality in which less than one-half of the low-income children are eligible.
- **Vision** — Statement of what the project intends to achieve. It describes aspirations for the future without specifying the means that will be used to achieve those desired ends.
- **Wants** — Wishes or desires of the target audience. These should be taken into consideration in determining the most appropriate solution or solutions to meet an identified need.

16.3 GRANT APPLICATIONS

In order to simplify the process of seeking support, there is a trend towards standardizing applications for grants. Many grantmakers in the private sector have adopted common grant application (CGA) forms to allow grant applicants to produce a single, standardized proposal for a specific community

---

Box 16.4 Sample CGA Form

Project/Program Abstract

1. Describe the proposed program.
2. Explain how it relates to the organization's mission.
3. Demonstrate the organization's capacity to carry out the program.
4. Indicate who will benefit from the program.

Organization Information

5. Provide a brief summary of the organization's mission, goals, programs, major accomplishments, success stories, and qualifications.
6. Show evidence of client and community support.
7. Describe the population served, including total number and geographic, demographic, and socioeconomic characteristics.
8. Provide information regarding the total number of paid and volunteer staff members.

Project/Program Description

9. Explain the significance and scope of the program and why your organization is qualified to carry it out.
10. Describe the expected outcomes and the indicators of those outcomes.
11. Describe the evaluation process and how the results will be used.
12. Document the size and characteristics of the population to be served.
13. Outline the strategy or methodology and timeline to be used in the development and implementation of the program.
14. What linkages or collaborations will be used?
15. How do you plan to involve the population you intend to serve in the design?
16. How does this program enhance the existing services in the community?

Funding Considerations

17. Describe plans for obtaining other funding needed to carry out the project, program or organizational goals, including amounts requested of other funders.
18. If the project or program is expected to continue beyond the grant period, describe plans for ensuring continued funding after the grant period.

Attachments

19. Attach a list of the organization's officers and directors; the organization's actual income and expense statement for the past fiscal year, identifying the organization's principal sources of support; the organization's projected income and expense budget for the current fiscal year, identifying the projected revenue sources; the organization's most recent audited financial statement including notes and IRS Form 990; and copies of the IRS federal tax exemption determination letters.

Source: Adapted from the Donors Forum of Wisconsin Common Application Form, revised March 2000. http://www. mu.edu/fic/common.html. Accessed July 6, 2004.

---

of funders (usually in a specific geographic area, such as a state or a large city). Increasingly, electronic versions of these forms will be available for grant seekers to download and enter their responses directly onto the form. Links to over a dozen CGA forms used in various regions of the U.S. are available on The Foundation Center Web site. A sample CGA appears in Box 16.4.

Through its grants Web site, the federal government provides a unified electronic "storefront" for its agencies to announce their grant opportunities and for potential applicants to find and apply

TABLE 16.2
Categories of Federal Grants

Agriculture	Employment, labor and training	Information and statistics
Arts	Energy	Law, justice, and legal services
Business and commerce	Environmental quality	Natural resources
Community development	Food and nutrition	Regional development
Consumer protection	Health	Science and technology
Disaster prevention and	Housing	Social services and income security
relief education	Humanities	Transportation

for grants. Launched in late 2003, www.grants.gov is a single, comprehensive Web site that contains information about finding and applying for all federal grant programs. The executive branch of the U.S. government has 26 grantmaking agencies that together award more than $350 billion annually to state and local governments, academia, nonprofit, and other organizations. The government's support is awarded through more than 900 grant programs in 21 categories. The categories are listed in Table 16.2.

HHS, which awards more than half of all the competitive grants from the federal government, is the lead agency for Grants.gov. The Find Grant Opportunities feature of the Web site allows grantseekers to search for information on available grant opportunities, using a number of criteria, including such key words as *obesity* and *schools*, or a specific agency, such as USDA or HHS. The Apply for Grants feature enables users to download, complete, and submit applications for grant opportunities offered by federal agencies. In sum, Grants.gov provides:

- A single unified platform for all federal agencies to announce their grant opportunities and for all grant applicants to find and apply for those opportunities
- A standardized manner of locating and learning more about funding opportunities
- A single, secure, and reliable source for applying for federal grants online
- A simplified grant application process with reduction of paperwork

16.3.1 GRANTWRITING

To write a successful application for external funding, one must start by understanding the *raison d'etre* of the prospective grantor organization. You may, for example, look at the funding agency's strategic plan, which establishes priorities and related goals and objectives to focus its investment of effort and resources over the plan period.

The two major government funding sources for nutrition in public health are the USDA and NIH. A strategic goal of the USDA is to improve nutrition and health by providing food assistance and nutrition education and promotion,[22] whereas the funding philosophy of NIH is to improve public health. The W.K. Kellogg Foundation (WKKF) (http://www.wkkf.org/) and the Robert Wood Johnson Foundation (RWJF) (http://www.rwjf.org/index.jsp) are among the most competitive private sector funders of nutrition causes. The WKKF mission is to help people help themselves through the practical application of knowledge and resources to improve their quality of life and that of future generations. The mission of RWJF is to improve the health and healthcare of all Americans through four goal areas: assure that all Americans have access to quality healthcare at reasonable cost; improve the quality of care and support for people with chronic health conditions; promoting healthy communities and lifestyles; and reducing the personal, social, and economic harm caused by substance abuse, such as tobacco, alcohol, and illicit drugs.

In general, the quality of a project is the factor that determines whether it is to be funded. The organization requesting support must also demonstrate to the funding agency that it has the means to accomplish the work, which includes both expertise and resources. The funding organization must be assured that (1) the principal investigator (PI) and his or her colleagues are qualified to do the work, and (2) the institution has equipment and personnel to support the proposed project and will allow the PI enough time to complete the required tasks.

16.3.1.1 Characteristics of the Successful Grant Application

Proposals succeed or fail for a number of reasons. Among these are:

- The strength, quality, and persuasiveness of the proposal
- The feasibility of the proposal, including but not limited to whether the project meets a clear community need, suggests a unique way to solve a well-defined problem, demonstrates community support, has access to a workforce that can see the project through to a successful completion, and has a well-planned budget
- How well the project fits the funder's mission and current funding interests
- The reputation, track record, and financial history of the institution requesting funds
- Competition: how many other requests the funder has received
- Funds and timing: how much money the funder has available in this cycle
- How well the funder knows and trusts the board and staff, if the agency requesting funds is a local NPO

16.3.2 PARTS OF THE PROPOSAL

A typical proposal contains eight parts and appendices: the proposal abstract or executive summary, introduction of the organization requesting support, the problem statement or needs assessment, project objectives, project methods or design to achieve the stated objectives, project evaluation, sustainability or future funding, and the project budget. Guidelines for writing proposals are available online. Refer to Grants.gov for specific details concerning the preparation of grant proposals for federal awards. Information about writing proposals for nongovernment funding is available in the Foundation Center (http://fdncenter.org/). Following are the nine parts:

16.3.2.1 Abstract or Executive Summary

Summarize the request clearly and succinctly. Like all summaries, it is written last, although it appears as the first section. It is given in proposals that are more than 15 pages long or if the funding organization requires a summary statement.

16.3.2.2 Introduction

Introduce the organization by stating its vision and mission, describe the agency's qualifications, and establish its credibility.

16.3.2.3 Statement of Need

The purpose of this section is to present the background and significance of the project by stating the problem to be investigated or needs to be met, providing the rationale for the proposed project, indicating the current state of knowledge relevant to the proposal, and suggesting the potential contribution of this project to the problem(s) addressed. Establish familiarity with recent research findings and use citations both to support specific statements and also to establish familiarity with all the relevant publications and points of view.

16.3.2.4 Goals and Objectives

The goals and objectives section of the proposal describes to the potential funder what will be achieved by the project. *Goals* are broad idealistic statements with a long-term outcome in mind. (Example: "The goal of this project is to improve the nutritional value of the food served in the New York City public school system."). Most proposals do not have more than three goals. For each goal, you may develop numerous corresponding *objectives*.

Objectives are specific statements that indicate to the reviewer exactly how you plan to achieve your goals. Objectives should challenge the institution to improve its functioning, expand its scope, or reach a larger target audience. They should stretch the current limits of the organization to bring about significant improvements that are important to the community. The best objectives have several characteristics in common. Well-written objectives are *s*pecific, *m*easurable, *a*chievable, *r*elevant, and *t*ime-bound (*smart*).

- *Specific.* Objectives state what is to be achieved. (Example: "There will be a reduction in the number of public schools in the district that sell soda and candy during regular school hours.")
- *Measurable.* Information concerning the objective can be collected, detected, or obtained from records. (Example: "There will be a 40% reduction in the number of public schools in the district that sell soda and candy during regular school hours.")
- *Achievable.* Not only is the objective possible, it is likely that the organization will be able to accomplish the task.
- *Relevant to the mission.* The objective fits into the overall mission of the funding organization as well as the mission of the organization that is applying for funding. In other words, the objective helps each organization achieve its mission.
- *Time-bound.* Each objective clearly indicates how much time it would take to accomplish the desired outcome. (Example: "By January 1, 2007 there will be a 40% reduction in the number of public schools in the district that sell soda and candy during regular school hours.")

There are several types of objectives. *Process objectives* may be used as intermediate markers of the organization's progress in attaining its overall goal. Process objectives measure the accomplishment of individual tasks completed as part of the implementation of a program. Examples of process objectives are provided:

By January 1, 2009, there will be a 50% or greater increase in the number of principals in the school district who agree to a ban on the sale of candy and sweetened soda water in school premises.

By September 1, 2009, there will be a 50% or greater increase in the number of schools in the district that do not sell candy and sweetened soda water on school premises.

In addition to process objectives, there are also *outcome objectives*, which measure the desired outcome of the proposed program. Examples of outcome objectives are provided:

By January 1, 2008, 100% of the principals in the school district will agree to a ban on the sale of candy and sweetened soda water on school premises.

By September 1, 2008, 100% of the schools in the district will not sell candy and sweetened soda water on school premises.

16.3.2.5 Methods

Describe methods and activities for addressing the identified problems and achieving the desired results. This part of the proposal enables the reader to visualize the implementation of the project. It should convince the reader that your agency knows what it is doing, thereby establishing the

---

Box 16.5 Credere

Credere, the Latin verb that means *to believe*, is the root of many words in English.

Credo	System of beliefs or principles
Credible	Capable of being believed
Credence	Something that establishes a claim to belief
Credential	Anything that provides basis for belief
Credit	Belief in the truth of something; trust
Credulous	Willing to believe or trust too readily
Incredulous	Disbelieving or skeptical
Incredulity	The state of being incredulous; disbelief
Incredible	Too implausible to be believed; unbelievable

---

credibility of the agency. It is helpful to conceptualize the methods section of a proposal as addressing the time-honored questions: How? When? Why? Where? Who?

- *How*: The detailed description of what will occur from the time the project begins until it is completed. The methods used to achieve the desired outcomes should match the objectives stated in the previous section. Include how the data will be collected, analyzed, and interpreted.
- *When*: The chronology of activities that must be performed to implement the project. A timetable for the project's activities presented in the form of a Gantt chart can illustrate both the order in which tasks are carried out and the length of time allotted for each activity. A Gantt chart is a bar graph that helps plan and monitor project development or resource allocation on a horizontal time scale.
- *Why*: This is the place to justify chosen methods, especially if they are new or unorthodox. Cite examples of successful use of the methods in previous projects and explain why the planned work will lead to the expected outcomes; describe any new methodology and its advantage over existing methodologies, and discuss the potential difficulties and limitations of the proposed procedures and alternative approaches to achieve the aims.
- *Where:* Indicate where the project will take place, which includes the location of administrative offices and areas designated for storage of sensitive documents, as well as settings for direct client contact.
- *Who*: Discuss the number of staff members, their qualifications and credentials (see Box 16.5), and the specific tasks assigned to each. Provide position descriptions for each paid staff member, indicating what percentage of time will be devoted to the project. Identify staff already employed by the organization and those to be recruited specifically for the project. (Details about individual staff members may be included here or in the appendix, depending on the length and importance of this information.)

Staffing refers to volunteers and consultants, as well as to paid staff. Describe volunteer activities to underscore the value added by the volunteers as well as the cost-effectiveness of the project.

Salary and project costs are affected by the qualifications of the staff. Indicate the practical experience required for key staff members, as well as their level of expertise and educational background. If individuals have already been selected to direct the program, summarize their credentials and include a brief biographical sketch in the appendix. A strong project director can help influence a grant decision.

Describe plans for administering the project, which is especially important in a large operation or if more than one agency is collaborating on the project. Identify the staff members who are responsible for financial management, project outcomes, record keeping, and reporting.

16.3.2.6 Evaluation

Present a plan to evaluate the degree to which the project's objectives are met (outcomes evaluation) and to improve the way the program works (process evaluation). Allocate 5 to 10% of the budget for activities related to evaluating the project. Consider budgeting for a statistician to assist with the planning and implementation of the evaluation component of the program. The value of a sound evaluation design cannot be overstated. Effective program evaluation helps to improve the program (process or formative evaluation) as well as determine the extent to which the program delivers on its promise (summative evaluation). Process evaluation provides information about the program while it is still in progress. It points to changes that might be needed to bring the project to a successful conclusion. Process evaluation focuses on program activities, outputs, and short-term outcomes. Summative evaluation, on the other hand, provides information on the project's efficacy (its ability to do what it was designed to do).

The WKKF supports the use of a "logic model"[23] to present the working of the program. A logic model uses words and/or pictures to (1) illustrate the sequence of activities proposed to bring about change and (2) demonstrate how these activities are linked to the results the program is expected to achieve.[24] A logic model can strengthen the case for investing in the proposed program as it captures in a single page what the program plans to do. Used correctly, it also helps to write the body of the proposal, clarify the services to be delivered, and streamline the evaluation process. For programs delivering primary and secondary prevention services, the logic model is a snapshot of the agency's primary services, short- and long-term goals, and intended outcomes of the services provided. It can be used as a guide to plan for new services or as the first step in planning for an evaluation of their services.

A review of current RFPs indicates that funders are requiring specificity and results, as indicated by their requests for "outcome-based evaluation," "best practices" programs, and "sustainable organizations." The logic model was developed to meet these requests.

Figure 16.1 shows the components of a generic program logic model. Each component is linked to the next in a conditional "if–then" relationship. In this paradigm, the term *output* substitutes for "objectives," *outcomes* replaces "short-term goals" and *impact* is used instead of "long-term goals." The components of the logic model are defined underneath each component's heading. Figure 16.2 is a sample program logic model for an initiative to eliminate the sale of food with no redeeming nutritional value in a local school district.

16.3.2.7 Future Funding

Describe a plan for sustainability of the project. Sustainability refers to the continuation of the program even after the initial funding has ended. The Foundation Center suggests its being prepared to demonstrate the long-term financial viability of the project to be funded and of the organization itself. Demonstrate that the project is *finite* (with a beginning, a middle, and an end) or that it is *capacity-building*, which means it will contribute to the future self-sufficiency of the organization, or that it will enable the agency to expand services that might generate revenue in the future, or that it will make the organization competitive for future external funding streams.[25]

16.3.2.8 Budget

Clearly delineate costs to be met by the grant. In longer proposals, a budget narrative will be provided along with the budget worksheet.

16.3.2.9 Appendices

The appendix includes materials to elaborate on any parts of the proposal. It also contains a list of the members of the agency's board of directors, a copy of the Internal Revenue Service (IRS) determination letter for 501(3)(c) organizations, financial documentation, and brief resumes of key staff.

Resources/ Inputs	→	Activities	→	Outputs (objectives)	→	Outcomes (short-term goals)	→	Impact (long-term goals)
Resources or *inputs* refers to funds, staff, community support, participants, e.g., funds requested from grantmaker as well as resources already available to the grantseeker		*Activities* refers to the methods used to accomplish goals, e.g., classes, counseling, training		*Outputs* refers to units produced by the program, e.g., number and type of clients served, number of events planned, number of policies developed		*Outcomes* refers to short-term indicators of progress towards the goal, e.g., collaborative partnerships		*Impact* refers to long-term program effects, e.g., economic self-sufficiency
PLANNED WORK				INTENDED RESULTS				

FIGURE 16.1 Components of a Program Logic Model.

Resources	Activities	Outputs	Outcomes	Goals
Funds to support program

School nutrition councils

Dietetic interns from local college

Local dental association | Develop consortium of stakeholders to coordinate all projects activities.

Enlist the support of school faculty and nurses by conducting training sessions to demonstrate the success of similar campaigns in other school districts.

Sponsor contests to help devise alternative streams of funding to replace revenue traditionally realized from sale of foods with no redeeming nutritional value.

Establish calendar of ongoing meetings with principals. | Within 1 year of the start of the program, all of the district principals will agree to a ban on the sale of candy and sweetened soda water on school premises. | Within 2 years of the start of the program…

None of the district schools will sell candy or sweetened soda water on school premises.

50% of the schools will be earning more money from alternative streams of fund-raising than previously earned from soda and candy sales. | All of the schools will be earning more money from alternative streams of fund-raising than they previously earned from soda and candy sales. |
| PLANNED WORK | | | INTENDED RESULTS | |

FIGURE 16.2 Sample program logic model for an initiative to eliminate the sale of food with no redeeming nutritional value in a local school district.

16.3.2.9.1 Project Narrative

The information in this section is abstracted from an RFP issued in 2004 by the AoA for a proposed *intervention* program.[26]

The project narrative is the most important part of the application as it will be used as the primary basis to determine whether or not your project meets the minimum requirements for the grant you are applying for. It should provide a clear and concise description of the project and might include the following components:

- Summary/abstract
- Problem statement
- Goal(s) and objective(s)
- Proposed intervention
- Special target populations and organizations
- Outcomes
- Project management
- Evaluation
- Dissemination
- Organizational capability

16.3.2.9.1.1 Summary/Abstract

This section should include a brief — not more than 300 words — description of the proposed project, including the goal, list of objectives, and the products to be developed. Detailed instructions for completing the summary/abstract are included in Attachment E of this document.

16.3.2.9.1.2 Problem Statement

This section should describe, in both quantitative and qualitative terms, the nature and scope of the particular problem or issue the proposed intervention is designed to address, including how the project will potentially affect the elderly population and their caregivers (including specific sub-groups within those populations), and possibly the healthcare and social services systems (e.g., the use of healthcare or nursing home services.)

16.3.2.9.1.3 Goals and Objectives

This section should consist of a description of the project's goals and major objectives. Unless the project involves multiple and complex interventions, it is better to have only one overall goal.

16.3.2.9.1.4 Proposed Intervention

This section should provide a clear and concise description of the intervention you are proposing to use to address the problem described in the problem statement section. You should also describe the rationale for using the particular intervention, including factors such as lessons learned from similar projects previously tested in your community or in other areas of the country and factors in the larger environment that have created the right conditions for the intervention (e.g., existing social, economic, or political factors that you will be able to take advantage of). Also note any major barriers you anticipate and how your project will be able to overcome those barriers. Be sure to describe the role and makeup of any strategic partnerships you plan to involve in implementing the intervention. Partnerships may be with other organizations, funders, and/or consumer groups.

16.3.2.9.1.5 Special Target Populations and Organizations

This section should describe how you plan to involve community-based organizations in a meaningful way in the planning and implementation of the proposed project. It should also describe how the proposed intervention will target disadvantaged populations, including limited-English-speaking populations.

16.3.2.9.1.6 Outcomes

This section of the project narrative must clearly identify the *measurable outcome* that will result from the project. It should also describe how the project's findings might benefit the field at large, for example, how the findings could help other organizations throughout the nation to address the same or similar

---

Box 16.6 Project Work Plan (Sample Format)

Goal:

Measurable Outcome(s):

Major Objectives	Key Tasks	Lead Person	Timeframe (Start and End Date by Month)
1.			
2.			
3.			
4.			

Note: Use as many continuation pages as necessary.

Source: Administration on Aging. Instructions for Preparing Competitive Grant Applications for the Aging Services Network Integrated Care Management Grants Program. Available at: http://www.sdcounty.ca.gov/cnty/cntydepts/ health/ais/ltc/media/AoA-04-08integratedcaregrant.doc. Accessed August 19, 2006.

---

problems. Give measurable outcomes in the work plan grid (see Box 16.6) in addition to any discussion included in the narrative and a description of how the project might benefit the field at large.

A "measurable outcome" is an observable end-result that describes how a particular intervention benefits consumers. It demonstrates functional status, mental well-being, knowledge, skill, attitude, awareness, or behavior. It can also show a change in the degree to which consumers exercise choice over the types of services they receive or whether they are satisfied with the way a service is delivered. Additional examples include a change in the responsiveness or cost-effectiveness of a service delivery system, a new model of support or care that can be replicated in the aging network, or new knowledge that can contribute to the field of aging. A measurable outcome is not a measurable "output," such as the number of clients served, the number of training sessions held, or the number of service units provided.

You should keep the focus of this section on describing what outcomes are anticipated and use the evaluation section that follows to describe how the outcomes will be measured and reported.

Your application will be scored on the clarity and nature of your proposed outcomes, not on the number of outcomes cited. It is totally appropriate for a project to have only one outcome that it is trying to achieve through intervention.

16.3.2.9.1.7 Project Management
This section should include a clear delineation of the roles and responsibilities of the project staff, consultants, and partner organizations and show how they will contribute to achieving the project's objectives and outcomes. It should specify who would have day-to-day responsibility for key tasks such as leadership of the project, monitoring of the project's ongoing progress, preparation of reports, and communication with other partners and funding organizations. It should also describe the approach that will be used to monitor and track progress on the project's tasks and objectives.

16.3.2.9.1.8 Evaluation
This section should describe the methods, techniques, and tools that will be used (1) to determine whether or not the proposed intervention achieved its anticipated outcomes, and (2) to document the "lessons learned" — both positive and negative — from the project that will be useful to people interested in replicating the intervention, if it proves successful.

16.3.2.9.1.9 Dissemination

This section should describe the method that will be used to disseminate the project's results and findings in a timely manner and in easily understandable formats to parties who might be interested in using the results of the project to inform practice, service delivery, program development, and/or policymaking, and especially to those parties who would be interested in replicating the project.

16.3.2.9.1.10 Organizational Capability Statement

Each application should include an organizational capability statement and resumes of key project personnel. The organizational capability statement should describe how the applicant agency (or the particular division of a larger agency that will have responsibility for this project) is organized, the nature and scope of its work and the capabilities it possesses. This description should cover capabilities of the applicant agency not included in the program narrative, such as any current or previous relevant experience or the record of the project team in preparing cogent and useful reports, publications, and other products. If appropriate, include an organization chart showing the relationship of the project to the current organization. Attach short resumes of key project staff only. Neither these nor an organizational chart will count toward the narrative page limit. Also include information about any contractual organization that might have a significant role in implementing the project and achieving project goals.

16.3.2.9.1.11 Work Plan

The project work plan should reflect and be consistent with the project narrative and budget. It should include a statement of the project's overall goal, anticipated outcomes, key objectives, and the major tasks or action steps that will be pursued to achieve the goal and outcomes. For each major task or action step, the work plan should identify the timeframes involved (including start- and end-dates), and the lead person responsible for completing the task. Use the sample work plan format included in Box 16.6.

16.3.2.9.1.12 Letters of Commitment from Key Participating Organizations
and Agencies

Include confirmation of the commitments to the project (should it be funded) made by key collaborating organizations and agencies in this part of the application. Any organization that is specifically named to have a significant role in carrying out the project should be considered an essential collaborator. Instructions will be provided on how to attach letters if the application is submitted electronically.

16.3.3 SMALL AWARDS

Sometimes a full grant proposal is not called for. When an unsolicited appeal is for a small amount of money (less than $1000), consider developing a solicitation letter in lieu of a full-scale proposal. A request for a contribution of $1000 or less hardly calls for more than a three or a four-page letter. To be effective, a letter proposal will cover essentially the same points as a full proposal but in considerably less space because must less money is being requested and a much more conservative product is expected as a result of the donation. Box 16.7 contains a summary of the components of an effective letter proposal.

Box 16.7 The Components of a Letter Proposal

1. Ask for the gift: The letter should begin with a reference to your agency's prior contact with the funder, if any. State why you are writing and how much funding is required from the particular foundation.
2. Describe the need: Briefly explain why there is a need for this project, piece of equipment, or whatever is being requested.

3. Explain what you will do: Provide enough detail to arouse the funder's interest. Describe precisely what will take place as a result of the grant.
4. Provide agency data: Acquaint the funder with the organization by providing its mission statement; a brief description of programs offered; the number of people served; and staff, volunteer, and board data, as appropriate.
5. Include appropriate budget data: The budget appears in the letter proper or in a separate attachment. It must clearly indicate the total cost of the project.
6. Close: Every proposal of any length needs a strong concluding statement. Include one or two concluding paragraphs. This is a good place to call attention to the future, after the grant is completed. If appropriate, outline some of the follow-up activities that might be undertaken to begin to prepare the funders for your agency's next request. This section is also the place to make a final appeal for the proposed project. Briefly reiterate what your organization expects to accomplish and why it is important. (At this point, a bit of emotion might make the letter even more persuasive.)
7. Attach any additional information required: The funder may need much of the same information to back up a small request as a large one. These are a board list, a copy of the applicant agency's IRS determination letter, financial documentation, and brief resumes of key staff.

When requesting information as to how to apply for a small amount of money, the response will include instructions that will provide guidance for writing the proposal. Box 16.8 contains a request posted in 2004 for two-page proposals for $2500 mini-grants for projects addressing women's health. The turnaround time for the proposal was just 2 weeks.

Box 16.8 Request for Mini Proposal

Request for Mini-Proposal from HHS Region 2 Office on Women's Health
Health mini-grants are available in the amount of $2500. FY 2004 priorities are for projects addressing women and heart disease, diabetes, cancer, HIV/AIDS, and minority women's health. There will be 15 awards. Prepare request on your organization's letterhead stationery and have it signed by an official of your organization. Requests should not exceed two pages in length. Provide all of the following in your request:

- Identification information: Organization's full name, mailing address, DUNS number, contact person's name, title, telephone number, fax number, e-mail address (for your organization to apply for a DUNS number free of charge, call 1-800-333-0505 or visit www.customerservice.dnb.com).
- Organization: Mission statement and recent project accomplishments.
- Proposed project: Goal of project, target population to be reached, approach that will be used to complete the project, time frame for completion of project (6 to 9 months), statement explaining how the project will help advance women's health.
- Product/deliverable: Identify the final product(s) that will be delivered to the HHS Region 2 Office on Women's Health.
- Budget: The budget requested, not to exceed $2500, with a brief explanation as to how funds will be used.

For further information, contact U.S. Department of Health and Human Services, Region II (NJ, NY, PR, VI), Office on Women's Health, 26 Federal Plaza, Room 3835, New York, NY 10278, Tel (212) 264-4628, Fax (212) 264-1324, E-mail: sestepa@osophs.dhhs.gov.

16.4 CONCLUSION

Seeking funding through grants can occupy a large part of a public health practitioner's work. Whereas many agencies at the federal level and private organizations provide funding, knowing the most appropriate agency to apply to for your particular program and needs can save a good deal of time and effort. In addition, it is extremely important to approach grant writing in an organized and deliberate, rather than a haphazard, albeit passionate, manner. Knowing exactly what you intend to do with the funds you receive — in other words, thoroughly planning before you even begin writing your grant — is very important to potential funders.

16.5 ACRONYMS

ACF	Administration for Children and Families
AHRQ	Agency for Healthcare Research and Quality
AoA	Administration on Aging
ATSDR	Agency for Toxic Substances and Disease Registry
CACFP	Child and Adult Care Food Program
CAM	Complementary or alternative medicine
CDC	Centers for Disease Control and Prevention
CFN	Community food and nutrition
CFPCGP	Community Food Projects Competitive Grant Program
CFSAN	Center for Food Safety and Applied Nutrition
CMS	Centers for Medicare and Medicaid Services
CRISP	Computer Retrieval of Information on Scientific Projects
CSBG	Community Services Block Grant
CSREES	Cooperative State Research, Education, and Extension Service
FDA	Food and Drug Administration
FNS	Food and Nutrition Service
FSIS	Food Safety and Inspection Service
FSP	Food Stamp Program
FY	Fiscal year
HHS	Department of Health and Human Services
HRSA	Health Resources and Services Administration
IHS	Indian Health Service
IRS	Internal Revenue Service
NCCAM	National Center for Complementary and Alternative Medicine
NCCDPHP	National Center for Chronic Disease Prevention and Health Promotion
NCMHD	National Center on Minority Health and Health Disparities
NHLBI	National Heart, Lung, and Blood Institute
NIA	National Institute of Aging
NICHD	National Institute of Child Health and Human Development
NIDCR	National Institute of Dental and Craniofacial Research
NIDDK	National Institute for Diabetes and Digestive and Kidney Diseases
NIH	National Institutes of Health
NINR	National Institute of Nursing Research
NPO	Nonprofit organization
NRI	National Research Initiative
NSLP	National School Lunch Program
OAA	Older Americans Act
OASH	Office of the Assistant Secretary of Health
OBSSR	NIH Office of Behavioral and Social Sciences Research

ODP	Office of Disease Prevention
OPHS	Office of Public Health and Science
PA	Program announcement
PHHSBG	Preventive Health and Health Services Block Grant
PI	Principle investigator
PSC	Program Support Center
RFA	Request for applications
RFP	Request for proposals
RWJF	Robert Wood Johnson Foundation
SAMHSA	Substance Abuse and Mental Health Services Administration
TEFAP	The Emergency Food Assistance Program
USDA	United States Department of Agriculture
WIC	Special Supplemental Nutrition Program for Women, Infants, and Children
WKKF	William K. Kellogg Foundation

REFERENCES

1. U.S. Government Manual Online, 2003–2004 Edition via GPO Access [wais.access.gpo.gov], pp. 220–232, DOCID:193760tx_xxx-41. Available at: http://frwebgate.access.gpo.gov/cgi-bin/getdoc.cgi?dbname=2003_government_manual&docid=193760tx_xxx-41. Accessed August 19, 2006.

2. U.S. Government Manual Online, 2003–2004 Edition via GPO Access [wais.access.gpo.gov], pp. 220–232, DOCID:193760tx_xxx-41. Available at http://www.gpoaccess.gov/gmanual/browse-gm-03.html. Accessed July 24, 2004.

3. Food and Drug Administration homepage. Available at: http://www.fda.gov/. Accessed July 28, 2004.

4. U.S. Department of Health and Human Services. Centers for Disease Control and Prevention homepage. Available at: http://www.cdc.gov/. Accessed July 28, 2004.

5. National Center for Chronic Disease Prevention and Health Promotion (NCCDPHP). Available at: http://www.scitechresources.gov/Results/show_result.php?rec=2144. Accessed July 27, 2004.

6. U.S. Department of Health and Human Services. Indian Health Service homepage. Available at: http://www.ihs.gov/. Accessed July 28, 2004.

7. U.S. Department of Health and Human Services. Administration for Children and Families homepage. Available at: http://www.acf.hhs.gov/. Accessed July 27, 2004.

8. U.S. Department of Health and Human Services. Administration for Children and Families. Community Service Block Grant. Available at: http://www.acf.hhs.gov/programs/ocs/csbg/index.htm. Accessed July 28, 2004.

9. U.S. Department of Health and Human Services. Administration for Children and Families. Community Food and Program, Grant award terms and conditions FY 2004. Available at: http://www.acf.dhhs.gov/programs/ocs/csbg/html/TERMS2004.htm. Accessed July 29, 2004.

10. U.S. Department of Health and Human Services. Administration of Aging homepage. Available at: http://www.aoa.gov/. Accessed July 28, 2004.

11. Older Americans Act Overview. Available at: http://aoa.gov/about/legbudg/oaa/legbudg_oaa.asp. Accessed July 28, 2004.

12. U.S. Department of Health and Human Services. National Institutes of Health homepage. Available at www.nih.gov. Accessed July 28, 2004.

13. National Institutes of Health. CRISP (Computer Retrieval of Information on Scientific Projects). Available at: http://crisp.cit.nih.gov/. Accessed June 30, 2005.

14. U.S. Department of Health and Human Services. National Institutes of Health National Institute of Digestive Diseases and Diabetes and Kidney Disease homepage. Available at: http://www.niddk.nih.gov/index.htm/. Accessed July 28, 2004.

15. NIDDK Sponsored-Research Centers. Available at: http://www.niddk.nih.gov/fund/other/centers.htm#ClinicalNutrition. Accessed July 28, 2004.

16. U.S. Department of Health and Human Services. National Institutes of Health. National Institute of Digestive Diseases and Diabetes and Kidney Disease. Obesity Prevention and Treatment Program. Available at: http://www.niddk.nih.gov/fund/program/M-Rlist.htm#obesprev. Accessed July 28, 2004.
17. U.S. Department of Health and Human Services. National Institutes of Health. National Heart, Lung, and Blood Institute homepage. Available at: http://www.nhlbi.nih.gov/index.htm/. Accessed July 28, 2004.
18. U.S. Department of Health and Human Services. National Institutes of Health National Institute on Aging homepage. Available at: http://www.nia.nih.gov/. Accessed July 28, 2004.
19. U.S. Department of Health and Human Services. National Institutes of Health. NIH Guide. Prevention and Treatment of Childhood Obesity in Primary Care Settings. Release date: July 20, 2004. RFA Number: RFA-HD-04-020. Available at: http://grants.nih.gov/grants/guide/rfa-files/RFA-HD-04-020.html/. Accessed July 28, 2004.
20. U.S. Department of Agriculture. Food Safety and Inspection Service Research Priorities. Available at: http://www.fsis.usda.gov/index.asp. Accessed July 26, 2004.
21. U.S. Department of Agriculture. Food and Nutrition Service Overview. http://www.fns.usda.gov/fns/menu/OVER.HTM. Accessed July 26, 2004.
22. U.S. Department of Agriculture. Office of the Chief Financial Officer. USDA Strategic Plan for FY 2002–2007. Available at http://www.usda.gov/ocfo/usdasp/pdf/sp02-02.pdf. Accessed July 6, 2004.
23. Anon. *Logic Model Development Guide*. W.K. Kellogg Foundation. Battle Creek, MI: January 2004. Available at: http://www.wkkf.org/Pubs/Tools/Evaluation/Pub3669.pdf . Accessed August 19, 2006.
24. University of Wisconsin Program Evaluation Unit. Available at: http://www.uwex.edu/ces/pdande/evaluation/evallogicmodel.html. Accessed July 27, 2004.
25. The Foundation Center. Proposal Writing Short Course. http://fdncenter.org/learn/shortcourse/prop1.html. Accessed July 11, 2004.
26. Administration on Aging. Instructions for Preparing Competitive Grant Applications for the Aging Services Network Integrated Care Management Grants Program. Available at: http://www.sdcounty.ca.gov/cnty/cntydepts/health/ais/ltc/media/AoA-04-08integratedcaregrant.doc. Accessed August 19, 2006.

Index